P9-CNB-963

Culture, Ethnicity, and Mental Illness

Culture, Ethnicity, and Mental Illness

Edited by

Albert C. Gaw, M.D.

Associate Professor of Psychiatry,
  Boston University School of Medicine
Lecturer on Psychiatry, Harvard Medical School
Staff Psychiatrist, Edith Nourse Rogers
  Memorial Veterans Medical Center,
  Bedford, Massachusetts, and
  Mount Auburn Hospital, Cambridge, Massachusetts

American Psychiatric Press, Inc.

Washington, DC
London, England

Note: The authors have worked to ensure that all information in this book concerning drug dosages, schedules, and routes of administration is accurate as of the time of publication and consistent with standards set by the U.S. Food and Drug Administration and the general medical community. As medical research and practice advance, however, therapeutic standards may change. For this reason and because human and mechanical errors sometimes occur, we recommend that readers follow the advice of a physician who is directly involved in their care or in the care of a member of their family.

Books published by the American Psychiatric Press, Inc., represent the views and opinions of the individual authors and do not necessarily represent the policies and opinions of the Press or the American Psychiatric Association.

Copyright © 1993 American Psychiatric Press, Inc.
ALL RIGHTS RESERVED
Manufactured in the United States of America on acid-free paper.
97 96 95 94 93   5 4 3 2
First Edition
American Psychiatric Press, Inc.
1400 K Street, N.W., Washington, DC 20005

Library of Congress Cataloging-in-Publication Data
Culture, ethnicity, and mental illness / edited by Albert C. Gaw.
    p. cm.
    Includes bibliographical references and index.
    ISBN 0-88048-359-8
    1. Minorities—Mental health—United States. 2. Psychiatry—Cross cultural studies.   3. Community psychiatry–United States.
    I. Gaw, Albert, 1939–
    [DNLM: 1. Mental illness—United States—Cross-cultural studies.
    2. Cross-Cultural Comparison. 3. Ethnic Groups—psychology.
    4. Mental Disorders—ethnology. 5. Psychotherapy—methods.
    WM 420 C968]
    RC451.5.A2C86   1992
    616.89'071—dc20
    DNLM/DLC   92-10686
    for Library of Congress   CIP

British Library Cataloguing in Publication Data
A CIP record is available from the British Library.

*This book is fondly dedicated
to my wife, Tina,
and my daughter, Julie,
and
to John Romano, M.D., and
George L. Engel, M.D.,
teachers par excellence*

Table of Contents

Section I:
Cultural Matrices of the
Psychiatric Encounter

Theoretical Considerations

Practical Considerations

Section II:
Culture and Clinical Care

Acknowledgments

This book has been 3 years in the making. No words are sufficient to convey my respect for and gratitude toward the 33 colleagues who have graced these pages and have helped expand our knowledge of cultural diversity in the treatment of mental illness.

There are 20 chapters and 8 glossaries of ethnic terms in this book. In addition to my glossary of Chinese terms, the following glossaries were prepared by these contributors for their chapters, and I thank them for their efforts. The glossaries for Chapters 3 and 8 appear after their respective chapters, and the rest appear at the back of the book.

Contributor	Chapter
Ronald C. Simons, M.D., M.A.	Culture-Bound Syndromes
Charles C. Hughes, Ph.D.	(Chapter 3)
James W. Thompson, M.D., M.P.H.	American Indians and
R. Dale Walker, M.D.	Alaska Natives (Chapter 8)
Patricia Silk-Walker, R.N., Ph.C.	
June S. Fujii, M.D.	Japanese Americans (Chapter 11)
Susan N. Fukushima, M.D.	
Joe Yamamoto, M.D.	
Luke I. C. Kim, M.D., Ph.D.	Korean Americans (Chapter 12)
Enrique G. Araneta, Jr., M.D.	Pilipino Americans (Chapter 13)
Cervando Martinez, Jr, M.D.	Mexican Americans (Chapter 15)
Ian A. Canino, M.D.	Puerto Ricans (Chapter 16)
Glorisa J. Canino, Ph.D.	

I also want to thank the following copyright owner and publisher for permission to adapt or reprint their work:

Leff J: Psychiatry Around the Globe, 2nd Edition. London, Gaskell Books, Royal College of Psychiatrists, 1988. By permission of the publisher.

Albert C. Gaw, M.D.

Contributors

Enrique G. Araneta, Jr., M.D.
Former Chief of Mental Hygiene Clinic, Veterans Administration
Outpatient Clinic, Jacksonville, Florida

F. M. Baker, M.D., M.P.H.
Associate Professor, Department of Psychiatry, University of
Maryland School of Medicine, Baltimore, Maryland

Eric G. Bing, M.D.
Robert Wood Johnson Clinical Scholar, Departments of Medicine
and Psychiatry, UCLA Medical Center, Los Angeles, California

Glorisa J. Canino, Ph.D.
Behavioral Sciences Research Institute, Office of Academic Affairs,
University of Puerto Rico School of Medicine, San Juan,
Puerto Rico

Ian A. Canino, M.D.
Associate Clinical Professor, Department of Psychiatry, College of
Physicians and Surgeons, Columbia University, New York,
New York

Christine Y. Chang, M.D., M.P.H.
Unit Co-Chief, Asian Pacific Inpatient Program, Santa Clara Valley
Medical Center, San Jose, California

Ching-Piao Chien, M.D.
Professor Emeritus of Psychiatry, University of California, Los
Angeles, California; Director, Taipei City Psychiatric Center,
Taipei, Republic of China

Javier I. Escobar, M.D.
Professor and Vice Chairman, Department of Psychiatry,
University of Connecticut School of Medicine, Farmington,
Connecticut

Francisco Fernandez, M.D.
Associate Professor of Psychiatry, Department of Psychiatry and
Behavioral Sciences, Baylor College of Medicine, Houston, Texas

June S. Fujii, M.D.
Assistant Clinical Professor of Psychiatry, UCLA Neuropsychiatric
Institute, Los Angeles, California

Susan N. Fukushima, M.D.
Assistant Clinical Professor of Psychiatry, UCLA Neuropsychiatric
Institute, Los Angeles, California

Albert C. Gaw, M.D.
Associate Professor of Psychiatry, Boston University School of
Medicine, Boston, Massachusetts; Lecturer on Psychiatry, Harvard
Medical School, Boston, Massachusetts; Staff Psychiatrist, Edith
Nourse Rogers Memorial Veterans Medical Center, Bedford,
Massachusetts, and Mount Auburn Hospital, Cambridge,
Massachusetts

Ezra E. H. Griffith, M.D.
Professor of Psychiatry and of African and Afro-American Studies,
Yale University; Director, Connecticut Mental Health Center, New
Haven, Connecticut

Charles C. Hughes, Ph.D.
Professor and Director, Graduate Programs in Public Health,
Department of Family and Preventive Medicine, University of Utah
School of Medicine; Professor, Department of Anthropology,
University of Utah, Salt Lake City, Utah

Ledro R. Justice, M.D.
Assistant Clinical Professor of Psychiatry, UCLA Neuropsychiatric
Institute, Los Angeles, California; Senior Psychiatrist, H. G. Stark
Youth Training School, California Youth Authority, Los Angeles,
California

Luke I. C. Kim, M.D., Ph.D.
Assistant Clinical Professor of Psychiatry, University of California,
Davis, School of Medicine, Davis, California

J. David Kinzie, M.D.
Professor of Psychiatry, Department of Psychiatry, Oregon Health
Sciences University School of Medicine, Portland, Oregon

James P. Krajeski, M.D.
Private Practice, San Francisco, California

Gregory B. Leong, M.D.
Assistant Professor of Psychiatry, UCLA School of Medicine; Staff
Psychiatrist, West Los Angeles Veterans Affairs Medical Center,
Los Angeles, California

Paul K. Leung, M.D.
Assistant Professor of Psychiatry, Department of Psychiatry,
Oregon Health Sciences University School of Medicine, Portland,
Oregon

Orlando B. Lightfoot, M.D.
Professor of Psychiatry, Boston University School of Medicine,
Boston, Massachusetts

Cervando Martinez, Jr., M.D.
Professor of Psychiatry, University of Texas Health Science Center,
San Antonio, Texas

Carol C. Nadelson, M.D.
Professor and Vice Chairman, Department of Psychiatry, Tufts
University School of Medicine, New England Medical Center,
Boston, Massachusetts

Donna M. Norris, M.D.
Clinical Instructor, Harvard Medical School; Senior Associate in
Psychiatry, Children's Hospital Medical Center and Judge Baker
Children's Center, Boston, Massachusetts

Pedro Ruiz, M.D.
Professor of Psychiatry, Department of Psychiatry and Behavioral
Sciences, Baylor College of Medicine, Houston, Texas

Patricia Silk-Walker, R.N., Ph.C.
Research Consultant, Department of Psychiatry, University of
Washington School of Medicine, Seattle, Washington

J. Arturo Silva, M.D.
Assistant Clinical Professor of Psychiatry, UCLA School of
Medicine; Staff Psychiatrist, West Los Angeles Veterans Affairs
Medical Center, Los Angeles, California

Ronald C. Simons, M.D., M.A.
Professor, Department of Psychiatry, and Adjunct Professor,
Department of Anthropology, Michigan State University, East
Lansing, Michigan

Jeanne Spurlock, M.D.
Clinical Professor of Psychiatry, George Washington University
School of Medicine and Health Sciences, and Howard University
College of Medicine, Washington, DC

James W. Thompson, M.D., M.P.H.
Associate Professor, Department of Psychiatry, University of
Maryland School of Medicine, Baltimore, Maryland

R. Dale Walker, M.D.
Professor, Department of Psychiatry and Behavioral Sciences,
University of Washington School of Medicine; Chief, Addictions
Treatment Center, VA Medical Center, Seattle, Washington

Joseph J. Westermeyer, M.D., M.P.H., Ph.D.
Professor and Head, Department of Psychiatry and Behavioral
Science, University of Oklahoma Health Sciences Center,
Oklahoma City, Oklahoma

Joe Yamamoto, M.D.
Professor of Psychiatry, Chief, Laboratory for Cross-Cultural
Studies, UCLA Neuropsychiatric Institute, Los Angeles, California

Veva Zimmerman, M.D.
Associate Dean and Associate Professor of Psychiatry, New York
University School of Medicine, New York, New York

Preface

This book attempts to examine the expression and treatment of mental illness in the context of culture. The emphasis is clinical, and the volume is intended to provide a cultural framework in the psychiatric care of ethnic patients in the United States for practitioners, students, and teachers of the mental health professions. It is my hope that the generic principle derived from such an approach can be generalized to enrich psychiatric care of all patients of different cultural and ethnic backgrounds.

In recent years, there has been a greater recognition and realization of the influence of culture in individual expression of mental distress, in psychiatric diagnosis and treatment, and in the delivery of mental health care community-wide.

Cultural concepts, values, and beliefs shape the way mental symptoms are expressed and how individuals and their families respond to such distresses. Cultural norms dictate when a cluster of symptoms and behaviors are labeled "normal" or "abnormal." Culture also determines the accessibility and acceptability of mental health services. Clearly, effective mental health care cannot be divorced from the cultural context in which the formation and expression of psychic distress occur; the coping strategies of the patients and their families and communities; and the diagnostic and therapeutic activities of the "healers."

Because the material on cross-cultural psychiatry is scarce and not readily cross-referenced in the literature, it is particularly important that we use an ethnic-specific focus and weave this in with a clinical care perspective in this book. With this in mind, this book is divided into two sections. The first section examines certain important cultural issues of the psychiatric encounter—key theoretical construct and major clinical themes. First, theoretical issues of the application of the concept of culture in clinical psychiatry and generic themes crucial in the understanding and practice of cross-cultural psychiatry are discussed. Charles Hughes, an anthropologist with a keen un-

This book was undertaken outside the regular working hours assumed by the editor as an employee of the U.S. Veterans Administration. The opinions expressed in each chapter are those of the individual authors and do not represent in any way the opinion of the U.S. government.

derstanding of the interface of anthropology and clinical psychiatry, expounds on the key theme that our present healing system (the Western system of psychiatric practice and scientific tradition as is commonly practiced) is a product of Western civilization and culture. When this Western system of mental health care is applied to patients of another ethnic background, one must be sensitive to areas of potential cultural variations, nuances, and/or differences that make the individual care of patients so interesting and challenging. Even items commonly used in the mental status examinations, such as a serial 7s examination, as Hughes pointed out, could be culturally biased. As psychotherapists are attuned to transference and countertransference phenomena, so must practitioners of cultural and cross-cultural psychiatry be attuned to personal biases that are embedded in one's cultural background. Hughes's chapter highlights the cultural sources of some of these biases and offers suggestions on ways of overcoming those cultural biases.

Having laid out the theoretical construct on how culture affects clinical psychiatry, the book proceeds to address several areas of the clinical encounter where culture is thought to play a prominent influence: psychiatric epidemiology, psychotherapy, culture-bound syndromes, and psychiatric assessment. Javier Escobar, a psychiatrist and psychiatric epidemiologist involved in the National Institute of Mental Health's Epidemiologic Catchment Area study, attempts to review current evidences on the influence of culture on mental illness by examining major contemporary community-based surveys of the incidences and prevalences of mental illness across national groups around the world. His chapter dwells on general evidences; specific epidemiologic data of individual ethnic groups such as African Americans or Chinese Americans are addressed in the respective chapters and are cross-referenced.

On the more mundane task of psychiatric diagnosis, Ronald Simons, a psychiatrist with training in anthropology, and Charles Hughes, co-authors of *The Culture-Bound Syndromes*, examine certain culture-specific disorders that are more likely to be encountered by practitioners in the United States and other industrialized countries. Diagnostic categories such as *koro, amok,* and *latah,* once thought rare, may increasingly be found in Western countries because of the ease of world travel and settlement of refugee populations in industrialized nations. The study of the culture-bound categories of mental illness demonstrates the need for the development of more scientifically valid diagnostic categories that are compatible across cultures in order to foster more valid comparative cross-cultural research.

Another issue examined in Section I is the whole realm of dynamic psychotherapy as it is applied to different ethnic patients in the United States. Joe Yamamoto, a seasoned clinician and researcher, and his colleagues of different ethnic backgrounds discuss important cultural context when conducting psychotherapy with varied minority patients. Their chapter illustrates how culturally relevant treatment procedures must incorporate understanding of the cultural antecedents in therapy.

Moving on to the more practical aspect of care, Joseph Westermeyer, a psychiatrist who has done extensive cross-cultural research in the Far East and in the United States, offers practical guidelines in the psychiatric assessment of patients of varied ethnic background. Guidelines to avoid major pitfalls, such as the effective use of an interpreter in the interview process, are suggested.

The second section of this book addresses expression of mental illness and the delivery of culture-sensitive mental health care in the context of identified minority cultural groups in the United States—namely, African Americans, American Indians and Alaska Natives, Asian Americans, and Hispanics. In addition, several chapters examine cultural aspects of some emerging issues in the psychiatric care of certain underserved and/or underrepresented populations in the United States: AIDS patients in minority populations, children, the ethnic elderly, women, and gay men and lesbians. The authors for each of these chapters are carefully selected to provide a blend of scholarship, a wealth of clinical experience, and a sensitivity to cultural issues. In keeping with the clinical focus of the book, contributors of the clinical chapters are all clinician-scholars who are expert in their fields.

For the sake of allowing comparison across chapters, contributors were advised to focus on five major areas where culture is thought to exert particular influence:

1. A brief history of the country of origin of the group, including values, religions, immigration experience in the United States, and pertinent demography;
2. Health beliefs and concepts of mental health and illness, including stigma of mental illness;
3. Epidemiology and expression of mental illness, including culture-specific category of illnesses;
4. Family response to the mental illness of one of its members; and
5. Practical suggestions on culturally appropriate treatment approaches and psychiatric care.

Finally, six glossaries of ethnic terms are provided at the end of the book for quick reference, and two are provided after Chapters 3 and 8.

Because of the limitations of publishing a one-volume study and the unavailability of certain authors, not all major minority and/or underserved populations in the United States could be selected for study. Likewise, major ethnic groups outside the identified minority groups in the United States are omitted. This omission should not be construed as a lack of interest on those groups or a paucity of research data. Rather, the study of selected groups should be seen only as a first step to address the phenomenon of mental illness and care from the perspective of culture on groups of patients whose cultural backgrounds present an obvious contrast to that of the "majority" European immigrant groups in the United States. One can hope that the principles culled from such a multidisciplinary and cultural approach can be equally applied to the care of other ethnic or racial groups as well.

The terms used in this book for the diverse ethnic and racial groups discussed were chosen from accepted current usage in the literature. As has always been the case with such terms, their usage evolves and new ones come into being, often seemingly overnight. The terminology used here—African American, Asian American, white, Hispanic, American Indian, Alaska Native, Pilipino, and so on—may indeed change. But the concern for cultural sensitivity we as clinicians have toward our patients will not alter. We can only hope that our awareness of ethnic and cultural diversity's challenges and rewards will be something that all our colleagues may one day share.

This book would not have come about without the hard work and patience of each contributor, and I am deeply grateful to each of them. Carol C. Nadelson, M.D., past President of the American Psychiatric Association and Editor-in-Chief of American Psychiatric Press, Inc., has been most encouraging and helpful throughout the preparation of this book. Pedro Ruiz, M.D., assisted in the organization of the book and the recruitment of contributors. Karen Mitzner, as initial editor, provided assistance in ensuring conformity in editorial style across chapters. The editorial staff of the American Psychiatric Press has shown immense patience and has been a delight to work with. And as ever, my wife, Tina, has been most understanding and supportive throughout the time I undertook to pull this book together.

Albert C. Gaw, M.D.

Section I:

Cultural Matrices of the Psychiatric Encounter

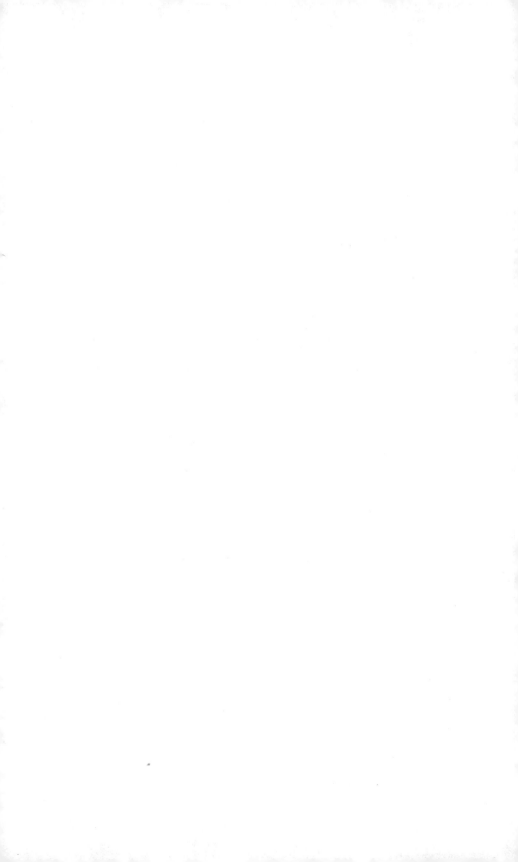

1 Culture in Clinical Psychiatry

Charles C. Hughes, Ph.D.

Interest in the relationship between psychiatry and "culture" is of long standing (e.g., Kluckhohn 1944). In this chapter, I consider only one set of such relationships: those between the practice of psychiatry and its cultural setting (and not, for example, the role of cultural factors in the etiology of psychiatric disorders). My basic assertion here is that the practice of psychiatry—*no matter where it is practiced*—is significantly influenced by its cultural setting. Although such influence is not explicitly recognized in the Western clinical protocol, that protocol is itself an artifact of the cultural structuring of human knowledge and behavior. And the structure is not, as often assumed, the pure yield of Western biomedical science—transcendent, objective, and free from the influences of a cultural system.

But how could the patient/psychiatrist relationship be influenced by culture? It is affected at several levels. For example, a cultural dimension is inherent in both the broad background patterns and the internalized expectations that guide social relationships, as well as in the interpersonal flow of behavior itself. Much of the patient's behavior is structured by his or her cultural or "ethnic" group affiliation, and so also is that of the clinician. Each is deeply influenced by bodies of belief that give form to the perceptually defined world and dictate norms for behavior. Accordingly, everyone has a conceptual "map" for understanding and interacting with the world. These beliefs may differ widely on many subjects, including models for the etiology of mental disorders, their symptomatic expressions, and their management. Such culturally relative belief systems can have important implications for diagnosis, management, and compliance with treatment, and therefore must be understood by clinicians.

The purpose of this chapter is to demonstrate the critical role a generic understanding of culture has in effecting the goals of clinical practice. But how to begin such a demonstration? The chapter itself conveys in considerable detail the numerous and pervasive ways a cultural system shapes and gives differential meaning to human behavior. But that in itself could be too

3

abstract, too exotic (perhaps too boring) to achieve the chapter's purpose. Therefore, placing the argument in a naturalistic context—that of the clinical encounter in the psychiatric examination—some intellectual goads to reflection and cultural self-awareness are suggested (Table 1–1). These may be taken as examples of questions to put to oneself in an attempt to reach an unclouded understanding of the patient and thereby prevent inadvertently insinuating one's own ethnocentric assumptions and standards into the treatment setting. Placed here, at the beginning, they also preview the chapter's detailed discussion.

More than a decade ago Engel (1977, 1980) wrote of the need to correct the reductionist limitations of a biological model for mental disorders. He proposed a "biopsychosocial" model for understanding disease (an orientation that includes what is here referred to as "culture"). Although often referred to in the literature, the model has had limited influence in the practice of psychiatry (Sadler and Hulgus 1990).

Some readers may think it unnecessary to be reminded that knowledge of a patient's cultural world is important in reaching a valid psychiatric diagnosis and in developing an appropriate treatment plan. After all, as Beiser (1985) has written, "Most psychiatrists would probably agree that culture affects clinical practice. . . . " (p. 130).[1] But how *does* culture "affect clinical practice"? Rarely in the literature can the interested reader find pragmatic answers to the question, "How can I avoid being insensitive to differences in language, values, behavioral norms, and idiomatic expressions of distress?"[2]

As Lin (1982), among others, has cogently observed:

> It would not be an exaggeration to state that the field of culture and psychiatry has been accorded only marginal attention by most psychiatrists. To some, it

---

[1]Note, however, that such awareness may not be as widely *operationalized* as Beiser (and a number of others) imply; this is acknowledged in the introduction to DSM-III-R (American Psychiatric Association 1987):

> Caution should be exercised in the application of DSM-III-R diagnostic criteria to assure that their use is culturally valid. It is important that the clinician not employ DSM-III-R in a mechanical fashion, insensitive to differences in language, values, behavioral norms, and idiomatic expressions of distress.

[2]One reason for the lack of answers may be that the diagnostic categories as structured in DSM-III-R are inimical to such exploration; for example, the term "culture" is not included in the index, and even such presumptively culturally influenced phenomena as "culture-bound syndromes" are not explicitly listed in either DSM-III-R or *The International Classification of Diseases, 9th Revision: Clinical Modification* (World Health Organization 1980).

may only represent a set of interesting travelogues dotted perhaps with certain psychiatric insights, while others may regard it as having no practical consequence for the mainstream of psychiatric activity, that is to say, for psychiatrists' daily diagnostic and therapeutic practice or their research into the nature of mental illness. We may say then that there is a general recognition that the field of cultural psychiatry exists, but beyond that, there appears to be only a vague awareness of its objectives or the scope and nature of its accomplishments. There is a sense of confusion as to its relationship to orthodox psychiatry and, in fact, there even seems to lurk a sense of doubt as to its ultimate practicality or usefulness. (p. 235)

(See boxed text, "Culture: Set or Subset?", for further comments on the treatment of culture as peripheral rather than central to clinical practice.)

Table 1–1.   Clinician's inquiry into his or her own cultural bias

- What about this patient's appearance or behavior makes me *think* that what I am seeing and hearing is pathology?
- What are the sources of the putative "pathologic" characterization?
- What label(s) am *I* subconsciously applying to this patient, and where did they come from?
- What social class or group am I *assuming* the patient belongs to, and what do I know about that? What are my own prejudices about that group, and where do such characterizations come from—childhood directives and role-modeling, family inculcated out-group attitudes, scanning of current events that may reinforce preexisting stereotypes?
- Other than "pathology," what other hypotheses come to mind to explain this unusual behavior and/or mentation?
- What other label could I use to describe this behavior instead of pathology?
- What are the circumstances of the *referral* (if a referral), and what is the descriptive *spoken* language used by other health care providers in conveying information about the patient?
- What labels and summary inferences are used in the patient's *chart* or in the referral? How many of the empirical observations such labels purport to reflect can I recreate from the written record (knowing that a medical record needs to be highly selective in the amount of data reported)? What do I know about the person or persons making such comments in the record?

Culture: Set or Subset?

Even when there is passing reference to "culture" in psychiatric texts, it is often assigned to a special category: chapters that speak of "social psychiatry" or "cultural psychiatry" after the conventional evaluation and diagnostic business of the field has been covered. As has been the case with the standard diagnostic manuals for some time, there is no generic index reference to or discussion of the semantic or ontologic status of the concept of "culture"—only special applications of the concept that appear to take for granted a fundamental understanding of what the term means (e.g., Kaplan and Sadock 1988; Lazare 1989). Such a structural omission in an index—a section of a book customarily designed to highlight salient conceptual areas—once again strongly implies that "culture" may be considered only a peripheral concept. When found at all, the chief reference usually is to "culture-bound syndromes," those unusual, "exotic," out-of-the-ordinary disorders in many non-Western societies and various ethnic groups in industrialized nations that defy a simplistic diagnostic categorization in terms of DSM-III-R and other classificatory schemes (Littlewood 1990; Simons and Hughes 1985 and Chapter 3 in this book).

But what is "cultural psychiatry" as contrasted to "psychiatry"? In what respects do they differ?

If viewed diagrammatically, as for example with a large circle representing "psychiatry," the conventional treatment assigns the domain of "cultural" or "social" psychiatry to a smaller, more constricted circle included within the broader field. However, from the *cultural constructionist perspective* informing this chapter, it is suggested that thinking about the relationship should be *reversed*, the larger circle representing the thesis expressed at the beginning of this chapter—namely, that quite aside from *etiology* of a disorder (which, of course, in particular instances may well be biologically based), psychiatric *practice* is *always* influenced by its cultural setting and does not exist in a cultureless vacuum. Psychiatry therefore becomes the "figure" against the "ground" of "culture."

"Culture": Concept and Referent

The received wisdom appears to be that the protocol guiding medical and psychiatric evaluation is inclusive and comprehensive in its incorporation of all relevant factors, including those included under the rubric of the concept of "culture." But, as demonstrated in what follows, when the full implications of the phrase "cultural factors" are explored, it is clear that the protocol falls far short of comprehensiveness.

Building upon a substrate of biological constraints and potentials, "culture" is a construct that captures a socially transmitted system of ideas— ideas that shape behavior, categorize perceptions, and (through language) give names and thereby a putative "reality" to selected aspects of experience. *[defini- tion]* Its fundamental locus is in underlying principles or tacit premises that structure the "assumptive world" of the person and the group. Such ideas are pervasive as well as persuasive (because many of them operate below a level of awareness, unexamined and taken for granted). Some years ago I formulated a definition that touches on the wide-ranging implications of "culture" as a programing system for behavior:

"A culture" is a learned configuration of images and other symbolic elements (such as language) widely shared among members of a given society or social group which, for individuals, functions as an orientational framework for behavior; and, for the group, serves as the communicational matrix which tends to coordinate and sanction behavior. (Hughes 1976, p. 13)

[↳ social norms stem from cultural premises]

Aside from mundane but vital survival skills—how to fashion a tool, cook food, build a shelter, and the like—a cultural process is the mechanism for conveying *values* through and across generations. As such, it lays a complex web of meanings, purposes, and ultimate ends across the continuous stream of human experience and perception. The philosopher Ernst Cassirer noted,

Between the receptor system and the effector system, which are to be found in all animal species, we find in man a third link which we may describe as the *symbolic system*. This new acquisition transforms the whole of human life. As compared with the other animals man lives not merely in a broader reality; he lives, so to speak, in a new dimension of reality. . . . Man cannot escape from his own achievement. He cannot but adopt the conditions of his own life. No longer in a merely physical universe, man lives in a symbolic universe. (Cassirer 1944, pp. 42–43)

The ecumenically-minded psychologist Jerome Bruner speaks in a similar vein:

> Cultures characteristically devise "prosthetic devices" that permit us to transcend "raw" biological limits. . . . [It] is culture, not biology, that shapes human life and the human mind, that gives meaning to action by situating its underlying intentional states in an interpretive system. (Bruner 1990, p. 34)

Culturally Influenced Behaviors

Aside from such lofty matters as meaning and transcendent ideals, a cultural system also specifies, in highly diverse ways, "normal" behavioral patterns (i.e., sanctioned, approved) for a great variety of daily needs. Two such biologically given activities that have figured prominently in Western psychological/psychiatric theorizing (as well as in everyday life, it must be remembered!) are sex and the eliminatory functions of defecation and urination. A clinician's awareness of the possibility that there might be widely contrasting cultural differences between the patient and him- or herself in this regard is therefore an important consideration in assessment.

Although at one level of analysis (that of phylogenetically given imperatives) human sexual drives are similar, in observed behavioral practice—and in meanings attached to their expression—they vary widely among societies around the world (Davis and Whitten 1987). Such variation is found in all aspects of sexual interest and expression: prepubertal sexual activity, self-masturbation, orgasm in sleep, petting and foreplay, premarital coitus, marital coitus, extramarital coitus, coital positions, orgasm in coitus, homosexual activity, sexual activity with animals, and paraphilias (Gebhard 1971). Cultural conceptions define what is permissible and what is forbidden; and ethnographic studies underscore that "large variations exist between different cultural groups in their patterns of sexual behavior. . . . Behavior which is discouraged and punished in one society may be tolerated in a second and encouraged and rewarded in a third" (Gebhard 1971, p. 206, reprinted in Hughes 1976. See also Ford and Beach 1952).

Wastes from metabolic processes—feces and urine—are also subject to highly diverse meanings and practices that range, on the one hand, from being considered casual acts prompted by both biological need and acceptability in the situation, to attitudes of esthetic distaste or religious and symbolic significance: "The aversion we feel to man's parts and functions, and especially to his principal excretory products, is something relatively new.

Primitive and ancient man felt differently about them. He accepted them, where we deny them" (Rosebury 1969, p. 108).

In societies where contagious magical beliefs prevail (i.e., the part contains the essence of the whole), a person is careful to hide feces or nail parings so that no evilwisher can obtain a sample and use it to engage in witchcraft. The Navajo are an example, and being aware that a patient with that background may hold such a belief could be very important in the clinical appraisal.

But feces and urine have been used for other purposes as well, such as in medical treatment. Among Eskimos and other Arctic peoples, human urine was employed in stanching the flow of blood from a cut; "feces and urine, as well as other excretory and secretory products of man and animals, were once extensively used by physicians in the treatment of disease" (Rosebury 1969, p. 138). In addition, "Feces, urine, and other products of man and animals were used as aphrodisiacs and antiaphrodisiacs . . . " (p. 120). Sometimes feces and urine are accorded a supernatural status beyond their use in witchcraft. The title of a classic compendium published a century ago and based on an extensive review of the ethnographic literature dealing with these matters conveys all: *Scatalogic Rites of All Nations. A Dissertation upon the Employment of Excrementitious Remedial Agents in Religion, Therapeutics, Divination, Witchcraft, Love-Philters, etc., in all Parts of the Globe* (Bourke 1891/1968).

Beyond sex and elimination, cultural processes markedly shape the behavioral and attitudinal aspects of many other mundane human activities, such as being born, dying, and being buried and mourned (Palgi and Abramovitch 1984). For example, also influenced by culture are the interpretation of visual perception and defining of "normal" geometric *form* (Segal et al. 1966). A cultural system dictates the appropriate uses of the language of the eyes and meaning of mutual gaze (Argyle and Cook 1976) and patterns of interpersonal etiquette and demeanor, especially status-dictated behavior toward people who belong to different castes (as in India) or that directed at strangers (e.g., Jewell 1952). Modes, occasions, and human objects of touch and fondling are culturally structured (Montagu 1972), as are ways of conveying affection (e.g., kissing on the lips—whether and how to do so; Pike 1976). Even the gestures and expression of emotion and pain are culturally prescribed (e.g., Eibl-Eibesfeldt 1972; La Barre 1947; Lutz and White 1986; Morris et al. 1979; Tao-Kim-Hai 1976; Zborowski 1969). And, as noted previously, the customary *behavioral* patterns for defecation do not escape the impress of culture, which also strongly influences the highly diversified selection of what things are eaten—and considered appropriate for human consumption. From the almost inexhaustible array of anything that grows, crawls, swims, slithers, runs, or is embedded in the ground (e.g., clay), "there is nothing edible, from roots to insects and whales, that some humans do not readily use as food" (Davenport 1945, p. 80; see also Messer 1984). And such dietary selections are not value- or affect-neutral, but are heavily invested with emotional reactions, both positive and negative (e.g., Lee 1957).

Even beyond generic language ability, in which diverse symbol systems convey culturally determined meanings, culture also assigns differences in language *behavior* between social castes, classes, or genders (e.g., Irvine 1985; Philips 1980). In fact, communication in all its other behavioral, perceptual, and interpretive modalities is deeply affected by its cultural context (e.g., Doob 1961).

The range and variety of culturally relative behaviors also includes internalized behavioral expectations about the meaning and uses of time (Gross 1984; Hall 1959); cognitive patterns for counting, weighing, and measuring objects (e.g., metric versus English), as well as the defining of acceptable spacing for interpersonal processes of various types, including speaking (e.g., Hall 1959); designation of customary geographic distances or spaces (e.g., Wallman 1965); wide variations in styles and symbolic meanings of clothing, hair patterns, cosmetic adornments, and bodily mutilations (Firth 1973; Roach and Eicher 1965; Schneider 1987); and sitting patterns and postures (Hewes 1955).

I must emphasize that such customs are not mere ethnographic exotica, for through the processes of socialization and internalization they become essential features of the inner core of personality and its consequent behavioral expressions.

Culturally Influenced Cognitive Systems

Behind such behaviors are intricate cognitive categorizing systems that often differ between Western and non-Western cultures (Casson 1983). Examples of such culturally based categories are "normality" and ideas of disease and its causation (e.g., Frake 1961). Also, conceptions of the body, its parts and processes, and in some instances (e.g., when working with Chinese patients) patients' perceptions of the body can make suggested therapies or invasive surgery in the mode of Western medicine difficult if not impossible. Another therapeutically relevant categorizing scheme is that used for classifying plants for food and medicinal use (e.g., Gunther 1973; Ortiz de Montellano 1975) as well as animals (e.g., Brown and

Witkowski 1982). Such schemes are at work even in terms of color, which may have important implications in a therapeutic setting. People in all cultures recognize the apparently phylogenetically programmed color domains of red, yellow, green, and blue (Berlin and Kay 1969). But there is great variation in selections made from the chromatic spectrum as expressed in specific language terms. This process of selection results in a delimited working sense of "colors" (e.g., Ray 1953, Lenneberg and Roberts 1956) and, therefore, different symbolic and behaviorally expressed meanings of such color designations in daily social life (e.g., Turner 1967).

Further, from the limitless possibilities provided by biological descent, cultures make different designations among genetically based ties of "kin." These serve as the basis for a wide array of socially designated forms of relationship, such as family, clan, and lineage. A clinician who loosely asks a patient about his or her "family" may therefore inadvertently define the scope of included relatives much more narrowly than the patient does. In numerous societies, for example, what are "cousins" in English concept and usage are called siblings and treated in accordance with the same norms.

Personal autonomy versus group identity. Of particular relevance for this chapter is the awareness that cultural systems shape the varying behavioral expressions of "personal autonomy" and profoundly influence the phenomenological processes that give it definition and boundaries. The inner core of one's self vis-à-vis relationships to others, for example—is it characterized by an inward-turning, self-exalting egoism? Or is it more centrifugal—reaching out, immersing and merging the self with the group, denying impulses toward individuation and separation of "self" from the collective other?

Cultural values that emphasize the essential aloneness of the person and exalt individualism as critically constitutive of self create one type of personality having profound implications for the clinical encounter. Appealing to the autonomy of such a patient—stressing the "right" as well as the responsibility of that patient to make his or her own decisions and build self-esteem around a narrow core of self—may, therefore, fit well with such a personal value matrix and make sense to the patient.

But cultural values that define the self or ideal person in a given society may be based on a very different model. In the socialization process, many human groups build toward the type of personality that puts the needs and considerations of the "environing group" above highly egoistic self-boundaries. A complex literature in "culture and personality" studies developed over a number of decades illustrates an alternative: the core of "self" is constituted by *identification with others* rather than narcissism.

The issue, then, regarding the qualities and meanings of the relationship of the person to the group is not simply one of abstract philosophical wonderment. For example, it can pose problems for the clinician who is ethically concerned with obtaining "informed consent" from a patient from a different culture. In a strongly hierarchical social and cultural system, it may not even occur to a patient that it is possible *not* to give consent (cf. Brody 1985; Hahn 1982; Lee 1959a, 1959b; Shweder and Bourne 1982). Also, cultures vary in the manner in which psychological introspection as contrasted to an externalization of problems is encouraged. For example, a cultural value frequently seen and exemplified in patients of Chinese cultural background is the tendency toward somatizing psychodynamic disturbances rather than acquiescing in the cultural legitimacy of psychological disorder per se (cf. Kleinman 1980; Kleinman and Mechanic 1981; Lin 1981; Niem 1989). This tendency may have its origin in the patient's culturally based sense of impropriety in disclosing his or her feelings and thoughts to a stranger—in this case, a therapist.

A final comment to underscore the clinical relevance of knowing the depth of the cultural structuring of a person's modes of adapting to the world. Consider, for example, a patient presenting with marked symptoms of depression, anxiety, hostility, or even somatic complaints. Such a patient may well be suffering the consequences of what has been termed "culture shock" (Oberg 1979, p. 43). Unless the far-reaching, culturally based psychodynamic implications are recognized, the patient's symptoms might well be imperfectly understood, erroneously diagnosed, and ineffectually treated. For personality development—in a larger conceptual context, "socialization" or "enculturation"—creates a predictable and therefore, in a fundamental sense, a rewarding pattern of expectations. But when that world of familiar objects, behavioral customs, events, and meanings is turned upside down, a variety of defense mechanisms comes into play to counteract a deep sense of disorientation and helplessness; "culture, in its broadest sense, is what makes you a stranger when you are away from home" (Bock 1970, p. ix). It is almost as if a *deculturalization* occurs that can lead to a sense of impotence and, if not infantilization, at least regressive reactive patterns when in an alien cultural world.

In general, the more "exotic" the alien society and the deeper one's immersion in its social life, the greater the shock. The outstanding features of culture shock include inability to make any sense out of the behavior of others or to predict what they will say or do. One's customary categories of experience are no longer useful, and habitual actions elicit seemingly bizarre responses. A friendly gesture may be treated as a threat, whereas a serious and sensible question provokes laughter or uncomprehending silence. (Bock 1970, pp. ix–x)

The literature on migration (e.g., Creed 1987; Helman 1990, pp. 266ff), refugee flight, sudden sociocultural change, foreign-culture assignments for business or other reasons (such as education, missionary activity, or volunteer work, as in the U.S. Peace Corps), and even that dealing with the return to one's own home culture after prolonged sojourn in another place (e.g., Uehara 1986) provides extensive documentation of such responses. Such a traumatic change in one's life-world is illustrated in this summary of a study of the profound readjustments necessary for Ethiopian Jewish immigrant adolescents into Israel.

[The patient was] a 15-year-old male from a very remote village, who had no formal education in Ethiopia. He was an only son, who worked to help his father. He immigrated to Israel on his own and began to adjust well to school and was enthusiastic about his studies. But his lack of grounding in educational skills began to affect him adversely and he fell behind in his studies; he became depressed, and considered himself a failure. He was homesick, angry, and subject to irritable temper outbursts. He suffered social ostracism and made suicide attempts. His treatment consisted of directed social support and individual help with his schoolwork (including Hebrew). After about 6 weeks he improved and was discharged in 6 months. (Ratzoni et al. 1988, p. 234)

A large number of recent studies have dealt with cultural disruption and consequent psychodynamic progression to trauma presented by refugees from Southeast Asia (e.g., Kinzie 1981; Lee 1988; Nguyen 1985).

Kinzie (1981) notes, "The following patient is typical of those seen in the clinic. Origin of their various symptom patterns corresponded to life changes."

L., a 40-year-old Vietnamese male, married, with two children, had a history of insomnia, decreased appetite, inability to concentrate, and pessimism about his ability to function in any job situation in the United States. He had been a successful secondary-school teacher in Vietnam and was the sole support of the family. L., his wife and family fled his country and had been in the United States for two years. He received training as an accountant but was unable or unwilling to find a job in this field. Subsequently he began looking for other training but was unable to concentrate on any job. Because of their financial situation, his wife started as a worker in an electronic plant. She became the sole wage earner and was away from home during the day while L. stayed with the children. His symptoms of depression became even more acute as his wife's employment caused a reversal of the family roles. Psychotherapy and antidepressant medicine helped him to recover from his depression and eventually enabled him to hold a job.

 Comment: This patient, who had functioned well in the past, had obviously suffered loss of position and status by coming to the United States. Nevertheless, he had adjusted fairly well in the first training program. When it was necessary for his wife to begin work, the shift in the family relationship created tension and lowered L.'s self-esteem with a subsequent depressive reaction. The changed life-style in this country undoubtedly contributed to the difficulty (Kinzie 1981, pp. 257–258).

It is clear that an overly hasty and too narrow diagnosis of posttraumatic stress disorder in DSM-III-R (American Psychiatric Association 1987) may well mask the pervasive nature of the difficulty and the scope of therapeutic steps required in adjusting to life in a different culture (e.g., Baxter 1988; Ratzoni et al. 1988). Whether or not preexisting pathology is involved, the person is obviously confronted with severe psychological challenges (Baron et al. 1983).

Semantic Scope and Depth

If the concept of culture is so important and its referents so pervasive, why then does it not figure more centrally in paradigms and protocols for the psychiatric encounter? What kind of a concept is this that would make it so difficult to include effectively in such an evaluation procedure?[3]

---

[3]"Culture" is an emergent concept. Its essential character relates to a matrix type of intuition, and attempting to comprehend what it means may seem as difficult as trying to grasp a cloud in the hand. Such a difficulty apparently beset compilers of a major compendium of behavioral science findings a generation ago when, in a manner revealing both frustration and befuddlement by this kind of idea as contrasted to the sharply specified "variables" dealt with in earlier chapters, they ended a short summary statement on the concept of *culture* by writing,

 [Almost] everything discussed in this book is conditioned by culture: ways of learning, types of personality, the organization of the family or the economy, the distribution of classes, the relations among ethnic groups. . . . [Almost] everything human is conditioned by culture . . . [by] the global character of culture. (Berelson and Steiner 1964, p. 643)

Culture is a *field concept*. It refers to the empirical matrix from which elements—factors or "variables"—may be selected and conceptualized for a given analysis. Culture is pervasive, not simply the compressed set of empirical variables frequently suggested in the literature (e.g., Moffic 1989, p. 686). But any concept—be it a field type or a more segmental one—must have an origin in data. The two kinds of data on which concepts of culture are based are behavior (what people do, say, and think), and artifacts (what they have made in the form of art, artifacts, architecture, and technology). To some, "culture" conceptualized in so holistic a manner may appear too formless, too shadowy, lacking neat boundaries or easily measured properties—and therefore not very useful. But recognizing culture's distinctive ontologic status and not forcing it into a Procrustean bed of "variables" does no violence to the process of enhancing understanding; on the contrary, it contributes greatly to that process.

Aside from culture, analytic concepts used in the behavioral sciences as points of entry for dissecting the perceived stream of observed behavior show considerable diversity in their semantic dimensions and levels or planes of abstraction. Is the scope and breadth and variety of the phenomena symbolized by the point-of-entry variables "birth order" or "age," for example, comparable in scope, depth, and pervasiveness in life-space to the range of the phenomena encompassed by "social class" or "culture" or even "life-style"? Hardly (see boxed text).

Yinger (1965) has developed a comprehensive approach to the several different behavioral domains using a field concept, and "gestalt" approaches in psychology well exemplify this particular perspective. Cartwright (1951), in an introduction to a collection of essays by Kurt Lewin, one of the major figures in the application of the concept of "field" to both individual and social psychology, conveys the gist of this approach in noting that for Lewin

[The most fundamental construct is] that of "field." All behavior (including action, thinking, wishing, striving, valuing, achieving, etc.) is conceived of as a change of some state of a field in a given unit of time. . . . In treating individual psychology, the field with which the scientist must deal is the "life space" of the individual. This life space consists of the person and the psychological environment as it exists for him. In dealing with group psychology or sociology, a similar formulation is proposed. One may speak of the field in which a group or institution exists with precisely the same meaning as one speaks of the individual life space in individual psychology. The life space of a group, therefore, consists of the group and its environment as it exists for the group. (p. xi)

Culture and Ethnicity

The root concept for the term "ethnicity" is culture. Ethnicity is a derivative concept that recognizes the in-group values conceptualized by a particular cultural group, such as "Italian Americans" or "French Canadians." In a pluralistic society in which a presumed collective unity is conveyed by a nation-state term that may well be more a nationalistic hope than probable fact (e.g., "Yugoslavia"), much of the operative force of the concept of culture as defined here is carried by the term "ethnicity." Of course, more refined distinctions are made by specialists in the field, but for purposes of this chapter the terms "culture" and "ethnicity" refer to the same generic process, a position well-explored by Cohen (1978). Of particular relevance in this regard for readers of this volume are the books *Cultural Conceptions of Mental Health and Therapy* (Marsella and White 1982) and *Cross-Cultural*

It is useful to consider the *metatheoretical* status of such concepts—to conduct a brief formal analysis in an attempt to discern some of the semantic assumptions that lie *behind* the overt terms.

A distinction can be made, for example, between concepts that appear to be, on the one hand, 1) "unit"- or organism-focused, that is, appropriate in characterizing some selected attribute of a *person;* and those that are 2) "environment"- or "field"-oriented. On the other hand, crosscutting those two dimensions are concepts that are 1) *diffuse* and wide-ranging and ramifying in their referents in the life-space of a given unit of application (either organism or environment); or 2) *segmental* or *focused* in semantic reference.

Thus, for example, the narrowly focused and unit-centered concept of *intelligence* may be contrasted with an environment-characterizing and *diffuse* concept such as "ghetto life"; or a unit-centered (in this case, personality) concept such as the type A personality—diffuse in its reference—may be contrasted with a type of variable that is *segmental* in referring to aggregate population characteristics, such as *median age* of a given group. (An earlier formulation of this approach is found in Leighton et al. 1963, pp. 182–184).

Counseling and Psychotherapy (Marsella and Pedersen 1981), as well as the other chapters in this book.

Cultural Matrices of the Psychiatric Encounter

There are several perspectives through which relationships between psychiatry and the concept of culture can be viewed. The first is the broad social structural background that sets the context for what is called here institutionalized (i.e., normatively sanctioned) behavior.

Institutionalized perspective. Psychiatry in the Western world derives from the broad stream of Euro-American culture, which generally is traced to Greek and other Mediterranean cultural antecedents. Western psychiatry is, then, simply one more illustration of the variety of responses human so-

---

These distinctions (obviously suggested as heuristic foci existing on continua and not as absolute, bounded categories) are illustrated in the following diagram:

Conceptual Matrix

	Unit-Centered	Environment-Centered
Diffuse	Age, gender, race, ethnic identity, "type A personality," etc.; "schizoaffective personality," "Health Belief Model," etc.	"Way of life," "social class," socioeconomic status, "urban" vs. "rural" residence, etc.
Segmental	Occupational role, birth order, voting rights, school class standing, etc.	Family composition, street address or neighborhood characterization, job conditions, etc.

The locus of "culture" in this framework is therefore in the "environment/diffuse" cell, referable to the *context* of behavior, in a manner similar to "field" in quantum physics (Pagels 1982).

---

cieties have made to disease and dysfunction. Its present form is clearly the product of *particular* historical developments and the cultural structuring of concepts of etiology, diagnosis, and treatment.

Lin comments on this in a review subtitled "A Chinese Perspective," noting the limitations of the Western ethnocentric vision of modern psychiatry:

> Modern psychiatry was born in the West, and as it grew it was moulded by specifically Western philosophical and scientific traditions; it developed as a child of Western culture. Considering, then, the prevalence of ethnocentrism and the untested presumption of clinical universality in modern psychiatry, it is not difficult to understand why unfamiliar psychiatric phenomena or folkloric healing practices aimed at mental disorders in non-Western cultures are regarded as foreign, primitive, uninteresting or even inferior. Quite simply they are considered as phenomena and practices isolated from the totality of the cultural contexts which shape them and serve to define their real significance. It is the challenge of cultural psychiatry to overcome the inertia of ethnocentrism while helping modern psychiatry to step beyond its boundaries, enriched by new materials, new perspectives and new insights. (Lin 1982, p. 235)

It is not only the sweeping influences of history that give shape to the modern practice of psychiatry. Other institutionalized features are involved as well, such as the culturally defined and culturally legitimated role of the practitioner in a medical context. In addition, the behavior expected of the person who is situationally defined in Western society as a "patient" is also institutionalized (e.g., Parsons 1951). For example, he or she has the obligation to be motivated and cooperate with the clinician in order to get well (to "follow doctor's orders"). Analogous directives for behavior of the patient exist in all societies, although frequently not only the patient but also the patient's family is expected to be fully compliant with and submissive to the unequivocally authoritarian stance of the healer.

In all societies, however, being a patient is ascribed—a special social role structured by its own constellation of norms and obligations. Furthermore, patients have particular cultural expectations about their health care system, whether that be in a "folk" society or a modern European state (cf. Payer 1988). And quite aside from folk cultures there are, even in psychiatry, different national cultural emphases in the diagnostic emphases and modes of evaluation of such disorders as schizophrenia (e.g., Helman 1990; Westermeyer 1988). In addition, of course, the patient may have made a conscious choice from the variety of institutionalized alternative healers who exemplify different modes of culturally based diagnoses and therapies. In some Western communities, the practitioner trained in Western allopathic medicine may be only one among a number of healers, such as *curanderos, espiritistas,* naturopaths, chiropractors, iridologists, or rolfers (and, of course, a number of others). Particularly useful discussions of patients' expectations of healers among defined ethnic groups in the contemporary United States are found in the *Western Journal of Medicine* (December 1983) and in Harwood (1981).

The sociopsychological relationship between clinician and patient occurs in a particular material and cultural context. In American society, this includes a hospital setting, which in itself can have baleful connotations for people from many different cultures (e.g., the Navajo). The material and cultural context for Western psychiatry also usually includes chairs or a couch, a desk, and other office appurtenances such as pens, writing pads, carpeted floor, particular types of lighting and office decoration, and a clock (a device for the mechanical marking of time into arbitrary segments—a concept decidedly unfamiliar in some cultures). Not all patients are comfortable in such surroundings, which may well create an underlying tension among, for example, patients from Southeast Asia. Not all peoples customarily sit on chairs; many squat, crouch, or sit on bended knee. Mainstream patients from different social class backgrounds may also feel uncomfortable in psychiatrists' offices. A sense of the familiar in terms of territory is very important in establishing a feeling of comfort and a lowering of vigilance and anxiety to the point that the patient feels safe in an unfamiliar space (cf. various chapters in Proshansky et al. 1970 and almost any issue of the *Journal of Environmental Psychology*).

Interpersonal and behavioral perspective.   What differences might it make in practice if a clinician operates in terms of one set of cultural assumptions and the patient lives in a different empirical, perceptual, and definitional world? To illustrate ethnocentrically created pitfalls that potentially could stand in the way of formulating a "culture-free" evaluation, let us look at an example of the typical—and suggested—clinical evaluation process.

Appearance and Behavior

A major text in the field illustrates the possible implications of using unexamined assumptions about "normal" appearance and behavior, assumptions that may be inappropriate for understanding the world of the patient.

The left-hand column is from Freedman and colleagues (1975, p. 729), and
the right-hand column raises questions about the possibly unconscious and
culturally determined criteria a clinician may be using in judging a patient.

The examiner's overall impression of the patient (attractive, unattractive)	[By whose—and what—criteria? How is "attractiveness" defined? Skin color, texture of hair, facial features, fullness or thinness of lips and bodily form?]
should be followed by a description of the patient's dress and grooming (careless, overly meticulous, bizarre),	[How defined? "Bizarre" according to what reference group standards—teenagers, cowboys, etc.? Is there a "uniform" that must be worn for the visit to the psychiatrist's office?]
unusual features in his physical appearance, facial expression (alert, dazed, perplexed),	[Numerous studies have shown that a visit to a healer—medical or psychiatric—is not a "normal" event; it is fraught with anxiety and, perhaps, "perplexity . . . "]
and eye contact (eyes open, avoids eye contact, stares directly into the examiner's eyes . . .)	[In some cultural and ethnic groups it is highly impolite to look directly into the eyes of another person, especially one in a power position, e.g., black or Asian populations; cf. Argyle and Cook 1976]

A more recent text (Lazare 1989) similarly speaks of the importance of observation of the patient's appearance and behavior as providing clues to
disorder.

The patient's appearance provides considerable information. Initial observations reveal important global characteristics. The sex, race, and apparent age are noted. Each of these features may have a bearing on the type of psychiatric problem encountered and its impact. (p. 164)

Dress and grooming are fundamental features of normal functioning. They break down in a variety of ways, usually in response to fairly serious changes in mental state. (p. 168)

[Could such a "breakdown" occur not only as a result of "serious changes in mental state" but also from drastic changes in *social* conditions, such as loss of job, homelessness, etc., and be a normal reaction to such an event?]

Manner of dress and condition of clothing, as well as grooming, may reveal much about the patient's state of mind. The neatness of the obsessive patient's dress and grooming is well known. Exotic or unusual clothing may reflect individual or eccentric style, perhaps grandiosity in the patient with mood disturbance, the delusional thinking of psychosis, or the provocativeness of the attention seeker. Soiled, disheveled clothing suggests unusual poverty, severe depression, psychosis, or coarse brain disease, as well as other medical illness. Soiled face, hands, nails, and skin tend to increase suspicion of more serious disturbances. (p. 168)

["Soiled," "disheveled"—how defined? How different from the clinician's own personal criteria? How to assess simply different—but "normal"—habits of personal hygiene, without grounding such an assessment in the context of the patient's daily normal round of activities and peer group expectations? For example, might not soiled face, hands, nails and skin be normal for a farm laborer or garage mechanic?]

[We] draw attention to particulars of dress, speech, locomotion, conversational style, and the like; we would add a strong caveat to avoid simplistic or formulaic inferences. Not all neat people are obsessive; not all emotionally intense patients are hysteric. The very essence of the psychodynamic method requires that we observe and record the here-and-now reality and then explore the less conscious meanings of these data on the basis of inferred unconscious dynamics of the patients. (p. 201)

[What are the operational criteria for "particulars of dress"? What is there about "speech" and "conversational style" that might arouse suspicion of pathology? After all, there are clear-cut (and "normal") differences, for example, in speech patterns between working class people and people of middle and upper socioeconomic strata with respect to such factors as the relative concreteness of terms used and specification of context of the action (cf. Bernstein 1966; Schatzman and Strauss 1966). Further, does the "here-and-now reality" go beyond the clinician's office? What about the *daily normal setting and routine* of the patient's life outside the consulting room?]

Thus whether or not a patient is dressed in an age-appropriate manner, removes his or her coat, keeps on dark glasses, and sits very close to or very far from the interviewer become signposts to begin building a diagnostic profile. (p. 201)

[But what if such "sitting close" is perfectly normal for the patient, e.g., a refugee from Salvador?

[In] Latin America the interaction distance is much less than it is in the United States. Indeed, people cannot talk comfortably with one another unless they are very close to the distance that evokes either sexual or hostile feelings in the North American. The result is that when they move close, we withdraw and back away. As a consequence, they think we are distant and cold, withdrawn and unfriendly. We, on the other hand, are constantly accusing them of breathing down our necks, crowding us, and spraying our faces. (Hall 1959, p. 164)]

Expression of affect. The expression of affect is also structured in significant ways by cultural conditioning. The impassive facial demeanor of many American Indians or Asians is an example. Many Mediterranean groups are ebullient, whereas the gestural and facial languages of the typical New Englander are constricted (e.g., Zborowski 1969). How, then, are such behaviors to be interpreted in terms of guidelines like these?

The patient may be neutral, displaying little or no feeling in telling his story or in replying to questions, or he may be fearful, perplexed, hostile, evasive, sarcastic, ingratiating, dramatic, seductive, or completely unresponsive, but rarely is any one of these attitudes consistently displayed. (Freedman et al. 1975, p. 732)

Thus, for therapeutic as well as diagnostic reasons, behaviors must be evaluated against a background of culturally or ethnically prescribed "normal" expectations. A particularly apt illustration is provided by Chang (1981).

In a clinical situation . . . a nurse gave a thorough explanation of the importance of a low-sodium diet to a female Asian patient, which the nurse felt the
patient understood. The patient had nodded and said "yes" throughout the
interchange. Later the nurse discovered that [in this patient's cultural frame of
reference] "yes" meant the patient was listening, and the kinds of foods they
had discussed were not included in the patient's usual diet and were not preferred foods. The patient simply did not want to be so impolite as to interrupt
(or disrupt) by saying "no" or by asking questions. (p. 264)

Symbolic, cognitive perspective.   Cognitive, conceptual, and categorizing
systems through socialization transform the biological offspring of a human
group into people with human status capable of operating in a shared symbol
world. As mentioned earlier, such categorizing ideas influence processes of
evaluation, diagnosis, and treatment that either overtly or subtly shape the
perceptions, interpretations, and meanings of both clinician and patient in
their interactions. For example, the conceptualized "cause" and, therefore,
the proper "cure" for a disorder usually differs between the biomedically
trained therapist and the patient, even though the latter may have some similarities in background to the clinician (e.g., being both white and middle
class).

Language.   Beyond being a communication device, language is of great importance as a categorizing (i.e., conceptual) system. It is the prime example
of the semantic reference for the term "culture" when that construct is defined as a system of symbols that programs much of behavior. Obviously,
communication across languages on matters of psychiatric concern (e.g.,
from Navajo to English) can be fraught with difficulties in interpretation,
even with use of a translator (e.g., Adair et al. 1988).

Even when a common language is spoken by the clinician and patient,
considerable cloudiness can arise from the level, style, and word choice of
the language used by the two speakers. There are well-documented region-
alisms as well as social class-based differences in language. These include
such important features as vocabulary, relative concreteness, and circumstan-
tiality (e.g., Bernstein 1966; Schatzman and Strauss 1966) and facility with
the use of the subjunctive ("it is as though"). Whether or not the patient's
mode of thinking is "literal" is not evenly distributed in terms of social class
standing (e.g., Al-Issa 1977, pp. 573–574, citing a number of studies). An
assessment of "literalness" as contrasted to "figurative" or metaphorical interpretation is important when judgments are made on the basis of the mental status examination (see Pittenger and Smith 1966).

The Clinical History and Mental Status Examination

Assessment of the patient's cognitive functioning is, of course, a critical part of the psychiatric interview. In its typical form, the evaluation is based on Western biomedical cultural assumptions and structuring, which may introduce major distortions into the validity of the findings. This skewing may occur not only with patients from cultural backgrounds different from those of the therapist, but also with patients who have the same general ethnic or cultural framework as the clinician.

For example, tests that rely on overly simplistic, culturally biased questions for assessing distortions or "unrealities" in perception—delusions, hallucinations, illusions—may yield false positives in assessing pathological states. Freedman and colleagues (1975) have proposed the following interview formula:

A few carefully phrased open-ended questions usually reveal the delusional thinking [of the patient] (does he believe something unusual is happening to him; does he feel that someone is trying to prevent him from succeeding or trying to cause him harm; does he think that he has a special mission to fulfill; does he perceive that someone has unusual power over him; does he believe that a supernatural force is controlling him; does he have strange or unusual experiences that are not easily explained). (p. 730)

Clinicians must be alert to patients' own constructions of their normal worlds (e.g., Al-Issa 1977; Sarbin 1967). Given the dilemmas, conflicts, uncertainties, and transempirical beliefs evident in modern pluralistic cultures, one can formulate answers to each of the questions of Freedman and colleagues (1975) that would place a given patient well within the bounds of "normal" functioning. For example, many devout religious believers throughout the world, such as those in fundamentalist Christian sects, are convinced that a supernatural force directs their lives; it is, after all, the sine qua non of religious thought! Is the belief of the Holiness People, the snake-handling Christian sect of the Appalachian region of the United States, that God directs them in their religious rites indicative of "irrational," disordered mentation any less (or more) than an African American patient's statement that someone is controlling his or her life through "rootwork"?

Orientation Assessment

For assessing orientation, it is agreed that degree of cognitive control of presumed commonplace facts is important, such as the ability to name individual items in various categories or classes like towns, fruits, or colors. Some suggested questions are: "What are the colors in the American flag? What is a thermometer? How far is it from Los Angeles to New York? What are the names of three countries in the Middle East?" (Freedman et al. 1975, p. 731)

Given the general population's considerable lack of knowledge of geography (including such information as names, locations of countries, and distances), concern must be raised about the validity of an assessment of "nonnormality" when questions of this nature are answered incorrectly. For example, in an international survey,

American adults scored lower in geographic literacy than those of Sweden, West Germany, Japan, France and Canada. ("A global test" 1988)

The survey sought to determine how many people could find 13 selected countries, Central America, and two bodies of water, the Pacific Ocean and the Persian Gulf, on an unmarked world map. . . . The survey . . . tested 10,820 adults in Canada, France, Italy, Japan, Mexico, Sweden, the United Kingdom, the United States and West Germany. . . .

Among American participants from the United States, no more than half those tested could answer correctly when asked to identify the country in which the Sandinistas and the contras are fighting; 52% were aware that the Soviet Union's war with rebel forces was in Afghanistan; 55% could identify South Africa as the country where apartheid is official government polity; only 24% could name four countries that officially acknowledge having nuclear weapons.

Although nearly 70% of Americans surveyed said the ability to read a map was absolutely necessary in today's world, more than a third could not pick out the westernmost city on a map or calculate the distance between two designated cities, given a mileage scale. ("Americans falter on geography test" 1988)

The class and ethnic bias inherent in asking such questions of people who may have no opportunity to travel because they are too poor is obvious— quite aside from the more fundamental issue of asking such questions of those who do not possess a fundamental geographic (spatial) sense of relationships for reasons other than pathology.

A similar caveat holds when testing memory and evaluating orientation with questions about current events (e.g., "Who is the President of the United States?" or "Who was the President before him?"; Freedman et al. 1975, p. 731). Polls of the public's knowledge of current affairs recurrently show discouraging results (e.g., Feinsilber 1990). However, ask an automobile mechanic, a computer repair technician, a farmer, or any number of other people about specific knowledge related to their daily life-worlds, and a different perspective on ability to recall specific facts may well emerge.

Sometimes a patient is asked to write out a list of responses to questions, or, prior to the interview, to read and complete a written assessment questionnaire such as the Cornell Medical Index (Brodman et al. 1949). For functionally illiterate patients, this source of data is obviously flawed. A national study notes that educational deficits in this regard are found in many normal adults in American society:

> Twenty million to 30 million American adults lack in basic skills, including reading, writing and problem solving. ("Bush is urged to give priority to fighting adult illiteracy" 1989)

The Serial 7s Test

Of long-standing reputation in the clinical examination has been the "serial 7s" test, used to assess mental acuity and the ability to concentrate. Yet one may question the implicit assumptions regarding pathology versus normality that have lain behind its extensive use.

> A number of studies seriously question . . . [its] validity [that is, the serial 7s test]. Smith . . . found errorless performance in only 42% of 132 normal subjects. Twenty-four percent of subjects made between 3 and 12 errors, and three subjects abandoned the test completely. Milstein et al. . . . studied more than 300 patients with severe psychiatric disorders and compared them to a matched sample of nonhospitalized patients. They found little diagnostic specificity and no evidence that subtraction of serial sevens was useful in detection of organic brain disease among psychiatric patients. These studies lead to the conclusion that this widely used test has not demonstrated its value to detect organicity or specific psychiatric syndromes. (Lazare 1989, p. 191)

And an earlier study by Smith (1967) reported,

> The 14 required errorless consecutive subtractions of sevens starting with 100 was shown by only 56 of 132 adults with above average education, socioeco-

nomic status, and presumably, general intelligence. . . . Since this study dealt with a highly selected and above-average population, a higher proportion of errors might be expected in a more representative population of normal adults. The results of the present study therefore suggest that . . . poor performances in the serial sevens test by well-educated as well as average adults may frequently have no pathological significance. (p. 80)

Given the low level of mathematical skills in the general U.S. adult population, including the ability to perform simple arithmetic, perhaps this is not surprising.

The rampant innumeracy of our high school students and of the educated public in general is appalling. . . . I'm not primarily concerned with esoteric mathematics here, only with some feel for numbers and probabilities, some ability to estimate answers to the ubiquitous questions: How many? How likely? . . . [They] ought to know roughly the population of the United States, the percentage of the world's population that is Chinese, the distance from New York City to Los Angeles, the odds of winning their state lottery and a host of other common magnitudes. (Paulos 1989, pp. 1, 16)

Ignorant and lacking in knowledge the patient may be; but is such lack of knowledge of this kind necessarily an indicator of pathology?

Overall, with regard not only to the serial 7s and memory tests but also to proverb interpretation (discussed in the next section), it has been remarked that

Clinicians who routinely administer serial sevens, memory tests, and proverb interpretations to assess higher intellectual functions must often wonder what meaning or practical value the results of these clinical tests have. . . . [There] has been surprisingly little systematic research to establish the value of such measures. Despite this lack of evidence, these tests remain widely used, not only by psychiatrists but by neurologists, internists, pediatricians, and others. Numerous medical specialty textbooks recommend them, yet fail to document the empirical basis for their use. . . . [We] describe many inadequacies in the assessment of mental status. (Keller and Manschreck 1981, p. 500)

Proverb Interpretation

A proverb is a compact metaphor, a veritable bundle of multiple meanings that expresses an assertion or commentary on life. Learned in a social context, it is commonly employed by individuals as a guide for decision making in human dilemmas. Indeed, as some have suggested (e.g., Goodwin and Wenzel 1979), a collection of proverbs may be regarded as a folk-derived codification of a particular group's mode of instruction in logical principles of thinking—a primer in practical reasoning:

> The proverb defines the situation and prescribes a response. . . . Characteristically, proverbs deal with the eternal and universal human concerns—love and money, family and friends, work and play—concrete problems that confront everyone. (p. 290)
>
> Taken as a body of conventional wisdom, proverbs serve the common run of humanity in the same way that a textbook on logic or argumentation serves the formally educated. Proverbs offer a general set of rational strategies for deliberating about life's problems. (p. 302)

The family of concepts and terms of the genus metaphor includes parables, similes, aphorisms, apothegms, fables, myths, maxims, and allegories. "Models," whether in science or art, are also metaphors. There is an enormous literature dealing with metaphoric and analogic thinking—the ability to see relationships expressed in different semantic and symbolic fields and often at different levels of abstraction (see Ortony et al. 1978; Turbayne 1970)—that is obviously clinically relevant. For this reason it has typically been used to assess a person's flexibility of mind and grasp of indirect meaning through interpretation of proverbs; for, in the words of Goodwin and Wenzel (1979), "The proverb moves the mind from the concrete image evoked by its familiar terms, through apprehension of the implicit metaphor, to a novel application to the problematic situation" (p. 291).

When used in the psychiatric examination, the degree of the patient's "success" (*as defined by the examiner*) in interpreting the proverb is commonly taken as an indication of "normal" cognitive functioning and of the person's ability to break out of the prison of literalness. The aim is to see how well a person functions in the world of *symbol* as contrasted to that of *sign*, the former being the distinctively human realm of a figurative, analogic construction of reality. This is important, for example, in the assessment of thinking that may appear to be schizoid.

But if the proverbs employed in such an assessment are based on a clinician's unexamined assumptions about the level of concordance between the "familiar terms" (perhaps familiar only to the clinician) and those of the patient, the tests may well be invalid. The patient may bring a distinctly different repertory of culturally structured "familiar terms" into the interpretation of the proverb. Clinicians must examine what assumptions are involved in the use of proverbs for assessing normality or pathology (e.g., the assumption of the universality of the vocabulary employed and the content-familiarity of the situation referred to, or the criteria for a "correct" interpretation). Clinicians must also determine whether the particular proverbs chosen for assessing mental flexibility are culture-bound. Further, one must ask if the use of proverbs as a mode of folk wisdom is evenly distributed in all societies or even **segments** of **any** society or social group? If not, how valid would be the presumption of pathology if this idiom is not part of the patient's routine cultural scene?

As recommended in major texts, "common" proverbs are to be employed (as follows):

> [It] is advisable to avoid asking the patient to interpret complex proverbs, particularly ones that are highly culture-dependent. Indeed, whenever possible, patients affiliated with an ethnic subgroup should be asked proverbs that are in common usage in that particular subculture. . . . Testing a patient's ability for abstract thinking by asking him to interpret a proverb is useful when the patient's intelligence is above average but is of questionable value otherwise. (Freedman et al. 1975, p. 731)

It may be suggested that a patient should *always* be asked to interpret only proverbs that make cultural sense to him or her. Yet, for many patients, what are "common" proverbs? Often, perhaps usually, they derive from a Euro-American cultural background. What if a patient—a "normal" patient—from another ethnic or cultural background has not been exposed to such proverbs, with their standardized "correct" interpretations?

To begin to grasp the difficulties involved in cross-cultural proverb interpretation, ask how well a mainstream American clinician would fare if told to interpret an African proverb, such as "The fowl has had its beak cut" (Zulu), meaning "By means of its beak, the fowl picks up food and also fights. With its beak cut, it would be altogether helpless"—an expression "also used of a talkative person who has been silenced" (Nyembezi 1963, p. 126). Another example is one from the "Uncle Remus" tales dealing with the African American experience in the South ("Hongry nigger won't w'ar his maul out") (Courlander 1976, p. 443).

A study conducted by two residents in psychiatric training demonstrates the point (Kim et al. 1977). One of the residents was from a Greek cultural background and the other from a Korean one. Each interpreted common proverbs from the other's ethnic culture, and significant "slippage" in meanings took place—and this at the level of professionals being trained in the same biomedical "culture" of psychiatry!

Even with patients from the same ethnic and cultural group, a "correct" interpretation may not be so easy to evaluate. The semantic variability in even commonly interpreted proverbs is illustrated in a study conducted among 80 college students in Texas who were asked the meaning of the familiar proverb, "A rolling stone gathers no moss." The students responded with three major types of interpretations:

1. A rolling stone gathering no moss is like a machine that keeps running and never gets rusty and broken.
2. A rolling stone is like a person who keeps on moving, never settles down, and therefore never gets anywhere.
3. A rolling stone is like a person who keeps moving and is therefore free, not burdened with a family and material possessions and not likely to fall into a rut. (Kirshenblatt-Gimblett 1981, p. 113)

Which interpretation is *incorrect?*

A number of other studies raise similar questions (e.g., Andreasen 1977). Selecting 10 proverbs familiar to subjects from the Euro-American cultural stream (e.g., "All that glitters is not gold" or "A stitch in time saves nine"), the researcher assessed the value of proverb interpretation in clinical intake situations and asked psychiatric residents and faculty members to rate the meanings as stated by a group of 44 patients (diagnosed with schizophrenia, manic depression, or depression) in terms of several conceptual dimensions (e.g., correctness or abstraction).

Based on the lack of discriminability shown among the three study populations, the author's analysis suggested that this test could not be considered either reliable or valid. She noted that "the use of proverb interpretation is firmly entrenched in psychiatric tradition. Yet its value in a clinical setting has never been carefully explored in a systematic or quantitative way" (p. 470), and concluded " . . . the validity of using proverbs in a clinical situation is somewhat questionable" (p. 471).

More recent research has borne out such caution (Penn et al. 1988). With a Black study population a commonly used proverb interpretation test that included proverbs familiar in the Anglo-American mainstream culture (e.g., "Where there's a will, there's a way") demonstrated that *familiarity* with the proverb increased responses, but respondents did not even attempt to interpret unfamiliar proverbs. How is nonresponsiveness to be interpreted? Is it necessarily flawed thinking? Or might it be a cautious, low-profile approach to a possibly embarrassing situation?

Further, the authors report that search of computerized bibliographic sources prior to their study demonstrated that there had been no comparable studies done for either Hispanic or African American populations, suggesting, therefore, that assumptions of universality of meaning for all ethnic groups are suspect. Given the numbers of patients from those ethnic groups who may seek mental health services, the implications of this deficit are clear.

Another authoritative source also suggests that use of proverbs to assess generalizability through analysis of similarities between two objects or interpretation of proverbs has shown low reliability and, as a measure of thought disorder, is confounded by level of intelligence (Lazare 1989, p. 193). Again, what is the clinician to make of an "inadequate" interpretation?

Culture and the Moment of Clinical Truth

Deficiencies of both commission and omission have been noted in psychiatric residency training and practice with respect to the concept of culture as applied in the clinical encounter (e.g., Gray et al. 1985; Moffic 1983, 1989). Such deficiencies can have long-range and critical implications for clinical practice (Beiser 1985), and some clinicians have written of programmatic attempts to rectify that situation (e.g., Faulkner et al. 1985; Foulks 1980; Moffic et al. 1988).

Deficiencies of commission arise from the medical training-based entrenchment of (or entrancement with) a biomedical reductionist paradigm, a paradigm that customarily pays slight attention to the role of psychosocial and cultural events in defining the parameters of the problem and developing a treatment plan.

Deficiencies of omission arise from a clinician's lack of systematic exposure to and practice in incorporating a culturally sensitive conceptual framework into the process of clinical appraisal. The process of evaluation is made even more problematic by potential limitations in applying *any* generalization if done uniformly, as noted by Lopez and Hernandez (1986):

> Although it is important to consider culture, it is important to do it well. Oftentimes the literature pertaining to cultural groups informs the clinician of specific cultural characteristics that pertain to specific cultural groups. Although this information can be helpful, it can also be misapplied. Cultural

groups are very heterogeneous and members are at different levels of acculturation and of different socioeconomic strata. . . . It is important for clinicians to
learn as much as possible about different cultural groups, but it is unlikely that
they will be able to learn the many subtleties of any given group. Therefore, it
may be equally important for them to learn how to properly assess the patient's
cultural background and its relationship to the clinical picture. As reported by
some of the respondents to the survey [in their study], finding out from the
patient, family, significant others, or colleagues what they view as cultural and
pathological is crucial. The more data one collects from these resources, the
fewer assumptions one will have to make as to what is and is not cultural. (p.
605)

However desirable it might be, it is usually not possible for a clinician to
take an extended period of graduate-level training in cultural anthropology
or another relevant discipline—although some, indeed, have done so. But an
episodic exposure during residency training or a few scattered weekend sessions attended to receive continuing medical education (CME) credit are not
likely, in themselves, to bring about a basic change in a clinician's fundamental conceptual frame of reference.

How can a clinician become better informed on cultural issues relevant to
his or her patients? I suggest that anyone can build upon personal background, the happenstances of foreign travel and/or research experience, relevant readings, as well as on cultural information gathered from the patient's
family (if that is possible). But, most important, the clinical encounter itself
can be used as a type of continuing education experience to begin developing
or enhancing a better operational understanding of the patient's "normal"
culturally shaped world; in short, one can "learn on the job." Such an approach builds upon what is perhaps the best of all learning aids: the percep-
tive question prompted by the empathetic, inquiring mind. A clinician must
seek out primary data and engage in a process of discovery, rather than simply impose on the patient a predefined assessment of problems as suggested
by a diagnostic manual or text-based directive.

In other words, the clinical encounter itself can be viewed as a natural
"laboratory" for gathering cultural data about the patient beyond *and behind*
what is presented. Kleinman and colleagues (1978) have suggested something akin to this with respect to the desirability of obtaining the patient's
own perceptions and definition of a disturbance; this is done by asking several short, focused questions that take the inquiry into the patient's world. In
a similar vein, the clinician can engage in the "flip side," so to speak, to that
approach. As the clinical encounter proceeds, he or she can conduct a serious, goal-oriented introspection directed at his or her culture-learning sen-

sitivities in order to get behind conventionally received labels. After all, the patient is always enjoined to develop insight with respect to his or her particular psychological blinders. Why shouldn't the clinician do so as well, and attempt to obtain a vicarious sense of the patient's particular cultural situation? Such an internal conversation can be a "mirror" that reflects one's own value positions; and the mental display may be effective in intercepting, early in its trajectory, the projection of one's own value judgments and ethnocentric interpretations onto the patient's world of assumptions. (Such an exercise recalls George Herbert Mead's influential theory of "symbolic interactionism"—"taking the role of the other"; Mead 1922/1964.)

Building, then, on the interaction with a patient, the clinician can in*tra*-act with his or her own thought processes and serve as a devil's advocate in something of the manner suggested by Gaines (1982) when he discusses the contributions of anthropology to understanding the construction of "clinical reality" (pp. 243ff). Further, a clinician can adopt the spirit of Stein's suggestion to use "the self as instrument . . . to be a *clinical ethnographer* in the service of patient care" (1982, p. 62).

Above all, during the patient encounter, the clinician might ponder questions like those in Table 1–1 and use the self-generated responses as windows into a deeper understanding of the patient's world.

Capturing the essence of this chapter, an incident from 1744 recounted by Benjamin Franklin conveys the tacit, self-justifying, and predictably parochial nature of one's own cultural world:

> Savages we call them, because their manners differ from ours, which we think the perfection of civility; they think the same of theirs.
>
> Perhaps, if we could examine the manners of different nations with impartiality, we should find no people so rude as to be without any rules of politeness; nor any so polite as not to have some remains of rudeness.
>
> The Indian men, when young, are hunters and warriors; when old, counselors; for all their government is by the counsel or advice of the sages; there is no force, there are no prisons, no officers to compel obedience, or inflict punishment. Hence, they generally study oratory; the best speaker having the most influence. The Indian women till the ground, dress the food, nurse and bring up the children, and preserve and hand down to posterity the memory of public transactions. These employments of men and women are accounted natural and honorable. Having few artificial wants, they have abundance of leisure for improvement in conversation.
>
> Our laborious manner of life, compared with theirs, they esteem slavish and base; and the learning on which we value ourselves, they regard as frivolous and useless. An instance of this occurred at the treaty of Lancaster, in Pennsyl-

vania, anno 1744, between the government of Virginia and the Six Nations. After the principal business was settled the commissioners from Virginia acquainted the Indians by a speech, that there was at Williamsburgh a college, with a fund, for educating Indian youth; and that if the chiefs of the Six Nations would send down half a dozen of their sons to that college, the government would take care that they should be well provided for, and instructed in all the learning of the white people.

It is one of the Indian rules of politeness not to answer a public proposition the same day that it is made: they think that it would be treating it as a light matter, and they show it respect by taking time to consider it, as of a matter important. They therefore deferred their answer till the following day: when their speaker began by expressing their deep sense of the kindness of the Virginia government, in making them that offer.

"For we know," says he, "that you highly esteem the kind of learning taught in those colleges, and that the maintenance of our young men, while with you, would be very expensive to you. We are convinced, therefore, that you mean to do us good by your proposal; and we thank you heartily. But you who are wise must know, that different nations have different conceptions of things; and you will therefore not take it amiss, if our ideas of this kind of education happen not to be the same with yours. We have had some experience of it; several of our young people were formerly brought up at the colleges of the northern provinces; they were instructed in all your sciences; but when they came back to us they were bad runners; ignorant of every means of living in the woods; unable to bear either cold or hunger; knew neither how to build a cabin, take a deer, or kill an enemy; spoke our language imperfectly; were therefore neither fit for hunters, warriors, or counselors; they were totally good for nothing. We are not, however, the less obliged by your kind offer, though we decline accepting it; and to show our grateful sense of it, if the gentlemen of Virginia will send us a dozen of their sons, we will take great care of their education, instruct them in all we know, and make men of them." (Franklin 1784, pp. 453–455)

References

Adair J, Deuschle KW, Barnett CR: The People's Health: Medicine and Anthropology in a Navajo Community. Albuquerque, NM, University of New Mexico Press, 1988

A global test. The Los Angeles Times, April 6, 1988, p II:6

Al-Issa I: Social and cultural aspects of hallucinations. Psychol Bull 84(3):570–587, 1977

American Psychiatric Association: Diagnostic and Statistical Manual of Mental Disorders, 3rd Edition, Revised. Washington, DC, American Psychiatric Association, 1987

Americans falter on geography test. The New York Times, July 28, 1988, p I:16

Andreasen N: Reliability and validity of proverb interpretation to assess mental status. Compr Psychiatry 18(5):465–472, 1977

Argyle M, Cook M: Gaze and Mutual Gaze. Cambridge, England, Cambridge University Press, 1976

Baron RC, Thacker SB, Leo G, et al: Sudden death among southeast Asian refugees: an unexplained nocturnal phenomenon. JAMA 250(21):2947–2951, 1983

Baxter C: Culture shock. Nursing Times 84(2):36–38, 1988

Beiser M: The grieving witch: a framework for applying principles of cultural psychiatry to clinical practice. Can J Psychiatry 30:130–141, 1985

Berelson B, Steiner G: Human Behavior: An Inventory of Scientific Findings. New York, Harcourt, Brace & World, 1964

Berlin B, Kay P: Basic Color Terms: Their Universality and Evolution. Berkeley, CA, University of California Press, 1969

Bernstein B: Elaborated and Restricted Codes: Their Social Origins and Some Consequences, in Communication and Culture: Readings in the Codes of Human Interaction. Edited by Smith A. New York, Holt, Rinehart & Winston, 1966, pp 427–441

Bock PK (ed): Culture Shock: A Reader in Modern Cultural Anthropology. New York, Knopf, 1970

Bourke JG: Scatalogic Rites of All Nations: A Dissertation upon the Employment of Excrementitious Remedial Agents in Religion, Therapeutics, Divination, Witchcraft, Love-Philters, etc., in all Parts of the Globe. Washington, DC, WH Lowdermilk and Company, 1891 [reprint edition published in New York, Johnson Reprint Corporation, 1968]

Brodman K, Erdmann AJ, Lorge I, et al: The Cornell Medical Index. JAMA 140:530, 1949

Brody E: Patients' rights: a challenge to western psychiatry. Am J Psychiatry 142(1):58–62, 1985

Brown CH, Witkowski SR: Growth and development of folk zoological life-forms in the Mayan language family. American Ethnologist 18:97–112, 1982

Bruner J: Acts of Meaning. Cambridge, MA, Harvard University Press, 1990

Bush is urged to give priority to fighting adult illiteracy. The New York Times, January 15, 1989, p I:20

Cartwright D (ed): Field Theory in Social Science: Selected Theoretical Papers by Kurt Lewin. New York, Harper & Brothers, 1951

Cassirer E: An Essay on Man: An Introduction to a Philosophy of Human Culture. New Haven, CT, Yale University Press, 1944

Casson R: Schemata in cognitive anthropology. Annual Review of Anthropology 12:429–462, 1983

Chang B: Asian-American Patient Care, in Transcultural Health Care. Edited by Henderson G, Primeaux M. Menlo Park, CA, Addison-Wesley, 1981, pp 255–278

Cohen R: Ethnicity: problem and focus in anthropology. Annual Review of Anthropology 7:379–403, 1978

Courlander H: A Treasury of Afro-American Folklore. New York, Crown, 1976

Creed F: Immigrant stress. Stress Medicine 3(3):185–192, 1987

Davenport C: The dietaries of primitive peoples. American Anthropologist 47:60–82, 1945

Davis DL, Whitten RG: The cross-cultural study of human sexuality. Annual Review of Anthropology 16:69–98, 1987

Doob L: Communication in Africa: A Search for Boundaries. New Haven, CT, Yale University Press, 1961

Eibl-Eibesfeldt I: Similarities and Differences Between Cultures in Expressive Movements, in Nonverbal Communication. Edited by Hinde R. Cambridge, England, Cambridge University Press, 1972, pp 297–312

Engel G: The need for a new medical model: a challenge for biomedicine. Science 196:129–136, 1977

Engel G: The clinical application of the biopsychosocial model. Am J Psychiatry 137(5):535–544, 1980

Faulkner LR, Kinzie JD, Angell A, et al: A comprehensive psychiatric formulation model. Journal of Psychiatric Education 9(3):189–103, 1985

Feinsilber M [Associated Press]: Survey discovers an information gap as younger Americans shun the news. The Salt Lake Tribune, June 28, 1990, p 6A

Firth R: Symbols: Public and Private. Ithaca, NY, Cornell University Press, 1973

Ford CS, Beach FA: Patterns of Sexual Behavior. New York, Harper & Brothers and Paul B. Hoeber, 1952

Foulks EF: The concept of culture in psychiatric residency education. Am J Psychiatry 137(7):811–816, 1980

Frake C: The diagnosis of disease among the Subanum of Mindanao. American Anthropologist 63:113–132, 1961

Franklin B: Remarks concerning the savages of North America (1784), in The Works of Benjamin Franklin, Vol II. Edited by Sparks J. Boston, MA, Tappan, Whittemore, and Mason, 1840, pp 453–460

Freedman A, Kaplan A, Sadock B: A Comprehensive Textbook of Psychiatry—II, Vol 1, 2nd Edition. Baltimore, MD, Williams & Wilkins, 1975

Gaines AD: Knowledge and practice: anthropological ideas and psychiatric practice, in Clinically Applied Anthropology: Anthropologists in Health Science Settings. Edited by Chrisman NJ, Maretzki TW. Dordrecht, Netherlands, D Reidel, 1982, pp 243–273

Gebhard P: Human sexual behavior: a summary statement, in Human Sexual Behavior: Variations in the Ethnographic Spectrum. Edited by Marshall DS, Suggs RC. Englewood Cliffs, NJ, Prentice-Hall, 1971, pp 206–217

Goodwin PD, Wenzel JW: Proverbs and practical reasoning: a study in socio-logic. The Quarterly Journal of Speech 65:289–302, 1979

Gray GE, Baron D, Herman J: Importance of medical anthropology in clinical psychiatry. Am J Psychiatry 142(2):275, 1985

Gross D: Time allocation: a tool for the study of cultural behavior. Annual Review of

Anthropology 13:519–558, 1984

Gunther E: The Ethnobotany of Western Washington: The Knowledge and Use of Indigenous Plants by Native Americans. Seattle, WA, University of Washington Press, 1973

Hahn R: Culture and informed consent: an anthropological perspective. in Making Health Care Decisions: The Ethical and Legal Implications of Informed Consent in the Patient-Practitioner Relationship, Vol 3: Appendices. Washington, DC, President's Commission for the Study of Ethical Problems in Medicine and Bio-medical and Behavioral Research, U.S. Government Printing Office, 1982, pp 37–62

Hall E: The Silent Language. New York, Doubleday, 1959

Harwood A (ed): Ethnicity and Medical Care. Cambridge, MA, Harvard University Press, 1981

Helman CG: Culture, Health and Illness, 2nd Edition. London, Wright, 1990

Hewes G: World distribution of certain postural habits. American Anthropologist 57:231–244, 1955

Hughes CC (ed): Custom-made: Introductory Readings for Cultural Anthropology. Chicago, IL, Rand McNally, 1976

Irvine J: Status and style in language. Annual Review of Anthropology 14:557–581, 1985

Jewell D: A case of a "psychotic" Navaho Indian male. Human Organization 11:32–36, 1952

Kaplan HI, Sadock BJ: Synopsis of Psychiatry: Behavioral Sciences Clinical Psychiatry. Baltimore, MD, Williams & Wilkins, 1988

Keller MB, Manschreck TC: The bedside mental status examination— reliability and validity. Compr Psychiatry 22(5):500–511, 1981

Kim S, Siomopoulos G, Cohen R: Verbal abstraction and culture: an exploratory study with proverbs. Psychol Rep 41:967–972, 1977

Kinzie JD: Evaluation and psychotherapy of Indochinese refugee patients. Am J Psychother 35(2):251–261, 1981

Kirshenblatt-Gimblett B: Toward a theory of proverb meaning, in The Wisdom of Many: Essays on the Proverb. Edited by Mieder W, Dundes A. New York, Garland Publishing, 1981, pp 111–121

Kleinman A, Eisenberg L, and Good B: Culture, illness, and care: clinical lessons from anthropologic and cross-cultural research. Ann Intern Med 88:251–258, 1978

Kleinman A: Patients and Healers in the Context of Culture: An Exploration of the Borderland Between Anthropology, Medicine, and Psychiatry. Berkeley, CA, University of California Press, 1980

Kleinman A, Mechanic D: Mental illness and psychosocial aspects of medical problems in China, in Normal and Abnormal Behavior in Chinese Culture. Edited by Kleinman A, Lin T. Dordrecht, Netherlands, D Reidel, 1981, pp 331–356

Kluckhohn C: The influence of psychiatry on anthropology in America during the last 100 hundred years, in One Hundred Years of American Psychiatry. Edited by Hall

JK, Zilboorg G, Bunker HA. New York, Columbia University Press, 1944, pp 589–617

La Barre W: The cultural basis of emotions and gestures. J Pers 16:49–68, 1947

Lazare A: Outpatient Psychiatry: Diagnosis and Treatment. Baltimore, MD, Williams & Wilkins, 1989

Lee D: Cultural factors in dietary choice. Am J Clin Nutr 5(2):166–170, 1957

Lee D: Individual autonomy and social structure, in Freedom and Culture. Edited by Lee D. Englewood Cliffs, NJ, Prentice-Hall, 1959a

Lee D: Personal significance and group structure, in Freedom and Culture. Edited by Lee D. Englewood Cliffs, NJ, Prentice-Hall, 1959b

Lee E: Cultural factors in working with Southeast Asian refugee adolescents. J Adolesc 11:167–179, 1988

Leighton AH, TA Lambo, CC Hughes, et al: Integration and disintegration, in Psychiatric Disorder Among the Yoruba: A Report from the Cornell-Aro Mental Health Research Project in the Western Region, Nigeria. Ithaca, NY, Cornell University Press, 1963, pp 182–184

Lenneberg E, Roberts J: The language of experience: a study in methodology. Supplement to International Journal of American Linguistics 22(2):1–33, 1956

Lin K: Traditional Chinese medical beliefs and their relevance for mental illness and psychiatry. in Normal and Abnormal Behavior in Chinese Culture. Edited by Kleinman A, Lin T. Dordrecht, Netherlands, D Reidel, 1981, pp 95–111

Lin T: Culture and psychiatry: a Chinese perspective. Aust N Z J Psychiatry 16:235–245, 1982

Littlewood R: From categories to contexts: a decade of the "new cross-cultural psychiatry." Br J Psychiatry 156:308–327, 1990

Lopez S, Hernandez P: How culture is considered in evaluations of psychopathology. J Nerv Ment Dis 176(10):598–606, 1986

Lutz C, White GM: The anthropology of emotions. Annual Review of Anthropology 15:405–436, 1986

Marsella AJ, Pedersen PB (eds): Cross-Cultural Counseling and Psychotherapy. New York, Pergamon, 1981

Marsella AJ, White GM (eds): Cultural Conceptions of Mental Health and Therapy. Dordrecht, Netherlands, D Reidel, 1982

Mead GH: A behavioristic account of the significant symbol, in Journal of Philosophy 19:157–163, 1922; and in Selected Writings, George Herbert Mead. Edited by Reck AJ. Indianapolis, IN, Bobbs-Merrill, 1964

Messer E: Anthropological perspectives on diet. Annual Review of Anthropology 13:205–249, 1984

Moffic HS: Sociocultural guidelines for clinicians in multicultural settings. Psychiatr Q 55(1):47–54, 1983

Moffic HS: Minimal cultural experiences in psychiatric training. Am J Psychiatry 146(5):686–687, 1989

Moffic HS, Kendrick EA, Reid L, et al: Cultural psychiatry education during psychiatric residency. Journal of Psychiatric Education 12(2):90–101, 1988

Montagu A: Culture and contact, in Touching: The Human Significance of the Skin. New York, Harper & Row, 1972, pp 253–331

Morris D, Collett P, Marsh P, et al: Gestures: Their Origins and Distributions. New York, Stein & Day, 1979

Niem TT: Treating Oriental patients with Western psychiatry: a 12-year experience with Vietnamese refugee psychiatric patients. Psychiatric Annals 19(12):648–652, 1989

Nguyen MD: Culture shock: a review of Vietnamese culture and its concepts of health and disease. West J Med 142(3):409–412, 1985

Nyembezi CLS: Zulu Proverbs. Johannesburg, South Africa, Witwatersrand University Press, 1963, p 126

Oberg K: Culture shock and the problem of adjustment in new cultural environments, in Toward Internationalism: Readings in Cross-Cultural Communication. Edited by Smith EC, Luce LF. Rowley, MA, Newbury House, 1979, pp 43–45

Ortiz de Montellano B: Empirical Aztec medicine. Science 188(4185):215, 1975

Ortony A, Reynolds R, Arter J: Metaphor: theoretical and empirical research. Psychol Bull 85(5):919–943, 1978

Pagels HR: The Cosmic Code: Quantum Physics as the Language of Nature. New York, Simon & Schuster, 1982

Palgi P, Abramovitch H: Death: a cross-cultural perspective. Annual Review of Anthropology 13:385–417, 1984

Parsons T: The Social System. Glencoe, IL, Free Press, 1951

Paulos JA: The odds are you're innumerate. The New York Times Book Review, January 1, 1989, pp 1, 16–17

Payer L: Medicine and Culture: Varieties of Treatment in the United States, England, West Germany, and France. New York, Henry Holt, 1988

Penn NE, Jacob TC, Brown M: Familiarity with proverbs and performance of a black population on Gorham's proverbs test. Percept Mot Skills 66:847–854, 1988

Philips S: Sex differences and language. Annual Review of Anthropology 9:523–544, 1980

Pike ER: The natural history of a kiss, in The World's Strangest Customs. London, Odhams Books, 1966, pp 11–19

Pittenger R, Smith H: A Basis For Some Contributions of Linguistics to Psychiatry. in Communication and Culture: Readings in the Codes of Human Interaction. Edited by Smith A. New York, Holt, Rinehart & Winston, 1966, pp 169–182

Proshansky H, Ittelson W, Rivlin L (eds): Environmental Psychology: Man and His Physical Setting. New York, Holt, Rinehart, & Winston, 1970

Ratzoni G, Apter A, Blumensohn R, et al: Psychopathology and management of hospitalized Ethiopian immigrant adolescents in Israel. J Adolesc 11:231–236, 1988

Ray V: Human color perception and behavioral response. NY Academy of Sciences, Transactions Series 2, 16:98–104, 1953

Roach ME, Eicher JB (eds): Dress, Adornment, and the Social Order. New York, Wiley,

1965

Rosebury T: Toilet training, in Life on Man. New York, Viking Press, 1969, pp 90–107

Sadler JZ, Hulgus YF: Knowing, valuing, acting: clues to revising the biopsychosocial model. Compr Psychiatry 31(3):185–195, 1990

Sarbin T: The concept of hallucination. J Pers 35:354–380, 1967

Schatzman L, Strauss A: Social Class and Modes of Communication. in Communication and Culture: Readings in the Codes of Human Interaction. Edited by Smith A. New York, Holt, Rinehart & Winston 1966, pp 442–455

Schneider J: The anthropology of cloth. Annual Review of Anthropology 16:409–448, 1987

Segal M, Campbell D, Herskovits M: The Influence of Culture on Visual Perception. Indianapolis, IN, Bobbs-Merrill, 1966

Shweder R, Bourne EJ: Does the concept of the person vary cross-culturally? in Cultural Conceptions of Mental Health and Therapy. Edited by Marsella AJ, White GM. Dordrecht, Netherlands, D Reidel, 1982, pp 97–137

Simons RC, Hughes CC (eds): The Culture-Bound Syndromes: Folk Illnesses of Psychiatric and Anthropological Interest. Dordrecht, Netherlands, D Reidel, 1985

Smith A: The serial sevens subtraction test. Arch Neurol 17:7880, 1967

Stein H: The ethnographic mode of teaching clinical behavioral science, in Clinically Applied Anthropology: Anthropologists in Health Science Settings. Edited by Chrisman NJ, Maretzki TW. Dordrecht, Netherlands, D Reidel, 1982, pp 61–82

Tao-Kim-Hai A: Orientals are stoic. The New Yorker, September 1957, pp 105ff

Turbayne C: The Myth of Metaphor. Columbia, SC, University of South Carolina Press, 1970

Turner V: Color classification in Ndembu ritual: a problem in primitive classification, in The Forest of Symbols: Aspects of Ndembu Ritual. Ithaca, NY, Cornell University Press, 1967, pp 59–92

Uehara A: The nature of American student reentry adjustment and perceptions of the sojourn experience. International J Intercultural Relations 10(4):415–438, 1986

Wallman S: The communication of measurement in Basutoland. Human Organization 24:236–243, 1965

Westermeyer J: National differences in psychiatric morbidity: methodological issues, scientific interpretations and social implications. Acta Psychiatr Scand Suppl 78:23–31, 1988

World Health Organization: The International Classification of Diseases, 9th Revision. Geneva, World Health Organization, 1980

Yinger JM: Toward a Field Theory of Behavior: Personality and Social Structure. New York, McGraw-Hill, 1965

Zborowski M: People in Pain. San Francisco, CA, Jossey-Bass, 1969

2 Psychiatric Epidemiology

Javier I. Escobar, M.D.

B ecause this book is devoted to cross-cultural issues in mental illness, with particular emphasis on the status of U.S. ethnic groups, a chapter on psychiatric epidemiology ought to reinforce such a perspective. Unfortunately, information on the presentation and prevalence of mental disorders among minorities in the United States is incomplete and, with few exceptions, the bulk of available data has been derived from anecdotal reports and comparative studies using "treated" samples.

To provide a not too lengthy and, I hope, a more factual review of the evidence, it was my intention to base this chapter on a compilation of those studies that adopted current scientific paradigms and utilized state-of-the-art methodologies. The handful of studies selected for this review sought to determine the prevalence of operationally defined psychiatric disorders in large community samples by using highly standardized procedures including structured diagnostic instruments. These studies have provided data on the distribution, correlates, and risk factors for a number of psychiatric disorders that may be applicable to some of the ethnic groups in the United States. The presentation of similar data gathered in other countries and cultures is intended to provide at least some peripheral information on those U.S. minority groups not included in the major North American surveys (i.e., Asian Americans and Puerto Ricans or other Latin Americans). Although these findings should not be generalized to U.S. ethnic minorities, these data may serve as an important frame of reference for future comparative studies, because they provide information on countries of origin for many U.S. immigrant groups.

Epidemiology: Definition and General Principles

Epidemiology is the branch of medicine that studies the distribution of diseases in populations. Epidemiological studies provide information on number of cases (the numerator in the ratio) present in a given setting (the denominator). Because it is expected that in each setting a constellation of factors may be operating, the prevalences obtained in different settings may be traced to various factors. The term "risk factors" is used to denote those factors that contribute to an increase in the prevalence of specific disorders, whereas "protective factors" are those that may attenuate or prevent a disorder's expression. By identifying prevalence, risk factors, and protective factors, epidemiological inquiry may provide etiological knowledge and lead to the implementation of preventive efforts.

Institutional Versus Community Studies

When exploring prevalences of a disorder, it is important to avoid reaching conclusions based on institutional or "treated" samples. Although such samples are almost always more accessible and convenient to use than large-scale survey samples, institution-based samples can be misleading about true prevalence. The use of available services is determined not only by the presence of a disorder, but also by factors that may be extraneous to it, such as cultural, financial, attitudinal, and educational factors. It is well documented, for example, that the prevalence of highly disabling conditions such as blindness would be greatly underestimated if only those individuals using health services were considered. Large-scale community surveys done on well-characterized, carefully sampled community populations are, therefore, essential for acquiring solid epidemiological evidence.

Psychiatric Epidemiology

In infectious and Mendelian disorders, cause and effect relationships can be easily drawn. Even for multifactorial medical disorders, such as hypertension, hyperlipidemia, and coronary artery disease, phenotypes can be characterized through rather simple measurements. Psychiatric illnesses, however, are extremely complex entities with variable natural histories and overlays with other disorders. Thus, in spite of recent nosologic and therapeutic advances, a majority of psychiatric conditions remain at the level of the syndrome. This situation is reminiscent of that of the difficulty of understanding the etiology of "mental retardation" prior to the recognition of Mendelian disorders (e.g., phenylketonuria), or of the "fever and polyarthritis" syndromic complex before the identification of infectious or autoimmune disorders. In view of the scarcity of systematic data available on many psychiatric disorders and in the absence of confirmatory "gold standards," current diagnostic systems such as DSM-III-R (American Psychiatric Association 1987) should be viewed as being largely drafts of categories in search of validity rather than definitive, unmodifiable entities. Therefore, premature closures of the nosology should be avoided.

Cross-cultural diagnosis in psychiatry. The cultural equivalence of psychiatric diagnoses has always been a matter of serious concern for psychiatric nosologists. Such factors as the subjective nature of clinical phenomena, the total reliance on anamnesis and mental status examination as sources of data, and the well-entrenched ("ethnocentric") notions of mental illness, among others, can introduce bias in numerous ways.

This was nicely documented by Simon and colleagues (1973), who convincingly demonstrated the powerful impact of race and observer bias in determining clinical diagnoses among North American psychiatric patients. In that study, it was reported that in spite of similar clinical presentations, diagnoses of schizophrenia were more likely to be given to African American patients. If there could be a silver lining for such an unfortunate occurrence, it was the observation made by the authors that once structured interviews were incorporated into the design, diagnostic differences across ethnic groups tended to disappear (Simon et al. 1973).

International cooperation in mental health spearheaded by the World Health Organization (WHO) that included major studies on schizophrenia (WHO 1975) and depression (Sartorius et al. 1980) demonstrated that it is possible to develop reliable instruments for diagnosis (i.e., structured diagnostic interviews) that can be translated and adapted to the various cultures to collect comparable data. In the WHO studies, universally valid syndromes could be identified among the patients recruited in many countries and cultures when study procedures (instruments and training of personnel) were standardized. Notwithstanding their "universal" qualities, interesting cross-cultural differences on the presentation and outcome of psychiatric disorders could also be documented in those studies (Sartorius et al. 1978, 1980).

Evolution of Psychiatric Epidemiology in North America

The pioneer epidemiological studies in North American psychiatry were the Stirling County Study in Canada (Leighton et al. 1963), the Midtown Manhattan study in New York (Srole et al. 1962) and the New Haven study

(Hollingshead and Redlich 1958). These studies took place in the 1950s when psychodynamic theories had an enormous influence on the field. At that time, diagnosis was viewed as a secondary task, but in view of the scarcity of therapies and their lack of specificity, diagnosis might have made little difference anyway.

It comes as no surprise that the official diagnostic system at the time, *Diagnostic and Statistical Manual: Mental Disorders* (DSM-I; American Psychiatric Association 1952) reflected that state of affairs. DSM-I as well as its successor, DSM-II (American Psychiatric Association 1968), had many shortcomings. The manuals offered no definition of concepts, displayed many ambiguous notions and terms subject to different interpretations, and failed to include solid data from well-designed follow-up studies. Because the diagnostic exercise required high levels of "clinical judgment," it was particularly vulnerable to observer bias.

In the next few sections, I first review briefly the major findings of the pioneer studies in epidemiological psychiatry. I then examine in more detail the factors that contributed to the modern era of this branch of psychiatry.

The Stirling County Study.   This study began in 1952 in Canada under the direction of Leighton and colleagues (1963). One thousand ten community respondents were randomly selected and interviewed with a survey instrument, the "Health Opinions Survey." This instrument included many questions related to general health and, in the case of psychiatric disorders, it paid particular attention to neurotic and psychophysiological disorders. Mental disorders were lumped into one of seven categories: organic brain syndromes, mental retardation, psychoses, psychoneuroses, and psychophysiological, psychopathic, or personality disorders.

Study clinicians reviewed responses to the survey questionnaires as well as all information available in medical and psychiatric records in order to determine whether a respondent fell into a diagnostic category. The results showed that 26% of the community respondents could be allocated to one of the seven diagnostic groups.

The Midtown Manhattan Study.   This study directed by Rennie and collaborators (Srole et al. 1962) took place in the 1950s in New York City. A total of 1,660 households were sampled, and at least one adult respondent per household was interviewed with a survey instrument, the "Home Interview Survey." This instrument asked about topics such as psychiatric symptoms, sociodemographic factors, personal history, and use of health services. The major goal of the study was the identification of cases after reviewing all information available. In identifying "cases," one suspects that clinicians may have paid more attention to information concerning each subject's level of disability than to the presence of specific symptoms or diagnoses.

The study indicated that 23% of respondents had mental health disorders resulting in major functional impairment. The task of identifying cases was made difficult by the abundant information available to the clinician making the judgment. As with the Stirling County Study, the almost absolute reliance on clinician judgment may have resulted in various types of observer bias.

The first New Haven Study by Hollingshead and Redlich (1958).   Although this study was one of treated prevalence and not a random community survey, it ought to be mentioned here in view of the significance of its findings. Their findings, which have been consistently supported by many epidemiological studies, showed that sociodemographic factors, such as social class, affect the frequency with which patients with certain mental disorders come to treatment settings and the type of treatment these patients receive. The relationship of social class to prevalence of mental disorders was particularly relevant in patients with schizophrenia.

The Modern Era of Psychiatric Epidemiology

As I emphasized previously, the early epidemiological studies were limited by the nosologies effective at the time, making the choice of diagnosis a matter of clinical judgment and, thus, vulnerable to observer bias. Other limitations of those studies included the lack of standardized assessments for diagnosis and the relatively small samples studied.

The list of factors paving the way toward the new epidemiological studies should be headed by nosological and instrumental developments in the field. Important roles have also been played by therapeutic advances such as the availability of more specific treatments like lithium, and even by economic and legal realities. For example, the third-party payors demanded a clearer description of the entities they were paying for. Frequently, court appearances by psychiatric expert witnesses resulted in conflicting messages, which brought awareness of a need for more replicable systems.

From a scientific perspective, key studies propelling the field into the new era of operational diagnosis were of three kinds: 1) those documenting the "infirmities" of the old systems in terms of reliability and validity, 2) those insinuating potential gains to be derived from new operational approaches, and 3) those providing methods for quantifying agreement in psychiatric diagnosis (Spitzer and Fleiss 1974).

Catalysts for the "New" Paradigms in Psychiatric Epidemiology

The U.S./U.K. diagnostic study. This study made it clear that problems in definition and standardization of mental disorders impaired clinicians' ability to communicate clinical experiences and to compare them cross-culturally. The study followed the observations of Kramer (1965) of discrepant admission rates for schizophrenia in the United States compared with those in England, and the likely contribution of diagnostic habits toward those trends. The U.S./U.K. study utilized the Present State Examination (PSE; Wing et al. 1974). It confirmed that in the United States schizophrenia was overly diagnosed and manic depressive illness grossly underdiagnosed, whereas in England the opposite was the case. It therefore appeared that the concept of schizophrenia was much more broadly defined in the United States than in England. Because standardized procedures (use of the PSE) and interviewer training decreased cross-cultural variation in diagnosis, it was likely that the original differences resulted from the way corresponding diseases were initially construed by psychiatrists. Thus, when a structured diagnostic instrument (PSE) was administered by homogeneously and rigorously trained psychiatrists, the agreement between diagnoses made in the two countries increased (Cooper et al. 1972).

Subsequently, researchers in the United States began to document that reliability of psychiatric diagnosis could be substantially enhanced by eliciting symptoms "atheoretically" using a structured format (e.g., by simply scoring symptoms as present or absent) and thus avoiding individual or "monolithic" school biases.

The St. Louis Group. The development of diagnostic criteria was first proposed by a group from Washington University and Renard Hospital in St. Louis. This group, led by Eli Robins, Samuel Guze, and George Winokur, had been engaged for many years in "naturalistic" follow-up studies to validate a handful of psychiatric syndromes. These studies branched out from pioneering efforts in the 1950s focusing on two major disorders—"neurocirculatory asthenia" (anxiety neurosis; Wheeler et al. 1950) and hysteria (Cohen et al. 1953). These studies were so detailed and sophisticated that they remain unsurpassed in the field.

The 12 diagnoses validated by the St. Louis group were first printed in the *Archives of General Psychiatry* in 1972, where they were introduced as "criteria for use in psychiatric research" (Feighner et al. 1972) and then compiled into a book, *Psychiatric Diagnosis* (Goodwin and Guze 1984). These criteria, better known as "Feighner's criteria," would become in more propitious times the single reference most widely quoted in the literature and would serve as the basis for the Research Diagnostic Criteria (RDC), also coauthored by Robins (Spitzer et al. 1978), which was the forerunner of DSM-III (American Psychiatric Association 1980).

Epidemiological Studies Using Structured Diagnostic Interviews/Operational Diagnoses

Studies in the United States. The "second" New Haven Study can be viewed as transitional, because it began in the old DSM-II (American Psychiatric Association 1968) era; but in its follow-up portions, it was linked to the "operational diagnosis" era. The study took place in the 1960s (Myers et al. 1971), and a community sample of 938 respondents was originally interviewed in households with a survey instrument that used DSM-II categories. This study found that overall prevalence of mental disorders was 16%.

Of the 938 original respondents to the study, 720 could be located and reinterviewed in the mid-1970s with a structured diagnostic interview, the Schedule for Affective Disorders and Schizophrenia (SADS; Endicott and Spitzer 1978). The SADS elicited data that were categorized using diagnoses operationally defined in the RDC, the immediate precursor of DSM-III. Results of the second set of interviews yielded an overall prevalence of mental disorders (RDC) of 18%, a proportion similar to that obtained in the pioneer studies. "Major" and "minor" depressions taken together were the most common RDC disorders: their prevalence was 7%. An important observation in this study was that, although only one-third of those individuals meeting criteria for depression had used psychiatric services, more than two-thirds sought help from nonpsychiatric health services for their psychiatric symptoms. This de facto mental health system would be emphasized repeatedly in future studies (Regier et al. 1978; Shapiro et al. 1984). No specific information was provided on ethnic distribution for these disorders, possibly because very few minority respondents were included in the study.

Studies outside the United States. Epidemiological studies with the PSE took place outside the United States in the 1960s and 1970s. Well-designed studies include those performed in Athens (Mavreas et al. 1986), Edinburgh (Dean et al. 1983), Canberra (Henderson et al. 1979), London (Bebbington et al. 1981), and Uganda (Orley et al. 1979). Table 2–1 shows the prevalences for anxiety and depressive syndromes in Edinburgh, London, and Canberra, together with those prevalences found in New Haven, Connecticut, by Weissman and colleagues (1980). As this table shows, the overall rates for these disorders in the four countries are similar.

Table 2–2 shows the prevalence rates for five PSE disorders in Uganda and Athens broken down by gender. It should be noted that, although Ugandans of both sexes have higher prevalences of depressive disorders than respondents from Athens, female respondents from Athens have a rate of anxiety disorders almost three times as high as that of their Ugandan counterparts.

Demographic correlates from these PSE studies indicate that alcoholism is a predominantly male disorder, whereas depressive and anxiety disorders have higher prevalences in females. In Greece, it was observed that those with low levels of education had higher rates of mental disorders than those with high educational levels, whereas respondents who were married had lower rates of disorder than those who were single, separated, widowed, or divorced (Mavreas et al. 1986). As this review continues, it will become apparent that these correlates appear as a common theme in most cultures studied.

Political "Catalyst": The President's Commission on Mental Health

The President's Commission, created by President Jimmy Carter in the 1970s to review the status of mental health in the United States, can be conceived as the political catalyst that ushered in the new psychiatric epidemiology (President's Commission on Mental Health 1978). As a first step, the commission encouraged input from experts in the field. A distillate of the scientific papers submitted to the commission appeared in a special issue of the *Archives of General Psychiatry* in June 1978. This issue

Table 2–1. Prevalence of anxiety and depressive disorders in four sites, defined according to PSE-CATEGO or RDC criteria (%)

Disorder	Edinburgh (PSE-CATEGO)	London (PSE-CATEGO)	Canberra (PSE-CATEGO)	New Haven (SADS-RDC)
Anxiety	3	4	3	3
Depression	9	7	7	8

Note. Rates were rounded to nearest integer.

reported on the status of research in epidemiology and mental health services in the United States. These reports, together with economic support from the Carter administration, provided the impetus for the important research to follow.

The two sets of reports (President's Commission on Mental Health 1978; Regier et al. 1978; Robins 1978) underlined the complexities inherent in this kind of research and provided a review of existing epidemiological studies. The review identified methodological problems affecting studies, outlined promising new strategies, and pointed to the desirability of systematically studying the prevalence and incidence of mental disorders, as well as the need for exploring the protective effect of supportive social networks and for evaluating available services. The commission's report also recognized the importance of pursuing research studies to examine the mental health needs of special populations, such as ethnic groups and their access to services. The Epidemiologic Catchment Area program (ECA) was one of the happy results of this presidential initiative.

The National Institute of Mental Health Epidemiologic Catchment Area Program (NIMH-ECA)

This study (Eaton and Kessler 1985; Regier et al. 1984), widely regarded as a landmark in psychiatric epidemiology (Freedman 1984), was a collaborative effort to apply common instruments to large population samples for diagnosis and use of health services. The NIMH-ECA interviewed close to 20,000 community respondents between 1978 and 1986 at five study sites. These were associated with The Johns Hopkins University in Baltimore,

Table 2–2.   Prevalence of psychiatric disorder (PSE-CATEGO) by gender in Uganda and Greece (%)

Disorder	Uganda (N = 221)		Greece (N = 489)	
	Males	Females	Males	Females
Schizophrenia and other psychoses	0.9	—	0.4	0.4
Mania	1.9	2.0	—	—
Anxiety	3.1	4.3	3.9	12.1
Depression	14.0	23.0	4.3	10.3
Alcoholism	—	—	2.6	0.0
Overall	24.0	27.0	9.0	23.0

Maryland; Duke University in Durham, North Carolina; The University of California in Los Angeles, California; Yale University in New Haven, Connecticut; and Washington University in St. Louis, Missouri.

The study was coordinated by the Division of Biometry and Epidemiology at the National Institute of Mental Health (NIMH). The selection of study sites was made on the basis of scientific merit of the submitted proposals while taking into account the availability of special populations of interest such as underserved ethnic minorities, the elderly, and residents from rural areas. The ECA design included two sets of interviews separated by 1 year: the first to provide information on prevalence and the second to provide information on the accretion of new symptoms (incidence). The survey included a diagnostic instrument, the Diagnostic Interview Schedule (DIS; Robins et al. 1981) as well as specific questions on use of health services, presence of physical illness, use of psychotropic medications, social support systems, and other variables.

The Diagnostic Interview Schedule (DIS).   The DIS is a highly structured diagnostic interview that was the key instrument used for case identification in the ECA surveys. It was developed by the St. Louis group under an NIMH contract specifically for the ECA study (Robins et al. 1981). It assesses specific criteria for 36 DSM-III categories through eliciting individual symptoms, assessing their severity, and using specific probes to exclude medical etiologies. Temporal cues make it possible to distinguish lifetime from current (within the past month) disorders. The instrument was translated and validated prior to its use on Hispanic respondents.

According to clinical comparisons, diagnoses made by trained lay interviewers using the DIS compared favorably with those made by clinicians in using a clinical interview format (Robins et al. 1981). However, when diagnoses made by lay interviewers using the DIS as part of the ECA surveys were compared with those made by clinicians at a later follow-up interview using other interview formats (e.g., SADS or PSE), there were only marginal levels of agreement shown for most diagnoses examined (Anthony et al. 1985; Helzer et al. 1985). Although many questions remain unanswered about the clinical equivalence of DIS-elicited syndromes, the DIS is perhaps the instrument that adheres most rigorously to DSM-III's operational rules. In my opinion, the DIS provides the best available "translation of DSM-III criteria into questions" (Robins 1989, p. 57).

The additional problems created when the DIS is translated and used in other countries or cultures will be discussed later in this chapter in the section "Instrument Translation and Adaptation."

Ethnic Minorities Included in the ECA Surveys

The selection of minority group respondents at most ECA sites was a random event, relative to their numbers in the general population. One exception was the large Hispanic sample selectively chosen in Los Angeles by "targeting" an area known to contain a high proportion of Mexican American respondents. Thus, 43% of the respondents in Los Angeles were Hispanic, compared with only 0.5%–2% at the other four sites. The proportion of African Americans relative to the total sample interviewed at the various sites was 4% in Los Angeles, 10% in New Haven, 19% in St Louis, 34% in Baltimore, and 36% in Durham (Leaf et al. 1991). Total numbers of Asian Americans interviewed at the various sites were unfortunately too low to perform meaningful prevalence estimates. Therefore, "ethnic" data in the ECA are restricted to African Americans, Hispanics (largely Mexican Americans), and a large and amorphous "White non-Hispanic" group.

ECA I results—prevalence of mental disorders at five sites. Table 2–3 presents 6-month prevalences for selected major disorders obtained at the various ECA sites. The data in the table indicate that there are remarkable similarities in the prevalence of most disorders examined at the five different sites, with the exception of phobic disorder. The higher prevalence of phobia observed in Durham and Baltimore may be partially related to the way interview questions were worded, and the relatively high propor-

Table 2–3. The Epidemiologic Catchment Area Study: 6-month prevalence of selected DSM-III disorders at five sites* (%)

DSM-III disorder	New Haven	Baltimore	St. Louis	Durham	Los Angeles
Schizophrenic/ schizophreniform	> 1	> 1	< 1	> 1	< 1
Major depressive	4	2	3	2	3
Phobic	6	13	5	14	6
Panic	< 1	1	1	< 1	1
Obsessive-compulsive	< 1	> 1	2	> 1	2
Alcohol	5	7	5	4	6
Drugs	2	3	2	1	2

* Modified from Burnam et al. 1987a.
Note. Rates have been rounded to nearest integer.

tion of African Americans and respondents from low socioeconomic backgrounds present at these sites.

Demographic correlates.   Secondary analyses of the ECA data that took sociodemographic factors into account consistently found higher prevalence rates of mental disorder among respondents who were younger than age 45, those who were unmarried (widowed, single, divorced, or separated), and those with low educational levels. Drug abuse or dependence and alcohol abuse or dependence were found to be predominantly diagnoses of male respondents in all age groups at all sites, whereas affective and anxiety disorders were found to be predominantly diagnoses of female respondents (Karno et al. 1987; Regier et al. 1988; Robins et al. 1984).

Urban versus rural populations.   In the Piedmont area of North Carolina, the ECA surveyors interviewed respondents in four rural counties (thought to be representative of the "rural South") as well as respondents residing in an urban area (the city of Durham). Comparisons of 6-month prevalence rates for major DSM-III disorders for rural and urban respondents shown in Table 2–4 indicate that, although the prevalence of most disorders did not differ significantly across rural and urban samples, urban residents compared with rural residents showed higher prevalences of major depression (2.4 versus 1.1), and drug abuse or dependence (0.2 versus 0.0). Conversely, rural respondents had higher prevalences of alcohol abuse or dependence than urban respondents (2.6 versus 2.2). When stratified by age, sex, race, and education, the prevalence of alcohol abuse or dependence was found to be particularly high among respondents with low levels of education (Blazer et al. 1985).

"Younger" versus "older" cohorts.   When "White non-Hispanic" ECA respondents are separated into different cohorts according to their date of birth, cumulative rates of depression show sharp increases in the case of respondents born after 1935, with those respondents born after 1955 showing the steepest slope (Klerman and Weissman 1989). Thus, the younger the cohort, the greater the probability of developing a major affective disorder. These data from the ECA are supported by those emerging from other North American studies as well as studies from Canada, New Zealand, and Germany (Klerman and Weissman 1989). Interestingly, however, these secular trends were not seen in the case of Mexican American ECA respondents, respondents from the Puerto Rican survey, or those interviewed in Korea using the same diagnostic format (Klerman and Weissman 1989). These findings suggest that factors unique to these countries or cultures may be playing a role in determining the secular trends.

Ethnicity and Prevalence of Mental Disorders in the ECA Data Set

Overall, African American respondents reported higher rates of lifetime or active disorders than whites or Hispanics. These differences have been largely attributed to effects of age and socioeducational factors (Robins and Regier 1991).

Schizophrenia. Prevalences of schizophrenia were found to be highest among African Americans, intermediate among "White non-Hispanics," and lowest among Hispanics. However, when analyses controlled for socioeducational status, most differences between ethnic groups disappeared (Keith et al. 1991).

Table 2–4.   Prevalence of specific mental disorders in rural and urban populations interviewed with the DIS in three countries (%)

DIS disorder	United States[a] (6-Month) Urban Areas	Rural Areas	Taiwan[b] (Lifetime) Urban (Taipei)	Small Towns	Rural Areas	Korea[c] (Lifetime) Urban Areas	Rural Areas
Schizophrenia/ schizophreniform	1.1	0.6	0.3	0.2	0.2	0.3	0.2
Major depressive	2.4	1.1	0.8	1.7	1.0	1.1	1.5
Dysthymic	1.6	1.8	0.9	1.5	0.9	0.2	1.5
Phobic	8.9	8.0	4.2	5.7	3.4	4.2	5.6
Obsessive- compulsive	1.5	2.7	0.9	0.3	0.5	0.9	0.5
Panic	—	—	0.2	0.3	0.1	0.2	0.3
Somatization			0.04	0.1	0.1	0.02	0.1
Alcohol[d]	2.2	2.6	4.5	9.8	7.4	4.9	9.8
Drugs[d]	0.2	0.0	0.1	0.0	0.1	0.1	0.2

[a] Blazer et al. 1985 (6-month prevalence rates).
[b] Hwu et al. 1989 (lifetime prevalence rates).
[c] Lee 1988 (lifetime prevalence rates).
[d] Abuse and dependence.

Affective disorders. "White non-Hispanic" respondents were found to have the highest lifetime rates of "Major Depression" (prevalences were 5% Whites, 4% Hispanics, and 3% African Americans), whereas prevalence of "Manic symptoms" was highest among African Americans, intermediate among "White non-Hispanics," and lowest among Hispanics (Weissman et al. 1991).

Anxiety disorders. Lifetime rates for phobic disorder (agoraphobia and simple phobia), were significantly higher among African American respondents compared with "White non-Hispanics" and Hispanics ($P < .05$). In the case of respondents with panic disorder, however, no ethnic differences were found (Eaton et al. 1991).

Addictive disorders. The prevalence of alcoholism for the various ethnic groups differed by age and sex. Thus, among younger males, prevalence of alcoholism was highest among Hispanic and "White non-Hispanic" respondents and lowest among African Americans, whereas in older males (age 45 or older) African Americans had the highest prevalences and "White non-Hispanics" the lowest (Helzer et al 1991). Prevalences of drug abuse by sex were 40% and 22% for African American males and females respectively, 36% and 26% for "White non-Hispanics," and 34% and 16% for Hispanics (Anthony and Helzer 1991).

Antisocial personality. This was the only Axis II diagnosis included in the DIS. Interestingly, no ethnic differences were found in the prevalence of this disorder, a finding in conflict with the consistent observation that minority groups are grossly overrepresented in incarcerated populations. The exact meaning of these findings remains unclear.

Somatization disorder. The highest prevalences of this disorder were found among African American women (0.8%), followed by African American men (0.4%), and may be related to their lower educational status. Surprisingly, Hispanics showed no increase in lifetime rates for the full diagnosis (Swartz et al. 1991). However, in Los Angeles, the prevalence of an abridged somatization construct was found to be higher in the case of Mexican American women relative to "White non-Hispanic" women, particularly in the older age groups, which is also possibly related to lower socioeducational indices (Escobar et al. 1987).

The Los Angeles ECA Study

In Los Angeles, our group (Karno et al. 1987) interviewed 1,305 Hispanic respondents. Because a large majority of these respondents (93%) were Mexican Americans, these data cannot be extrapolated to other Hispanic groups in the United States. For the comparative analyses, Mexican American respondents were compared with a sample of "White non-Hispanics" interviewed in the same catchment areas. Analyses of the data yielded more similarities than differences in the prevalence of disorders across these two groups. There were only a few ethnic differences observed in lifetime prevalence rates. These included a higher prevalence of alcohol abuse or dependence but lower prevalences of drug abuse or dependence and major depression among Mexican American males compared with their non-Hispanic counterparts, a somewhat higher prevalence of phobia and dysthymia among Mexican American women over the age of 40, and a lower prevalence of drug and alcohol disorders for Hispanic women of any age group compared with non-Hispanic women (Karno et al. 1987).

Mexican Americans, country of birth, and psychiatric disorder. Of the Mexican American respondents interviewed in Los Angeles, about 60% were first-generation Mexican Americans (born in Mexico), whereas the remaining 40% were born in the United States. When lifetime prevalences of DSM-III disorders for these two groups were compared, we found surprising differences (Karno et al. 1987). Mexico-born Mexican Americans had consistently lower prevalences than their U.S.-born counterparts for most disorders examined. These differences were particularly pronounced in the case of respondents with substance use disorders (see Table 2–5). Explanations for the differences between the two groups are offered in the next section.

Acculturation. This concept refers to the sociocultural changes that take place when individuals originating in one culture move to a new culture. High levels of acculturation imply a high degree of assimilation or identification with the new culture; low levels of acculturation indicate that most traditional cultural values are retained. Mexican American respondents in the Los Angeles-ECA (LA-ECA) survey were allocated to "high," "medium," or "low" acculturation groups based on responses to an acculturation scale (Burnam et al. 1987b). When lifetime prevalences of mental disorders were compared across acculturation groups, no significant differences could be found (Burnam et al. 1987b).

The findings of the LA-ECA study were quite contrary to the findings in the voluminous literature on immigration and mental disorder. How can one explain the LA-ECA findings that level of acculturation did not affect prevalence rates of mental disorders, whereas country of birth greatly influenced such rates in an unexpected direction? Potential explanations include 1) a "selective-migration" theory that proposes the migration of rather robust, resilient individuals from Mexico to the United States, and 2) conjectures that, compared with U.S.-born minorities, recent immigrants have a less drastic perception of discrimination, minority status, or deprivation in their new environment. It is also possible that some of the differences between the LA-ECA findings and those of other studies may be related to cultural or linguistic artifacts of the instrumental measures (the DIS). These potential biases will be discussed in more detail in the section "Instrument Translation and Adaptation."

ECA II results—incidence of mental disorders at four sites.   Because the ECA included two waves of interviewing 1 year apart, it is possible to estimate the number of new cases appearing during a 1-year observation period. Eaton and colleagues (1989) have provided preliminary incidence estimates for seven disorders with a relatively high prevalence at the ECA sites. These incidence analyses excluded one of the original sites: Yale University.

Table 2–5.   Lifetime prevalence of selected DSM-III disorders for Mexican American respondents born in Mexico or in the United States[a] (%)

DSM-III disorder	Mexican American respondents		
	Mexico-born	U.S.-born	Significance
Major depressive	3	7	< .001
Dysthymic	3	6	< .01
Phobic	10	17	< .001
Obsessive-compulsive	1	2	NS
Panic	1	1	NS
Alcohol[b]	14	24	< .0001
Drugs[b]	3	8	< .0001
Antisocial personality	3	4	NS

[a] Modified from Burnam et al. 1987b.
[b] Abuse or dependence.
Note.   Rates have been rounded to the nearest integer.

In calculating "first" incidence for each disorder, Eaton and colleagues (1989) included in the numerator respondents who met criteria for the disorder for the first time in their lives during the observation period. The denominator included only those respondents who started the 1-year observation period without prior history of the disorder. A difficult methodological problem encountered in estimating incidence in the ECA data set was the observation that 1-year prevalence rates for most disorders declined from wave 1 to wave 2, and that this decline may simply be due to the effect of being interviewed a second time.

Results of these preliminary incidence analyses indicated that among men, major depression and alcohol and drug disorders had a peak incidence in the youngest group (ages 18 through 29). Although for women, substance use disorders also peaked in the youngest group, the incidence of depression reached its highest point in the middle-aged groups (ages 30 through 64). In the case of both sexes, panic disorder had its highest incidence in the middle-aged group (ages 30 through 44), whereas phobic and obsessive compulsive disorders had less clear profiles.

These observations on incidence of panic disorder are in conflict with naturalistic studies consistently showing that the disorder starts in early adulthood (early 20s). The figures on panic disorder may be due to "contamination" with major depression, a frequent comorbid occurrence. The diagnostic data included in the analyses did not utilize a system of hierarchies. Instead, all diagnoses for which the respondent met criteria were included in the findings. Interestingly, the relationship of age to incidence of disorder was very similar for respondents with major depressive, panic, and phobic disorders (Eaton et al. 1989).

Other DIS Epidemiological Studies in North America

The Hispanic HANES.   The Hispanic Health and Nutrition Examination (H-HANES) was conducted by the National Center for Health Statistics (NCHS) to gather data on the physical and mental health status of Hispanic Americans (Moscicki et al. 1987). This study was one in a series of periodic surveys conducted by NCHS since 1962 in which the major component is a physical examination. The H-HANES took place between 1982 and 1984 and included multistage, stratified samples of U.S. Hispanics drawn from several geographical areas: Mexican Americans from five Southwestern states (N = 3,500), Cuban Americans from the Miami area (N = 900), and Puerto Ricans from the New York City area (N = 1,300). In addition to being given a physical examination, these respondents were interviewed with the depressive disorders section of the DIS. They also completed a self-rating instrument, the Center of Epidemiological Studies Depression Scale (CES-D; Radloff 1977).

The Hispanic groups differed in terms of demographic factors. From a socioeconomic perspective, the most disadvantaged among the Hispanic respondents were the Puerto Ricans. For example, 36% of Puerto Ricans versus 27% of Mexican Americans and 19% of Cuban Americans were at or below the poverty level. Puerto Ricans were more likely to be unemployed; 50% of Puerto Ricans, 39% of Mexican Americans, and 32% of Cuban Americans reported no current employment. Also, Puerto Rican respondents were less likely to be married; 51% of Puerto Ricans were married, compared with 69% of Cuban Americans and 71% of Mexican Americans.

DIS and CES-D data showed that Puerto Rican respondents had a significantly higher prevalence of major depressive disorders and higher levels of depressive symptoms than the other groups. As can be seen in Table 2–6, lifetime prevalence rates of major depressive disorders were 9% for Puerto Ricans and 4% each for Mexican Americans and Cubans. In the CES-D, 28% of Puerto Ricans, 13% of Mexican Americans, and 9% of Cuban Americans met the criteria for having a disorder (Moscicki et al. 1987). As will be seen

Table 2–6.   Lifetime prevalence of selected DSM-III disorders among Hispanic populations both inside and outside the United States* (%)

DSM-III disorder	Mexican Americans			Puerto Ricans		Peruvians	Cubans
	USA	Mex.	H-HANES	PR	H-HANES	Lima	H-HANES
Depression	3	7	4	2	9	7	4
Dysthymia	3	6		5		4	
Panic	1	1		2		2	
Phobic	11	13		12		16	
Obsessive-compulsive	2	2		3		5	
Alcohol	14	24		13		17	
Drugs	2	8				< 1	

* Data in this table have been modified from several sources: Burnam et al. 1987a; Canino et al. 1987; Hagashi et al. 1985; Moscicki et al. 1987.
Note.   Rates have been rounded to the nearest integer. USA = Born in the United States; Mex. = Born in Mexico; PR = Born in Puerto Rico.

later in this chapter, despite similar demographic characteristics, the prevalence of major depressive disorders for mainland Puerto Ricans was also significantly higher than that of Puerto Ricans living in Puerto Rico.

The Canadian Study. In this study (Bland et al. 1988a), 3,258 community respondents, all urban dwellers in Edmonton, Alberta, were interviewed between 1983 and 1986 with a survey instrument that included the DIS. A majority of the respondents (more than 90%) were catalogued as "White." Specific data on ethnicity were not collected, which represents a major omission in view of the multicultural composition of the Canadian society.

Lifetime prevalence rates for Canadian respondents are shown in Table 2–7. As can be seen in the table, the overall prevalence rates for most disorders were very similar to those found at the ECA sites, except that the rates of alcohol abuse and dependence and major depression tended to be higher in Canada than in the United States.

The demographic correlates of mental disorder in Canada were very similar to those previously detailed in the ECA surveys. In Canada, men also had higher prevalences of alcohol disorders; women had higher prevalences of affective, anxiety, and somatoform disorders; and unmarried respondents (widowed, separated, single, or divorced) had higher

Table 2–7.   Lifetime prevalence of major DSM-III disorders in Edmonton*

DSM-III disorder	Prevalence (%)
Schizophrenia/schizophreniform	< 1
Major depressive	9
Dysthymic	4
Panic	< 1
Phobic	9
Obsessive-compulsive	3
Somatization	0
Antisocial personality	4
Alcohol abuse or dependence	18
Drug abuse or dependence	7

* Modified from Bland et al. 1988a.
Note. Rates have been rounded to the nearest integer.

prevalences for most disorders compared with those respondents who were currently married (Bland et al. 1988b).

Epidemiological Studies with the DIS in Latin America

The Puerto Rican Survey.   This study (Canino et al. 1987) took place in Puerto Rico in the 1980s. It utilized methodologies very similar to those of the ECA surveys to interview respondents ages 17 through 64 from rural and urban areas with a Spanish version of the DIS adapted for local usage. The demographic characteristics of the sample were similar to those described in the 1980 U.S. census for the whole island. Of the 1,551 respondents interviewed, about two-thirds were urban residents, one-half were younger than age 35, 40% had less than 10 years of education, and 60% were living below the U.S. poverty level. Indeed, Puerto Rico's per capita income is less than one-half that of Mississippi, the poorest U.S. state. Regarding language, most respondents (more than 60%) were monolingual Spanish speakers.

In view of these factors, and because of the widely held belief that Puerto Ricans exhibit far greater levels of symptoms than other U.S. populations, the expectation was that prevalence rates of mental disorders in the island would exceed those documented on the mainland. The results surprisingly showed that prevalence rates for most disorders among respondents in Puerto Rico were not different from those found at the ECA sites in the mainland (see Table 2–6).

As was also true in the ECA survey, the data from the Puerto Rican survey showed that prevalence rates of mental disorders in men compared with women were higher among the less-educated respondents, who also showed higher rates of alcoholism, whereas women had a higher prevalence of affective and anxiety disorders. Interestingly, however, prevalence rates for somatization disorder were identical for male and female respondents in Puerto Rico, a finding at variance with that of the ECA and Canadian studies and also contrary to clinical lore.

The Peruvian Study.   In this study (Hagashi et al. 1985), which was financed by a Japanese grant and included Japanese coinvestigators, community respondents ($N = 808$) of a slum area in Lima, Peru, were interviewed with the Spanish version of the DIS. Preliminary results indicated that more than 40% of respondents met criteria for at least one DIS–DSM-III disorder throughout their lifetimes, a rate far higher than that reported in most other settings. The prevalence rates for specific DSM-III disorders are shown in

Table 2–6. It should be noted from the table that, compared with other Latin American or Hispanic groups, the rates for obsessive-compulsive disorder and antisocial personality are higher among respondents in Peru. These findings are difficult to interpret but may be related to problems with instrument adaptation and cross-cultural equivalence, both semantic and conceptual.

DIS Epidemiological Studies in Asia

In the absence of epidemiological data in the United States for the various Asian American groups, it is important to scrutinize studies recently completed in Taiwan and Korea to at least provide some hints on particular mental health trends for these ethnic groups.

The Taiwanese study. This study took place between 1982 and 1986 and used a Chinese version of the DIS (Hwu et al. 1989). A total of 11,004 community respondents—5,005 in the capital city (Taipei), 3,004 in two small towns, and 2,995 in six rural villages—were interviewed. The overall prevalences of DIS–DSM-III disorders among respondents were 16% in Taipei, 28% in the small towns, and 21% in the rural areas, rates all lower than those found in other DIS studies.

Table 2–4 shows the lifetime prevalence rates for specific psychiatric disorders in Taiwan. It should be noted that the rates for most disorders tend to be lower than those reported in the United States, Canada, Latin America, and Korea; also, the small towns, compared with Taipei and the rural areas, had higher prevalences of several disorders. This finding may be related to the low educational status and high levels of social upheaval present in these townships (Hwu et al. 1989).

Demographic correlates were similar to those of other DIS studies. Thus, alcohol abuse and drug related disorders as well as antisocial personality were more common among men, whereas affective/anxiety disorders were more common among women. In view of the low prevalences found in Taiwan, questions can be raised concerning whether the DSM-III criteria are applicable in Taiwan, or whether Taiwanese respondents suffer from disorders different from those included in the ECA surveys.

The opportunity to test this latter hypothesis arose when two additional diagnoses, generalized anxiety disorder and psychophysiologic disorder, were added to the DIS. The results were that psychophysiologic disorder was the most common diagnosis in Taiwan with lifetime prevalences of 9% in Taipei, 10% in small towns, and 7% in rural areas. Generalized anxiety disorder was the second most common, with prevalences of 3% in Taipei, 9% in small towns, and 6% in rural areas (Hwu et al. 1989). These two diagnoses may be the DSM-III categories closest to *The International Classification of Diseases, 10th Revision* (ICD-10; World Health Organization 1992) category of "neurasthenia," traditionally one of the most common diagnoses reported in non-Western societies (Kleinman 1982).

The Korean study. This study also took place in the mid-1980s. More than 3,000 Seoul area and rural respondents were interviewed with a Korean version of the DIS (Lee 1988). The results of this survey indicated that, overall, 40% of the respondents met criteria for at least one Lifetime DIS–DSM-III diagnosis. This rate was almost twice as high as that seen in Taiwan and higher than the average overall rate reported for the ECA study sites.

The rates for specific disorders in Korea are shown in Table 2–4. As can be seen in the table, prevalence rates for most disorders in Korea are higher than those reported for Taiwan. Note that rates for most disorders in Taiwan and Korea were very similar in urban and rural areas. Higher rates of alcohol abuse or dependence and affective disorders were seen among rural Koreans compared with their urban counterparts.

Discussion

From the perspective of international psychiatry, a major accomplishment of the new epidemiological studies was that they reaffirmed that it was indeed possible to perform large-scale epidemiologic surveys in different countries and cultures using standard methodologies. Data from these international studies indicated that there were remarkable similarities in the prevalence of psychiatric disorders in different countries and cultures. The overall prevalence defined as any DIS–DSM-III disorder present over a lifetime averaged 34% in the United States, 34% in Canada, 28% in Puerto Rico, 41% in Peru, 22% in Taiwan, and 40% in Korea. The range at the various U.S. sites was 30%–40%. Although the prevalence of specific disorders was also lower for the Taiwan samples compared with those at other sites, prevalences and distributions for the major DSM-III disorders were remarkably similar across most international sites surveyed.

Many investigators, particularly the proponents of a biological diathesis, may find it reassuring that the presentation and prevalence of disorders defined in Western biomedical terms show such uniformity. They may be tempted to conclude that such consistency is proof that these mental disorders are indeed universal and biologically driven phenomena. Those of us who are culturally oriented psychiatrists suspect, however, that some of this congruence may be artifactual. From this cross-cultural perspective, psychiatric disorders are viewed as the aggregate contribution of biological, psychological, and social factors. Therefore, similarities in prevalence rates raise serious questions concerning diagnostic and instrumental equivalence in view of the disparate geographical, ethnic, linguistic, educational, and economic conditions present at the different sites. Thus, a sensitive and valid measure should have at least theoretically yielded more discrepant rates to coincide with the unique risk/protective factors operating in each culture. Kleinman (1987) has brought about an awareness of the strong bias of Western psychiatrists toward demonstrating cross-cultural similarities and universals in mental illness. He has also argued that applying a diagnostic category developed for a specific cultural group to another cultural group constitutes a "category fallacy" (Kleinman 1987, p. 452).

However, more practically, the consistent findings obtained in the various studies regarding a relatively uniform distribution of disorders by gender, educational, and marital status, suggest the measures may have validity. For example, in most countries surveyed, DIS diagnostic data indicated that alcohol and drug abuse were found predominantly among men, whereas anxiety and affective disorders were found predominantly among women. At every site, low educational levels implied higher rates, whereas being currently married was related to lower rates of psychiatric disorder.

Among the few findings from these epidemiological studies suggesting that cultural factors may affect the prevalences of disorders, one can name the lack of cohort effect on rates of affective illness among Los Angeles Mexican Americans, Puerto Ricans, and Koreans, and the absence of a gender effect for somatization disorder in Puerto Rico (Canino et al. 1987; Klerman and Weissman 1989). These findings provide interesting leads to be pursued in second-generation studies. For example, an ongoing study is currently exploring whether "protective"factors such as social support systems may play a role in determining the direction of the cohort effects mentioned above (Ellen Frank Ph.D., personal communication, December 1991).

Methodological Strategies

In efforts to enhance the scope of ethnic research, the following should be taken into account.

Instrument translation and adaptation.   A well-known problem in psychiatric research is that of translating and adapting instruments developed in a particular country or culture for use in a different country or culture. Karno and colleagues (1985) and Canino and colleagues (1987) have underlined the difficulties in adapting the DIS for use among Spanish-speaking Mexican American and Puerto Rican respondents. Even though the translation/validation steps incorporated in the Los Angeles and Puerto Rico surveys provided confidence about the validity of the data obtained in those populations, a number of questions remain regarding the proper interpretation and extrapolation of these findings.

Assessing the various types of diagnostic and instrumental validity prior to engaging in cross-cultural research.   After acknowledging problems in translating and adapting the DIS for use among Peruvian respondents of low socioeconomic status, Flaherty and colleagues (1988) articulated a comprehensive step-by-step procedure into the process of translating and adapting instruments to be used in a new cultural setting. Full implementation of the various steps is viewed by the authors as a prerequisite to guarantee that use of the instrument in the new culture may indeed provide useful data. The procedure involves awareness and proper assessment of five different forms of validity—"content," "semantic," "technical," "criterion," and "conceptual," each implying a number of specific tasks (Flaherty et al. 1988). Unfortunately, cross-cultural research has not yet adopted these excellent recommendations.

Educational and linguistic artifacts.   Our group (Escobar et al. 1986) and that of Canino and colleagues (1987) demonstrated that scores in the Mini-Mental State Examination (MMSE; Folstein et al. 1975)—the instrument used in the various epidemiological surveys to elicit cognitive disturbance—are influenced by ethnicity and language, and result in a high number of false-positive cases when used in Hispanic populations, particularly among respondents with low educational levels.

Ethnicity and responses to clinical instruments.   Another important issue needing clarification is the differing ways ethnic groups may respond to clinical instruments and interviewing formats. For example, in a study of Hispanic and non-Hispanic white schizophrenic patients with a self-rating instrument (Hopkins Symptom Checklist—90 [SCL-90]; Derogatis 1983) and an interviewer-administered instrument (DIS), we observed that there were cultural differences in the responses to these instruments. Thus, although Hispanics provided consistent responses to questions on psychopathology regardless of format, non-Hispanic white respondents were more likely to acknowledge and endorse symptoms when questions were asked in the self-rating format, but tended to "deny" these same symptoms when asked about their presence during a face-to-face interview (Randolph et al. 1985). This interesting dimension that may affect the type and quality of clinical data elicited remains unexplored in most epidemiological and cross-cultural studies.

Conclusion

The epidemiological studies reviewed here allow only a glimpse at the mental health picture of U.S. minorities. Even the ECA study (Eaton and Kessler 1985; Regier et al. 1984), the most ambitious undertaking in psychiatric epidemiology ever performed in this country, came far short in its ethnic scope. Obviously, practical limitations in the sampling process and geographical regions chosen restricted the "analyzable" ethnic minorities to a handful of African American respondents in the South and Northeast and a small pocket of Mexican Americans in California. Also, although the H-HANES (Moscicki et al. 1987) included the largest Hispanic subgroups (Mexican Americans, Puerto Ricans, and Cubans), the information elicited on psychiatric status was extremely limited. Thus, with the exception of Mexican Americans and Puerto Ricans (thanks to the Puerto Rican study [Canino et al. 1987]), other large Hispanic subgroups such as Cubans or Central and South American immigrants remain to be studied. In the case of Asian Americans, no reliable information is available either, because no large-scale survey has included representative samples of this group, and only very limited inferences can be made from the studies performed in the Asian countries.

In a multicultural society like the United States, minority status is more often linked to economic and social disadvantages of a group rather than numerical realities or degree of cultural allegiance. This restrictive view of ethnic minority tends to exclude from due consideration many other cultural groups that may also display a tendency to preserve their original heritage (i.e., language, religion) and experience differing degrees of assimilation into North American society (i.e., Eastern and Western Europeans, Arabs, Hasidic Jews, and many others). At least theoretically, these groups could also serve as important sources of data when assessing the impact of cultural background on the form and prevalence of mental disorders.

Unfortunately, in these times of budgetary constraints, funding for ambitious epidemiological undertakings that would attempt to answer many of the questions posed here may not be feasible. However, I do not think it is too unreasonable to conclude that we may not be quite ready yet to go for the "definitive" study that would lead to etiological assumptions and preventive interventions. Indeed, the field of psychiatry is in need of further scientific growth, particularly regarding its nosological and etiological dimensions. Simply stated, this implies that in order to fully profit from all the "ideal" refinements in design and methodologies previously outlined, the field awaits the development of new scientific "paradigms." These new "paradigms" would, I hope, move us past the old "demoralization/stress" model and into more objective and replicable contingencies that would promote a clearer definition and demarcation of syndromes by using, for example, specific "gold standards" (e.g., biological "markers") that could be reliably identified in all countries and races.

From a more practical and "optimistic" perspective, I would like to propose that ethnic researchers in this country become more cognizant of some of the relative advantages and benefits conferred by membership into the distinct ethnocultural groups. To this date, it seems to me that we have been almost exclusively concerned with "disadvantages" such as poverty, discrimination, low educational levels, or other physical, mental, or social "infirmities" and may have neglected potentially important hints on advantages. For example, in the case of Hispanic Americans, evidence is beginning to accumulate that in spite of their economic and educational "disadvantages," some relative advantages may also be present. Among these are the relatively low prevalences for most psychiatric disorders among, for example, Mexican Americans with low levels of acculturation (Burnam et al. 1987b), the low indices of suicide for Hispanic Americans compared with whites (Earls et al. 1990), and the absence of cohort effects in the prevalence of affective disorders among Mexican Americans and Puerto Ricans (Klerman and Weissman 1989). In the case of general health, an example would be the relatively high longevity rates in Puerto Rico; Puerto Rican females have a life expectancy of 78.9 years, compared with 78.4 years for the female population of the United States (Health United States 1991, p. 74). Another perceived advantage would be the rather favorable morbidity and mortality health statistics for Mexican Americans relative to other ethnic groups (Health United States 1991).

These interesting "contrasts" warrant further study in a search for unique biological (e.g., genetic) or social factors that may have a "protective" value and therefore could become important components in preventive strategies.

References

American Psychiatric Association: Diagnostic and Statistical Manual: Mental Disorders. Washington, DC, American Psychiatric Association, 1952

American Psychiatric Association: Diagnostic and Statistical Manual of Mental Disorders, 2nd Edition. Washington, DC, American Psychiatric Association, 1968

American Psychiatric Association: Diagnostic and Statistical Manual of Mental Disorders, 3rd Edition. Washington, DC, American Psychiatric Association, 1980

American Psychiatric Association: Diagnostic and Statistical Manual of Mental Disorders, 3rd Edition, Revised. Washington, DC, American Psychiatric Association, 1987

Anthony JC, Helzer JE: Syndromes of drug abuse and dependence, in Psychiatric Disorders in America. Edited by Robins LN, Regier DA. New York, Free Press, 1991

Anthony JC, Folstein, M, Romanovsky, AJ, et al: Comparison of lay diagnostic interview schedule and a standardized psychiatric diagnosis. Arch Gen Psychiatry 42:667–676, 1985

Bebbington P, Hurry J, Tenant C, et al: Epidemiology of mental disorders in Camberwell. Psychol Med 11:561–579, 1981

Bland RC, Orn H, Newman SC: Lifetime prevalence of psychiatric disorders in Edmonton. Acta Psychiatr Scand 77(suppl 338):24–32, 1988a

Bland RC, Newman SC, Orn H: Period prevalence of psychiatric disorders in Edmonton. Acta Psychiatr Scand 77(suppl 338):33–42, 1988b

Blazer D, George LK, Landerman R, et al: Psychiatric disorders: a rural urban comparison. Arch Gen Psychiatry 42:651–656, 1985

Burnam MA, Hough RL, Escobar JI, et al: Six-month prevalence of specific psychiatric disorders among Mexican-Americans and non-Hispanic Whites in Los Angeles. Arch Gen Psychiatry 44:687–694, 1987a

Burnam MA, Hough RL, Karno M, et al: Acculturation and lifetime prevalence of psychiatric disorders among Mexican-Americans in Los Angeles. J Health Soc Behav 28(1):89–102, 1987b

Canino GJ, Bird HR, Shrout PE, et al: The prevalence of specific psychiatric disorders in Puerto Rico. Arch Gen Psychiatry 44:727–735, 1987

Cohen ME, Robins E, Purtell JJ, et al: Excessive surgery in hysteria. JAMA 151:977–986, 1953

Cooper JE, Kendell RE, Gurland BJ, et al: Psychiatric diagnoses in New York and London. London, Oxford University Press, 1972

Dean C, Surtees PG, Sashidharan SP: Comparison of research diagnostic systems in an Edinburgh community sample. Br J Psychiatry 142:247–256, 1983

Derogatis L: SCL-90-R Manual II. Towson, MD, Clinical Psychometric Research, 1983

Earls F, Escobar JI, Manson S: Epidemiological and cultural considerations in studying suicide and suicidal behavior in minority groups, in Suicide Over the Life Cycle: Understanding Risk Factors, Assessment and Treatment. Edited by Blumenthal S,

Kupfer DG. Washington, DC, American Psychiatric Press, 1990

Eaton WW, Kessler LG (eds): Epidemiologic Field Methods in Psychiatry: The NIMH Epidemiologic Catchment Area Program. New York, Academic Press, 1985

Eaton WW, Kramer M, Anthony JC, et al: The incidence of specific DIS/DSM-III mental disorders: data from the NIMH Epidemiologic Catchment Area Program. Acta Psychiatr Scand 79:163–178, 1989

Eaton WW, Dryman A, Weissman MM: Panic and phobia, in Psychiatric Disorders in America. Edited by Robins LN, Regier DA. New York, Free Press, 1991

Endicott J, Spitzer RL: A diagnostic interview: the Schedule for Affective Disorders and Schizophrenia. Arch Gen Psychiatry 35:837–844, 1978

Escobar JI, Burnam A, Karno M, et al: Use of the mini-mental state examination (MMSE) in a community population of mixed ethnicity: cultural and linguistic artifacts. J Nerv Ment Dis 174:607–614, 1986

Escobar JI, Burnam MA, Karno M: Somatization in the community. Arch Gen Psychiatry 44:713–718, 1987

Feighner JP, Robins E, Guze SB, et al: Diagnostic criteria for use in psychiatric research. Arch Gen Psychiatry 26:57–63, 1972

Flaherty JA, Gaviria FM, Pathak D, et al: Developing instruments for cross-cultural psychiatric research. J Nerv Ment Dis 176(5):257–263, 1988

Folstein MF, Folstein SE, McHugh PR: Mini-Mental State: a practical method for grading the cognitive state of patients for the clinician. J Psychiatr Res 12:189–198, 1975

Freedman DX: Psychiatry epidemiology counts. Arch Gen Psychiatry 41:931–933, 1984

Goodwin DW, Guze SB: Psychiatric Diagnosis. New York, Oxford University Press, 1984

Hagashi S, Perales A, Sogi C, et al: Prevalencia de vida de trastornos mentales en independencia (Lima, Peru). Anales de Salud Mental 1:206–222, 1985

Health United States, 1990. Hyattsville, MD, U.S. Department of Health and Human Services, March 1991

Helzer JE, Robins LN, McEvoy LT, et al: A comparison of clinical and diagnostic interview schedule diagnoses: physician re-examination of lay interviewed cases in the general population. Arch Gen Psychiatry 42:657–666, 1985

Helzer JE, Burnam MA, McEvoy LT: Alcohol abuse and dependence, in Psychiatric Disorders in America. Edited by Robins LN, Regier DA. New York, Free Press, 1991

Henderson S, Duncan-Jones P, Byrne DG, et al: Psychiatric disorders in Canberra. Acta Psychiatr Scand 60:355–374, 1979

Hollingshead AB, Redlich FC: Social Class and Mental Illness. New York, Wiley, 1958

Hwu HG, Yeh EK, Chang LY: Prevalence of psychiatric disorders in Taiwan defined by the Chinese diagnostic interview schedule. Acta Psychiatr Scand 79:136–147, 1989

Karno M, Burnam A, Escobar JI, et al: The Spanish language version of the diagnostic interview schedule, in Epidemiologic Field Methods in Psychiatry: The NIMH Epidemiologic Catchment Area Program. Edited by Eaton WW, Kessler LG. New York, Academic Press, 1985

Karno M, Hough RL, Burnam MA, et al: Lifetime prevalence of specific psychiatric disorders among Mexican-Americans and non-Hispanic Whites in Los Angeles. Arch Gen Psychiatry 44(8):695–701, 1987

Keith S: Schizophrenic disorders, in Psychiatric Disorders in America. Edited by Robins LN, Regier DA. New York, Free Press, 1992, pp 33–52

Kleinman A: Neurasthenia and depression: a study of somatization and culture in China. Cult Med Psychiatry 6:117–190, 1982

Kleinman A: Anthropology and psychiatry: the role of culture in cross-cultural research on illness. Br J Psychiatry 151:447–454, 1987

Klerman GI, Weissman MM: Increasing rates of depression. JAMA 261(15):2229–2235, 1989

Kramer M: Classification of Mental disorders for epidemiologic and medical care purposes: current states, problems and needs, in The Role and Methodology of Classification in Psychiatry and Psychopathology (Public Health Service Publ #1584). Edited by Katz MM, Cole JO, Barton WE. Washington, DC, U.S. Government Printing Office, 1965

Leaf PJ, Myers JK, McEvoy LT: Procedures used in the Epidemiologic Catchment Area Study, in Psychiatric Disorders in America. Edited by Robins LN, Regier DA. New York, Free Press, 1991

Lee CK: The nationwide epidemiological study of mental disorders in Korea, in Proceedings of the Third Scientific Meeting of the Pacific Rim College of Psychiatrists. Tokyo, Human Research, Inc., 1988

Leighton DC, Harding JS, Macklin DB, et al: Psychiatric findings of the Stirling County Study. Am J Psychiatry 119:1021–1026, 1963

Mavreas VG, Beis A, Mouyies A, et al: Prevalence of psychiatric disorders in Athens: a community study. Social Psychiatry 21:172–181, 1986

Moscicki EK, Rae DS, Regier DA, et al: The Hispanic health and nutrition examination study: depression among Mexican-Americans, Cuban-Americans and Puerto-Ricans, in Health and Behavior Research Agenda for Hispanics (Research Monograph Series No. 1). Edited by Gavira AM, Arana JD. Chicago, IL, University of Illinois at Chicago, 1987

Myers JK, Lindenthal JJ, Pepper MD: Life events and psychiatric impairment. J Nerv Ment Dis 152:149–157, 1971

Orley J, Blitt DM, Wing JK: Psychiatric disorders in two African villages. Arch Gen Psychiatry 36:513–570, 1979

President's Commission on Mental Health: Report to the President. Washington, DC, U.S. Government Printing Office, 1978

Radloff LS: The CES-D Scale: a self report depression scale for research in the general population. Applied Psychological Measurement 1:385–401, 1977

Randolph ET, Escobar JI, Paz DH, et al: Ethnicity and reporting of schizophrenic symptoms. J Nerv Ment Dis 173:332–340, 1985

Regier DA, Goldberg ID, Taube CA: The de facto U.S. mental health services system. Arch Gen Psychiatry 35:685–693, 1978

Regier DA, Myers JK, Kramer M, et al: The NIMH epidemiologic catchment area program. Arch Gen Psychiatry 41:934–941, 1984

Regier DA, Boyd JH, Burke JD, et al: One-month prevalence of mental disorders in the United States based on five epidemiologic catchment area sites. Arch Gen Psychiatry 45:977–986, 1988

Robins LN: Psychiatric epidemiology. Arch Gen Psychiatry 35:697–702, 1978

Robins LN: Diagnostic grammar and assessment: translating criteria into questions. Psychol Med 19:57–68, 1989

Robins LN, Regier DA (eds): Psychiatric Disorders in America. New York, Free Press, 1991

Robins LN, Helzer JE, Croughan J, et al: National Institute of Mental Health Diagnostic Interview Schedule: its history, characteristics, and validity. Arch Gen Psychiatry 38:381–389, 1981

Robins LN, Helzer JE, Weissman MM, et al: Lifetime prevalence of specific psychiatric disorders in three sites. Arch Gen Psychiatry 41:949–958, 1984

Sartorius N, Jablensky A, Shapiro R: Cross cultural differences in the short term prognosis of schizophrenic psychoses. Schizophr Bull 4:102–113, 1978

Sartorius N, Jablensky A, Gulbinat W, et al: WHO Collaborative Study: assessment of depressive disorders. Psychol Med 10:743–749, 1980

Shapiro S, Skinner EA, Kessler LG, et al: Utilization of health and mental health services. Arch Gen Psychiatry 41:971–987, 1984

Simon RJ, Fleiss JL, Gurland BJ, et al: Depression and schizophrenia in hospitalized black and white mental patients. Arch Gen Psychiatry 28:509–512, 1973

Spitzer RL, Fleiss JL: A re-analysis of the reliability of psychiatric diagnoses. Br J Psychiatry 125:341–347, 1974

Spitzer RL, Endicott J, Robins E: Research diagnostic criteria. Arch Gen Psychiatry 35:773–782, 1978

Srole L, Langer TS, Michael ST, et al: Mental health in the metropolis: the Midtown Manhattan Study. New York, McGraw-Hill, 1962

Swartz M, Landerman R, George LK, et al: Somatization disorder, in Psychiatric Disorders in America. Edited by Robins LN, Regier DA. New York, Free Press, 1991

Weissman MM, Myers JK, Thompson WD: Depression and its treatment in a U.S. urban community. Arch Gen Psychiatry 38:417–421, 1980

Weissman MM, Livingston-Bruce M, Leaf PJ, et al: Affective disorders, in Psychiatric Disorders in America. Edited by Robins LN, Regier DA. New York, Free Press, 1991

Wheeler EO, White PD, Ried WE, et al: Neurocirculatory asthenia (anxiety neurosis, effort syndrome, neurasthenia). JAMA 142:878–889, 1950

Wing JK, Cooper JE, Sartorius N: The Measurement and Classification of Psychiatric Symptoms. New York, Cambridge University Press, 1974

World Health Organization: Schizophrenia: A Multinational Study. Geneva, World Health Organization, 1975

World Health Organization: The International Classification of Diseases, 10th Revision. Geneva, World Health Organization, 1992

3 Culture-Bound Syndromes

Ronald C. Simons, M.D., M.A.
Charles C. Hughes, Ph.D.

The term "culture-bound syndrome" is used to denote any of certain recurrent, locality-specific patterns of aberrant behavior and experience that appear to fall outside conventional Western psychiatric diagnostic categories. Most of these patterns are indigenously considered to be "illnesses," and most have local names. Older and less frequently used terms that refer to more or less the same set of patterns are "ethnic psychoses" and ethnic neuroses (Devereux 1956, p. 34), "atypical culture-bound reactive syndromes" (Yap 1974, p. 56), and "exotic psychotic syndromes" (Arieti and Meth 1959, pp. 556–559). Though examples of the major diagnostic categories of DSM-III-R (American Psychiatric Association 1987) and ICD-10 (International Classification of Diseases 1992) are ubiquitous (schizophrenia and bipolar illnesses, for example, being found throughout the world), any given culture-bound syndrome is found in one, or at most a few, of the world's societies.

We consider the culture-bound syndromes to be folk diagnostic categories—categories that supply coherent meanings to certain recurrent and remarkable sets of experiences and observations. Western scientific diagnoses and diagnostic systems are, of course no less "bound" by a particular culture. The syndromes referred to as "culture-bound" are called so only because the cultures they are bound to are foreign to the ordinary cultural expectations of the Western clinician or investigator; hence, their shaping by cultural determinants is more visible.

Certain behaviors and experiences that are the signs and symptoms of the culture-bound syndromes occur in many unrelated cultural settings. However, in different cultural settings they may be interpreted, and thus experienced, in disparate ways. In culturally differing settings, they also may be sorted into quite different categories. These ways of understanding and of

75

sorting are based, in large part, on locality-specific ideas of personhood, autonomy, vital essence, supernatural beings, illness, transgression, and health—in short, the matter and the forces that constitute the experienced universe. Therefore, it is important in considering any instance of a culture-bound syndrome to consider not only the elements of the presented behavior and observations that are significant in the Western scientific system, but also the elements that are considered important by patients and those about them. The "culture-bound syndromes" are especially clear examples of the need to explore the "patient's explanatory model" of disease (Kleinman et al. 1978, p. 256). When a clinician demonstrates that he or she can accept a patient's definition of his or her situation, the likelihood of appropriate and effective intervention is vastly increased.

Although a single manifestation of almost any culture-bound syndrome may include all or most of the diagnostic criteria sufficient for a Western diagnosis, sortings by the folk categories are somewhat different, and elements considered significant in one diagnostic system may be not be attended to by the other. Instances of aberrant behavior that would be sorted by a Western diagnostician into several diagnostic categories (including "other" and "no psychiatric diagnosis") may be incuded in a single folk category, and instances that would be sorted by a Western diagnostician into one category may be sorted into several in a non-Western diagnostic system. Thus, there is no one-to-one equivalence of any culture-bound syndrome with any DSM or ICD diagnostic classification.

Syndrome Names

It is easy to be confused by the multiplicity of names that have been used to refer to various culture-bound syndromes. Not only are there English names (e.g., Arctic hysteria, brain fag), French names (e.g., boufée delirante aigue), Danish names (e.g., angst, as in kayak angst), and names taken from other European languages, but there are also many names taken from non-Western languages as well, such as amok (Malay/Indonesian), pibloktoq (Eskimo), and phii pob (Thai). Differing transcription conventions give different spellings for the same term, and most syndromes have more than one name.

Because there are many more names than syndromes and because the lack of consistency in terminology has hindered systematic comparative study, one of us (C. C. H.) developed a glossary or synonymy to aid in sorting out the behavioral similarities that transcend the labels employed (1985). In it,

185 syndromes are listed. Each entry in the glossary is organized under four headings. The first (A.) lists alternative spellings of the same term and syndromes with other (folk) names that appear to exhibit essentially the same pathology or behavior as the key entry. The published sources of the particular spelling(s) for names are also given when available. The second heading (B.) gives information on either the geographic location of the group in which the term is found or the general cultural context if a simple geographic localization is not possible (e.g., "Hispanic cultures"). Under the third heading (C.) are listed commonly reported symptoms and signs, and under the last (D.), a selection of the more important references.

Here are sample entries adapted from the book for *amok* (Simons and Hughes 1985, p. 476), *koro* (pp. 485–486), and *latah* (p. 486).

1. *Amok*

A. *ahade idizi be* (Newman 1964); *cafard* (Yap 1951, p. 319); *cathard* (Kiev 1972 p. 86); *soudanite, pseudonite* (Kiev 1972, p. 86; Yap 1951, p. 319); *mal de pelea* (Rothenberg 1964; Yap 1974, p. 98); *colera* (Yap 1974, p. 98); *iich'aa* (Yap 1974, p. 77, p. 99); *gila mengamok* (Chen 1970, p. 207); *ngamok* (Schmidt 1964, p. 148); *gila besi* (Schmidt 1964, p. 149)

B. Malaysia, Indonesia

C. dissociative episode(s); outburst(s) of violent and aggressive or homicidal behavior directed at people and objects; persecutory ideas; automatism; amnesia; exhaustion and return of consciousness following the episode (for *amok* runners who are not killed during the episode)

D. Kiev (1972); Murphy (1973); Teoh (1972); van Loon (1926/1927); van Wulfften Palthe (1936, pp. 529–531); Yap (1974); and chapters by Arboleda-Florez, Burton-Bradley, Carr, and Westermeyer in Simons and Hughes (1985)

2. *Koro*

A. *shook yong, show yang* (van Wulfften Palthe 1936, p. 533); *shuk yang* (Pfeiffer 1982, p. 210); *su yang* (Yap 1951, p. 317); *suo yang*; *suk yeon* (Yap 1964); *suk yeong* (Yap 1974, p. 98); *rok-joo* (Keshavan 1983); *jinjinia bemar* (Dutta 1983; Nandi et al. 1983; Rosenthal and Rosenthal 1982)

B. South China; Chinese and Malaysian populations in Southeast Asia; Assam (Hindus)

C. intense and sudden anxiety that the penis (or, for females, the vulva and breasts) will recede into the body; the penis is held by the victim or someone else, or devices are attached to prevent its receding

D. Dutta (1983); Jilek and Jilek-Aall (1977); Lin et al. (1981, pp. 255–256); Nandi et al. (1983); Ngui (1969); Rosenthal and Rosenthal (1982); Tan (1981 pp. 375–376); van Wulfften Palthe (1936, pp. 532–538); Yap (1964, 1965); and chapters by J. G. Edwards, J. M. Edwards, Ifabumuyi and Rwegellera, and Leng in Simons and Hughes (1985)

3. Latah

A. *Latha* (Ionescu-Tongyonk 1977, p. 154); *imu* (Yap 1951, p. 318); *ikota* (Yap 1952, p. 516); *ilota; ihota; mali-mali* (Yap 1951, p. 318); *myriachit* (Yap 1974, p. 97); *yaun, young-dah-te* (Yap 1974, p. 97); *bah-tsi, bah tschi* (Yap 1974, p. 97); *amurakh* (Czaplicka 1914, p. 320); *jumping Frenchman* (Yap 1951, p. 319); *pibloktoq* (Yap 1974, p. 97); *misala* (Yap 1951, p. 319)
B. Malaysia and Indonesia
C. hypersensitivity to sudden fright or startle; hypersuggestibility; echopraxia; echolalia; dissociative or trancelike behavior
D. Aberle (1952); Czaplicka (1914, pp. 307–325); de la Tourette (1884); Murphy (1973, 1976); van Loon (1926/1927); van Wulfften Palthe (1936, pp. 531–532); Yap (1952); and chapters by Kenney, Ohnuki-Tierney, and Simons in Simons and Hughes (1985)

Sorting by Descriptive Detail (Into Taxa)

As the glossary shows, there are syndromes with different names from a variety of cultures that are essentially the same set of behaviors, culturally elaborated in somewhat different ways. *Imu, myriachit,* and *latah,* for example, are defined by a group of attributes, experiences, and behaviors (hyperstartling, matching, and command obedience) found in a variety of unrelated cultures (Simons 1980). Further, sometimes isolated instances of the pattern of behavior that constitutes a culture-bound syndrome occur in areas far from those where the named and elaborated syndrome is endemic. The term "orphan cases" has been suggested to refer to such instances (Simons 1988). The anthropological and transcultural psychiatric literature contains many papers debating whether orphan cases are properly considered instances of the syndrome with which their constituent behaviors correspond. Certainly, to the extent that any syndrome is defined by the particular local *meaning* attached to it, orphan cases cannot be considered examples of that syndrome.

However, in many instances, the descriptive resemblances are too strong to discount; sometimes, not only the gross outlines of the behaviors but even their fine details match those of a syndrome that elsewhere has been named and culturally elaborated. This is all the more remarkable in view of the disparate cultural settings in which the orphan cases occur and the disparate local meanings attached to them. For this and other reasons, some authors (Prince and Tcheng-Laroche 1987; Simons 1985) have suggested that it is most useful to define each culture-bound syndrome in terms of the behaviors of which it is constituted, independent of the meanings locally assigned to those behaviors. This suggestion is, of course, for definitional and classificatory purposes only. As with other psychiatric nosologic entities, a full understanding of any given syndrome requires attention to the cultural setting in which it occurs.

To circumvent the terminologic confusion inherent in asking whether an out-of-culture instance of genital retraction and fear of death is *koro* or if an instance of hyperstartling and mimesis is *latah,* it has been suggested that names be assigned to the descriptively similar symptom groups—for example, "The Startle-Matching Syndromes" for *latah* and syndromes descriptively like it; "The Genital Retraction Syndromes" for *koro* and syndromes like it; and "The Sudden Mass Assault Syndromes" or "Sudden Mass Assault Syndrome With Homicide" or "SMASH Syndromes" (Westermeyer 1982) for *amok* and its out-of-culture orphan cases. The general term suggested for a grouping of descriptively similar syndromes is a "taxon" (plural: "taxa" [Simons 1985]). When syndromes are sorted by their constituent behaviors and experiences, it is useful to have some general term for each taxon that is not bound to a specific culture area and a specific cultural elaboration (Simons 1985; Westermeyer 1982).

The pattern of commonalities and differences across cultures within a taxon may suggest etiologic factors (e.g., those leading to a predisposition to hyperstartle in the startle-matching syndromes). Culture-bound syndromes are increasingly being considered for inclusion in world diagnostic schemata such as the ICD. When they are included, we suggest that, to the extent possible, the taxa rather than the individual, locally named syndromes be given taxonomic status.

Illnesses of Attribution

Because there has been no single agreed-upon, rigorous definition of "culture-bound syndromes," the folk illnesses that have been considered such at one time or another differ not only descriptively but also in their conceptualizations. Most include some specific out-of-the-ordinary behaviors or experiences, but the symptoms of some are quite unspecific, like "fatigue," "worry," or "inability to carry out ordinary routines." These latter folk illnesses are not unified by their constituent behaviors and experiences but rather by the attribution of a variety of unrelated debilitated states to some specific cause.

Susto, for example, is a folk diagnosis commonly made in Latin American Hispanic countries. It denotes tiredness and debility attributed to an antecedent fright or startle. That is, someone experiencing lassitude and inability to carry out expected functioning in any one of a number of ways might attribute this to some frightening or startling experience and thus diagnose the difficulty as *susto.* The fright or startle may have occurred as long as 30 years before the emergence of symptoms. The person frightened or startled may not be the person who later develops *susto;* it may be his or her child or another family member (Klein 1978; Rubel et al. 1984).

Research has revealed that the variety of states considered instances of *susto* is extremely heterogenous and includes a number of infectious diseases, heavy parasitic infestations, and various other disorders (Rubel et al. 1984). No single consistent behavioral syndrome was found to characterize a person suffering from *susto.* The diagnosis of *susto* is not made on the basis of a symptom complex or syndrome, but only on the retrospective judgment that any of a variety of afflictions has been "caused" by an antecedent fright or startle. How this process works is well described in a number of papers (e.g., Crandon 1983). Cognate syndromes in other parts of the world are known by local terms (including *espanto, saladera, lanti, mogo laya, haak-tsan,* and others (see Simons and Hughes 1985 and Wikan 1989). Because properly speaking there is no *susto* syndrome, we have suggested that *susto* and the other illnesses that are defined only by a presumed cause no longer be considered culture-bound syndromes (Simons and Hughes 1985).

A Note on "Possession"

Though the term "possession" often comes up in discussions of the culture-bound syndromes, possession per se is not a syndrome. Possession is an explanation of the observation that people sometimes break out of their world of ordinary social routine into a dissociated or often ecstatic state. Possession is the indigenous interpretation of the altered state as the result of having been taken over by some culture-specific other, often a deity, spirit, deceased relative, or historical personage. The actual events that have been considered as instances of possession are of several different kinds. Possession may be the indigenous explanation of a psychotic state, but sometimes "possessed" behavior is simply the playing out of a socially prescribed role. There is a considerable literature discussing the periods of altered consciousness prescribed for certain social and ceremonial occasions (e.g., Crapanzano and Garrison 1977; Prince 1968). In the glossary of culture-bound syndromes one of us compiled (Hughes 1985), some reference to possession can be found in about one-tenth of the 185 entries. Thus, possession may be used to explain both the behaviors and experiences that constitute elements of certain culture-bound syndromes and also trances or other altered states that occur as desired and expected parts of a group's rituals or ceremonies.

Culture-Bound Syndromes of Western Societies

A number of authors have pointed out that recurrent patterns of culturally shaped aberrant behavior that are indigenously considered pathological but that have no place in official diagnostic taxonomies occur in Western as well as non-Western scocieties. These authors suggested that they be considered "culture-bound syndromes" of Western culture. Candidates for culture-bound syndrome status in the recent psychological anthropology literature include "obesity" (Rittenbaugh 1982), "anorexia nervosa" (Nasser 1988), "the type A behavior pattern" (Helman 1987), "nerves" (Davis and Whitten 1988), and "petism" (a single person, usually elderly, sharing a radically untidy household with a rather large menagerie of dogs or cats [Simons 1981]).

In every society there are culturally constructed patterns of behavior whose origins and expressions are traceable to particular values and normative emphases. Moreover, people in every society categorize events, including episodes of illness and out-of-the-ordinary behavior. Thus, it is reasonable to examine Western industrialized societies for behavioral and psychopathological complexes comparable in structure and function to the culture-bound syndromes found elsewhere in the world. Whether any or all of the patterns listed above are most usefully thought of in this way is currently a subject of considerable debate.

"Culture-Bound Syndromes" and the Western Clinician

Increasingly, immigration to the United States, Canada, Australia, and much of Western Europe is from developing countries. As the world continues to shrink, travel and extended stays by non-Westerners in Western countries for educational and business reasons have become increasingly common. There is also a heightened appreciation of the need to provide adequate health care to Americans from disadvantaged ethnic and cultural groups. It is therefore likely that most practitioners will see patients who manifest the symptoms of a culture-bound syndrome and already bear an indigenous diagnosis and some ideas about its etiology and appropriate treatment. It thus becomes increasingly important for Western-trained psychiatrists to become familiar with the concept of the culture-bound syndromes and at least a few of the syndromes themselves. What follows is a brief description of some of the culture-bound syndromes that a Western practitioner is most likely to encounter.

Ataque de nervios.   A number of studies have shown that 30%–80% of Puerto Ricans in the New York City area seek help from local folk healers known as *espiritistas,* specialists in mental health (Garrison, 1977 p. 392). Many consult for episodes of *ataque de nervios,* an out-of-consciousness state explained as resulting from the presence of malevolent spirits. Interpreted by observers as involuntary behavior, it is "a culturally recognized, acceptable cry for help or an admission of inability to cope, and family and friends are required by norms of good behavior to rally to the aid of the ataque victim and relieve the intolerable stresses" (Garrison 1977, p. 389).

A typical episode was described by Garrison (1977):

> [M]. . . was sitting at her bench in a handbag factory in New York's garment district, where she had worked for four years. Suddenly, to the surprise of those around her, she began to scream and tear her clothes from her chest. She ran to the window, apparently trying to throw herself through it. When restrained, she fell to the floor in an unconscious state, with her whole body twitching. (p. 383)

M. was taken to a nearby clinic and referred for psychiatric hospitalization. When tests did not reveal an organic explanation for her attack, her condition was ascribed to spiritual causes.

Guarnaccia and colleagues (1989) have also described a "typical" *ataque de nervios:*

> . . . trembling, heart palpitations, a sense of heat in the chest rising into the head, difficulty moving limbs, loss of consciousness or mind going blank, memory loss, a sensation of needles in parts of the body (paresthesia), chest tightness, difficulty breathing (dyspnea), dizziness, faintness, and spells. Be-

haviorally, the person begins to shout, swear and strike out at others. The person then falls to the ground and either experiences convulsive body movements or lies "as if dead." (p. 280)

Brain fag. Clinicians treating students from Africa may encounter brain fag, a syndrome originally described and labelled by Prince (1960) from his work in Nigeria. Persons complaining of brain fag report difficulties in concentrating, remembering, and thinking, often stating that their brains are "fatigued." Although sensory disturbances in other parts of the body are also found, the principal symptoms of brain fag center on the head and neck: pain, pressure or tightness, blurring of vision, and a sensation of heat or burning. Intellectual functions are impaired, with difficulty in reading, remembering, and understanding. Other symptoms sometimes reported include the feeling of worms crawling in the head. At times there is also excessive fatigue and anxiety (Prince 1985).

Although most of those who complain of brain fag are students, in Nigeria at least, people other than students are sometimes affected (Makanjuola 1987). Similar symptomatology has been described from many parts of Africa and from other areas of the developing world (Morakinyo 1980, 1985).

This pattern of symptoms is similar to a disorder known in traditional Nigerian (Yoruba) nosology, *ori ode* ("Hunter in the Head"), which is characterized by a variety of somatic complaints, including sensations of an organism crawling in the brain, palpitations, and noises in the ears (Makanjuola 1987; Prince 1964). The word *ori* refers both to one's head and to one's spiritually prescribed destiny. In Nigerian folk belief, noises in the ears are ascribed to the voice of an enemy calling out one's name for malevolent purposes. It is useful for a clinician who encounters a patient complaining of brain fag to inquire after his or her ideas about its etiology and to ask specifically about witchcraft.

Falling-out. Falling-out or blackout is a disorder seen in certain ethnic populations in the southeastern United States, especially reported from the Miami, Florida, area. It is a seizurelike affliction affecting southern African Americans and Afro-Caribbeans (e.g., Bahamians and Haitians, the latter group sometimes referring to it as "indisposition"). Typically there is a sudden collapse, sometimes without warning, but sometimes preceded by feelings of dizziness or "swimming" in the head. The eyes are usually open, but the person says that he or she cannot see and, although hearing and understanding surrounding events, is powerless to move. During the falling-out there is no convulsive behavior, tongue-biting, bladder or bowel incontinence, or other symptoms suggestive of a true seizure (Weidman 1979).

One study reports that in 23% of Bahamanian households one or more members reported blackout spells. Among southern African Americans, 10% of the households were so afflicted (Weidman 1979), significantly more than members of other groups (Lefley 1979, p. 113). Episodes of falling-out were interpreted by researchers as a way for people to respond to traumatic events or situations, ranging from accidents, robberies, and personal assaults to more deeply ingrained problems deriving from a worldview fearful of what life would present from day to day.

Ghost sickness. Although there appears to be no term in Navajo specifically designating this affliction, ghost sickness is well known among the Navajos. It is believed to be a disorder caused by the action of witches and malevolent supernatural powers (Kaplan and Johnson 1964, p. 212) in which the victim feels overwhelmed by the forces of evil.

Symptoms include weakness, loss of appetite, dizziness, fainting, and a feeling of suffocation. Having bad dreams may be reported, as well as a sense of confusion, danger, futility, and dread. As reported in one account, "The chief symptoms of ghost sickness are fainting or the loss of consciousness, delirium (lost [one's] mind for a while), bad dreams (fall dreams or dreams [in which one] waste[s] away and [is] dead), or terror (especially at night)" (quoted in Kaplan and Johnson 1964, pp. 212–213). Presenting symptoms may also include those of many of the physical illnesses diagnosed by Western medicine. Like *susto,* ghost sickness may be an illness of attribution rather than a true syndrome.

Traditional Navajo treatment rituals are structured in conformance with the Navajo worldview. The Navajo recognize, for example, that if "Evil" is struggling for control of a person's very being, it must be counterbalanced by a stronger force acting on his behalf. Traditionally that stronger force is the healer ("Singer," as translated into English) using the powerful symbolism of ceremony that includes smoking, emetics, and other cleansing and purificatory procedures.

Hwa-byung. Several hundred thousand Koreans have immigrated to the United States over the past 40 years, settling predominantly on the West Coast (Liu 1986, p. 156). Thus, there is an increasing likelihood that a clinician will at some time encounter a patient presenting with the symptoms of *hwa-byung,* a disorder distinctively conceptualized and labelled in traditional Korean culture. Lin (1983) has discussed the typical configuration of symptoms presented by patients with this syndrome, which centers most prominently on, but is not limited to, epigastric pain. The pain is attributed to a mass in the upper abdomen that the patient fears will lead to death.

Other common symptoms include excessive tiredness and insomnia, acute panic, fear of impending death, loss of appetite, digestive disorders, dyspnea, palpitation, and muscle aches and pains. *Byung* refers to "sickness" and *Hwa* to "fire" and "anger." In Korean medical culture (as in many other traditional Asian medical systems), "fire" (one of the basic elements constituting the structure of "reality") and "anger" are related. Illness is believed to result from the imbalance or lack of harmony among the basic elements. Etiological beliefs underscore anger as the precipitant of this illness, and in Lin's (1983) cases, depression engendered by negative life circumstances appears often to be related to numerous somatic symptoms.

Lin noted that, although this symptom complex is not frequently mentioned in the psychiatric literature, "This does not mean . . . that *hwa-byung* is a rare condition. Most Korean health professionals are familiar with the condition . . . " (1983, p. 106).

Taijin kyofusho.   Also referred to as "anthropophobia," this condition is found in Japan. *Taijin* is an adjective referring to "interpersonal," and *kyofusho* means "phobia" or "fear." As noted by Kleinman (1988), "Patients feel guilty about embarrassing others with their behavior . . . rather than fearful of others' criticisms" (pp. 45–46). *Taijin kyofusho* includes patients who in Western diagnostic systems would be diagnosed as having anxiety or obsessive-compulsive reactions, neurasthenia, or social phobia. Patients complain that their bodies, its parts, or its functions displease or are offensive to other people: appearance, odor, facial expressions, or movements. So severe and debilitating is this disorder that social support groups have developed to aid victims (Takahashi 1975).

The disorder is especially prevalent among young people. Sufferers experience their worst bouts of symptoms in interpersonal situations. Though some social anxiety for some persons is probably ubiquitous in the world's cultures, it has been suggested that it is especially frequent and debilitating in Japan because of the emphasis in Japanese culture on the importance of proper behavior and demeanor in all situations and social contexts (Tanaka-Matsumi 1979, pp. 232–233).

Traditional therapy for *taijin kyofusho* occurs in the context of a ritual setting and includes a variety of physiological applications (e.g., sweating and massage), behavioral restrictions (e.g., diet), and social support.

Voodoo death. Though anecdotal evidence abounds, it has been much debated whether people have actually died simply because they believed with certainty that someone else put a death spell on them. A case report of a conference from the Department of Pathology at Johns Hopkins Medical School describes a patient who had been admitted with shortness of breath and episodes of chest pain and syncope of 1 month's duration. She was given a thorough medical workup and, aside from relatively minor problems, the physical findings were unremarkable. Manifestly terrified, the patient had been "hexed" since birth and was doomed to die before her 23rd birthday—in fact, she did die the day before her 23rd birthday (Clinico-Pathologic Conference 1967).

Also known by such terms as hex, root-work, and numerous other terms (in Spanish, *mal puesto*), belief in witchcraft—the power of other people to bring about misfortune, disability, and death through "spiritual" (read: "psychological") mechanisms—has been well-nigh universal in human history. The common thread in its distribution appears to be a profound loss of hope, an engulfing sense of impotence, and an inability to change a foretold course of events. In its social consequences, it is often characterized by the phenomena Engel referred to as the "giving-up—given-up complex" (Dimsdale 1977; Engel 1968, 1970). In some reported cases, the cause of death has been dehydration or starvation from water or food refusal (Cannon 1942).

Among some African Americans, a distinction is made between "natural" diseases (afflictions that can be expected as a result of "God's plan") and "unnatural" diseases, those that represent disharmony, conflict with God's will, and evil (Snow 1974). Witchcraft affliction—the "hex" that may lead to voodoo death—falls in the latter category. Because "unnatural" diseases are believed to emanate from evil powers (e.g., the "Devil"), a physician suggesting therapy that does not explicitly take into account the patient's explanatory model can well be frustrated by noncompliance and failure. For example, in developing an effective treatment plan, it may be critical for a clinician to recognize the significance and power of a patient's need to guard his or her fingernail and hair clippings, or the reasoning behind his or her fearfulness on finding that a piece of clothing has been snipped off.

Wacinko. Recognized as a distinctive syndrome by native practitioners among the Oglala Sioux, *wacinko* includes symptoms of anger, withdrawal, mutism, and immobility and has been cited as an illness leading to suicide. Analyzed as a culturally structured and named reaction to disappointment and interpersonal problems, the syndrome is often treated by traditional healers. One psychiatrist who has worked with such patients noted: "Some behavior patterns that are well known within a culture are enigmas to outsiders. The patient who can consult a healer who understands him is fortunate indeed" (Lewis 1975, p. 755).

Wind illness. The term "wind illness" is a translation of *p'a-leng,* a disorder found in Chinese populations. It is based on the humoral theory of the dynamics of nature and human well-being, a theory that explains why so many human goals and values, such as good health and good fortune, are frustrated when essential natural and supernatural elements (*yin/yang*) are out of balance. The disorder is characterized by a morbid fear of the cold, especially of the wind, as a factor in upsetting the optimum balance of forces. In a typical case a patient develops

> . . . culturally specific fear of being cold . . . which correlates with a belief that
> he is losing yang and is thus in a state of weakness and susceptibility to illness.
> He treats himself by keeping warm, avoiding potential chill, taking tonics, and
> eating "hot" food. He wears several layers of clothing at all times and in all
> seasons, keeps many blankets on his bed, and has his windows shut tightly
> even in hot weather. (Kleinman 1980, p. 164)

Although *p'a-leng* is a Chinese syndrome, the idea that human actions can upset some natural balance and thus cause disease is widespread. For example, the idea that a person's good health requires "hot" and "cold" elements to be in balance is also found in Latin American societies that derive from Mediterranean cultures (which in turn may have been influenced by similar ideas from India and China). Wind illness is also "one of the most common complaints in South-East Asian societies" (Eisenbruch 1983, pp. 323–326).

Conclusion

The principal theme of most discussions of the "culture-bound syndromes" is that such disorders represent symptom patterns that are linked in some definitive manner to the particular cultural setting in which they occur. Because they are so bizarre from the conceptual perspective of Western biomedicine, however, they are often dismissed from serious analysis and therefore, inadvertently, from effective therapeutic intervention. These disorders appear to exist in a twilight zone of psychiatric diagnosis and may be regarded merely as exotic "instances of *deviant* deviance" (Hughes 1985, p. 3; emphasis in original). To almost everyone, the behavior and expectations developed in one's own culture appear "natural" or "logical," whereas those derived from other cultures appear unnatural, culture-specific, or arising from abnormal conditions. However, as Murphy pointed out, "The time is overdue when the relationship between cultural backgrounds and psychopathology or forms of therapy in developed countries should be more formally examined, and when we should cease thinking that our behavioural expectations are all 'natural,' not requiring re-examination" (1977, pp. 370–371).

Most clinicians are more likely to consider "culture" in the explanation of a presenting patient's problem when he or she is from a cultural setting other than the clinicians' own. However "cultural factors are a substantial part of every disorder and not a descriptive, picturesque component" (Alarcon 1983, p. 104). Though all psychiatric illnesses are culture-bound, the term "culture-bound syndrome" is used in a more restricted sense. The subset of psychiatric illnesses called the culture-bound syndromes are those found only in circumscribed cultural areas. Though culture shapes all illness behavior, it is always potentially revealing to ask why any given syndrome appears there and not here, or here and not there. What is it about the beliefs and practices of a group that results in one of its members exhibiting a pattern of behavior the group itself considers aberrant—aberrant in an expected and meaningful way, different from the aberrant behavior of members of other groups?

In recent years, awareness of cultural diversity and of the role of culture in all illness has greatly increased. Because of the insights into the relationship between individual psychopathology and culturally determined practices and beliefs that the study of the culture-bound syndromes provides, interest in these syndromes has grown exponentially in the past several years. We believe that it is likely to continue to grow and that further study of the culture-bound syndromes will continue to yield fresh insight into questions basic to all of anthropology and psychiatry.

References

Aberle DA: Arctic hysteria and Latah in Mongolia. New York Academy of Sciences 14(7):291–297, 1952

Alarcon RD: A Latin American perspective on DSM-III. Am J Psychiatry 140:102–105, 1983

American Psychiatric Association: Diagnostic and Statistical Manual of Mental Disorders, 3rd Edition, Revised. Washington, DC, American Psychiatric Association,

1987

Arboleda-Florez J: *Amok,* in The Culture-Bound Syndromes: Folk Illnesses of Psychiatric and Anthropological Interest. Edited by Simons RC, Hughes CC. Dordrecht, Netherlands, D Reidel, 1985, pp 251–262

Arieti S, Meth JM: Rare unclassifiable, collective, and exotic psychotic syndromes, in American Handbook of Psychiatry, Vol I. Edited by Arieti S. New York, Basic Books, 1959, pp 546–563

Burton-Bradley BG: The *Amok* syndrome in Papua and New Guinea, in The Culture-Bound Syndromes: Folk Illnesses of Psychiatric and Anthropological Interest. Edited by Simons RC, Hughes CC. Dordrecht, Netherlands, D Reidel, 1985, pp 251–262

Cannon WB: Voodoo Death. American Anthropologist 44:169–181, 1942

Carr JE: Ethno-behaviorism and the culture-bound syndromes: the case of *Amok,* in The Culture-Bound Syndromes: Folk Illnesses of Psychiatic and Anthropological Interest. Edited by Simons RC, Hughes CC. Dordrecht, Netherlands, D Reidel, 1985, pp 199–223

Chen PCY: Classification and concepts of causation of mental illness in a rural Malay community. Int J Soc Psychiatry 16:205–215, 1970

Clinico-Pathologic Conference—Case Presentation. Johns Hopkins Medical Journal 120:186–199, 1967

Crandon L: Why *susto?* Ethnology 22:153–167, 1983

Crapanzano V, Garrison V (eds): Case Studies in Spirit Possession. New York, Wiley, 1977

Czaplicka MA: Pathology, in Aboriginal Siberia: A Study in Social Anthropology. Oxford, Clarendon Press, 1914, pp 307–325

Davis L, Whitten RG: Medical and Popular Traditions of Nerves. Soc Sci Med 26:1209–1221, 1988

de la Tourette GG: *Jumping, Latah,* and *Myriachit.* Archives de Neurologie 8:68–74, 1884

Devereux G: Normal and abnormal: the key problem of psychiatric anthropology, in Some Uses of Anthropology: Theoretical and Applied. Edited by Casagrande JB, Gladwin T. Washington, DC, Anthropological Society of Washington, 1956, pp 23–48

Dimsdale JE: Emotional causes of sudden death. Am J Psychiatry 134(12):1361–1366, 1977

Dutta D: *Koro* epidemic in Assam. Br J Psychiatry 143:309–310, 1983

Edwards JG: The *koro* pattern of depersonalization in an American schizophrenic patient. Am J Psychiatry 126:1171–1173, 1970

Edwards JG: The *Koro* pattern of depersonalization in an American schizophrenic patient, in The Culture-Bound Syndromes: Folk Illnesses of Psychiatric and Anthropological Interest. Edited by Simons RC, Hughes CC. Dordrecht, Netherlands, D Reidel, 1985, pp 165–168

Edwards JM: Indigenous *Koro,* a genital retraction syndrome of insular southeast Asia:

a critical review, in The Culture-Bound Syndromes: Folk Illnesses of Psychiatric and Anthropological Interest. Edited by Simons RC, Hughes CC. Dordrecht, Netherlands, D Reidel, 1985, pp 169–191

Eisenbruch M: "Wind illness" or somatic depression?—a case study in psychiatric anthropology. Br J Psychiatry 143:323–326, 1983

Engel GL: A life setting conducive to illness—the giving-up—given-up complex. Ann Intern Med 69(2):293–300, 1968

Engel GL: Sudden death and the "medical model" in psychiatry. Canadian Psychiatric Association Journal 15(6):527–537, 1970

Garrison V: The "Puerto Rican syndrome" in psychiatry and espritismo, in Case Studies in Spirit Posession. Edited by Crapanzano V, Garrison V. New York, Wiley, 1977, pp 383–449

Guarnaccia P, Rubio-Stipec M, Canino G: Ataques de nervios in the Puerto Rican Diagnostic Interview Schedule—the impact of cultural categories on psychiatric epidemiology. Cult Med Psychiatry 13:275–295, 1989

Helman CG: Heart disease and the cultural construction of time: the type A behaviour pattern as a western culture-bound syndrome. Soc Sci Med 25:969–979, 1987

Hughes CC: Culture-bound or construct-bound?: the syndromes and DSM-III, in The Culture-Bound Syndromes: Folk Illnesses of Psychiatric and Anthropological Interest. Edited by Simons RC, Hughes CC. Dordrecht, Netherlands, D Reidel, 1985, pp 3–24

Ifabumuyi OI, Rwegellera GGC: Koro in a Nigerian male patient: a case report, in The Culture-Bound Syndromes: Folk Illnesses of Psychiatric and Anthropological Interest. Edited by Simons RC, Hughes CC. Dordrecht, Netherlands, D Reidel, 1985, pp 161–163

International Classification of Diseases: 10th Revision: Clinical Modification, Vol 1. Washington, DC, U.S. Department of Health and Human Services, Public Health Services, Health Care Financing Administration, 1992

Ionescu-Tongyonk J: Transcultural psychiatry in Thailand: a review of the last two decades. Transcultural Psychiattry Research Review 14:145–162, 1977

Jilek W, Jilek-Aall L: A Koro epidemic in Thailand. Transcult Psychiat Res Rev 14:57–59, 1977

Kaplan B, Johnson D: The social meaning of Navaho psychopathology and psychotherapy, in Magic, Faith, and Healing—Studies in Primitive Psychiatry Today. Edited by Kiev A. New York, Free Press, 1964, pp 203–229

Kenney MG: Paradox Lost: The Latah problem revisited, in The Culture-Bound Syndromes: Folk Illnesses of Psychiatric and Anthropological Interest. Edited by Simons RC, Hughes CC. Dordrecht, Netherlands, D Reidel, 1985, pp 63–76

Keshavan MS: Epidemic psychoses, or epidemic Koro? Br J Psychiatry 148:100–101, 1983

Kiev A (ed): Transcultural Psychiatry. New York, Free Press, 1972

Kirmayer LJ: The place of culture in psychiatric nosology: taijin kuofusho and DSM-III-R. J Nerv Ment Dis 179(1):19–28, 1991

Klein J: *Susto*—the anthropological study of diseases of adaptation. Soc Sci Med 12:23–28, 1978

Kleinman A: Patients and Healers in the Context of Culture: An Exploration of the Borderland between Anthropology, Medicine, and Psychiatry. Berkeley, CA, University of California Press, 1980

Kleinman A: Rethinking Psychiatry: From Cultural Category to Personal Experience. New York, Free Press, 1988

Kleinman A, Eisenberg L, Good B: Clinical lessons from anthropologic and cross-cultural research. Ann Intern Med 88:251–258, 1978

Lefley H: Prevalence of potential falling-out cases among the black, Latin and non-Latin white populations of the city of Miami. Soc Sci Med 13B:113–114, 1979

Leng GA: *Koro*—a cultural disease, in The Culture-Bound Syndromes: Folk Illnesses of Psychiatric and Anthropological Interest. Edited by Simons RC, Hughes CC. Dordrecht, Netherlands, D Reidel, 1985, pp 155–159

Lewis TH: A syndrome of depression and mutism in the Oglala Sioux. Am J Psychiatry 132(7):753–755, 1975

Lin KM: *Hwa-byung:* a Korean culture-bound syndrome? Am J Psychiatry 140(1):105–107, 1983

Lin KM, Kleinman A, Lin T: Overview of mental disorders in Chinese cultures: review of epidemiological and clinical studies, in Normal and Abnormal Behavior in Chinese Culture. Edited by Kleinman A, Lin T. Dordrecht, Netherlands, D Reidel, 1981, pp 237–272

Liu WT: Health Services for Asian Elderly. Research on Aging 8(1):156–175, 1986

Makanjuola ROA: *Ori ode:* a culture-Bound disorder with prominent somatic features in Yoruba Nigerian patients. Acta Psychiatr Scand 75:231–236, 1987

Morakinyo O: The *brain-fag* syndrome in Nigeria—cognitive deficits in an illness associated with study. Br J Psychiatry 146:209–210, 1985

Morakinyo O: A psychophysiological theory of a psychiatric illness (the *brain fag* syndrome) associated with study among Africans. J Nerv Ment Dis 168(2):84–89, 1980

Murphy HBM: History and the evolution of syndromes: the striking case of *Latah* and *Amok*, in Psychopathology: Contributions From the Biological, Behavioral, and Social Sciences. Edited by Hammer M, Salinger K, Sutton S. New York, Wiley, 1973, pp 33–53

Murphy HBM: Notes for the theory on *Latah*, in Culture-Bound Syndromes, Ethnopsychiatry, and Alternate Therapies. Volume IV of Mental Health Research in Asia and the Pacific. Edited by Lebra WP. Honolulu, HI, University Press of Hawaii, 1976, pp 3–21

Murphy HBM: Transcultural psychiatry should begin at home. Psychol Med 7:369–371, 1977

Nandi DN, Banerjee G, Saha H, et al: Epidemic *Koro* in West Bengal, India. Int J Soc Psychiatry 29(4):265–268, 1983

Nasser M: Eating disorders: the cultural dimension. Soc Psychiatry Psychiatr

Epidemiol 23:184–187, 1988

Newman PL: "Wild Man" behavior in a New Guinea highland community. American Anthropologist 66:1–19, 1964

Ngui PW: The *Koro* epidemic in Singapore. Aust N Z J Psychiatry 3:263–265, 1969

Ohnuki-Tierney E: Shamans and *Imu* among two Ainu groups—towards a cross-cultural model of interpretation, in The Culture-Bound Syndromes: Folk Illnesses of Psychiatric and Anthropological Interest. Edited by Simons RC, Hughes CC. Dordrecht, Netherlands, D Reidel, 1985, pp 91–110

Pfeiffer WM: Culture-bound syndromes, in Culture and Psychopathology. Edited by Issa IA. Baltimore, MD, University Park Press, 1982, pp 201–218

Prince R: The *brain fag* syndrome in Nigerian students. Journal of Mental Science 106:559–570, 1960

Prince R: Indigenous Yoruba psychiatry, in Magic, Faith, and Healing—Studies in Primitive Psychiatry Today. Edited by Kiev A. New York, Free Press, 1964, pp 84–120

Prince R (ed): Trance and Possession States. Montreal, R.M. Bucke Memorial Society, 1968

Prince R: The concept of culture-bound syndromes: *anorexia nervosa* and *brain-fag*. Soc Sci Med 21(2):197–203, 1985

Prince R, Tcheng-Laroche F: Culture-bound syndromes and international disease classifications. Cult Med Psychiatry 11:3–19, 1987

Rittenbaugh C: Obesity as a culture-bound syndrome. Cult Med Psychiatry 6:341–361, 1982

Rosenthal S, Rosenthal PA: *Koro* in an adolescent: hypochrondriasis as a stress response. Adolesc Psychiatry 10:523–530, 1982

Rothenberg A: Puerto Rico and aggression. Am J Psychiatry 120:962–970, 1964

Rubel AJ, O'Nell CW, and Collado-Ardón R: *Susto*: a folk illness. Berkeley and Los Angeles, CA, University of California Press, 1984

Schmidt KE: Folk psychiatry in Sarawak: a tentative system of psychiatry of the Iban, in Magic, Faith and Healing. Edited by Kiev A. New York, Free Press of Glencoe, 1964, pp 139–155

Simons RC: The resolution of the *latah* paradox. J Nerv Ment Dis 168:195–206, 1980

Simons RC: A review of the culture-bound syndromes. Paper presented at the annual meeting of the Society for the Study of Culture and Psychiatry, Mt. Hood, Oregon, 1981

Simons RC: Sorting the culture-bound syndromes, in The Culture-Bound Syndromes: Folk Illnesses of Pychiatric and Anthropological Interest. Edited by Simons RC, Hughes CC. Dordrecht, Netherlands, D Reidel, 1985, pp 25–38

Simons RC: Sorting the culture-bound syndromes into descriptively similar taxa. Presented as part of the symposium on Culture-Bound Syndromes and DSM-III at the annual meeting of the American Psychiatric Assocation, Montreal, May 1988

Simons RC, Hughes CC (eds): The Culture-Bound Syndromes: Folk Illnesses of Psychiatric and Anthropological Interest. Dordrecht, Netherlands, D Reidel, 1985

Snow LF: Folk medicine beliefs and their implications for care of patients—a review based on studies among black Americans. Ann Intern Med 81(1):82–96, 1974

Takahashi T: A social club spontaneously formed by ex-patients who had suffered from anthropophobia (taijin kyofu [sho]). Int J Soc Psychiatry 2(2):137–140, 1975

Tan E-S: Culture-bound syndromes among overseas Chinese, in Normal and Abnormal Behavior in Chinese Culture. Edited by Kleinman A, Lin T. Dordrecht, Netherlands, D Reidel, 1981, pp 371–386

Tanaka-Matsumi J: *Taijin kyofusho*—diagnostic and cultural issues in Japanese psychiatry. Cult Med Psychiatry 3:231–245, 1979

van Loon FHG: *Amok* and *Lattah*. Journal of Abnormal and Social Psychology 21:434–444, 1926/1927

van Wulfften Palthe PM: Psychiatry and neurology in the tropics, in Clinical Textbook of Tropical Medicine. Batavia, NY, G Kolff, 1936, pp 526–538

Weidman HH: *Falling-out:* A diagnostic and treatment problem viewed from a transcultural perspective. Soc Sci Med 13B:95–112, 1979

Westermeyer J: *Amok*, in Extraordinary Disorders of Human Behavior. Edited by Freidmann C, Faguet R. New York, Plenum, 1982, pp 173–190

Westermeyer J: Sudden mass assault with grenade: an epidemic *Amok* form from Laos, in The Culture-Bound Syndromes: Folk Illnesses of Psychiatric and Anthropological Interest. Edited by Simons RC, Hughes CC. Dordrecht, Netherlands, D Reidel, 1985, pp 225–235

Wikan U: Illness from fright or soul loss: a north Balinese culture-bound syndrome? Cult Med Psychiatry 13: 25–50, 1989

Yap PM: Mental diseases peculiar to certain cultures: a survey of comparative psychiatry. Journal of Mental Science 97:313–327, 1951

Yap PM: The *Latah* reaction: Its pathodynamics and nosological position. Journal of Mental Science 98(413):515–564, 1952

Yap PM: *Suk-Yeon* or *Koro*—a culture-bound depersonalization syndrome. Bulletin of the Hong Kong Chinese Medical Association 16(1):31–47, 1964

Yap PM: *Koro*—a culture-bound depersonalization syndrome. Br J Psychiatry 111:43–50, 1965

Yap PM: Comparative Psychiatry: A Theoretical Framework. Edited by Lau MP, Stokes AB. Toronto, Ontario, University of Toronto Press, 1974

Selected Glossary of
Ethnic Terms for Folk Illnesses

Pronunciation guides for the following terms are based on the authors' language familiarity (e.g., Spanish and French) and in a number of other instances, upon consultation with native speakers (e.g., Navajo, Korean, Mandarin and Cantonese Chinese). In the absence of native speakers, pronunciation data were derived from ethnographic specialists (e.g., for indigenous terms from eastern Siberia or the Oglala Sioux Indians) and national embassy personnel from countries in which the given term is used (e.g., Thailand, Indonesia, Malawi, Burma). In some instances, such inquiry resulted in the addition of a synonym for the given term (e.g., *rok-jit* for *rok-joo*). When definitive sources have not been available, the straightforward English transcription as found in the literature is provided (e.g., *mogo laya,* a term of the Huli people of Papua New Guinea). It is not uncommon in non-Western languages for structural tonality to convey meaning, not simply situational or dramatic emphasis (e.g., Navajo, Chinese, most African languages). Where appropriate, verbal commentary approximates such an intonational pattern; see the Glossary of Chinese Terms for further discussion.

Ahade idizi be [a-ha'-de i-di'-zi be]
Navajo term denoting dissociative outburst of violent or aggressive behavior, sometimes with persecutory ideas; similar to the well-known *amok* (Malay).

Amurakh [a-moo-rakh']
Yakut word (eastern Siberia) meaning "sensitive" or—in closely related groups—"complaint" or "shudder." Common symptoms are echolalia and echopraxia, and sometimes coprolalia. Cognate terms in other aboriginal Siberian groups are *irkunii* (Yukaghir), *olan* (Tungus), *menkeiti* (Koryak), and *imu* (Ainu). Symptoms are similar to the Malay *latah.*

Angst [ongst]
Anxiety, dread, anguish. From German and Danish. See *kayak angst*.

Bah tschi [bah'-see]
Thai term denoting episode of dissociative, mimetic behavior in which the person is highly suggestible. (*Bah* is a colloquial expression for "crazy.") There is a falling tone on the first syllable, which is emphasized. Term is comparable to *latah* (Malay). (In a related expression, one may say that a person is *bah-bah bawbaw* [ba-ba'-bawh-bawh], or "not all there.")

Boufée delirante [boo-fay' day-lee-rawnt']
A syndrome observed in West Africa and Haiti. This French term refers to a sudden outburst of aggressive and agitated behavior, marked confusion, psychomotor excitement, and sometimes visual and auditory hallucinations or paranoid ideation.

Cafard (or **cathard**) [ka-fawr']
Putatively a Polynesian term referring to acute outburst of homicidal violence followed by exhaustion; preceded by brooding.

Colera [ko-lay'-raw]
Spanish word referring to episode of various physiological symptoms (e.g., nausea, vomiting, fever); severe temper tantrum; and dissociative behavior. Sometimes compared with *amok*, which may include violent and homicidal behavior and persecutory ideation. (See also *gila mengamok*.)

Espanto [ace-pawn'-tow]
An alternative Spanish term for *susto*, meaning "fright."

Gila besi [gee'-lah bay'-see]
Indonesian term (Sarawak; Iban people). *Gila* is the generic term for insanity ("mad [from disease, infatuated]"). *Gila besi* refers to a violent outburst ("craziness").

Gila mengamok [gee'-lah men'-gah-mok]
Malay term. *Gila mengamok* is the localized term for *amok* or *amuck,* in which a person suddenly begins an indiscriminant homicidal spree (in pre-European times using a dagger or machete, in modern times using firearms or hand grenades) and continues until he or she is overpowered or killed.

Haak-tsan [hawk^2-tsaan^1]
A Cantonese term referring to the syndrome known in other places as *susto. Haak* has a rising inflection (2nd tone—see Glossary of Chinese Terms for explanation of tonality); the second element—*tsan*—has a high, even tone (1st tone).

Hwa-byung [hwa-byoong']
A Korean folk syndrome literally translated into English as "anger sickness." A variety of symptomatic expressions: insomnia, excessive fatigue, acute panic, morbid fear of impending death, dysphoric affect, indigestion, anorexia, dyspnea, palpitation, generalized pains and aches, feeling of a mass in the epigastrium. Attributed to suppression of anger.

Iich'aa [eech aaw; no inflection]
Navajo word translated as "moth craziness" and referring to epileptiform behavior, loss of self-control, and fits of violence and rage. Sometimes compared with *amok* (see *gila mengamok*).

Ikota [ee-koh'-tah] or ilota
Aboriginal Siberian term referring to hypersensitivity to startle and suggestibility, with a dissociative episode followed by an amnesic reaction. Often considered same disorder as *amurakh* and *latah.*

Imu [ee'-moo]
Ainu term (Sakhalin and other islands north of Japan) referring to hypersuggestibility, dramatic startle response, dissociative behavior; often grouped with *amurakh* and *latah.*

Jinjinia bemar
Assamese (south Asian group). Term referring to condition known elsewhere in South and East Asia as *koro* (Malay) or *suk yeong* or cognate terms (Chinese), in which a male grasps his penis out of intense fear that it will retract into his body and cause death.

Kayak angst [ka'-ee-yak ongst]
Intense fear of capsizing and drowning associated with going out on the open sea in a kayak. *Kayak* is an Eskimo (Inuit) term referring to the now well-known canoe that is skin-covered and wooden-framed, with an opening for the hunter allowing him to be tied into the boat to prevent water from coming in. The Greenlandic indigenous term for an attack of intense anxiety and fear while out on the sea is *nangiarpok* [nong'-ee-ar-pok] (alternatively *nangiarnek*) [nong'-ee-ar-nek].

Latah [law'-taaw]
Malay term denoting hypersuggestibility and hypersusceptibility to a startle reaction. See also *amurakh* or *imu*.

Mal de pelea [mall day pay-lay'-aa]
Puerto Rican (Spanish) term referring to outburst of violent, often homicidal behavior comparable to the Malay term *amok*. See entries for *ahade idizi be, cafard, colera, iich'aa,* or *gila mengamok*.

Mal puesto [mall poo-ay'-stow]
Spanish term for condition of believing one is bewitched; alternative term is *brujería*. Multiple psychological and somatic problems explained as caused by ensorceling activity by another person.

Misala [mee-sah'-lah]
Malawian (eastern Africa) term for condition known elsewhere as *latah*—dissociative, hypersuggestible behavior. See *latah*.

Mogo laya [mo-go law-yaw]
Huli (indigenous Papua New Guinea group) term that refers
to behavioral and psychological consequences of intense
startle or fright; see *susto*.

Myriachit [mee-ryeh'-cheet]
A term used by one of the aboriginal Siberian groups meaning
hysteria and convulsions, or Arctic hysteria. Term is similar
to that for symptoms found elsewhere labelled
latah—hypersuggestibility and dissociative behavior.

Ngamok [nah'-mok]
Indonesian term. Alternative rendering of *amok*; see *gila mengamok*.

P'a-leng [pah⁴-lung³]
Mandarin Chinese term. The first word—*p'a*—has a dropping
inflection (4th tone—see Glossary of Chinese Terms for
explanation of tonality); the second element—*leng*—at first
drops and then rises (3rd tone). The phrase means "morbid
fear of the cold." Symptoms include loss of vitality and feeling
of the need to wear excessive clothing.

Phii pob [pee-pob']
Thai term for the belief that one is possessed by a spirit, or
that a living person has the power to possess others in this
way. First syllable is pronounced with a soft *p* and means
"ghost" or "spirit." Second syllable is pronounced with a hard
p and means "possessive" or "to be possessed by."
Accompanied by numbness of limbs, falling (sometimes with
convulsions); unconsciousness; and sometimes clenched fists
and bodily rigidity or shouting, screaming, weeping, and
confused speech.

Rok-joo [rowk'-jew]
Thai term for syndrome in Malay called *koro* (Chinese,
suo-yang)—intense fear that a man's penis will recede into the
abdomen and cause death. First syllable means "diseased";
second syllable is a colloquial term for "penis." A related term
is *rok-jit* [rowk'-jiht], or "mental disease."

Saladera [sawl-a-day'-raw]
Alternative local term (Peruvian) for *susto*. (See following entry.)

Susto [soos'-tow]
Widespread Spanish term designating various somatic and psychological symptoms the etiology for which is attributed to a traumatic incident, which may have been experienced by the victim or another person close to the person (such as a child). The core belief is that the frightening event dislodged the victim's spirit or soul from the body. Other Spanish terms used for the same phenomena are *espanto, espasmo, pasmo,* and *miedo.*

Taijin kyofusho [ta-ee-jeen' ki-yo-foo-sho']
(Literally, *taijin* = face-to-face; *kyofu* = fearful; *sho* = syndrome). Japanese term for what has been termed "anthropophobia": intense anxiety in the presence of other people; fearfulness that one's bodily appearance, odor, or behavior is offensive. Symptoms include blushing, evasive facial gestures, timidity.

Wacinko [wah-chin'-ko]
Oglala Sioux term for syndrome of withdrawn, overly sensitive, sometimes suicidal behavior.

Yaun [yawn] (alternative term **young-dah-te** [yong-dah-tay'])
Burmese term for symptom complex elsewhere known as *latah*—dissociative behavior prompted by sudden startle and hypersuggestibility.

4 Cross-Cultural Psychotherapy

Joe Yamamoto, M.D.
J. Arturo Silva, M.D.
Ledro R. Justice, M.D.
Christine Y. Chang, M.D., M.P.H.
Gregory B. Leong, M.D.

A s the number of people in the United States who are from diverse cultural backgrounds has grown, cross-cultural therapy has become an increasingly important concern. There has been a prevalent myth in the past that America is a melting pot: "America is God's crucible, the great Melting-Pot where all the races of Europe are melting and reforming!" (Zangwill 1909, p. 37). In the 1990s, there is an appreciation that America is multicultural, that we will not all melt into one pot, and that we Americans are shaped by diverse and distinct ethnic and cultural backgrounds. These cultures may be African, American Indian, Asian, Latin American, or European, but we are all Americans.

Engel (1977) emphasized the diversity in psychiatry in describing his approach to the etiology of psychiatric disorders and their manifestations when he coined the term "biopsychosocial." Because of the multicultural nature of our changing America, we believe that Engel's concept should now be expanded to explicitly include culture: that is, we advocate a "biopsychosociocultural" approach to mental and emotional illnesses.

In this chapter, we focus on the psychotherapy of patients from diverse backgrounds. Therapists who treat patients in this cross-cultural milieu should be aware of the cultural issues that may affect the therapeutic process.

It is possible to make some general distinctions between traditional and Western cultures, such as that of the mainstream in the United States. Leff (1988) provides an interesting discussion of such differences, which are sum-

This study was supported in part by the National Research Center on Asian American Mental Health (NIMH #R01 MH44331).

marized in Table 4–1. Such general social characteristics, of course, may not apply in the case of all individuals from these groups, because there are intragroup variations that depend in large part on the particular culture from which a patient comes.

The general differences between traditional and Western cultures can be illustrated by comparing the values and traits of Japanese and American cultures as is done in Table 4–2. We note that, in these cultural terms, the Chinese, the Koreans, and the Vietnamese are similar to the Japanese. That is, they are all traditional cultures and are thus tied to the past in terms of factors such as ancestor worship and the belief in the importance of maintaining historical traditions while developing into modern industrialized societies.

There are also similarities between Asian cultures and Hispanic American culture, as noted by Acosta and Evans (1982):

> The family has traditionally been one of the most valued and proud aspects of life among Hispanic Americans. A great deal of importance has typically been placed on preserving family unity, respect, and loyalty, and the family tends to be a source of strength for Hispanic Americans.

Table 4–1.   Polar attributes of traditional and modern societies

Traditional society	Modern society
Group-oriented	Individual-oriented
Extended family	Nuclear family
Income-producing linked to kinship ties	Income-producing independent of kinship ties
Economic functions nonspecialized	Economic functions specialized
High mortality, high fertility	Low mortality, low fertility
Status determined by age and position in family	Status achieved by own efforts
Relationships between kin obligatory	Relationships between kin permissive
Relationships determined by role and position in family	Relationships determined by individual choice
Arranged marriages	Choice of marital partner
Individuals can be replaced by others filling same roles	Individuals unique and irreplaceable
Extensive classification terminology for distant relatives	Restricted classification terminology for close relatives only
Behavior to specific kin prescribed	Great variation in kin behavior

Source.   Leff 1988, p. 79.

The family structure is usually hierarchical with special respect and much authority given to the husband and father. The wife and mother is often obedient to her husband and also receives respect and much emotional reward from the children. Sex-role identification for the Hispanic American is thus much stricter than that of the general population of the United States. However, many of these traditional sex-role characteristics may also be found among the poor and the rural in our country. As Hispanic Americans move up the socioeconomic ladder to more middle-class levels and as more assimilation of Anglo life-styles occurs, sex-role delineations become less strict. (p. 55)

The family also plays a crucial role in other American cultural groups. For example, the importance of the family for African Americans has been described by Bass and colleagues (1982) as follows:

Five characteristics or strengths . . . lead toward survival, advancement, and stability of [African] American families: adaptability of family roles, strong kinship bonds, strong work orientation, strong achievement orientation, and strong religious orientation. (p. 85)

In addition to the value systems we have described above, sexual identity, social class, rural or urban residence, and regional differences within the United States may all affect the patient-therapist relationship. Cultural factors may also pose challenges for the therapist treating a patient with a mental illness, as may other factors such as generation and social class (Gordon 1964). Because of the diverse backgrounds patients bring to the treatment setting, therapists must be aware of the difficulties the immigrant or minority patient may have in achieving active empathy. The clinician must also be prepared for the special countertransference problems such a patient may evoke (Yamamoto and Chang 1988).

Ethnicity and Traditional Medicine

In this chapter, we focus on the cultural backgrounds of non-European ethnic patients in the United States. Asians in America have come from a number of countries that are populated by many diverse ethnic groups. Each group of Asians—Japanese, Chinese, Indians, Koreans, Vietnamese, Laotians, Cambodians, Pilipinos, and Pacific Islanders, among others—has unique characteristics. Nonetheless, there are similarities among them, such as an emphasis on traditional ways, on the family, and on interdependence. (Latin Americans likewise come from Mexico and Central and

South America and share similarities such as language, religion, and traditional cultural values.) For simplicity and clarity, we will discuss the cultural characteristics of traditional, unacculturated Asians, although we
acknowledge that many Asian American families have now been in America
for three or four generations.

Knowledge of the following traditional Eastern medical beliefs can be
helpful in improving the treatment compliance of immigrant Asian patients.
First, Asians tend to perceive Western medicines as "too strong." Second,
under the rubric of traditional Asian medicine, mental illness is treated according to an infection model; once the patient is better, he or she feels
"cured" or "healed" and no longer believes that medicines need be continued. The Western model of continuing care and medication is rather novel,
and educating patients and their families is therefore crucial.

Further, therapists need to understand that Asian patients may believe in
the traditional Chinese categories of "hot and cold theory" (Wallnofer and
von Rottauscher 1965), as the following case illustrates.

A young Laotian woman suffering from a major depressive episode was prescribed nortriptyline, which was supplied in capsules of yellow or orange. She
refused to take this medication because of the color of the capsules. She be-

Table 4–2.   Comparison of cultural values and traditions

American civilization		Japanese civilization
Individualism	v.	Familism
Independence	v.	Interdependence
Protestant ethic: emphasis on work, science and technology; human ability to control the environment; religious support of human endeavors toward economic and material progress	v.	Confucian ethics: loyalty between lord and subordinates; intimacy between father and sons; propriety between husband and wife; order between elder and junior; trust between friends
Present and future orientation	v.	Past, present, and future orientation
Tolerance of differences	v.	Tolerance for similarities
Emphasis on self-fulfillment, self-development	v.	Emphasis on interpersonal relationships
Emphasis on individual achievement	v.	Emphasis on group achievement
Emphasis on newness, change	v.	Emphasis on newness and change in the context of tradition

Source. Yamamoto 1982, pp. 84–85.

lieved that her mental illness was caused by too much heat in her body, and, therefore, that the correct medication should be a "cold" color. She eventually accepted doxepin, which is supplied in blue-green capsules.

Finally, patients who practice coining and cupping as healing methods should be warned that those practices might be acceptable for adults but not for children, because of the bruising and marks that are left from the treatments. There have been several cases of parents being investigated for suspected child abuse because they had performed coining on their children. In the practice of coining, oil is applied to the back and chest, the skin massaged until warm, and the edge of a coin rubbed on the skin until bruises occur (Gellis and Feingold 1976; Yeatman et al 1976). In cupping, hot suction cups are applied to the skin and may also cause bruises (N. Nguyen, P. H. Nguyen, L. Nguyen, Coin Treatment in Vietnamese Families: Traditional Medical Practice vs. Child Abuse [unpublished data], February 1988; Quock and Louie 1986).

In the following sections, we provide brief reviews of what, in our experience, may be central cross-cultural issues for patients from major ethnic groups in the United States. These include issues of group identity and of value systems stemming from traditional societies.

Thus far, we have mentioned those from ethnic groups that have immigrated to America from Europe, Africa, Latin America, and Asia. But American Indians also face special problems. Although American Indian tribes have diverse cultural backgrounds, they are stereotyped by Americans in highly specific and negative ways. Therefore, therapy undertaken with any member of an American Indian tribe must be performed with careful consideration of the specific culture of that tribe. The therapist who treats a patient from a given American Indian tribe should make every effort to understand the cultural heritage of the patient and should understand the patient's ecology, which also is known to influence the culture as well as the individual development of the patient.

Although Asians and Hispanics in America may easily identify with their culture and country of ancestry and/or origin, such comfort is not so easily obtained for many African Americans (Haley 1976). The term "African American" denotes derivation from a continent, not a country. Moreover, this general identification is externally imposed, as is alluded to by Stuckey (1987):

During the process of their becoming a single people, Yorubas, Akans, Ibos, Angolans, and others were present on slave ships to America and experienced a common horror—unearthly moans and piercing shrieks, the smell of filth and the stench of death, all during the violent rhythms and quiet coursings of ships at sea. As such, slave ships were the first real incubators of slave unity across cultural lines, cruelly revealing irreducible links from one ethnic group to the other, fostering resistance thousands of miles before the shores of the new land appeared on the horizon—before there was mention of natural rights in North America. (p. 3)

African Americans continue to be perceived as representing a common cultural background, and this perception can pose a barrier to therapy if a therapist attempts to "treat" a stereotype instead of the patient before him or her. Banks (1989) points out that "one of the most important characteristics of African Americans today is their intra-group variation" (p. 65). Moreover, some Afro-Caribbeans have had the advantage of being permitted to maintain cultural ties.

Once in America, slaves were treated as inferior in status to whites. For instance, Wilkinson (1970) notes,

> Early American myths . . . held that black persons were inherently inferior to whites. In present-day America, the genetic basis for inferiority is being replaced with a sociopathological basis caused by the oppressiveness of slavery and the failure to rectify the ills that followed this subjugation. (p. 1089)

This history leads us to the issue of racism, which is prevalent and affects all the ethnic groups that belong to the defined minority groups in the United States, including African Americans, Asian Americans, Latin Americans, and American Indians. The prevalence of overt racism has decreased to some extent since the era of the civil rights movement of the 1960s and the leadership of Martin Luther King, Jr. However, racism still persists and may enter the psychotherapeutic picture. Moreover, those therapists who are racists may be correctly perceived as prejudiced by their patients (Yamamoto et al. 1967, 1968).

We cannot adequately consider all the various permutations of therapists and patients in terms of cultural background, social class, postimmigration generational status, language differences, and problems related to mistaken assumptions about one another. But we can say, in general, that American therapists have a Western-centric point of view (Roland 1988). One psychiatrist (Kinzie 1985) has highlighted this issue in his description of the values of American therapists:

> Mental health professionals are dominated by value systems of clinical humanistic psychology which promote self-aggrandizement and self-satisfaction,

autonomy and rejection of authority, relativity in values, situational ethics, apology (rather than restitution), and avoidance of long-term relationships and responsibility. (p. 48)

Although some would argue that Kinzie greatly magnifies the issue of American therapists' values, such values need to be considered when treating so-called cross-cultural patients, because these values pose potential pitfalls to successful treatment.

The relevance of ethnicity in the immigrant population cannot be underemphasized because of dissimilarities among minorities, even those often categorized together, such as Asian Americans. For example, Koreans and Chinese have distinct differences in behavior that are related to distinct cultural values. Koreans have been known to have substantial problems with alcoholism. As such, they are known to have drinking habits that are substantial and even comparable to those of American males (Yamamoto et al. 1988). Indeed, such a pattern may have a biological basis: 50% of the Han Chinese lack aldehyde dehydrogenase isoenzyme 1, an enzyme involved in the metabolism of alcohol, whereas only 25% of Koreans do (Goedde et al. 1984).

Generational Experiences Affecting Psychotherapy

Intergenerational differences in ethnic groups are often the products of different experiences in the objective world. But even if an experience, such as a great tragedy, is shared by a culture, it may produce different effects in those who undergo it, depending on their age and level of individual development. For example, a young child who loses his parents is likely to experience problems associated with mistrust. Adults who lose family and culture may have special problems associated with generativity—that is, the ability to establish and guide the next generation (Erikson 1980).

Intergenerational differences are especially important to many ethnic minorities who reside in the United States. These variations may signify cultural differences associated with various degrees of acculturation (or lack thereof) to the dominant society. Intergenerational differences may also arise from experiences to which members of a specific age-defined cohort may have been exposed and which, therefore, serve to differentiate different groups. For example, an historic event of major proportions, the economic debacle known as the Great Depression, has been shown to exert long-lasting influences on worldview and mental health among those who lived through it (Elder 1974, 1979).

The historical experience of African Americans has greatly affected them as a group. But the racist oppression they have endured has varied in kind and severity across generations, from the agonies of slavery to the humiliation and poverty of segregation, to the great economic and social hardships of the current period. As Spurlock (1982) points out, "Characteristics of a cultural grouping are shaped, in part, in response to the broader environment. . . . Justice (personal communication 1979) suggests that characteristics and problems of [African] Americans are highly related to experiences of exclusion" (p. 167).

The cultural experiences endured by various other ethnic groups have also marked them with significant generational differences. These differences appear especially when the historical stresses endured are moderate to severe (Kessner and Caroli 1981). Some groups have experienced such severe stresses that they have threatened to destroy the very fabric of their societies. An example is the Holocaust, during which many Jews perished and experienced untold suffering (Gilbert 1985).

More recently, the Khmer Rouge regime was responsible for the deaths of a significant proportion of the Cambodian people. Along with this genocide, there was extensive torture, starvation, and the inevitable destabilization of many families and major social structures (Becker 1986; Ngor 1987). These experiences led to the development among Cambodians of posttraumatic stress disorder, depression, and other severe stress-induced disorders (Bochnlein et al. 1985; Gong-Guy 1987; Kinzie et al. 1984, 1986; Mollica et al. 1987; Sack et al. 1986).

Thousands of Cambodians who suffered at the hands of the Khmer Rouge have immigrated to this country. The problems faced by these people are likely to vary, depending in part on the stages of emotional development of those who experienced losses. Some of these people may be traumatized to such an extent that denial of the stressful experience also causes them to repress the more positive aspects of the sociocultural milieus in which they were raised and in which, unfortunately, they sustained their traumatic experiences.

Case Study of Generational Trauma in a Vietnam Veteran

There are a myriad of tragic examples of events that created severe generational trauma. For the United States, the Vietnam War is the foremost modern example of such an event. It created emotional scars carried by many to this day.

The following case study of a Vietnam veteran illustrates some of the generational and ecological aspects that may become important in therapy.

Mr. G. is a 34-year-old Puerto Rican Vietnam veteran who was hospitalized after he had beaten his girlfriend and his son. During the night of the beatings, he had awakened from a nightmare associated with war trauma and had been unable to recognize them, believing them to be Vietcong. Mr. G. also experienced flashbacks and intrusive thoughts which reminded him of the war trauma he had experienced in Viet Nam. He tended to be hyperalert and was suspicious of other people in general.

Mr. G. lived in the continental United States and made many efforts to avoid contacting his family. He was ashamed to do so because he believed that he was a "weak man" for being ill and for being unable to support his son. After his symptoms diminished somewhat while he was hospitalized, subsequent outpatient treatment with amitriptyline and behavioral therapy by a white therapist proved unsuccessful.

At this point, an Hispanic therapist assumed care of Mr. G. and initiated a biopsychosociocultural approach utilizing a life-span orientation to his therapy. From a biological point of view, Mr. G. responded moderately well in that his flashbacks, nightmares, insomnia, and hyperalertness diminished with antidepressant pharmacotherapy. He was also encouraged to engage in a life-review therapeutic approach in which he reexamined the life he had lived before his traumatic war experiences. Although he initially saw his early life as a "waste of time," he slowly began to appreciate that his family had cared for him despite limitations he may have had as a child and as an adolescent.

Part of the therapy involved encouraging Mr. G. to recall specific ecological areas such as various cities in Puerto Rico, including his home town, in an effort to allow him to recall early experiences. The psychotherapist used independently researched material from the geographical area and cultural milieu in which the patient was raised. Some of these materials (such as photographs) were used in therapy to enable Mr. G. to recall the many positive aspects of his early life.

In this way, the negative schema that Mr. G. had developed as a result of his traumatic war experiences were slowly changed into more positive schemata. As he regained a more positive view of himself, he began to communicate more with his family through telephone calls. Eventually, he was able to share his psychiatric difficulties with his family. He then allowed his brother to visit him. Eventually, he agreed to return to live in Puerto Rico, close to his family, where he planned to receive further psychiatric help.

It is obviously very important that therapists who treat members of extremely traumatized ethnic groups take into account not only the cultural background and level of individual development of the patients, but also the specific ecological and historical milieus to which they were exposed at specific periods of their lives (Silva and Liederman 1986). For example, self-isolation is a more likely response of individuals who were exposed to the massive stresses of the Pol Pot regime during their childhood years compared to those without analogous experiences at similar ages (Sack et al. 1986). The origin of such behavior needs to be taken into account when evaluating these individuals for treatment. Their somewhat distant behavior should not be interpreted as the "cultural norm," because it may have been developed as a result of their traumatic war experiences.

Demographic Factors

Race, class, sex, and ethnicity all affect behavior, values, and attitudes toward therapy in significant ways, as the following brief treatment of these factors suggests.

In assessing African Americans, it is important to understand that "differences are not necessarily deviances" (Spurlock 1982, p. 166).

> Non-[African American] therapists may have difficulty understanding successful coping styles which do not fit white middle-class norms. Because their environmental realities may be quite different, [African American] patients' coping mechanisms may go unnoticed. . . . The ability to deal with single parenthood, poverty, and other environmental and social stresses is often an indication of ego strength which should be noted. (Block 1981, p. 189)

It is well for clinicians to allow for class differences in assessing and treating all groups.

> Most poor and working-class people want the same things as other Americans, namely, the American Dream. This includes education, a decent job, suitable housing, and treatment with respect and consideration in one's day-to-day activities. However, there may be differences in the priorities people place on attaining this dream. For example, there are people who persevere despite the obstacles, disadvantages, and odds against them. There are others who do not persevere and who settle for some different version of the dream. This seems to suggest that despite the fact that there are similarities in aspirations between the working class and the middle and upper classes, we must look at the past history of these people. If someone has been a graduate student, then a course of treatment which includes long-term therapy geared toward the solution of

the intrapsychic conflicts would seem reasonable because of the experience of long-term education. In contrast, a working-class person with less education may view such a proposal as being interminable, irrelevant, and financially impossible. This is an aspect that we need to consider. Although many people agree with the American Dream and speak of the importance of long-term therapy and the understanding of internal conflicts, we have to see if people place a high enough priority upon it to expend the necessary time and energy to accomplish it. (Yamamoto et al. 1982)

Among Asians, there are rapid generational changes, more swift among the females than among the males because of the tendency of the males to want to cling to the more traditional values of the East. As is pointed out later in this chapter, Confucian values tend to be sexist and favor the men. The women, on the other hand, quickly learn about the American values of equal rights for women, become more independent, and show their previously hidden strengths. They are more often able to get jobs because they are more readily accepted by whites.

The large recent influx of Koreans into Los Angeles illustrates this point. Koreans are different from the Chinese and Japanese of previous immigrant generations in that they adapt to American ways much more quickly. When immigrant Koreans become United States citizens, they frequently adopt American first names. The fact that perhaps 25% of Koreans in Korea are Protestant Christians also hastens the acculturation process in some ways. Most Korean Americans—70%—are Protestant Christians and attend church regularly (Hurh and Kim 1984). However, it should be noted that the churches they attend are ethnic Korean churches, and there is therefore a great deal of sociocultural support in these havens.

For Japanese Americans, the acculturation process has been noted to have occurred very rapidly. By the second and third generations, the cultural values of Japanese families in the United States are mostly American, with an estimated 10% of traditional values being maintained (Yamamoto and Wagatsuma 1980). Indeed, recent trends have shown that Asian Americans tend to out-marry in very large numbers as a result of acculturation in the second and third generations (Kitano et al. 1984). Nonetheless, Asians maintain their close-knit family ties much longer than mainstream Americans (Yamamoto and Wagatsuma 1980).

One important factor in assessing ethnicity is variation in skin color among groups such as African Americans, Hispanics, and American Indians. With the pervasive influence of the aesthetic values of the mainstream society, members of minority groups not infrequently come to value physical norms more consonant with those of whites than of their own group. This process has significant consequences for the self-concept and self-esteem of minority individuals who may decide to pursue aesthetic ideals that are incongruent with their own culture and perhaps biologically inaccessible. These issues need to be carefully explored in therapy. Furthermore, the minority patient's views about skin color may also have important transference value. For example, the skin color of the therapist, regardless of the therapist's ethnicity, may cause the patient to view the therapist in a relatively more positive or negative light.

Language

Language plays a very important role in psychotherapy. The need for effective communication in the therapeutic situation is best appreciated when therapist and patient do not share a common language and therapy with the aid of translators is either slow and inaccurate, or not infrequently destructive or impossible (Carillo 1978). However, even when both therapist and patient are bilingual in the same languages, the implications of language for psychotherapy are likely to be important. For example, some bilingual patients may utilize one of their languages in a defensive way, preferring to speak in the language that enables them to become emotionally divorced from issues important in understanding their psychiatric difficulties (Marcos 1976).

Code switching, the process of making a partial or total language shift, must also be looked at in the context of the therapeutic intervention (Pitta et al. 1978). When a therapist initiates switching from one language to another, he or she may introduce cognitive and affective cues that may signal a new framework of meaning for the patient. A skillful therapist must make an attempt to identify the major effects of code switching on a patient, because this process may affect psychotherapy substantially. For example, a therapist may facilitate the therapeutic process by allowing some bilingual patients "to approach material in the second language which would be too threatening or emotionally charged in the primary language" (Pitta et al. 1978, p. 255).

The therapist must pay attention to the same process when it is presented by the patient. Code switching may not simply signal emotional distancing. Russell (1988), referring to Burling, points out that "Such switching is used not only as a rhetorical device to give greater emphasis but as a sign of intimacy as well" (p. 35). Russell (1988) emphasizes that "clients who code-switch during a session are sending a potent message that astute clinicians cannot afford to ignore" (p. 35).

Even in initial interviews between clinicians and patients before therapy begins, language can have important consequences. For example, Marcos (1976) found that bilingual patients whose native language was Spanish, if interviewed in English rather than Spanish, were rated as being more mentally ill, less emotionally detached, and having less contact with the interviewer.

Language discrepancies between therapists and patients whose native language is English can also affect diagnosis and treatment. For example, clinicians may have negative perceptions of African Americans who are not articulate in Standard English (SE). This may be a significant problem. Russell (1988) citing Valentine, observes that "In fact, many types of African American (nonstandard) English exist, originating out of the African diaspora cultures of the West Indies, Guyana, and Suriname" (p. 35).

The Black Nonstandard English (BNE) of the urban centers of the United States is just one of the many nonstandard English (NE) dialects, such as Louisiana Cajun, Hawaiian pidgin, Southern, New England, Bostonian, and Brooklynese. All of these various types of NE can have an effect on the therapeutic relationship; a client speaking Hawaiian pidgin, for example, may be "viewed and assessed differently from his or her SE [Standard English]-speaking counterparts" (Comas-Diaz 1988, p. 35).

The credibility of a psychotherapist can have important implications for all phases of the therapeutic process, and language may affect the credibility of the clinician. Although the available literature is far from clear, there are indications that language factors may affect the psychotherapist's stature in the patient's eyes (Russell 1988). For example, Lambert and associates (1960) found in a comparison of French and English spoken-language that both English and French listeners from Canada scored French speakers lower on several measures of credibility, such as perceived leadership, self-confidence, and intelligence. Such negative community-wide stereotypes may adversely affect the course of therapy.

Identification with the therapist is likely to be an important factor in the way that patients relate to the psychotherapist. Although patients' perception of similarities to their therapists are multifactorial, language appears to be an important factor in this respect. When both patient and therapist are similarly bilingual and share a common native language and culture, the psychotherapist may use the original language. In the process, the therapist provides a powerful message that he or she can understand the patient, because they share a common set of cultural experiences that may lead to a better therapeutic alliance (Russell 1988; Silva and Liederman 1986). Nevertheless, care should be taken to identify both transference and countertransference reactions as a result of these impressions, because both positive and negative reactions can be expected (Munoz 1979).

In summary, although language is generally acknowledged to be an important factor in initial interviews with a patient and in its influence on the outcome of therapy, much remains to be discovered. Nevertheless, the therapist is likely to find that language will need to be considered in order to make psychotherapy as effective as possible.

Diagnosis

There are many difficulties in formulating appropriate diagnoses when evaluating patients from immigrant populations. One such example is identifying depressive disorders in Asians. Asians often display only somatic symptoms of depression, such as insomnia, anorexia, weight loss, and difficulty in concentrating while not endorsing a dysphoric mood (Yamamoto et al. 1985a). Yet the prevalence of major depression can be substantial in Asian American populations (Yamamoto et al. 1985b). Moreover, the patient may not always be the best source of information concerning his or her disorder. We would certainly recommend that the family be included in the evaluation of first-generation immigrants from Asia and Latin America, because these patients often function more as part of a unit rather than as individuals (Roland 1988; Yamamoto and Chang 1988).

Clinicians may also fail to recognize dysphoria and depression in the African American patient. Substance abuse and problems with impulse control, including conduct disturbance and apparent sexual irresponsibility, may be the outward expressions of deeply seated struggles in functioning. Adebimpe (1981) has argued,

> Factors that could contribute to misdiagnosis [of African Americans] were the social and cultural distance between patient and clinician, stereotyping of [African American] psychopathology, false-positive symptoms, biased diagnostic instruments, and the combined effects of various sources of diagnostic error. (p. 167)

The following account by Dash (1989) pertaining to African American teenage pregnancy suggests the need for careful clinical exploration. African American teenage pregnancy and parenthood may not just mean character pathology manifested by poor impulse control, ignorance, and antisocial behavior. Deeper problems associated with self-esteem must be considered by clinicians while assessing teenage parents.

> I found that the girls, far from being passive victims, were often equal—or greater—actors than their boyfriends in exploring sexuality and becoming pregnant. The girls were as often the leaders in their desire to have a child as the boys were. I did not find one adolescent couple where both partners were ignorant about the results of sexual activity without the use of contraception.
>
> In time it became clear that for many girls in the poverty-stricken community of Washington Highlands, a baby is a *tangible* achievement in an otherwise dreary and empty future. It is one way of announcing: I *am* a woman. For many boys in Washington Highlands the birth of a baby represents an identical rite of passage. The boy is saying: I *am* a man.
>
> The desire for a child was especially acute among adolescents who were doing poorly in school. They knew implicitly and had been told explicitly that they were not likely to graduate from high school. These were the youths, ages fifteen to seventeen and still in the seventh grade, who were at highest risk to get pregnant or father a child. While the better students strove for a diploma, the poorer students achieved their form of recognition with a baby.
>
> If the crisis of black teenage parents were simply a matter of ignorance, then it might be a relatively easy problem to solve. But poor academic preparation that begins in elementary school, the poverty that surrounds them, and social isolation from mainstream American life motivate many of these boys and girls to have children. (Dash 1989, pp. 9–10)

Treatment

In the therapy of unacculturated immigrant populations, one has the advantage of using the family as a part of the treatment team, starting with the evaluation. The family may offer advantages in terms of encouragement and compliance in keeping the therapeutic appointment. The family may also help the patient adhere to the dosage regimen of psychotropic medications. This means that not only the patient but also the family must have sufficient information about therapy. Both need to understand the potential benefits of the recommended treatment regimen, possible alternative treatment, possible side effects of the medication, problems that may accrue with premature interruption of therapy, and finally, strategies for dealing with the stigma of mental illness labeling.

In most Asian families, it is assumed that the family knows best and will participate in the therapeutic process. For example, if a therapist initiates a treatment regimen that includes proper nutrition, exercise, and recreational activities, appropriate methods of relaxation, and psychotropic medications, the family should be educated in the rationale for this plan. The family can be a positive, constructive force in assisting the patient to achieve therapeutic goals.

The family has an important impact on the development of effective forms of therapy. Cultural patterns are firmly tied to the family, and the family unit is one of the basic structures through which culture is transmitted. Furthermore, culture and identity are closely associated, and their healthy interplay often takes place within the microenvironment of the family. The extent to which people feel secure with their identities also influences their abilities to interact with others in a productive and healthy way (Cobbs 1972).

Given the central aspect that ethnocultural factors play in understanding families, it should not be surprising that psychotherapy is also influenced by family factors. Among Mexican American families, for example, the parents are expected to be given a great degree of respect by their children, and attention is carefully paid to familial hierarchy and interdependence. Thus, therapeutic approaches likely to be intelligible and therefore effective in these families are those that are centered around redefining familial difficulties in interactional terms involving parents and children (Falicov 1982).

Liberman reported that while training patients in an assertiveness training program, a young Hispanic man went home and asserted himself with his father, who promptly blackened the patient's eye. This is an example of how assertiveness training should be tempered with an understanding of cultural values, which might include properly respectful behavior towards one's father in Hispanic cultural terms (R. Liberman, personal communication, February 1988).

In therapy with Asian patients, as with many ethnic minority patients, an important issue is empowerment. Minority patients often feel they cannot speak up or assert themselves. Despite improving race relations, minorities often express that they still feel as if they are "second-class citizens." Refugee immigrants, in particular, might not assert themselves in situations in which they may have been wronged because of fear of authority, fear of deportation, or fear of giving a bad reputation to the rest of their compatriots.

For many Asian patients, the World War II internment of American Japanese, both legitimate resident aliens and United States citizens, is a grim reminder of bigotry and racism in this country. The following case illustrates that the impact of the relocation camp experience has even affected the internees' children, who were born long after the war was over.

A 25-year-old Japanese American male came to therapy for generalized anxiety. In the course of treatment, it was learned that an important conflict for him was the relocation camp experience of his parents. It was a topic that was never discussed in the family, yet the losses suffered by the parents were clear to the patient. He felt angered but unable to rectify the injustice. In addition, any unfair treatment, no matter how small, that he himself received at work was perceived as a major setback. He felt that his boss did not give him recognition for his work, and that his white co-workers were given the promotions instead. However, he also felt that he could not speak up for fear of retribution. He clearly felt that he was left out of the "Boys' Club" because he was Asian.

A discussion of the usual duration of therapy is indicated, because most people—and particularly Asians as well as some socially disenfranchised American groups—expect a cure and relief to occur immediately. This issue is especially important when the patients have disorders that require treatment over several months or years, such as schizophrenia and affective disorders.

Issues involving countertransference are very important in the psychotherapy of minorities. These partially emanate from the fact that these patients may find themselves in treatment with therapists from the majority culture. Although a few therapists may experience serious difficulties in treating minority patients due to their own racist views, many of the relevant issues may be more subtle. For example, some mainstream therapists do not feel comfortable dealing with minority patients who are relatively uneducated and inarticulate. Lack of understanding by a therapist may also lead him or her to provide such a patient with a less optimal form of therapy. For example, a patient may need individual therapy but may only be provided with pharmacotherapy on the mistaken assumption that the patient is not psychologically sophisticated.

When therapist and patient are of the same cultural background, important countertransference factors may ensue. This frequently occurs with Asian and Hispanic therapists who may inadvertently accept the authority role assigned to them by the patient. In these situations, the therapist may confuse subtle knowledge of the culture with knowledge about the patient.

The Concept of Empathy Among Asian Patients

Confucius (552–479 B.C.) has greatly influenced values in the Orient. Confucius taught the precept of "human heartedness," which seems close to the

Western concept of empathy. According to the Confucian view, human beings are social creatures, bound to their peers by *jen,* or human heartedness, in the five relationships: 1) sovereign and subject, 2) parent and child, 3) elder and younger brothers, 4) husband and wife, and 5) friend and friend. Of these, the relationship among Asians between parent and child, filial piety, may be best known to Westerners. Li is the etiquette and ritual that makes these relationships function smoothly. In Confucian doctrine, correct conduct proceeds from human heartedness and from an internal sense of virtue and ethics, not by compulsion (Herbert 1950).

Taoism, another major influence in Asia, had its beginnings in the third century B.C. The central belief in Taoism is in the natural flow and progression of *yang* into *yin,* that is, of life into death, and of the reverse from *yin* to *yang*—that is, from death into life. The ideal state is that of a newborn child, who is free from desire and striving. The elements of the earth, the directions on a compass, and the attributes of a human being are all interrelated, and the movements of all these must be balanced in the *yin-yang* theory (Saso and Chapell 1977).

The emphasis in Confucianism and Taoism on harmonious relationship and consideration of the family and kinship is also reflected in Japanese culture. The Japanese place a special emphasis on empathy as an essential part of interdependence in human relationships (Lebra 1984). Empathy among Asians is directly related to interpersonal sensitivity. Lebra (1984) writes, "For the Japanese, empathy (*omoiyari*) ranks high among the virtues considered indispensable for one to be really human, morally mature, and deserving of respect. I am even tempted to call Japanese culture an *omoiyari* culture" (p. 38).

We believe that the concept of empathy for Asians may be somewhat different from the Western concept. In this context, suffice it to say that empathy is, for the Easterner, a very acute sensitivity to the feelings of others. The roots of the conceptual differences lie in the family structures and in the manners in which children are raised in the West and in the East. In traditional Eastern families, relatives live very close together. For example, the traditional Japanese family does almost everything together, from bathing, sleeping, and eating to playing. There are often especially strong bonds between the mother and her children, because many Japanese fathers may be very involved in work-related activities. Fathers may maintain strong relationships with colleagues at work; even occasionally on Sundays, the family day, these men may be involved in a company golf tournament.

The bonds among family members are central to the teachings of Confucius. The importance of harmony between "superior" and subject, parent and child, elder and younger, husband and wife, and friend and friend, is taught so well that it becomes instinctive to children of Asian heritage.

There is a cultural difference between Asians and Americans in the value of verbal communication versus intuitive communication. An example of this difference is illustrated by the treatment of dinner guests in Japanese homes. In Japan, the host gives a great amount of thought and planning as to which foods and dining experience the guest would enjoy. Dinner is prepared in response to the host's perception of what the guest would appreciate.

The phrase "active empathy" was coined to emphasize that intuitive understanding is not the only important aspect of interpersonal relationships among traditional Asians (Yamamoto 1980). The relevance of this new phrase was that not only should a therapist who treats an Asian patient be intuitively empathic, he or she must also communicate actively an appreciation of the patient's and the family's situation and how the therapist plans to be helpful on these grounds. Many Asians are not aware of the relevance of therapy for the treatment of their emotional difficulties. Thus, they need to be actively involved and educated about psychotherapy, because many expect the hands-on methods of the medical model.

Matching Patient and Therapist

The initial tendency is to match an Asian patient with an Asian therapist, but such a random procedure has many pitfalls. If assignments are made in an agency, the patient should be asked if he or she prefers an Asian therapist. Otherwise, the practice may be construed as discriminatory. Further, some Asian nations have had a long history of hostile relations. Chinese and Japanese, Japanese and Koreans, Chinese and Vietnamese, Vietnamese and Cambodians—all have been at war with each other during this century and in centuries past.

For example, an older Chinese patient might not be able to overcome feelings of anger if he or she lived under Japanese rule in China in the 1930s. The Asian client who sees an Asian therapist may easily develop an unhealthy transference by idealizing or identifying too quickly with the therapist, or at the opposite extreme, feeling negatively toward the therapist. For example, a young Chinese woman seeking therapy was assigned to a Japanese woman therapist of similar age. The patient immediately felt uncomfortable and said she thought the therapist was "too much like" her. She terminated treatment after the initial session. On the other hand, the patient may place undue expectations of empathy and similitude on the therapist because they are of the same race, and he or she can be disappointed when the therapist may not have had experiences that enable easy identification with the patient.

Conclusion

It is important for therapists to understand that immigrant and minority patients are a highly diverse group. These patients range from individuals who have been greatly influenced by the teachings of Confucius to those who practice Christianity, Buddhism, animism, or other Eastern religions or philosophical systems. Socioeconomic class and generational differences also influence their behavior powerfully. It is recommended that psychiatrists and other mental health professionals try to meet the patient on his or her own ground (i.e., on a culturally syntonic basis).

In planning therapy for immigrants and other minorities, in general, a new model needs to be constructed that not only includes an awareness of the cultural differences and the importance of the native languages and NE, but also of new and improved methods of intervention. We use the word intervention (rather than therapy) advisedly in order to highlight the importance of avoiding the stigma of psychiatric disorder. Therefore, we suggest that appropriate psychotherapeutic planning must devise approaches to be used in the community with an educational emphasis, with medical treatment as necessary, and appropriate community follow-up. We believe that help in the community setting, such as in churches, will increase the utilization of relevant help and diminish the tragic underutilization of mental health services by immigrants from Asia and Latin America.

Finally, in relation to empathy and transference in the treatment of new immigrants, we need to highlight the importance of the family, especially in those who are not acculturated to the majority culture. Because these are a majority of the newcomers, there are complicated issues related to empathy and transference. Most American therapists are trained to be empathic with an individual. With immigrants, one needs to learn to be empathic with both the individual and his or her family. This presents a double problem, because some therapists may wish to adhere to the models with which they have been trained.

Current American conceptions of family therapy are far from what we would recommend for traditional immigrant families. We believe that these families require much more structure in therapy than American families. The therapist must be willing to be the learned teacher and to lead the way to active interventions, including direct instructions on how to help the family cope with the patient's illness. Transference is also complicated, because the therapist deals with either components of a family system or the entire family. Because two or three generations of family members may be younger than, the same age as, or older than the therapist, the possibilities for countertransference problems are many. In addition, the change from the passive, expectant role of the traditional American psychotherapist to that of the more actively empathic role needed with immigrants may lead some therapists to feel insecure, especially because the patient's expectations are of instant insight and magic medicine. We believe that all of these factors make the role of the psychiatrist for immigrants more challenging and complicated, but nonetheless much more rewarding: It is possible to be flexible and creative in adapting therapeutic approaches to the unique features of each family and patient. This wide variety of people, cultures, and therapeutic adjustments makes multicultural therapy highly interesting and stimulating.

References

Acosta FX, Evans LA: The Hispanic-American patient, in Effective Psychotherapy for Low-Income and Minority Patients. Edited by Acosta FX, Yamamoto J, Evans LA. New York, Plenum, 1982, pp 51–82

Adebimpe VR: Overview: White norms and psychiatric diagnosis of Black patients. Am J Psychiatry 138:279–285, 1981

Banks JA: Black youth in predominantly White suburbs, in Black Adolescents. Edited by Jones RL. Berkeley, CA, Cobb and Henry, 1989, pp 65–77

Bass BA, Acosta FX, Evans LA: The Black American patient, in Effective Psychotherapy for Low-Income and Minority Patients. Edited by Acosta FX, Yamamoto J, Evans LA. New York, Plenum, 1982, pp 83–108

Becker E: When the War is Over: The Voices of Cambodia's Revolution and Its People. New York, Simon & Schuster, 1986

Block CB: Black Americans and the cross-cultural counseling and psychotherapy experience, in Cross-Cultural Counseling and Psychotherapy. Edited by Marsella AJ, Pederson PB. New York, Pergamon, 1981, pp 177–194

Bochnlein JK, Kinzie JD, Ben R, et al: One year follow-up study of posttraumatic stress disorder among survivors of Cambodian concentration camps. Am J Psychiatry 142:956–959, 1985

Carillo C: Directions for a Chicano psychotherapy, in Family and Mental Health in the Mexican American Community. Edited by Casas JM, Keefe SE. Los Angeles, CA, Spanish Speaking Mental Health Research Center, 1978, pp 143–156

Cobbs PM: Ethnotherapy in groups, in New Perspectives on Encounter Groups. Edited by Solomon LN, Berzon B. San Francisco, CA, Jossey-Bass, 1972, pp 383–403

Comas-Diaz L, Griffith EEH (eds): Clinical Guidelines in Cross-Cultural Mental Health. New York, Wiley, 1988

Dash L: When Children Want Children. New York, William Morrow, 1989

Elder G: Children of the Depression. Chicago, IL, University of Chicago Press, 1974

Elder G: Historical change in life patterns and personality, in Life-Span Development and Behavior, Vol 2. Edited by Baltes PB, Brim OG Jr. New York, Academic Press, 1979, pp 117–159

Engel GL: The need for a new medical model: a challenge for biomedicine. Science 196:127–137, 1977

Erikson EH: Growth crises of the healthy personality, in Identity and the Life Cycle. Edited by Erikson E. New York, WW Norton, 1980, pp 51–107

Falicov CV: Mexican families, in Ethnicity and Family Therapy. Edited by McGoldrick M, Pearce JK, Giordano J. New York, Guilford, 1982, pp 134–163

Gellis SS, Feingold M: Pseudobattering in Vietnamese children. Am J Dis Child 130:857–858, 1976

Gilbert M: The Holocaust, A history of the Jews of Europe During the Second World War. New York, Henry Holt, 1985

Goedde HW, Benkmann HG, Kriese L, et al: Aldehyde dehydrogenase isozyme deficiency and alcohol sensitivity in four different Chinese populations. Hum Hered 34:183–186, 1984

Gong-Guy E: The California Southeast Asian mental health needs assessment (a monograph published under California State Department of Mental Health Contract #85-76282A-2)). Oakland, CA, Asian Community Mental Health Services, 1987

Gordon MM: Assimilation in American Life. New York, Oxford University Press, 1964

Haley A: Roots. Garden City, NY, Doubleday, 1976

Herbert EA: Confucian Notebook. London, Butler and Tanner, Ltd, 1950

Hurh WM, Kim KC: Korean Immigrants in America: A Structured Analysis of Ethnic Confinement and Adhesive Adaptation. Cranbury, NJ, Fairleigh Dickinson University Press, 1984

Kessner T, Caroli BB: Today's Immigrants, Their Stories, A New Look at the Newest Americans. New York, Oxford University Press, 1981

Kinzie JD: Cultural aspects of psychiatric treatment with Indochinese refugees. Am J Soc Psychiatry 5(1):47–53, 1985

Kinzie JD, Frederickson RH, Ben R, et al: Posttraumatic stress disorder among survivors of Cambodian concentration camps. Am J Psychiatry 141:645–650, 1984

Kinzie JD, Sack WH, Angell RH, et al: The psychiatric effects of massive trauma on Cambodian children, I: the children. Journal of the American Academy of Child Psychiatry 25:370–376, 1986

Kitano HHL, Yeung WT, Chai L, et al: Asian-American interracial marriage. Journal of Marriage and Family, February 1984, pp 179–190

Lambert WE, Hodgson RC, Gardner RC, et al: Evaluation reactions to spoken languages. Journal of Abnormal and Social Psychology 60:44–51, 1960

Lebra TS: Japanese Patterns of Behavior. Honolulu, HI, University of Hawaii Press, 1984

Leff J: Psychiatry Around the Globe, 2nd Edition. London, Gaskell Books, Royal College of Psychiatrists, 1988

Marcos LR: Bilinguals in psychotherapy: language as an emotional barrier. Am J Psychother 30:552–560, 1976

Mollica RF, Wyshak G, Lavelle V: The psychosocial impact of war trauma and torture on Southeast Asian refugees. Am J Psychiatry 144:1567–1572, 1987

Munoz JA: Difficulties of a Spanish-American psychotherapist. Am J Orthopsychiatry 51:646–653, 1979

Ngor H: A Cambodian Odyssey. New York, Macmillan, 1987

Pitta P, Marcos LR, Alpert M: Language switching as a treatment strategy with bilingual patients. Am J Psychoanal 38:255–258, 1978

Quock CP, Louie J (eds): Proceedings of the First Asian American Health Forum, New York, August 21–23, 1986. Washington, DC, Public Health Service, U.S. Department of Health and Human Services, 1986

Roland A: In Search of Self in India and Japan: Toward a Cross-Cultural Psychology. Princeton, NJ, Princeton University Press, 1988

Russell DM: Language and psychotherapy: the influence of nonstandard English in clinical practice, in Clinical Guidelines in Cross-Cultural Mental Health. Edited by Comas-Diaz L, Griffith EEH. New York, Wiley, 1988, pp 33–68

Sack WH, Angell RH, Kinzie JD, et al: The psychiatric effects of massive trauma on Cambodian children, II: the family, the home, and the school. Journal of the American Academy of Child Psychiatry 25:377–393, 1986

Saso M, Chapell DW: Buddhist and Taoist Studies I. Honolulu, HI, University Press of Hawaii, 1977

Silva JA, Liederman PH: The life-span approach to individual therapy: An overview with case presentation, in Life-Span Development and Behavior, Vol 7. Edited by Baltes PB, Featherman D, Lerner RM. Hillsdale, NJ, Erlbaum, 1986, pp 113–134

Spurlock J: Black Americans, in Cross-Cultural Psychiatry. Edited by Gaw A. Littleton, MA, John Wright-PSG Pub Co, 1982, pp 163–178

Stuckey S: Slave Culture: Nationalist Theory and the Foundations of Black America. New York, Oxford University Press, 1987

Wallnofer H, von Rottauscher A: Chinese Folk Medicine. New York, Bell Publishing Co, 1965

Wilkinson CB: The destructiveness of myths. Am J Psychiatry 126(28):1087–1092, 1970

Yamamoto J: Psychotherapy for Asian Americans, in The Plenary Session on Culture and Psyche in Korea. Seoul, The Korean Neuropsychiatric Association, 1980, pp 40–48

Yamamoto J: Consideration of creativity in Japan. Scientific Bulletin 7(2):84–87, 1982

Yamamoto J, Chang CY: Empathy and transference in the therapy of Asian Americans. Paper presented at the 4th Scientific Meeting of Pacific Rim College of Psychiatrists, Hong Kong, December 4–9, 1988

Yamamoto J, Wagatsuma H: The Japanese and Japanese Americans. J Operational Psychiatry 11(2):120–135, 1980

Yamamoto J, James QC, Bloombaum M, et al: Racial factors in patient selection. Am J Psychiatry 124(5):630–636, 1967

Yamamoto J, James QC, Palley N: Cultural problems in psychiatric therapy. Arch Gen Psychiatry 19:45–49, 1968

Yamamoto J, Acosta FX, Evans LA: The poor and working-class patient, in Effective Psychotherapy for Low-Income and Minority Patients. Edited by Acosta FX, Yamamoto J, Evans LA. New York, Plenum, 1982, pp 31–50

Yamamoto J, Yeh EK, Loya F, et al: Are American psychiatric outpatients more depressed than Chinese outpatients? Am J Psychiatry 142:1347–1351, 1985a

Yamamoto J, Machizawa S, Araki F, et al: Mental health of elderly Asian Americans in Los Angeles. Am J Soc Psychiatry 5(1):37–46, 1985b

Yamamoto J, Yeh EK, Lee CK, et al: Alcohol abuse among Koreans and Taiwanese, in Cultural Influences and Drinking Patterns: A Focus on Hispanic and Japanese Populations (Research Monograph No 19 [DHHS Publ No ADM-88-1563]). Edited by Towle LH, Harford TC. Washington, DC, U.S. Government Printing Office, 1988, pp 135–175

Yeatman GW, Shaw C, Barlow MJ, et al: Pseudobattering in Vietnamese children. Pediatrics 58(4):618–619, 1976

Zangwill I: Melting Pot. New York, Macmillan, 1909, Act One, p 37

5 Cross-Cultural Psychiatric Assessment

Joseph J. Westermeyer, M.D., M.P.H., Ph.D.

To understand patients and their problems, psychiatrists rely heavily on shared language (both nonverbal communication and spoken language), communication style, and other features of a culture. Patients' cultural and religious beliefs, values, behavior, and even dress and grooming can be important factors in a psychiatric evaluation. If a psychiatrist does not share a patient's culture, the task of psychiatric assessment becomes more challenging. If the psychiatrist has little or no knowledge of the patient's culture, the task may seem overwhelming (Adebimpe 1981).

My goal in this chapter is to make the task less daunting by presenting concepts, information, and procedures that will help the psychiatrist to manage this effort as a kind of special assessment. This process is analogous to other special assessments, such as child, disability, family, forensic, or gerontological assessments. Each special assessment has its particular body of knowledge, emphases and nuances; each is also based on certain generic aspects of psychiatric assessment.

As with all special assessments, psychiatrists begin from a strong position of considerable advantages, which include their knowledge of psychopathology, their skills in facilitating communication and establishing rapport, and their experience with a variety of people and behaviors. The importance of understanding the patient and the patient's individual perspectives, a core value in the psychiatry field, stands the clinician in good stead. General life experience, a broad education, medical school experience with diverse ethnic groups, and the ethnic diversity of colleagues may further enhance the psychiatrist's ability to acquire skills in cross-cultural assessment.

Cultural Concepts

Culture is a broad term referring to total social organization, technology, and shared beliefs and customs of a people. One may conceive of the histor-

125

ical Athenians, pre-Columbian Sioux, contemporary Americans, Mexicans, Chinese, or Nigerians as possessing a culture. Within most of these cultural units exist various "ethnic subgroups" that possess their own histories, language (or dialects), beliefs, and traditions that distinguish them from others within the culture. In some cultures, such as the United States, the Commonwealth of Independent States, China, Malaysia, Yugoslavia, and many countries of Africa, no one ethnic group is in the majority. Ethnic groups come to share culture with one another through common systems of government, public education, mass media, shared language or lingua franca, communication systems, the workplace and the market place, methods of transportation, and other shared artifacts and experiences.

Ensocialization is the process by which children learn to live, function, and survive in a social group. During the preschool and elementary school years, a child's basic ethnic identity, values, norms, and relationships are established. Even intensive and lengthy exposure later in adolescence or adulthood cannot fully replicate ensocialization into a culture during childhood. Outside of the culture gained during childhood, one is forever an alien to some extent. It is possible for a person to learn the elements of more than one culture if one has parents from different cultures or grows up in more than one culture. But even then, one culture tends to predominate. Because any two cultures conflict in some ways, the child must choose (or be guided in choosing) one way or the other. For example, the following case report illustrates a contradictory cultural message an American Indian child received because his parents were from two different tribes.

> A boy with a Pueblo mother and a Navajo father lived close by his maternal grandparents but often visited his paternal grandparents. His mother's parents fed him venison, made a deerskin dance costume for him, and taught him to participate in the biannual sacred Deer Dance. His paternal grandparents taught him that the deer was a taboo animal, one whose hide and flesh should never be touched.

In a multiethnic society such as America's, children learn their ethnic identities at home among their families and relatives. If a child lives in a predominantly ethnic community or region, the local political system, church, school, recreational pastimes, and other institutions may reinforce this ethnic identity. As more commonly occurs in the United States, the preschool child begins watching television (largely a dominant cultural rather than ethnic minority mass medium), plays with children of other ethnic groups, and visits mainstream cultural recreation facilities (e.g., Disneyland).

Attendance at public school, participation in extracurricular activities, and friendships across ethnicities further emphasize shared culture.

Acculturation occurs when two cultures in contact come to adopt beliefs, values, and practices from one another. An example is the influence that Cuban refugees have had on the Miami area, and vice versa. More commonly, an individual or a small in-migrating group experiences changes imposed by a much larger established community. The experience of these sudden changes—which may involve climate, diet, dress, language, social status, social network, occupation, values, norms, and laws—is sometimes referred to as "culture shock."

The degree of culture shock is related to 1) the extent of the differences between the two cultures in such features as their histories, religions, technologies, and languages, 2) the geographic distance between the new and old communities, and 3) the age of the migrant. In general, the greater the cultural differences, the longer the distance between the two cultures, and the more advanced the age of the migrant, the more difficult the adjustment (Westermeyer 1989a, 1989b).

An "ethnic" child entering a school of the dominant culture can be thought of as undergoing acculturation. The child may fail if unable to achieve productive adult status in the majority culture or may successfully adapt to the dominant culture.

Values are the concepts, moral goods, and desirable ends or goals to which a people attach positive emotional valance. One culture's soldiers risk death to ensure freedom of religious worship for their people; another culture's soldiers will risk death to see that their religion is the people's exclusive one. One ethnic group may attach prestige to acquiring material goods; another may attach prestige to giving them away. For example, the American Indian ceremonial *potlatch* consists of dispersing acquired good as a means of establishing high status.

Because values are largely unconscious, severe problems can occur in the clinical arena if clinician and patient assume that they possess common values when in fact theirs are markedly different. A clarification of values is frequently needed in cross-cultural assessment. An example of such a case would be a depressed Asian refugee couple, seen at a psychiatric clinic, who wanted to reestablish a polygynous household that had been forcibly separated by immigration officials.

Norms are the guidelines that define socially acceptable behavior. Each culture and each ethnic group has ideal norms—limits that are prescribed verbally, which may or may not coincide with actual behavioral norms, or limits as they exist in fact. For example, members of a group may decry intoxication or out-of-wedlock pregnancy, yet the group may have high rates of both. For the purposes of psychiatric interviewing, it is important to know which behaviors in a culture or ethnic group have norms that diverge in their ideal and actual forms.

Identity refers to the emotional and conceptual merging of self with others. Culture and ethnicity forge an individual's developing identity as girl or boy, youth and adult, family member, and ethnic group member. In a multiethnic or multiracial family, children may develop their own special identities. For example, a 6-year-old child born to a white mother and an African American father identified her mother as white and her father as black. She had developed her own identity, which she labeled as "tan," that included elements of both races and ethnicities.

Cross-Cultural Communication

Lingua Franca and Dialect

Most cultures have a single major language or lingua franca, such as English in the United States. This may or may not be the language spoken in the home. The patient's first language is usually the one he or she is able to speak most easily and comfortably. Moreover, this language is the one most available for emotional expression. Use of a patient's second language with a therapist may distort the clinical findings in a number of ways. For example, the severity of the patient's condition may be accentuated if the patient's language facility is undermined by use of a second language; or as the patient relates events without attendant emotional coloring, the severity of the patient's condition may be minimized (Berkanovic 1980; Kline et al. 1980; Peck 1974).

In a given country, relatively isolated groups spread out over broad distances often speak different "dialects." Even within the same geographic region, ethnic groups may have different dialects based on differences in their histories, former languages, value systems, life-styles, and worldviews. Slang expressions, idioms, and proverbs—those means of expression most reflective of feeling and attitude—may be mutually unintelligible among ethnic groups who speak the same language.

The psychotherapist working cross-culturally can urge patients to speak colloquially in their dialect. If the therapist does not understand a patient's expression, this is an excellent opportunity to learn more about the patient by asking him or her for clarification.

Translation, Interpretation, and Bilingual Workers

Translation is the exchange of the denotative meaning of a word, phrase, or sentence in one language for the same meaning in another language. At times, the clinician wants a word-for-word translation (for example, when testing for orientation to time and place or for serial 7s). The term "interpretation" emphasizes the exchange of connotative meaning between languages so that both affect and meaning are conveyed.

Especially in psychiatric interviewing, full interpretation can be crucial to an accurate understanding of the patient. An interpreter's failure to appreciate the patient's distress or viewpoint can lead to misunderstanding at best or to a fatal outcome at worst (Berkanovic 1980; Del Castillo 1970; Marcos 1979; Marcos et al. 1973). An example of a misleading translation, albeit not one in a clinical setting, was Khrushchev's words, quoted to the American press as "We [the Russians] will bury you [the Americans]." This was taken as an ominous threat of war. A less literal, and less ominous, translation of Khrushchev's Russian idiom "We will attend your funeral" is "We will succeed, and our system will outlive yours."

Nonverbal communication, a critical feature of psychiatric assessment, can vary widely from one culture to another and one ethnic group to another. An anthropologist (Hall 1959) initiated a field called "proxemics," the study of social and interpersonal nonverbal behavior. Hall demonstrated the influence of ethnicity on such aspects of communication as eye contact, gesticulation, body envelope, and interpersonal touching. Even signals of emotional state, such as facial muscle tension and galvanic skin response, can differ greatly across cultures (Lieblich et al. 1973; Uchiyama et al. 1981).

A translator might be able to translate well between two languages but be only fair or even poor at interpreting a patient's verbal and nonverbal communication. Further, a person might be able to interpret for medical purposes but be inept at dealing with the strong feelings, disturbing behavior, or taboo topics that ensue during psychiatric evaluation. For these reasons, an interpreter should be specially trained to psychiatric work, rather than merely to medical or social interpreting (Sabin 1975).

The patient often cathects initially to the interpreter as a cultural peer with whom verbal and nonverbal communication can be established, rather than to the clinician. For this reason, the psychiatric interpreter should ideally be part of the psychiatric team. In this role, such an interpreter is often referred to as a bilingual psychiatric worker. Besides interpretation, a bilingual psychiatric worker often assumes other roles, such as outreach worker, case manager, crisis intervenor, and psychiatric educator (e.g., regarding prognosis, treatment alternatives, and pharmacotherapy).

In the clinical context, translation is usually sequential. That is, the patient speaks, followed by the translator, then the clinician, and then the translator again. This process requires extra time, but it has the advantage of providing a respite during which the psychiatrist can reflect on the last response, observe the patient's and translator's behaviors, and consider the best and most economical phrasing for the next question or statement. Some professional translators do concurrent translation, which speeds up the process considerably. However, concurrent translations are primarily denotative, and they tend to fatigue the translator in 20 to 30 minutes. For these reasons, they are better used for clerical information or for follow-up medical checks rather than for diagnostic interviews (Marcos et al. 1973; Westermeyer 1990).

The patient's cathexis to the bilingual worker leads to an additional transference relationship besides the patient-psychiatrist transference (Marcos 1979; Westermeyer 1990). Likewise, the translator-patient countertransference also exists. Although patient-translator relationships are generally positive and therapeutic, the psychiatrist must be alert to problems in these relationships. Difficulties can arise from social class or ethnic differences between the patient and the translator. The translator may be embarrassed by the patient's psychopathology and attempt to make the patient appear "normal" to the psychiatrist. Perhaps worst of all, these difficulties may also lead to breaks in confidentiality (Sabin 1975).

For maximum efficiency, a trusting, mutually cooperative relationship must exist between the bilingual worker and the psychiatrist. Depending on the background of the bilingual worker, it is possible that such a relationship will not be easily or rapidly established. Especially if the worker comes from a culture unfamiliar with psychiatric concepts, methods, and care, several months may be needed for a trusting relationship to develop. After a period of using this team approach and experiencing together the improvement or recovery of several patients, both partners in the patient's treatment ordinarily rely on one another's skills, much like a surgeon and a surgical assistant (Westermeyer 1990).

One skill in psychiatric interviewing involves phrasing questions in such a way that a patient either acknowledges the presence of a symptom or denies it if it is absent. In this context, psychiatric translators must learn to avoid asking leading questions. Moreover, sensitive questioning must be learned regarding hallucinations, delusions, suspiciousness, hostility, suicidal feelings, ideas, plans, and other subjects. Furthermore, translators must be sensitive to dialect differences that may distort intended meaning in questions and typical responses (Westermeyer 1990).

Some of the difficulties in translation and interpretation arise from the cultural and linguistic differences in expressions in various languages for emotional and mental experiences. For example, English has many more words to describe anxious feelings compared with the Thai-Lao languages. English terms referring to anxiety include "tense," "uptight," "nervous," "anxious," and "jittery." In the Thai-Lao languages it is possible to describe anxiety, but it would take a paragraph to do so (i.e., "Do you have a feeling that is like fear, but there may be nothing specific to be fearful about; your heart may speed up; you may feel lightheaded; you may perspire"; and so forth). On the other hand, the Thai-Lao languages has a greater panoply of terms to describe sadness or depression, including the literally translated terms "lost-heart," "fallen-heart," "screaming-heart," "little heart," "a horrible, empty feeling in the chest," and others. Such terminological differences partially explain the common occurrence of wide variance in the amount of time an interpreter takes to translate a clinician's question or statement, depending on the feelings being discussed (Kline et al. 1980; Westermeyer 1990).

Physiological and somatic terms such as headache, constipation, insomnia, or poor appetite are usually translated directly and easily. Even with these terms, however, translation problems may occur. For example, some languages do not distinguish between "sickness" and "pain." Moreover, for some languages there may be unwanted connotations for what appear to English speakers to be objective terms. For example, in some cultures, "becoming weak" may be a euphemism for the anticipation of dying (Edgerton and Karno 1971; Nichter 1981).

Although we know relatively little about cross-cultural evaluation regarding many symptoms, it is possible that cultures assign differing weights to symptoms that accompany psychiatric disorder (Kinzie et al. 1982; Leff 1974). For example, headache may be cause for greater concern in some cultures than in others. Translation problems may also occur when bodily processes or sexuality are being discussed. There are obfuscating euphemisms in some languages for terms such as urination, defecation, masturbation, or sexual intercourse.

A sensitive issue in translation may arise from the use in many languages of personal pronouns that imply a particular hierarchical relationship between speaker and listener. Examples of such words in archaic English are "sire" (for addressing royalty), "you" (for formal but egalitarian address), and "thou" (for familiar address). Some languages have several such terms. Depending on what language is being translated, it may be useful for a clinician to know which terms the patient and interpreter are employing (Nichter 1981; Schmidt 1965; Westermeyer 1987a).

Psychopathology and Culture

Somatic presentations or somatization occur frequently in the cross-cultural context. Several factors may account for patients' presenting with physical symptoms of emotional disorders. Some cultures may not endorse seeking help for mental or emotional problems but may judge somatic problems socially acceptable. Another factor that may contribute to a somatic presentation is a patient's reluctance to entrust a clinician from another culture with much personal information, especially if the patient is not on his or her own cultural turf. Refugees appear more apt to somatize than others.

To delineate the patient's condition under such circumstances, the psychiatrist should probe first for physiological symptoms that may accompany psychiatric disorders (e.g., sleep disturbance, loss of appetite, weakness, constipation, tachycardia, palpitations, lightheadedness, headaches, visual or auditory problems, abdominal or skeletal pain, muscle contractions or tics, urinary frequency, loss of menstruation, and impotence). Once these symptoms have been explored in a deliberate and empathetic fashion, the physician may then ask about psychological symptoms, including worry, prevailing sadness or rage, tearfulness, problems with concentration or memory, loss of enjoyment, fears, crying spells, feelings of helplessness or worthlessness, and hallucinations. Finally, social symptoms can be addressed, such as irritability with others, social withdrawal, family arguments, loss of friends, and suspiciousness or mistrust of others (Eitinger 1959; Hes 1958; Nichter 1981; Westermeyer 1989a).

Paranoid symptoms, like somatization, are also encountered more frequently than usual when the patient is in an alien social context (Duff and Arthur 1967; Edwards 1972; Kendler 1982). This pattern of occurrence may be related to the high prevalence of suspiciousness (perhaps adaptive) that migrants demonstrate in a new environment (Kendler 1982; Kino 1951; Prange 1959; Westermeyer 1989b). Refugees or those who have escaped repressive regimes or survived concentration camps are especially apt to feel insecure or threatened in a new and unfamiliar setting (Eitinger 1959; Mezey 1960; Pedersen 1949; Tseng 1969; Westermeyer 1989c). Paranoid symptoms—from suspiciousness or mistrust, to projection of evil intent, to frank delusions or hallucinations—may accompany virtually any psychiatric disorder and are not peculiar to delusional disorder or schizophrenia.

There are many tactics a clinician may use to deal with the paranoid symptom complex. One is to spend extra time in establishing rapport. Another is to have a family member or friend serve as a collateral source of information. A bilingual worker of the patient's own ethnic group, who has already met with the patient and established a relationship, may also facilitate trust. Finally, discussing the patient's suspiciousness or mistrust, including rational explanations for its presence (or its unlikelihood), may be productive.

Epidemiological distribution of certain psychiatric disorders varies little among cultures or ethnic groups. For example, schizophrenia and mania tend to have stable rates around the world (Westermeyer 1989c), although migrating groups as well as groups with considerable out-migration have been found to have increased rates of affective disorder, schizophrenia, and other disorders in several studies (Dean et al. 1981; Eitinger 1959; Kimura et al. 1975; Krupinski 1967; Malzberg 1964; Odegaard 1932). Among ethnic groups in the United States, affective and anxiety disorders tend to have quite constant crude rates but somewhat different age-specific and sex-specific rates (Regier et al. 1984).

Rates of psychoactive substance use disorders have fluctuated greatly over time, as well as from one culture or ethnic group to another (Bennett and Ames 1985; Prince 1968; Roberts and Myers 1954; Shore et al. 1973; Tseng and McDermott 1981). Mental retardation may also differ considerably among groups, presumably due to such factors as prenatal and natal care, physical health, or volatile inhalant abuse (Westermeyer 1987b, 1988a; Westermeyer et al. 1989).

Among refugees and other migrants, rates of most forms of psychopathology have been found to be higher after migration as compared with rates for cohorts in their countries of origin. The risk of depression incurred with migration is elevated for the first several years. Substance abuse tends to increase several years after resettlement, and schizophrenia may occur either sooner or later following migration (Krupinski et al. 1973; Williams and Westermeyer 1986).

Pathoplasticity refers to the variable manifestations of a given pathological process (in this case, the psychopathological process). Psychotic delusions across cultures are constant in form (e.g., paranoid, grandiose, and somatic) but pathoplastic in content. For example, whites may fear that the Mafia or the CIA is after them; rural African Americans and Afro-Caribbeans may believe that someone is killing them with a curse or "roots"; and Asians may believe that an ancestor ghost is tormenting them (Gaw 1982; Marsella and White 1982; Westermeyer 1988b). Because of this pathoplastic content, it may be important for a clinician to determine whether a particular fixed idea is a culturally supported belief or experience, or an idiosyncratic belief not shared by peers.

Psychiatric disorders involving any kind of conduct or behavior are apt to show 1) variable rates over time, 2) different rates from one group to another, and 3) considerable pathoplastic differences in symptom manifestations. Examples include conduct disorder, pathological gambling, psychoactive substance use disorders, eating disorders, episodic dyscontrol or sudden assault syndromes, acute florid psychosis, and various hysterical conditions (Collomb 1965; Friedman and Faguet 1982; Gift et al. 1985; Shan-Ming et al. 1984). A therapist needs to appreciate the clinical epidemiology of behavioral disorder if he or she is to function effectively in treating patients. For example, pathological gambling occurs predominantly among men in the United States, but it is a frequent malady among women from certain areas of Asia.

Culture-bound syndromes (e.g., *latah, amok,* Arctic hysteria) may present confusing problems for clinicians. In fact, most of these so-called syndromes are culture-related rather than culture-bound, as Simons and Hughes discuss in Chapter 3 of this book. Such syndromes occur in many cultures, albeit with widely disparate rates of occurrence (Friedman and Faguet 1982; Simons 1980; Simons and Hughes 1985; Westermeyer 1982). These complexes include symptoms that accompany a wide variety of psychiatric disorders (e.g., social withdrawal, assaultiveness, suicide attempt, and agitation). Therefore, it is important not to simply assign a diagnosis of culture-related syndrome and pass it off as a benign or self-limited condition. Psychiatric conditions presenting as a culture-related syndrome can range from adjustment difficulties to affective disorders, anxiety disorders, schizophreniform disorders, or organic disorders (Westermeyer 1982). Psychiatrists must exert as much care in conducting a psychiatric assessment with patients who have these conditions as with any others and not simply turn these patients over to a folk healer (as sometimes occurs).

The Doctor-Patient Relationship

When the patient's culture or ethnicity differs from that of the psychiatrist, there are many potential sources of misunderstanding or poor rapport. To reduce the risks of such problems, adequate time must be devoted to facilitation and clarification in the psychiatric interview; confrontation or interpretation should be delayed until rapport is established. Clinical workers of a patient's race or ethnicity can greatly allay the patient's concerns and help assure that the consultation is conducted in a timely fashion (Westermeyer 1989b; Westermeyer et al. 1976).

Cultural transference, a term coined by Spiegel (1976), refers to the feelings and attitudes a patient may have for the clinician's ethnic group (or groups, because many Americans are themselves multiethnic). The patient may or may not be aware of these feelings or attitudes, which may have their basis in historical relationships between the ethnic groups of the patient and the psychiatrist, ethnic attitudes the patient learned as a child, or adverse experience the patient may have undergone.

Cultural countertransference—the feelings and attitudes of the psychiatrist toward a patient's culture—may influence the clinician's interaction with the patient (Spiegel 1976; Westermeyer 1989b). As with the patient, the clinician's ethnic identities, attitudes, and values are apt to be characteristics of which he or she is not fully aware. Their unconscious nature, and thereby their unquestioned validity, can make these cultural assumptions especially troublesome for the doctor-patient relationship. Psychiatric education, training, and supervision (described later in this chapter) are key to overcoming these inhibitors of valid clinical assessment.

Privacy needs differ considerably from one culture to another. Americans and, especially Americans of European heritage, tend to be at one end of the spectrum, being considerably more concerned that family members and friends not know their personal secrets. But for many of the world's peoples, there is often an expectation that the family (rather than the individual) is the repository of privacy. Thus, the patient and the family may expect to see the psychiatrist together. This arrangement may be quite helpful in reassuring the patient, in providing abundant collateral information, and in facilitating family assessment and education. However, family participation may pose a problem if the patient wants to convey information in private. In such an instance, creative patients may call the therapist by phone, slip him or her a note, come early to a session, or return to retrieve a "forgotten" piece of apparel.

The ideal doctor-patient relationship does vary from one culture to another (Portela 1971; Shuval et al. 1967). In some cultures, patients may concurrently seek the care of several clinicians and folk healers. This can result in harm for the patient if several doctors are consulted concurrently without informing each of them. Such problems may often be averted by instructing the patient and the family concerning the importance of complete knowledge regarding other physicians, medications (including folk herbal nostrums), and therapists (including folk healers).

The Mental Status Exam

Appearance appropriate for a visit to a physician's office differs widely around the world. Daily shaving, hair grooming, or even bathing are not universal customs. Moreover, nonverbal communication, such as eye contact and gesticulation, can show vast cross-cultural variability (Westermeyer 1987a; Winkelmayer et al. 1978).

Orientation tasks can also differ with culture (Escobar et al. 1986). There are several calendars in use around the world besides the Georgian calendar, which is officially used in the United States and dates back to the birth of Christ. For example, the Buddhist calendar dates back to the Lord Buddha. It may be important in a cross-cultural assessment to remember that several day cycles besides the 7-day week also exist, although the latter has been standard in most areas over recent decades. Even schemata for counting floors in a building vary: the French *rey de chausée* is the American first floor, and the French first floor is the American second floor. (American hotels are the only ones to omit the thirteenth floor, incidentally—a datum demonstrating our own cultural myth orientation.)

Memory tasks can be influenced by the terms and language used. Addition and subtraction tasks are fairly uniform across cultures, if the patient is educated. Even among illiterate patients, former merchants in currency-based economies can usually add and subtract simple numbers rapidly and with great skill (Westermeyer 1987a, 1989b).

A person's general intelligence and fund of information depend to a considerable extent on education and past experience. To test mental function adequately in an illiterate hunter-farmer or homemaker-gardener can strain the creativity of psychiatrists not familiar with such people and their life-style and lead to a substandard assessment (Schmidt 1965; Westermeyer 1989b). Conversely, literate patients from any culture can be more readily evaluated by psychiatrists whose life experience has been limited to dealing with literate people. Highly educated persons are often more similar to one another despite cultural differences than they are to their own ethnic peers, because education shapes information, experience, attitudes, and beliefs. The culturally informed psychiatrist should be able to assess an animist, monotheist, or atheist, as well as the individual steeped in Taoism-Confucianism, the philosophical thought of Aristotle and Aquinas, the psychological theories of Descartes, James, and Freud, or the political philosophy of Marx and Lenin.

Sociocultural and Ethnic Assessment of Patients

Social history, a core element in medical evaluation, includes sociocultural assessment. The traditional social history format consists of family background, parental occupations and social roles, birthplace, childhood, education, training, sexual-marital history, recreation and hobbies, avocations and special social roles, significant life events, religious affiliation and practice, residences and migrations, self-identities and association memberships, and like factors. These categories provide a superb format for pursuing the patient's ethnicity and cultural affiliation. The key element is the psychiatrist's interest and sensitivity in obtaining relevant data and in being able to perceive the cultural dimensions of the data obtained.

Certain problems in cultural assessment have become evident to me from supervising psychiatric residents and acting as a consultant to other psychiatrists in cross-cultural cases. Two common problems are as follows:

- Sociocultural data on immigrants prior to their arrival in the United States are often scant or absent. Patients are treated, from a history-taking perspective, as though their lives began with their arrival in the United States.
- Data on "cultural mainstream" matters are routinely obtained (e.g., years of formal education, marital status), whereas ethnic-specific data are usually absent (e.g., attendance at religious or ethnically affiliated schools, secular or religious marriage ceremony, ethnic affiliation of the patient's spouse and children).

Deficits in clinical assessment across cultures are remediable through education, training, and supervision. Once trained, a therapist can proceed through an assessment with the cognitive framework, awareness, and skill that become automatic parts of the clinical psychiatrist's armamentarium. Without such background, the culturally naive clinician often avoids ethnic-specific data collection because of negative attitudes and a lack of skills. Such a clinician may see the patient's ethnic affiliations or identities as irrelevant to the clinical problem, or he or she may believe ethnic matters should be avoided because they are too personal, emotionally loaded, or taboo.

Typical questions that should be considered in sociocultural assessment include the following:

- What are (were) your parents' ethnic backgrounds? Were these similar or different? If different, how did your parents deal with each other's cultural differences?
- Have you lived in other countries or in ethnic American subgroups? If so, at what time(s) in your life, and for how long?
- What is your primary language? How do you spend your available time and disposable income? In what groups do you hold membership?
- Do you and your spouse share ethnicity?
- Do you esteem or not esteem your own ethnic group, and why?
- What elements of your ethnicity are important to pass on to your children?

Among immigrants and internal migrants, it is important to ascertain the nature of the migration—voluntary (for marriage, job advancement, or education) or involuntary (to escape war, political repression, or prejudice, or because of lack of work), precipitous or planned, and into a welcoming or rejecting community of relocation (Berry et al. 1987).

Obtaining Culturally Sensitive Psychological Consultation and Testing

Psychiatrists are apt to turn to psychologists for assistance in those cases in which the diagnosis is unclear. Because this is especially apt to occur in cross-cultural cases, psychological consultation is often sought. Thus, psychiatrists should know how to proceed with obtaining and interpreting psychological consultation.

A first task is to find a cross-culturally trained and experienced psychologist. The local state psychological association can refer clinicians to people with such skills. Although there are not many cross-cultural psychologists, their numbers are growing. There is sufficient interest in the field that a journal, *The Journal of Cross Cultural Psychology,* has been established.

No psychological test is completely culture-free, although some tests are more culture-fair than others. For example, the Porteus Maze and Bender-Gestalt tests are known as relatively culture-fair tests (Westermeyer 1989b). However, even these tests require familiarity with paper-and-pencil tasks and may thus not tap into the abilities of illiterate patients. Creative and knowledgeable psychologists can devise methods for getting at such abilities (even if in a gross fashion) without paper and pencil (Butcher and Garcia 1978). At the other end of the spectrum are instruments for the assessment of personality or psychopathology, such as the Minnesota Multiphasic Personality Inventory (MMPI; Hathaway and McKinley 1989). As originally devised, the MMPI includes numerous items that are strongly culture-bound. However, even the MMPI can be adapted to other cultures, even very dissimilar ones, through a process that is technical and requires a good deal of time and care in renorming the items and restandardizing the test (Butcher 1985; Butcher and Pancheri 1976; Cheung 1985). The practical problem is that most tests have been translated, renormed, and restandardized into only a limited number of languages.

Several self-rating scales have been widely translated into numerous languages, such as the Symptom Checklist—90 (SCL-90 [Derogatis et al. 1971]) and the Zung Depression Scale (Westermeyer 1986; Zung 1975). The process for translation and restandardization of these more content-obvious items is easier than for the personality tests. Psychiatrist-rated scales depend on a culturally sensitive psychiatrist (and a skilled translator, if the patient and psychiatrist do not share a language). Self-rated scales and psychiatrist-rated scales have shown strong reliabilities in cross-cultural context (Chien 1978; Kinzie and Manson 1987; Westermeyer 1986).

Special Considerations

The time required for cross-cultural assessment and diagnosis often exceeds that needed for other evaluations. This reality must be acknowledged and addressed. Cross-cultural evaluations place extra demands on the schedules of busy clinicians, and extra time translates into extra cost.

Cost is greater for cross-cultural evaluations for reasons other than the extra time involved in these assessments. Consultation with cultural psychologists involves additional cost; moreover, translators, interpreters, or bilingual workers add to expenditures for care. Migrants, refugees, and members of disadvantaged minority groups tend to enter treatment only after a disorder has become severe; this adds to the difficulty of the assessment and, hence, to the expense.

Intraethnic differences must be considered and recognized. Patient care may be imperiled if assessment deteriorates into mere ascriptions of ethnic stereotypes. No one person—whether patient or clinician—bears all the trappings of a culture or ascribes to every norm or value of the group. Individual assessment remains the mandatory counterbalance to stereotyping. Subjected to careful analysis, intraethnic variability usually exceeds interethnic variability (Abad and Boyce 1979; Butcher and Pancheri

1976; Kinzie and Manson 1987; Tsuang 1976).

Interethnic individuals and families have been and continue to be a prominent feature of the American scene, and in other multiethnic societies as well. Intermarriage is perhaps the most common venue for this phenomenon, but cross-ethnic adoption and foster care are also sources at the family level. At the social or national level, immigration and migration also produce interethnic mixtures in individuals and families. For clinical purposes, the goal is to assess creatively each unique individual and familial interethnic composition—a sometimes daunting but always interesting task. Features of the psychiatrist's own ethnicity may even become apparent in the patient once positive transference is established—one means by which a transcultural "melting pot" of cultures is accomplished.

Education and Training

The first step in training consists of lectures or courses aimed at informing students, residents, and practitioners in the numerous life-styles that make up human experience. A simple awareness of different child-raising methods, marriage forms, social organization, and worldviews contributes greatly toward removing ethnocentric blinders. Personal experiences through travel, education, or residence among other ethnic groups can greatly augment cognitive experiences.

Seminars provide an opportunity for enhancing ethnic self-awareness in the setting of a small, mutually supportive group. Moffic and colleagues (1987, 1988) have developed a seminar format for fostering such enlightenment among psychiatric residents, and Lefley and Pedersen (1986) have prepared a text addressing programmatic aspects of cultural psychiatry training. Skilled supervision in cross-cultural assessment and treatment is a key strategy in preparing psychiatrists for this challenging task.

In a developing field like cultural psychiatry, continuing education is needed to keep abreast of new concepts and methods. A growing number of texts are available for background reading and consultation (i.e., Bennett and Ames 1985; Friedman and Faguet 1982; Gaw 1982; Marsella and White 1982; Simons and Hughes 1985; Westermeyer 1989a, 1989b). Relevant research reports, case studies, and literature reviews occur in many journals but are particularly common in the following: *Acta Psychiatrica Scandinavica, American Journal of Alcohol and Drug Abuse, American Journal of Psychiatry, British Journal of Psychiatry, Culture, Medicine and Psychiatry, International Migration Review, Journal of Nervous and Mental Disease, Social Psychiatry,*

Social Science and Medicine, and *Transcultural Psychiatric Research Reviews.* Affiliation with the American Association of Social Psychiatry (AASP) or the Society for the Study of Psychiatry and Culture (SSPC) provides collegial contacts as well as annual conferences. Various universities, medical centers, and professional societies provide training in cultural psychiatry, depending on local interest, need, and resources. As in other areas of psychiatry, the study of cultural psychiatry is a lifelong pursuit enhancing a clinician's clinical expertise, personal insight, and social awareness.

References

Abad V, Boyce E: Issues in psychiatric evaluations of Puerto Ricans: a socio-cultural perspective. Journal of Operational Psychiatry 10:28–39, 1979

Adebimpe VR: Overview: White norms and psychiatric diagnosis of Black patients. Am J Psychiatry 138:279–285, 1981

Bennett LA, Ames GM (eds): The American Experience With Alcohol: Contrasting Cultural Perspectives. New York, Plenum, 1985

Berkanovic E: The effect of inadequate language translation on Hispanics' responses to health surveys. Am J Public Health 70:1273–1276, 1980

Berry JW, Kim V, Minde T, et al: Comparative studies of acculturative stress. International Migration Review 21:491–511, 1987

Butcher JN: Current developments in MMPI use: an international perspective, in Advances in Personality Assessment, Vol 4. Edited by Butcher JN, Spielberger CD. Hillsdale, NJ, Lawrence Erlbaum, 1985

Butcher JN, Garcia R: Cross-national application of psychological tests. Personnel and Guidance 56:472–475, 1978

Butcher JN, Pancheri P: A Handbook of Cross National MMPI Research. Minneapolis, MN, University of Minnesota Press, 1976

Cheung FM: Cross-cultural considerations for the translation and adaptation of the Chinese MMPI in Hong Kong, in Advances in Personality Assessment, Vol 4. Edited by Butcher JN, Spielberger CD. Hillsdale, NJ, Lawrence Erlbaum, 1985

Chien CC: Application of self rating symptoms to psychiatric outpatients. Bulletin of the Chinese Society for Neurology and Psychiatry 4:47–56, 1978

Collomb M: Boufees delirantes en psychiatrie Africaine. Psychopathologie Africaine 1:167–239, 1965

Dean G, Downing M, Shelly E: First admission to psychiatric hospitals in south-east England in 1976 among immigrants from Ireland. BMJ 282:1831–1833, 1981

Del Castillo JC: The influence of language upon symptomatology in foreign-born patients. Am J Psychiatry 127:242–244, 1970

Derogatis LR, Covi L, Lipman RS, et al: Social class and race as mediator variables in neurotic symptomatology. Arch Gen Psychiatry 25:31–40, 1971

Duff DF, Arthur RH: Between two worlds: Filipinos in the U.S. Navy. Am J Psychiatry 123:836–843, 1967

Edgerton RB, Karno M: Mexican-American bilingualism and the perception of mental illness. Arch Gen Psychiatry 24:286–290, 1971

Edwards AT: Paranoid reactions. Med J Aust 1:778–779, 1972

Eitinger L: The incidence of mental disease among refugees in Norway. Journal of Mental Sciences 105:326–328, 1959

Escobar JI, Burman A, Karno M, et al: Use of the Mini-Mental State Examination (MMSE) in a community population of mixed ethnicity. J Nerv Ment Dis 174:607–614, 1986

Friedman CTH, Faguet RA: Extraordinary Disorders of Human Behavior. New York, Plenum 1982

Gaw A (ed): Cross-Cultural Psychiatry. Littleton, MA, John Wright-PSG Pub Co, 1982

Gift TE, Strauss JS, Young Y: Hysterical psychosis: An empirical approach. Am J Psychiatry 142:345–347, 1985

Hall ET: The Silent Language. Garden City, NY, Doubleday, 1959

Hathaway SR, McKinley JC: Minnesota Multiphasic Personality Inventory—2. Minneapolis, MN, University of Minnesota, 1989

Hes JP: Hypochondriasis in Oriental Jewish immigrants: a preliminary report. Int J Soc Psychiatry 4:18–23, 1958

Kendler KS: Demography of paranoid psychosis (delusional disorder): a review and comparison with schizophrenia and affective illness. Arch Gen Psychiatry 38:890–902, 1982

Kimura SD, Mikolashek PI, Kirk SA: Madness in paradise: psychiatric crises among newcomers in Honolulu. Hawaii Med J 34:275–278, 1975

Kino FF: Alien's paranoid reaction. Journal of Mental Sciences 97:589–594, 1951

Kinzie JD, Manson SM: The use of self-rating scales in cross-cultural psychiatry. Hosp Community Psychiatry 38:190–196, 1987

Kinzie JD, Manson SM, Vinh DT, et al: Development and validation of a Vietnamese language depression rating scale. Am J Psychiatry 139:1276–1281, 1982

Kline F, Acosta FX, Austin V, et al: The misunderstood Spanish-speaking patient. Am J Psychiatry 137:1530–1533, 1980

Krupinski J: Sociological aspects of mental ill-health in migrants. Soc Sci Med 1:267–281, 1967

Krupinski J, Stoller A, Wallace L: Psychiatric disorder in East European refugees now in Australia. Soc Sci Med 7:31–49, 1973

Leff JP: Transcultural influences on psychiatrists' rating of verbally expressed emotion. Br J Psychiatry 125:336–340, 1974

Lefley HP, Pedersen PB: Cross-Cultural Training for Mental Health Professionals. Springfield, IL, Charles C Thomas, 1986

Lieblich I, Kugelmass S, Ben-Shakhar G: Psychophysiological baselines as a function of race and ethnic origin. Psychophysiology 10:426–430, 1973

Malzberg B: Mental disease among native and foreign-born Whites in New York State,

1949–51. Mental Hygiene 48:478–499, 1964

Marcos LR: Effects of interpreters on the evaluation of psychopathology in non-English-speaking patients. Am J Psychiatry 136:171–174, 1979

Marcos LR, Urcuyo L, Kesselman M, et al: The language barrier in evaluating Spanish-American patients. Arch Gen Psychiatry 29:655–659, 1973

Marsella AJ, White GM (eds): Cultural Conceptions of Mental Health and Therapy. Dordrecht, Netherlands, Reidel, 1982

Mezey AG: Personal background, emigration and mental disorder in Hungarian refugees. Journal of Mental Sciences 106:618–627, 1960

Moffic HS, Kendrick EA, Lomax JW, et al: Education in cultural psychiatry in the United States. Transcultural Psychiatric Research Review 24:167–187, 1987

Moffic HS, Kendrick EP, Reid K, et al: Cultural psychiatry education during psychiatric residency. Journal of Psychiatric Education 12:90–101, 1988

Nichter M: Idioms of distress, alternatives in the expression of psychosocial distress: a case study from South India. Cult Med Psychiatry 5:379–408, 1981

Odegaard O: Emigration and insanity: A study of mental disease among the Norwegian born population of Minnesota. Acta Psychiatrica et Neurologica Suppl 4:1–206, 1932

Peck EC: The relationship of disease and other stress to second language. Int J Soc Psychiatry 20:128–133, 1974

Pedersen S: Psychopathological reactions to extreme social displacements (refugee neurosis). Psychoanal Rev 36:344–354, 1949

Portela JM: Social aspects of transference and countertransference in the patient-psychiatrist relationship in an underdeveloped country: Brazil. Int J Soc Psychiatry 17:177–188, 1971

Prange AJ: An interpretation of cultural isolation and alien's paranoid reaction. Int J Soc Psychiatry 4:254–263, 1959

Prince R: The changing picture of depressive syndromes in Africa. Canadian Journal of African Studies 1:177–192, 1968

Regier DA, Myers JK, Kramer M, et al: The NIMH Epidemiological Catchment Area program. Arch Gen Psychiatry 411:934–941, 1984

Roberts BM, Myers JK: Religion, national origin, immigration, and mental illness. Am J Psychiatry 110:759–764, 1954

Sabin JE: Translating despair. Am J Psychiatry 132:197–199, 1975

Schmidt KE: Communication problems with psychiatric patients in the multilingual society of Sarawak. Psychiatry 28:229–233, 1965

Shan-Ming Y, Zhao XD, Yuzhan C, et al: The frequency of major psychiatric disorder in Chinese inpatients. Am J Psychiatry 141:690–692, 1984

Shore JH, Kinzie JD, Hampson JL, et al: Psychiatric epidemiology of an Indian village. Psychiatry 36:70–81, 1973

Shuval JT, Antonovsky A, Davies DM: The doctor-patient relationship in an ethnically heterogeneous society. Soc Sci Med 1:141–154, 1967

Simons RC: The resolution of the Latah paradox. J Nerv Ment Dis 168:195–206, 1980

Simons RC, Hughes CC (eds): The Culture-Bound Syndromes: Folk Illnesses of Psychiatric and Anthropological Interest. Dordrecht, Netherlands, D Reidel, 1985

Spiegel JP: Cultural aspects of transference and countertransference revisited. J Am Acad Psychoanal 4:447–467, 1976

Tseng WS: A paranoid family in Taiwan: a dynamic study of folie à famille. Arch Gen Psychiatry 21:55–65, 1969

Tseng WS, McDermott JF: Culture, Mind and Therapy: An Introduction to Cultural Psychiatry. New York, Brunner/Mazel, 1981

Tsuang MT: Schizophrenia around the world. Compr Psychiatry 17:477–481, 1976

Uchiyama K, Lutterjohann M, Shah MD: Crosscultural differences in frontalis muscle tension levels: an exploratory study comparing Japanese and Westerners. Biofeedback Self Regul 6:75–78, 1981

Westermeyer J: Amok, in Extraordinary Disorders of Human Behavior. Edited by Friedman CTH, Faguet R. New York, Plenum, 1982

Westermeyer J: Two self rating scales for depression among Hmong refugees: assessment in clinical and nonclinical samples. J Psychiatr Res 20:103–113, 1986

Westermeyer J: Cultural factors in clinical assessment. J Consult Clin Psychol 55:471–478, 1987a

Westermeyer J: The psychiatrist and solvent-inhalant abuse: recognition, assessment and treatment. Am J Psychiatry 144:903–907, 1987b

Westermeyer J: National difference in psychiatric morbidity: methodological issues, scientific interpretations and social implications. Acta Psychiatr Scand 78(suppl 344):23–31, 1988a

Westermeyer J: Some cross cultural aspects of delusions, in Delusional Beliefs. Edited by Oltmanns TF, Maher BA. New York, Wiley, 1988b, pp 212–229

Westermeyer J: Mental Health for Refugees and Other Migrants: Social and Preventive Approaches. Springfield, IL, Charles C Thomas, 1989a

Westermeyer J: The Psychiatric Care of Migrants: A Clinical Guide. Washington, DC, American Psychiatric Press, 1989b

Westermeyer J: Paranoid symptoms and disorders among 100 Hmong refugees: a longitudinal study. Acta Psychiatr Scand 80:47–49, 1989c

Westermeyer J: Working with an interpreter in psychiatric assessment and treatment. J Nerv Ment Dis 178:745–749, 1990

Westermeyer J, Tanner R, Smelker J: Staff integration at a neighborhood health center. Urban Health 5:43–48, 1976

Westermeyer J, Bouafuely M, Neider J: Somatization among refugees: an epidemiological study. Psychosomatics 30:34–43, 1989

Williams C, Westermeyer J (eds): Refugee Mental Health in Resettlement Countries. New York, Hemisphere, 1986

Winkelmayer R, Gottheil E, Exline RV, et al: The relative accuracy of U.S., British, and Mexican raters in judging the emotional displays of schizophrenic and normal U.S. women. J Clin Psychol 34:600–608, 1978

Zung WWF: A self-rating depression scale. Arch Gen Psychiatry 12:63–70, 1975

Section II:

Culture and Clinical Care

6 Psychiatric Care of African Americans

Ezra E. H. Griffith, M.D.
F. M. Baker, M.D., M.P.H.

The clinical management of African American patients is a potentially satisfying but demanding aspect of mental health care. This requires basic knowledge of the history of African Americans in the United States and some appreciation of their treatment at the hands of whites over the years. This does not mean a willingness to establish a connection to African American patients that in turn excludes similar linkages to white patients. But it does mean that clinicians must be flexible and aware of the unique status and experiences of African Americans in order to be helpful to them in the therapeutic context. In this chapter, we outline areas of which clinicians should be aware as they undertake treatment of these patients.

Background

Definition, Identification, and Variability

The African American population of the United States is a heterogeneous group of individuals who may speak other languages in addition to English. They have different ethnic heritages and skin color. In the early part of this century, they were called Negroes or people of color. As a result of the civil rights activity of the 1960s and the "Black-is-beautiful" movement, many of these people preferred simply to be called blacks, although some preferred the designation Afro-American. Because the former terminology refers explicitly to skin color and excludes any reference to cultural heritage, some have found it inadequate, preferring to be called African Americans (Baker 1987; Pinderhughes 1989). However, "black," "Afro-American," and "African American" continue to be used interchangeably to denote nonwhites born in the United States who are descendants of African slaves, as well as

147

recent immigrants from the West Indies, Brazil, and a host of other countries, including those in Africa.

The ancestors of African Americans were Africans who lived in tribal communities located predominantly in West Africa. Their cultural values (Pinderhughes 1982; Wylie 1971) emphasized family ties that included the extended family, focused on the good of the community, and accentuated respect for older folk, because elders provided knowledge and wisdom to the younger generations. These tribal communities were well developed, with their own languages, traditions, role definitions, and governing bodies.

Explorations of the North American continent and its subsequent economic exploitation required cheap labor and resulted eventually in the use of slaves. Africans became the primary focus of the slave trade. Chattel slavery in the United States was a system that dehumanized individuals in countless ways, including the intentional division of family units and the separation of parents from their young children. With the defeat of the South in the Civil War, the progeny of these Africans began a fight to obtain an equal place in American society.

The devaluation of people of African heritage still exists as a pervasive, institutionalized pattern within American culture. Although identified and confronted during the 1960s and the 1970s, there has been considerable recent activity making it clear that racial prejudice is still a strong force in the United States. The murders in New York City of African Americans by whites crying racial epithets are dramatic testimony to the persistence of racial hatred and isolation that are strong enough in this country to produce acts of racial violence (French 1989). The court decision that practically absolved Los Angeles Police Department officers of any responsibility for beating Rodney King—a decision that fueled the 1992 Los Angeles riot—also confirmed African Americans' belief that racial discrimination is not yet a thing of the past and that such discrimination continues to influence judicial opinions. On a very large scale, African Americans also continue to suffer the extremes of economic victimization and to complain of a resurgence in political conservatism, as recent attempts to roll back civil rights legislation and other legislative and affirmative action gains have met with some success.

None of this should be construed as suggesting that no gains have been made in the quest for equality. Considerable progress has occurred, resulting in a clear heterogeneity of educational, economic, and social subclasses of African Americans. In essence, some African Americans have made it, and others have not. Consequently, they vary not only in skin color and in ethnic heritage, but also in political party allegiance, socioeconomic status, educational background, and religious affiliation.

Key Political Events

During their history in the United States, African Americans have experienced events that have had a collective and long-term impact on the evolution of their place in American society and their relationship to whites. Blacks saw freedom from slavery in the United States in the mid-nineteenth century. Their emancipation was followed by a period of expansion of their political and economic rights, evidenced by the election of blacks to the U.S. Congress and the legislatures of several states. A period of conservatism soon set in. Earlier gains were eroded, and segregation laws throughout the South were enacted. Following World War I came the Red Summer, so named because black soldiers returning from war were assaulted and lynched by white mobs fearful of armed black men who had been treated as equals abroad. These events led many Southern blacks looking for greater economic and educational opportunities to migrate to cities like Chicago and New York. During World War II, black men served in segregated units, and black women found improved employment opportunities in industry supporting the war effort.

The refusal of Rosa Parks to give up her seat on a segregated bus to a white man in 1955 marked the beginning of the passive resistance movement headed by Dr. Martin Luther King, Jr.—a movement joined by many other civil rights leaders and organizations. The Black Revolution of the 1960s directly confronted institutional racism and saw the rise in influence of militant blacks who spanned the spectrum from the revolutionary Black Panthers to the proponents of passive resistance led by Dr. King (Wilcox 1974). The affirmative action initiatives of the 1970s attempted to redress the consequences of several generations of racial bias in education and employment.

Population Distribution

Although significant numbers of African Americans were brought to the southern United States during the period of chattel slavery, some of them lived as free individuals who worked as artisans and craftsmen in other regions of the nation, particularly the Northeast. After Reconstruction, African Americans sought greater opportunities outside of those Southern states that restricted their education and economic advancement. In the early 1900s, the great Northern migration of blacks began. In the 1990s, African Americans are resident throughout the contiguous United States in rural and suburban as well as urban settings. Although biases may result in African Americans being viewed solely as inner-city dwellers who work in service-oriented jobs, African American employment actually spans the full range of jobs in the American workplace.

Large numbers of African Americans are currently concentrated in inner-city areas, such as Detroit, Los Angeles, and New York City. Some of these cities have also absorbed many black immigrants from the Caribbean and South and Central America. Beginning in the 1980s, some middle-class African American families began a reverse migration to the Southern hometowns of their parents and grandparents. This relocation was intended to remove their children from the stresses of substance abuse problems, high crime, and deteriorating educational systems in the large urban centers outside the South.

Current Demographic Data

Acknowledged inaccuracies exist in U.S. Bureau of the Census data about African Americans. The data are flawed because enumerators were afraid to enter urban neighborhoods and, therefore, often did not perform interviews directly. Despite the institution of mailed census forms, problems have persisted. Not all forms were received by intended recipients, because mail was stolen or removed from mailboxes. Some individuals did not respond because of their concern about the uses to which the data might be put. Still others were worried that the forms might be used to compromise their immigration status.

African Americans number about 28,878,000 people and make up 12% of the population of the United States (National Center for Health Statistics 1987a). Fifty-three percent are female, and 47% are male. Forty-nine percent of African American women are estimated to be in the childbearing years between ages 15 and 44. Although African American males outnumber African American females at birth, in the age range between 15 and 24, there is a reversal in this pattern (National Center for Health Statistics 1987a). Women begin to outnumber men as a result of the loss of African American adolescents and young adult men to homicide, suicide, and substance abuse (Baker 1989; Poussaint 1972). This sex difference is sustained throughout the life cycle, with accidents and medical problems (particularly obesity, hypertension, cerebrovascular disease, diabetes, and cancer) contributing to the loss of African American men in subsequent years (Task Force on Black and Minority Health 1986).

The U.S. Bureau of the Census (1980) reported that almost 30% of African Americans were living below the poverty level, compared with only 9.4% of white Americans. The average number of individuals per African American family was 3.72 versus 3.9 in white families. Among African Americans, there were 1,568,417 female-headed households (i.e., without a husband present) and with children under age 18. For whites, 3,166,397 were raised in female-headed households and with children under age 18.

Life expectancy for blacks improved during the period from 1900 to 1985. African American women born in 1900 had a life expectancy of 33.5 years; African American women born in 1985 may expect to live 73.5 years. An African American man born in 1900 lived only 32.5 years; in contrast, an African American man born in 1985 can expect to live to 65.3 years (National Center for Health Statistics 1987a).

Epidemiologic Studies

Simon and colleagues (1973) reported one of the few studies that compared the diagnoses of African American and white patients in a state hospital. On admission, research psychiatrists, using the Research Diagnostic Criteria (Spitzer et al. 1978), evaluated patients and assigned them psychiatric diagnoses. These diagnoses were compared with the discharge diagnoses made by the treating psychiatrist. The researchers found that African American patients were more likely to be diagnosed by their clinicians as having schizophrenia rather than a major depressive disorder. Bell and colleagues (1985) emphasized the misdiagnosis of African American patients as having schizophrenia who in fact had an organic brain syndrome related to alcohol abuse. These authors noted that the pattern of drinking at an early age, as well as the tendency for heavier alcohol consumption by African American men compared with African American women, increased the risk for organic brain syndromes in African Americans. Baker (1988b) suggested that research on the prevalence of dementia in African American elders needed to assess whether the prevalence of alcohol dementia was higher in these populations because of the patterns of alcohol use documented by previous studies.

Bell and Mehta (1979) and Jones and colleagues (1981) reported on the misdiagnosis of African American patients as having schizophrenia who in fact had manic-depressive disorder. These authors noted that African American patients showing symptoms of psychosis with mood changes were diagnosed too frequently as schizophrenic, without other diagnoses being considered.

There were no published studies in the psychiatric literature that reported for any age cohort on the prevalence of disorders such as anxiety disorder, phobia, and panic disorder in a population-based, representative sample of African Americans before the Epidemiologic Catchment Area (ECA) Survey, which was carried out in five U.S. cities (Easton and Kessler 1985). In preparation for an American Psychiatric Association Task Force Report on Ethnic Minority Elders, the ECA data tapes were obtained, and the data on African Americans, Hispanics, whites, and others from the five cities were pooled. The 6-month prevalence of disorders among community residents age 18 and older for all age and ethnic groups was obtained for the five cities studied (New Haven; Baltimore; St. Louis; Durham, North Carolina; and Los Angeles).

African Americans were found to have a higher 6-month prevalence rate for cognitive impairment, drug abuse, panic attacks, and phobia. The African American prevalence rates across all age groups for major depression and schizophrenia among community residents were lower than those of whites but higher than those of Hispanics. The ECA data demonstrate that the rates of psychiatric disorder in community resident African Americans differ from those of other ethnic groups. Further, the types of psychiatric disorders identified in a representative sample of African Americans by a standardized interview, not unexpectedly, differ from the diagnoses observed in inpatient samples, which in general are not representative. Furthermore, clinicians in inpatient settings evaluate and treat patients who are more seriously ill. Nevertheless, Williams (1986) has expressed caution about placing too much faith in these ECA data on African Americans because of the small number of cases on which the prevalence rates were based.

The existing research data on the misdiagnosis of African Americans in hospital settings should alert clinicians to review carefully a patient's medical records for a description of the presenting symptoms of the psychiatric illness, as well as to obtain a description of the illness from the African American patient and his or her family. More careful review of the patient's complaints and serious attention to the documented course of the illness should lead to more exact assignments of diagnostic labels.

Jackson (1967, 1971, 1975, 1988) reported on the rural African American elder population of Durham, North Carolina. She emphasized the "quadruple jeopardy of being old, poor, black, and female" (Jackson 1975, p. 16) and described the severe poverty and absence of resources for older African Americans. The higher 6-month prevalence rates for certain psychiatric disorders in African Americans age 50 and older noted in the ECA data at the Durham site compared with the other four cities suggest that clinicians should consider the impact of a rural environment on African Americans, especially because treatment resources are likely to be less available.

The significantly higher prevalence of cognitive impairment in African Americans may be hypothesized as being caused primarily by substance abuse and impairment in attention and registration resulting from anxiety, phobias, panic attacks, and medical problems such as diabetes mellitus, a disease that has increased fourfold among African Americans between 1963 and 1985 (National Center for Health Statistics 1987b). The role of accidents involving head trauma, a third cause of cognitive impairment, must also be considered in the evaluation of African American patients (Task Force on Black and Minority Health 1986).

Clearly, further evaluation of these findings is indicated. The public health implications of these preliminary data are clear. There is an obvious need to improve screening in African American community populations for cognitive function and for the spectrum of anxiety disorders as well as to review the diagnostic labels assigned to African American psychiatric patients who have been hospitalized.

Myths and Realities About Mental Health and Mental Illness in African Americans

Bell and colleagues (1983) summarized the myths and stereotypes that resulted from racism and that influenced diagnoses, treatment, and research decisions. During Reconstruction, census figures were falsified to show an increase in the incidence of mental illness in African Americans who had "lost the benefits of slavery" (Deutsch 1944). For blacks who were truly mentally ill in the 1800s, access to care was often a problem. Prudhomme and Musto (1973) noted that only a few Northern mental hospitals admitted African Americans, who were then kept in segregated units. The majority of psychiatrically ill African Americans were admitted to almshouses or placed in jail.

Psychiatric literature in the early 1900s characterized African Americans as "too emotional, sexually promiscuous, lazy, in need of authority, criminally inclined, and unintelligent" (Bevis 1921, p. 71). Wilson and Lantz (1957) summarized several reports written between 1868 and 1952 that emphasized how African Americans were either too inferior or lacked the intrapsychic framework to become depressed. An enduring bias in favor of diagnosing psychiatrically ill African Americans as schizophrenic was also documented by Evarts (1914), Frumkin (1954), Fisher (1969), and Cannon and Locke (1977). In a classic paper, Simon and colleagues (1973) showed

there was diagnostic bias in admissions to state and county mental hospitals—white men tended to be diagnosed as alcoholic and African American
men as schizophrenic. In psychiatric units in general hospitals, African
American men and women were more often diagnosed as schizophrenic in
contrast to white men and women, who were more often diagnosed as
having depressive disorders. Unfortunately, racism in the United States has
influenced psychiatric diagnosis as well as the locus of treatment of African
American patients.

The institutional bias against African Americans with psychiatric disorders resulted in their families' serving as an important resource for these
patients. These families were forced to tolerate unusual behavior and to care
for their mentally ill family members at home until the patients became too
violent.

The mental health needs of African Americans are influenced by the socioeconomic realities of their existence. In a study of African American families in Dallas, Lewis and Looney (1983) documented that families above the
poverty level could function well. In contrast, African American families at
or below the poverty level were so stressed by concerns with survival that
they degenerated into a dysfunctional family pattern in reaction to these ongoing stresses. When such a family had a member with a psychiatric illness,
relatives would require the skills of a multidisciplinary team of psychiatrist,
psychiatric nurse, social worker, and vocational/rehabilitation counselor to
deal with that family member. Although the middle-class family clearly has
more resources and more knowledge about ways of obtaining treatment, con-
tinuity of care and involvement of significant others in treatment planning
are still important elements in stabilizing the family in need (Baker 1988a).

Stigmatization of the Mentally Ill African American

African Americans have had a tradition of beliefs regarding mental illness
that are similar in some ways to those of Mexican Americans, who ascribe
some psychiatric disorders to *susto* (magical fright or soul loss) and *mal
puesto* (hex; Martinez 1988).

Some blacks have believed earnestly in the power of the hex to cause
psychological and somatic illness, which has led them to use voodoo for
therapy (Jordan 1975). It seems reasonable to assume that such explanatory
beliefs are an offshoot of African sociohistorical antecedents. Newer immigrants, such as the West Indians, have also brought their own views of
mental illness as a disorder that derives from the hex phenomenon. Conse-

quently, for blacks who hold these beliefs, psychiatrists may not be consulted, except as a last resort after other forms of therapeutic intervention have failed. *Banks' article*

The hex explanation places the responsibility for mental illness outside of the patient and the family, which has the advantage of ameliorating the stigma. Among many blacks, mental illness is, in general, highly stigmatizing, and the individual is seen as "going off," "having trouble," or "not being right in the head." Although these terms have been used to describe disorganized behavior arising from psychotic illness or toxic delirium, they have also been used to describe aberrant behavior in persons with mental retardation. From the 1920s through the 1940s, African Americans with psychiatric disorders were often kept hidden or were sent away to family members who lived in the South or on farms.

Only with the advent of the community mental health centers (CMHCs) and the increased emphasis in the media on psychiatric disorders has the attitude within the African American community changed. The description of psychiatric illness on television, in the movies, and in advertisements for psychiatric hospitals has led to a more open discussion of psychiatric disorders in American society in general. The revelations by political, movie, and sports personalities of the diagnosis and treatment of their psychiatric disorders has increased the acceptance of these "invisible" illnesses. African Americans who live in rural and urban areas and of varying socioeconomic status have an increasing understanding of the specific behavioral changes and attitudes that are consistently linked to particular psychiatric disorders. This enhanced knowledge tends to facilitate the connection of the patient to the treating clinician.

Folk, Traditional, and Mainstream Psychiatric Care

Ness and Wintrob (1981) have pointed out that all societies find their own unique ways of contending with physical and mental illness. Generally, these responses evolve within specific cultural contexts to form systems of folk healing. The African American tradition of folk medicine reflects the knowledge of plants and herbs that African ancestors applied to the indigenous plants of the American continent. The use of sassafras tea as an herbal beverage, willow leaves in tea to treat fever, and dampened mullen leaves to heal skin lacerations are examples of this "old knowledge" that is carried on today mainly by older blacks. During the 1800s and 1900s, parasitic infections were a concern because of poor public sanitation, and spring tonics were used to "flush the system" of children to prevent and cure their infestation with worms. This use of herbal medicine is still referred to as "doctoring."

The "working of roots" involved the use of plant roots to prepare potions that were employed to bring about either good or evil. In this folk belief system, illness was thought to be produced or life events influenced by selecting and/or combining specific plant roots. Although a belief in the "working of roots" is seen frequently in African American communities in rural Southern areas, it is known at all socioeconomic levels in the African American community. Although the woman who "works roots" bears some similarity to the "old woman" of voodoo, the "working of roots" remains a separate belief system and is thought not to involve animal sacrifice or the reading of bones (Jordan 1975).

Ness and Wintrob (1981) reported it is a common belief that "working roots" on someone with the intention to harm can cause the victim to manifest psychiatric symptoms that include delusions, persecutory hallucinations, anxiety, and agitation. Obviously, the effectiveness of the curse is related to the victim's strength of belief in the power of the root-working.

Blacks also use other traditional systems for psychological care. Baer (1984) has published an incisive ethnographic analysis of the Black Spiritual Movement. This sect, formed around 1923 to meet the healing needs of its black members, utilized syncretic beliefs and rituals from Protestantism, Catholicism, and even voodoo. Similarly, Griffith and colleagues (1984) analyzed a Wednesday night meeting in a black church and demonstrated how churchgoers were using that particular service to meet their psychological needs and desires to feel better. Such research is powerful evidence of African Americans' use of community institutions other than orthodox medical systems for their psychological benefit.

In addition to the use of spiritual rituals and church services, African American pastors are also used for psychotherapeutic care. These pastors may constitute in many cases a triage system in the African American community, because they may be the first point of consultation for individuals under stress who are seeking solace and a way to cope. Personal but nonsystematic observation suggests that African American females use these systems of care more often than African American males. This notion deserves greater study.

Classic psychiatric care did not exist for the African American with psychiatric illness until the desegregation of state hospitals (Malzberg 1963; Prudhomme and Musto 1973). In an agrarian society, people who were psychotically ill could wander the land and were accepted as "a little touched in the head." With the industrialization of American society and the growth of major cities, tolerance of unusual or bizarre behavior declined, and the schizoid life-style of a hermit or recluse was no longer possible. The presence of CMHCs has certainly provided a locus of care in the community for the African American patient, who is, in general, likely to be poor or have marginal resources for psychiatric and medical care (Adams 1950; Spurlock 1969, 1982). But the CMHCs have not meant that all blacks have given up using their traditional or folk systems. The modern clinician must learn to be patient and nonjudgmental when presenting some doubting black patients with a modern biomedical explanation of the cause of their presenting complaints.

Furthermore, psychiatric care of the African American continues to be fraught with landmines. In addition to the problems of bias in diagnosis, the myths and stereotypes often held by the psychiatric treatment team may make African American patients afraid, which may result in overmedication, particularly of male patients (Baker 1988a). Moreover, misdiagnosis of alcoholic hallucinosis (Bell et al. 1985) as schizophrenia could commit the patient to years of ineffective treatment with antipsychotic agents and increase the patient's risk for developing tardive dsykinesia.

Concepts of Mental Health and Mental Illness

Pride in the ability to survive in a largely hostile, racist environment and the ability to endure adversity are strengths thought to be characteristic of many African Americans. The African Americans resident in North America today are the descendants of individuals who survived the crossing of slave ships to the Americas, chattel slavery, legalized segregation in the United States, as well as the lynchings, beatings, and murders that occurred time and again throughout the United States. Added to these ills is the oppression of poverty, which has been a chronic stressor in the lives of many African Americans. Nevertheless, African Americans have needed, like individuals in other cultures, a belief system that enables them to understand why they have been afflicted with such sustained suffering. We posit that the earliest explanatory models used by African Americans have relied principally on notions of mystical causation (such as fate), animistic causation (such as gods and spirits), or magical causation (such as witchcraft). These explanatory notions have also been used by African Americans to explain mental illness (Ness and Wintrob 1981). However, scientific theories have now begun to enjoy greater popularity as a means of explaining psychiatric illness. But even some of this change has been diluted by the recent immigration to the United States of blacks from the Caribbean and South America, who still hold traditional notions attributing aberrant behavior to all but scientifically determined causes.

Similarly, many African Americans see the maintenance of good mental health as depending on a person's ability to stay in harmony with the magico-religious world. Good health is supposed to result from having a close walk with God or with other spirits, and biology and modern medicine are not seen as having the predominant role in determining illness or health. However, many blacks see no contradiction in using both prayer and modern medicine to help them confront illness.

Rubin and Jones (1979) carried out a detailed analysis of the clinical presentation of a 52-year-old Bahamian black man who sought care at a Florida hospital. Following an accidental acute intoxication episode from the pesticide parathion, the patient began to have multiple complaints, including sequences of "falling-out" (losing consciousness). Rubin and Jones pointed out that the patient viewed the poisoning accident as a time of physical weakness when magical poisoning could easily occur. Because the patient did in fact have psychiatric symptoms following the accident, he assumed that magic was at work, most likely because someone was working roots on him. He subsequently lost a job he had held for 24 years, and female companions stopped visiting him. He saw this as further evidence of magical intervention. He began to have auditory hallucinations, which he interpreted as the work of spirits seeking his death. The spirits were also seen as causing his blackout spells.

The authors described how the patient began to improve only after the treatment team realized the nature of the framework that the patient was using to understand and interpret his own sickness. At that point, the team sanctioned the patient's use of a folk healer, who participated in ceremonies intended to counter the magic being worked against the patient, whose condition then improved. However, this is not to suggest that in situations where such folk healers are unavailable, clinicians should attempt to carry out such religious rituals themselves.

Psychopathology

Culture-Related Syndromes

Although other ethnic groups have specific and well-described culture-bound syndromes, such as *amok* among Malayans, typical culture-bound patterns are much less often reported for African Americans. However, it is also possible that observers have paid relatively little attention to delineating unique clinical presentations among blacks. A research group at the University of Miami School of Medicine (Lefley 1979) has suggested that "falling-out," here defined as lapsing into a state of semiconsciousness, may be a presentation characteristic of many blacks. The researchers thought it could represent an "extreme method of denial and escape from an unbearable environment" (p. 123).

Major Classic Disorders

Classic mental illnesses do occur among blacks. Authors have raised specific concerns about misdiagnosis, inadequate treatment, and poor long-term management of blacks with psychiatric disorders (Fisher 1969; Helzer 1975; Johnson 1975; Pierce 1974; Spurlock 1975). Major depression and bipolar illness also are found in African American populations (Bell and Mehta 1979; Jones et al. 1981; Raskin et al. 1975). Specific national data on the prevalence of affective disorders for African Americans ages 18 through 64 in institutional settings have not yet been extracted from the ECA data tapes.

Several studies (Cassem 1988; Rosenthal et al. 1987) have reported an increasing incidence of depressive illness in association with medical problems in the elderly. Therefore, the prevalence of major depressive disorders in older African Americans may equal, if not exceed, the prevalence rates of about 33% in samples of black and white medical outpatients (Kukull et al. 1986; Nielson and Williams 1975; Rosenthal et al. 1987) or 25%–28% in medical inpatients (Derogatis et al. 1983; Moffic and Paykel 1975; Rodin and Voshart 1986).

Because stoicism and denial of illness are particularly common in African American patients, clinicians should make a systematic review of the following before concluding that these individuals are not depressed: neurovegetative signs; outlook for the future; identification of specific persons or events having given pleasure in the past, and determination of whether these continue to currently provide pleasure; and, finally, level of productivity. Other questions should address whether these patients are still active in their community churches or as caregivers for younger family members.

The presence of bipolar disorder in African Americans has been established by the work of Bell and Mehta (1979) and Jones and colleagues (1981). Other authors (Helzer 1975; Spurlock 1975) have also provided data that negate the myth that African Americans could not and did not become depressed.

A disparity between the prevalence of schizophrenia and of manic-depressive disorder in England and the United States (Cooper et al. 1972) was confirmed by the *International Collaborative Study of Schizophrenia* (Taylor and Abrams 1978). Although African Americans were regarded as too jovial to be depressed or too impoverished to experience object losses (Prange and Vitols 1962), these biased perspectives were countered by data on the presentation of affective illness in African Americans (Adebimpe 1981b; Bell and Mehta 1979; Jones et al. 1981).

One study documented diagnostic bias (Raskin et al. 1975). African American and white patients were screened for the presence of depressive symptoms by two clinicians prior to entry into a multihospital collaborative study of depression sponsored by the National Institute of Mental Health. The clinical features of depression were similar for both samples. Although the authors controlled the sample for age, sex, and social class, white patients were diagnosed more often as depressed, and African American patients were diagnosed more often as having some form of schizophrenia. The authors of this study found it difficult to explain these diagnostic differences. Adebimpe (1981b) emphasized the importance of psychiatrists' knowing about these results and suggested that social and cultural distance between patients and clinicians, stereotyping of African American psychopathology, false-positive symptoms, biased diagnostic instruments, and interaction of these factors all contributed to misdiagnosis.

Another factor influencing diagnosis is the interpretation of psychotic symptoms. Too frequently, American psychiatrists diagnosed these symptoms as pathognomonic of paranoid schizophrenia. Fortunately, Taylor and Abrams (1978) have shown there has been an increasing examination of psychiatric diagnosis by American psychiatrists and a move to standardize diagnosis. Studies by Vitols and colleagues (1963), Liss and colleagues (1973), Sletten and colleagues (1982), and Singer (1977) demonstrated that hallucinations and delusions occurred more frequently among African Americans in the populations studied by these authors. These findings led Adebimpe (1981a) to caution against making the diagnosis of schizophrenia in an African American patient solely on the basis of hallucinations and delusions, because these symptoms are also seen in cases of mania, psychotic depression, chronic alcoholism, and acute organic brain syndrome.

In addition to the need to avoid misdiagnosing alcohol abuse syndromes as schizophrenia, clinicians should always do their best to check for a history of substance abuse in African American patients. Phencyclidine (PCP) abuse remains a concern, particularly in Washington, DC, and Los Angeles (Fauman 1976). The epidemic use of "crack," a cocaine derivative, throughout the continental United States results in various clinical presentations, including paranoid psychosis and depressive symptoms during the "crash" (Gawin and Kleber 1986). The practice of "speedballing"—using a mixture of cocaine and heroin to produce a sustained euphoria and to avoid the cocaine "crash"—is increasingly becoming a pattern of abuse. If an individual complaining of paranoid ideation and Lilliputian hallucinations (visual hallucinations of little people) has a resolution of symptoms within 2 hours without psychopharmacologic intervention, the patient, in all likelihood, has manifested a cocaine psychosis (Goldfrank et al. 1981). Clearly, a diagnosis of schizophrenia is inappropriate in such a case.

Suicidal ideation may be a manifestation of several psychiatric illnesses, including affective disorder, schizophrenia, and adjustment disorder, as well as substance abuse. Thus, suicide may be viewed as the final common pathway of several disorders. However, there also tends to be a substantial correlation for some subgroups of African Americans between suicide and factors such as poverty, unemployment, and racism. It has proven difficult to identify the exact mechanisms that lead a particular person to decide to end his or her life.

Griffith and Bell (1989) showed that black males between the ages of 25 and 34 represent the group most affected by the phenomena of suicide and homicide. Black females are, relatively speaking, better protected against these kinds of death. Why there is this substantial difference between black males and females is a matter for conjecture, because there has been no empirical work on this subject.

Furthermore, black males between 25 and 34 years of age are also likely to engage in substance abuse and, in turn, to become infected with human immunodeficiency virus (HIV). Griffith and Bell (1989) have therefore suggested that preventive and therapeutic efforts must be aimed specifically at this group, especially if there is to be significant progress in reducing the black homicide rate. In addition, Baker (1989) has suggested that preventive psychiatric intervention focus on suicide attempters while they are still in the emergency room.

Mortality statistics related to alcoholic cirrhosis among blacks are alarming (Herd 1985; Task Force on Black and Minority Health 1986). The cirrhosis mortality rate for African American males ages 25 to 34 was 10 times that for white males of the same ages. When the cirrhosis mortality rate for all ages was reviewed comparing African Americans and whites, African Americans had twice the mortality rates of whites. Although African American women were more likely than African American men to be abstainers (Gary and Gary 1985), black women who did drink were more likely to be heavy

drinkers and to participate in binge drinking. Although rivaled by the escalating use of cocaine, alcohol abuse and dependence remain a central focus
of substance abuse in the African American community (Primm and Wesley
1985).

It is important to note that alcohol abuse in the African American community does not represent an age-old pattern. During the 1840s and 1850s,
abstinence from alcohol was synonymous with freedom from slavery and
moral uprightness; slavery and demon rum both were seen as examples of
moral depravity (Herd 1985). It was not until Reconstruction and the association of the temperance cause with African American disenfranchisement
and white supremacy that African Americans withdrew from the temperance
cause (Herd 1985). The migration of blacks in the 1920s and the 1930s during Prohibition and the Great Depression resulted in African Americans' becoming more involved in the production, sale, and consumption of alcohol.
Alcohol became a public health problem in the black community with the
employment of African American entertainers in Northern clubs and "speak-
easies" and their involvement in the "nightlife."

Cirrhosis was identified as one of the six causes of excess deaths in African
Americans between 1979 and 1981 (Task Force on Black and Minority
Health 1986). For males and females age 45 and under, cirrhosis was responsible for 4.9% of the excess deaths observed in African Americans compared
with whites. In African American males and females age 70 and under, cirrhosis was responsible for 3.7% of the excess mortality. It is therefore obvious
that alcohol dependence remains a concern for the African American community.

Although substance abuse, psychotic illness, and affective illness can all
produce changes in cognitive functioning, blacks are at increased risk for
fixed deficits in cognitive functioning because of multi-infarct dementia and
alcoholic dementia. This increased risk is attributable to the prevalence of
obesity, diabetes, hypertension, and alcohol abuse in the population (National Center for Health Statistics 1987a; Task Force on Black and Minority
Health 1986).

Although international (Rocca et al. 1986) and national studies with African American samples (Folstein et al. 1985; Schoenberg et al. 1985) have
shown a similar prevalence for clinically diagnosed Alzheimer's disease, the
data from the national studies have suggested a higher prevalence of vascular
dementia (multi-infarct dementia) in African Americans. Baker (1988b)
posed the question of whether prevalence studies will demonstrate a higher
rate of alcoholic dementia and multi-infarct dementia in African American
populations and at younger ages than in the general population. Given our

knowledge of the pattern of alcohol abuse, particularly among African American males, and the pattern of obesity, diabetes, and hypertension in African American females, these hypotheses seem reasonable. Because these dementias are preventable with changes in specific behavioral patterns, epidemiologic studies are indicated to clarify the extent to which morbidity and mortality due to these causes can be decreased.

Family Response to Mental Illness of Its Members

The black family is thought to have evolved from blacks' West African heritage, in which the welfare of the community superseded that of the individual. In addition, African cultures emphasized the importance of children (Pinderhughes 1989). The grandchild was seen as the fruition of the grandparents' generation (Wylie 1971). The African American family remains an extended family, and unrelated persons may be adopted or absorbed into it (Martin and Martin 1978; Stack 1974).

The African American family is evolving. Most families must come to terms with pressures of survival (Pinderhughes 1982) and many with being marginally stable economically (Coner-Edwards and Spurlock 1988). Although characterized as a tangle of pathology by Moynihan (1965), subsequent studies of the black family have addressed the biases inherent in generalizing from poor welfare families to all African American families (Coner-Edwards and Spurlock 1988; Hill 1971; Hines and Boyd-Franklin 1982; Johnson 1982; Pinderhughes 1982). The myth of the universality of the African American matriarchy has been exploded by these authors. Mullings (1985) provided an excellent review of the debate concerning the structure and function of the African American family.

Chattel slavery disrupted the family unit of parents and children, as well as the extended family, by auction and by death. African American family units during slavery were composed of biologically related and nonbiologically related individuals who joined together to provide support, care, and comfort as well as survival skills and key information (Gutman 1976). Johnson (1982) noted that such units continued during Reconstruction. They were the forerunners of the present-day African American extended family (Coner-Edwards and Spurlock 1988).

The intergenerational support of the African American extended family must be noted (Hines and Boyd-Franklin 1982). Often, elders in the family provide the wisdom of their years of experience, maintain a favored role as family historians, and are productive and useful members of the family

(Baker 1982). The lower rates of suicide among older African Americans in contrast to white Americans may reflect black elders' enhanced self-esteem, continued usefulness, and sense of a meaningful existence derived from the family role of elder. However, caution should be exercised in arriving at such interpretations, because national data suggest that suicide among blacks over age 65 may be on the increase (Griffith and Bell 1989).

Egalitarian relationships in the parental dyad have been identified by Hines and Boyd-Franklin (1982) and Lewis and Looney (1983). Further evidence against the myth of the universality of the "black matriarchy" is found within the recent work of Lewis and Looney (1983), who reported on well-functioning working-class African American families. These families were living at slightly above the poverty level and were involved in church and Scouting as important outlets and avenues for socialization of family members. The researchers noted that when survival became the focus of family life, African American families moved toward more rigid role definition, with the male setting family policy and making decisions.

In general, Spurlock (1969), Pinderhughes (1973), Norton (1983), and Pierce (1974) noted that, too often, observers were ignoring the influence of racism, social status, and poverty on the observed patterns of black family function and structure. These authors suggested that black families took on dysfunctional structures and function because of a heightened preoccupation with survival, and that these structures were not true of families who were better off. This does not mean that families headed by black women are necessarily dysfunctional. We wish to indicate only that the great stresses of poverty, racism, and sexism on these families often have pathological repercussions on family structure and function. Lawson (1986) has emphasized the need to study further the impact on African American families of providing care for a chronically mentally ill family member while bearing the additional burdens of racism and scarce economic resources.

Choice of Treatment

Choice of treatment provider differs, depending in part on the patient's age. Younger cohorts are more likely to seek psychiatric treatment at outpatient psychiatric clinics in their community or, if financially able, through private care. Older African Americans, in contrast, are more likely to consult friends, ask a neighbor who is a nurse about symptoms, and visit a local pharmacist. Only if there is no improvement in symptoms will the African American elder tend to seek treatment in a formal health care setting, more usually from a family practitioner or an internist (Baker 1989). The difference in providers chosen by younger versus older blacks may possibly be largely explained by the historical differences in their experiences of racism.

Although segregation ended in some American cities in the 1950s, African American elders still recall white society's negative attitudes toward blacks and the infantilization and disrespect that they were shown. However, younger blacks may view health care as a right and are therefore willing to confront those health care professionals whom they consider less responsive to their needs or disrespectful in their treatment of African American patients.

Clinicians are also grounded in their own developmental experience, which is a function of age. The older clinician may wonder about the ability of African American patients to pay for services and may doubt that African Americans have the necessary skills to engage effectively in insight-oriented psychotherapy (Baker 1988a). Younger clinicians may view all African Americans as the products of the "cycle of poverty." This stereotype may be so strong that some clinicians may fail to establish the specific educational level, employment history, and friendship and social network of the patient as they attempt to relate to him or her as "a brother" or "a sister" rather than as a member of the patient-therapist dyad.

Adams (1950) defined primary concerns in the interaction between the white therapist and the African American patient and warned of the danger of focusing on their differences. However, not only are there pitfalls for white therapists working with blacks, but countertransference issues between therapists and patients of the same race may also prevent the formation of a therapeutic alliance.

Although African American patients approach a health care institution with anticipatory anxiety, several authors have documented that what is required for successful psychotherapy with an African American patient is simply an empathic, sensitive, inquiring, and concerned therapist (Bell et al. 1983; Bradshaw 1978; Jones et al. 1982; Spurlock 1982).

The therapist providing psychiatric care to African American patients needs to recognize the potential impact of socioeconomic factors on patients. Access to care is often restricted by the patient's lack of insurance or the type of insurance. Because of concern about the potential cost of care and a possible dislike of interacting with health care systems, the African American patient may be likely to seek care later in the course of his or her illness and to have some restrictions on the resources that can be mobilized. Although the African American extended family is a key resource and can provide crucial support for the patient, it may not be enough—particularly if the family is stressed by the economics of basic survival.

An additional concern for the treating clinician is the historic pattern of misdiagnosis. An African American patient with a 25-year history of "schizophrenia" may have had his or her long-standing alcohol abuse ignored or a cyclical pattern of illness unidentified. It is crucial to review all the available records as well as to interview available family members, by telephone if necessary, to characterize the symptoms that make up the patient's psychiatric illness. Frequently, to develop an appropriate treatment plan, the task of the mental health professional becomes that of a retrospective diagnostician.

Although questions have arisen about whether the therapeutic levels of psychoactive medications differ for African American patients (Baker 1988a), there are to date no published studies that resolve the questions. While it is recognized that the African American population contains the gene for sickle cell anemia, the impact of hemoglobin S on lithium carbonate excretion by a patient with bipolar disorder and with sickle cell trait or sickle cell anemia remains unknown (Shader 1982). Studies have shown that high-dose neuroleptics can result in toxic states (Mayer et al. 1980), thereby producing a worsening of psychotic symptoms. The frequency with which this occurs in African American patients, who are more likely to receive higher doses of neuroleptics in acute care settings, is unknown.

Because African Americans are a heterogeneous group with various educational, occupational, and social network resources, only general comments can be made about the type or form of psychotherapy or treatment interventions they may need. It is important to acquire specific knowledge of the patient rather than to work from false assumptions. The therapist needs to ask the patient about his or her educational level, current occupation, and prior medical and psychiatric treatment history and must also clarify the specific roles of those accompanying the patient to the initial interview. The evaluating therapist should recognize that the African American person is attending to nonverbal behavior and will pick up evidence in the therapist of any anxiety, discomfort, or rejection.

If the patient perceives the therapeutic environment as hostile and non-supportive, he or she may leave and not return to treatment. Geller (1988) recently provided a framework for helping therapists explore their stereotypic ways of thinking about black patients, particularly during the evaluation phase of treatment. Geller showed how clinicians, in dealing with a black patient, may maximize the possibility of adverse effects from the environment on the patient. They may prematurely anticipate the patient's dropping-out from treatment and inadvertently characterize the black patient as inarticulate, incompetent, and unsophisticated. All of those suggestions may simply express the therapist's wish not to be close to the black patient and may ultimately spell disaster for treatment. Russell (1988) has additionally warned that some therapists may be prejudiced against blacks who use Black Nonstandard English and that such therapists may feel alienated from these patients in the long run.

If the focus of treatment is on developmental tasks and the reworking of maladaptive patterns, individual psychotherapy may be indicated. After the initial evaluation of two or three sessions, it is important that the therapist review findings in understandable language with the patient, discuss the prescribed treatment plan and its length. If there is a specific precipitant of a sudden decompensation in effective coping strategies, then brief treatment may be indicated. Once a successful therapeutic alliance has been established and therapeutic benefit has been attained, further work will be feasible. As has been suggested above, it is the establishment of a fruitful alliance between therapist and patient that may be fraught with difficulty.

When psychotic or affective illness is the focus of treatment, the black patient's extended family should be involved in the initial evaluation and at relevant stages of the treatment. Although significant tension may exist between the patient and family members or close friends, the therapist with family and group psychotherapy training and experience can use therapeutic skills to put the issues on the table, gather a firsthand assessment of the patient's significant relationships, and inform everyone about the current understanding of the illness, its course, and the proposed treatment. It will be helpful to the therapist to know the specific resources that exist for a given family for respite from a setting with intensely expressed emotion, as one example, and the specific family members who are more likely to precipitate a relapse.

For some patients, the addition of assertiveness group training to other forms of treatment may be beneficial. As patients learn specific assertiveness techniques, they can implement them in situations in which they have been silent, withdrawn, or inarticulate though angry. In the psychotherapeutic process, African American patients can develop effective mechanisms for verbalizing their feelings and conveying their concerns. This new sense of mastery can be incorporated into therapy as well as into daily interactions.

Where indicated, more than one modality of treatment (e.g., individual, family, group, and pharmacologic modalities) should be considered to facilitate maximum improvement of the patient. Because of the heterogeneity of the African American population in heritage, social support networks, education, and socioeconomic status, it is inappropriate for any therapist to assert that there is a "best treatment" that is applicable to all African American patients. The decision for a specific therapeutic regimen should depend on the assessment, the diagnosis, and the wishes of the patient and his or her family.

Conclusion

The African American individual brings the strengths of an African heritage, including the cultural asset of the extended family and the stoicism and survival skills learned in America, to the management of psychiatric illness. Racial bias may complicate the evaluation, diagnosis, and treatment of black patients. But such problematic pitfalls are much better appreciated today than 25 years ago. With an awareness of and sensitivity to these issues, clinicians should find the treatment experience with blacks to be challenging and most interesting.

We have reviewed here the macrohistory of African Americans in the United States so as to facilitate an understanding of how African Americans of different ages view health care institutions, define mental illness, and seek treatment. Obviously, many areas remain where there is substantial lack of empirical data to support clinical hypotheses. We hope that we have emphasized the need for research to fill these gaps in knowledge.

References

Adams WA: The Negro patient in psychiatric treatment. Am J Orthopsychiatry 20:305–310, 1950

Adebimpe VR: Hallucinations and delusions in black psychiatric patients. J Natl Med Assoc 73:517–520, 1981a

Adebimpe VR: Overview: white norms and psychiatric diagnosis of black patients. Am J Psychiatry 138:279–285, 1981b

Baer HA: The Black Spiritual Movement. Knoxville, TN, University of Tennessee Press, 1984

Baker FM: The black elderly: biopsychosocial perspective within an age cohort and adult development context. J Geriatr Psychiatry 15:227–239, 1982

Baker FM: The Afro-American life cycle: success, failure, and mental health. J Natl Med Assoc 73(6):625–633, 1987

Baker FM: Afro-Americans, in Clinical Guidelines in Cross-Cultural Mental Health. Edited by Comas-Diaz L, Griffith EEH. New York, Wiley, 1988a, pp 151–181

Baker FM: Dementing illness and black Americans, in The Black American Elderly. Research on Physical and Psychosocial Health. Edited by Jackson JS. New York, Springer, 1988b, pp 215–233

Baker FM: Black youth suicide: literature review with a focus on prevention, in Report of the Secretary's Task Force on Youth Suicide, Vol 3: Prevention and Interventions in Youth Suicide (DHHS Publ No ADM-89-1623). Washington DC, U.S. Government Printing Office, 1989, pp 3:177–3:195

Bell C, Mehta H: The misdiagnosis of black patients with manic-depressive illness. J Natl Med Assoc 72:141–145, 1979

Bell CC, Bland IJ, Houston E, et al: Enhancement of knowledge and skills for the psychiatric treatment of black populations, in Mental Health and People of Color. Edited by Chunn JC, Dunston PJ, Ross-Sheriff F. Washington, DC, Howard University Press, 1983, pp 205–237

Bell CC, Thompson JP, Lewis D, et al: Misdiagnosis of alcohol related organic brain syndromes: Implications for treatment, in Treatment of Black Alcoholics. Edited by Brisbane FL, Womble M. New York, Haworth Press, 1985, pp 45–65

Bevis MW: Psychological traits of the Southern Negro with observations as to some of his psychoses. Am J Psychiatry 18:67–78, 1921

Bradshaw MH: Training psychiatrists for working with blacks in basic residency training programs. Am J Psychiatry 135:1520–1524, 1978

Cannon M, Locke B: Being black is detrimental to one's mental health: myth or reality? Phylon 38:408–428, 1977

Cassem EH: Depression secondary to medical illness, in American Psychiatric Press Review of Psychiatry, Vol 7. Edited by Frances AJ, Hales RE. Washington, DC, American Psychiatric Press, 1988, pp 256–273

Coner-Edwards AF, Spurlock J: Black Families in Crisis: The Middle Class. New York, Brunner/Mazel, 1988

Cooper JE, Kendell RE, Gurland BJ: Psychiatric Diagnosis in New York and London: A Comprehensive Study of Mental Hospital Admissions. London, Oxford University Press, 1972

Derogatis LR, Morrow GR, Fetting J, et al: The prevalence of psychiatric disorders among cancer patients. JAMA 249:751–757, 1983

Deutsch A: The first U.S. census of the insane (1840) and its use as pro-slavery propaganda. Bull Hist Med 15:469–482, 1944

Easton WE, Kessler LG (eds): Epidemiologic Field Methods in Psychiatry. New York, Academic Press, 1985

Evarts AB: Dementia praecox in the colored race. Psychoanal Rev 1:338–403, 1914

Fauman B: Psychiatric sequelae of phencyclidine abuse. Clinical Toxicology 9:529–538, 1976

Fisher J: Negro and white rates of mental illness: reconstruction of a myth. Psychiatry 32:428–446, 1969

Folstein M, Anthony JC, Parhad I, et al: The meaning of cognitive impairment in the elderly. J Am Geriatr Soc 33:228–235, 1985

French HW: Hatred and social isolation may spur acts of racial violence, experts say. The New York Times, Monday, September 4, 1989, p 31

Frumkin RM: Race and major mental disorders. Journal of Negro Education 23:97–98, 1954

Gary LE, Gary RB: Treatment needs of black alcoholic women, in Treatment of Black Alcoholics. Edited by Brisbane FL, Womble M. New York, Haworth Press, 1985, pp 97–114

Gawin FH, Kleber HD: Abstinence symptomatology and psychiatric diagnosis in cocaine abusers. Arch Gen Psychiatry 343:107–113, 1986

Geller J: Racial bias in the evaluation of patients for psychotherapy, in Clinical Guidelines in Cross-Cultural Mental Health. Edited by Comas-Diaz L, Griffith EEH. New York, Wiley, 1988, pp 112–134

Goldfrank L, Lewin N, Weisman RS: Cocaine. Hospital Physician 17:26–44, 1981

Griffith EEH, Bell CC: Recent trends in suicide and homicide among blacks. JAMA 262:2265–2269, 1989

Griffith EEH, Young JL, Smith DL: An analysis of the therapeutic elements in a black church service. Hosp Community Psychiatry 35:464–469, 1984

Gutman H: The Black Family in Slavery and Freedom. New York, Pantheon, 1976

Helzer J: Bipolar affective disorder in black and white men. Arch Gen Psychiatry 32:1140–1143, 1975

Herd D: We cannot stagger to freedom. A history of blacks and alcohol in American politics, in The Yearbook of Substance Use and Abuse, Vol 3. Edited by Brill L, Winick C. New York, Human Sciences Press, 1985, pp 141–186

Hill R: The Strengths of Black Families. New York, Emerson Hall Publishers, 1971

Hines PM, Boyd-Franklin N: Black families, in Ethnicity and Family Therapy. Edited by McGoldrick M, Pearce JK, Giordano J. New York, Guilford, 1982, pp 84–107

Jackson JJ: Social gerontology and the Negro: a review. Gerontologist 7(3):168–178, 1967

Jackson JJ: The blacklands of gerontology. Aging and Human Development 2:156–171, 1971

Jackson JJ: Plight of older black women in the United States. Black Aging 1:12–20, 1975

Jackson JJ: Social determinants of the health of aging black populations in the United States, in The Black American Elderly: Research on Physical and Psychosocial Health. Edited by Jackson JS. New York, Springer, 1988, pp 69–98

Johnson JE: The Afro-American family: A historical overview, in The Afro-American Family: Assessment, Treatment, and Research Issues. Edited by Bass BA, Wyatt GE, Powell GJ. New York, Grune & Statton, 1982, pp 3–12

Johnson JT: Alcoholism: a social disease from a medical perspective, in Textbook of Black-Related Diseases. Edited by Williams RA. New York, McGraw-Hill, 1975, pp 639–654

Jones BE, Gray BA, Parson EB: Manic-depressive illness among poor urban blacks. Am J Psychiatry 185:654–657, 1981

Jones BE, Gray BA, Jospitre J: Survey of psychotherapy with black men. Am J Psychiatry 139:1174–1177, 1982

Jordan WC: Voodoo medicine, in Textbook of Black-Related Diseases. Edited by Williams RA. New York, McGraw-Hill, 1975, pp 715–738

Kukull WA, Koepsell TD, Inui TS, et al: Depression and physical illness in elderly general medical clinic patients. J Affect Disord 10:153–162, 1986

Lawson WB: Chronic mental illness and the black family. American Journal of Social Psychiatry 6:57–61, 1986

Lefley HP: Female cases of falling-out: a psychological evaluation of a small sample. Soc Sci Med 13B:115–116, 1979

Lewis JM, Looney JG: The Long Struggle: Well-Functioning Working Class Black Families. New York, Brunner/Mazel, 1983

Liss JL, Weiner A, Robins E, et al: Psychiatric symptoms in white and black inpatients. Compr Psychiatry 14:475–481, 1973

Malzberg B: Mental disorders in the U.S., in The Encyclopedia of Mental Health, Vol 3. Edited by Deutsch A, Fishman H. New York, Franklin Walts, 1963, pp 1051–1066

Martin EP, Martin JM: The Black Extended Family. Chicago, IL, University of Chicago Press, 1978

Martinez C: Mexican-Americans, in Clinical Guidelines in Cross-Cultural Mental Health. Edited by Comas-Diaz L, Griffith EEH. New York, Wiley, 1988, pp 182–203

Mayer SE, Melmon KL, Gilman AG: The dynamics of drug absorption, distribution, and elimination, in Goodman and Gilman's The Pharmacological Basis of Therapeutics—Sixth Edition. Edited by Gilman AG, Goodman LS, Gilman A. New York, Macmillan, 1980, pp 1–27

Moffic HS, Paykel ES: Depression in medical inpatients. Br J Psychiatry 126:346–353, 1975

Moynihan D: The Negro Family: The Case for National Action. Washington, DC, U.S. Department of Labor, 1965

Mullings L: Anthropological perspective of the Afro-American family, in The Black Family: Mental Health Perspectives. Edited by Fulliove MT. San Francisco, CA, Rosenberg Foundation, 1985, pp 11–21

National Center for Health Statistics: Health. United States. 1987. Washington, DC, U.S. Government Printing Office, 1987a

National Center for Health Statistics: Prevalence of known diabetes among black Americans, in Advance Data from Vital and Health Statistics (DHHS Publ No PHS-87-1250). Hyattsville, MD, U.S. Public Health Service, 1987b

Ness RC, Wintrob RM: Folk healing: A description and synthesis. Am J Psychiatry 138:1477–1481, 1981

Nielson AC, Williams TA: Depression in ambulatory medical patients. Br J Psychiatry 126:346–353, 1975

Norton DG: Black family life patterns, the development of self, and cognitive development of black children, in The Psychosocial Development of Minority Group Children. Edited by Powell GJ. New York, Brunner/Mazel, 1983, pp 181–193

Pierce CM: Psychiatric problems of the black minority, in American Handbook of Psychiatry—Second Edition Revised and Expanded. Volume 2. Edited by Caplan G. New York, Basic Books, 1974, pp 512–523

Pinderhughes C: Racism and psychotherapy, in Racism and Mental Health. Edited by Willie CV, Kramer BM, Brown BS. Pittsburgh, PA, University of Pittsburgh Press, 1973, pp 61–121

Pinderhughes E: Afro-American families and the victim system, in Ethnicity and Family Therapy. Edited by McGoldrick M, Pearce JK, Giordano J. New York, Guilford, 1982, pp 108–122

Pinderhughes E: Understanding Race, Ethnicity, and Power. New York, Free Press, 1989

Poussaint AF: Why Blacks Kill Blacks. New York, Emerson Hall Publishers, 1972

Prange AJ, Vitols MM: Cultural aspects of the relatively low incidence of depression in southern Negroes. Int J Soc Psychiatry 8:104–112, 1962

Primm BJ, Wesley JE: Treating the multiply addicted black alcoholic. Alcoholism Treatment Quarterly 2:155–178, 1985

Prudhomme C, Musto DF: Historical perspective on mental health and racism in the United States, in Racism and Mental Health. Edited by Willie CV, Kramer BM, Brown BS. Pittsburgh, PA, University of Pittsburgh Press, 1973, pp 25–55

Raskin A, Crook TH, Herman KD: Psychiatry history and symptom differences in black and white depressed inpatients. J Consult Clin Psychology 43:73–80, 1975

Rocca WA, Amaducci LA, Schoenberg BS: Epidemiology of clinically diagnosed Alzheimer's Disease. Ann Neurol 19:415–424, 1986

Rodin G, Voshart K: Depression in the medically ill: an overview. Am J Psychiatry 143:696–705, 1986

Rosenthal MP, Goldfarb NJ, Carlson BL, et al: Assessment of depression in a family practice center. J Fam Pract 25:143–149, 1987

Rubin JC, Jones J: Falling-out: a clinical study. Soc Sci Med 13B:117–127, 1979

Russell DM: Language and psychotherapy: the influence of nonstandard English in clinical practice, in Clinical Guidelines in Cross-Cultural Mental Health. Edited by Comas-Diaz L, Griffith EEH. New York, Wiley, 1988, pp 33–68

Schoenberg BS, Anderson DW, Haerer AF: Severe dementia. Prevalence and clinical features in a biracial U.S. population. Arch Neurol 42:740–743, 1985

Shader RI: Cultural aspects of mental health care for black Americans: Cultural aspects of psychiatric training, in Cross-Cultural Psychiatry. Edited by Gaw A. Littleton, MA, John Wright-PSG Pub Co, 1982, pp 187–199

Simon RJ, Fleiss JL, Gurland BJ, et al: Depression and schizophrenia in black and white mental patients. Arch Gen Psychiatry 28:509–512, 1973

Singer BP: Racial Factors in Psychiatric Intervention. San Francisco, CA, R and E Research Associates, 1977

Sletten J, Schuff S, Altman H, et al: A statewide computerized psychiatric system:

demographic, diagnostic, and mental status data. Int J Soc Psychiatry 18:30–40, 1982

Spitzer RL, Endicott J, Robins E: Research Diagnostic Criteria: rationale and reliability. Arch Gen Psychiatry 35:773–782, 1978

Spurlock J: Should the poor get none? Journal of the American Academy of Child Psychiatry 8:16–35, 1969

Spurlock J: Psychiatric states, in Textbook of Black-Related Disease. Edited by Williams RA. New York, McGraw-Hill, 1975, pp 688–704

Spurlock J: Black Americans, in Cross-Cultural Psychiatry. Edited by Gaw A. Littleton, MA, John Wright-PSG Pub Co, 1982, pp 163–178

Stack C: All Our Kin. New York, Harper & Row, 1974

Task Force on Black and Minority Health: Report on the Secretary's Task Force on Black and Minority Health. Volume V: Homicide, Suicide, and Unintentional Injuries. Washington, DC, U.S. Department of Health and Human Services, 1986

Taylor HA, Abrams R: The prevalence of schizophrenia: a reassessment using modern diagnostic criteria. Am J Psychiatry 135:945–948, 1978

U.S. Bureau of the Census: Detailed Population Characteristics. U.S. Summary, Section A. Washington, DC, U.S. Government Printing Office, 1980

Vitols MM, Waters HG, Keeler MH: Hallucinations and delusions in white and Negro schizophrenics. Am J Psychiatry 120:472–476, 1963

Wilcox P: Positive mental health in the black community: the black liberation movement, in Racism and Mental Health: Essays. Edited by Willie CV, Kramer BM, Brown BS. Pittsburgh, PA, University of Pittsburgh Press, 1974, pp 463–524

Williams DH: The epidemiology of mental illness in Afro-Americans. Hosp Community Psychiatry 37:42–49, 1986

Wilson D, Lantz E: The effect of cultural change in the Negro race in Virginia as indicated by a study of state hospital admissions. Am J Psychiatry 14:25–34, 1957

Wylie FM: Attitudes toward aging and the aged among black Americans: some historical perspectives. Aging and Human Development 2:66–70, 1971

7 Separation and Loss in African American Children: Clinical Perspectives

Donna M. Norris, M.D.
Jeanne Spurlock, M.D.

hildren's responses to separation and loss have been studied and reported in the psychiatric literature for more than five decades (Burlingham 1944; Robertson 1952; Spitz 1945, 1946). These reports have concerned children who have lost their parents or siblings because of illness or violence and/or the stresses of wars. Most of these studies, however, have considered the effects of separation and loss primarily for children of the dominant racial group in the United States. There has been little reported on the effects of separation and loss for the African American child in this country. It is our hypothesis that there are special circumstances for the African American family that mandate a more in-depth investigation and evaluation of African American children's perception of losses and separations. We believe that America faces a crisis for the future of African American youth, because they are continually bombarded with violence, as if in war.

The early studies of attachment have related primarily to the infant's connection to the maternal figure and the young child's anxiety resulting from threats or anticipated threats of abandonment. It is now recognized that an understanding of mourning is essential when conducting therapeutic work with children (Bowlby 1982; Sekaer 1987).

Furman (1983) has defined the tasks of bereavement as "1) understanding and accepting the reality of the death . . . 2) mourning, that is the internal process of adaptation to the permanent unavailability of the deceased love object, and 3) resuming functioning in accord with one's state in life" (pp. 242–243). For children to be able to manage these restorative processes, it is necessary for them to have certain interpersonal, familiar, and/or professional supports so that they may move successfully toward reorganization from one phase of mourning to the next. It is recognized that environmental stability is one important component for optimal progress.

For African American children, the factor of culture adds a special dimension to the therapeutic work done by mental health professionals (Spurlock 1985). Looff (1979) also has discussed the importance of understanding sociocultural traits of a people in order to work effectively with its children. As he noted, the expected personality development or ego functions of the child are dependent upon what is expected and permitted by the child's culture.

There may be subtypes within a culture that have importance but are not readily identified by outsiders. It must be understood that not all people who live in the ghetto are of the ghetto (Rainwater 1970). All individuals in the ghetto may share poor economic circumstances as well as the daily reminders of their victimization by a racist society, but they may differ significantly in their values and/or their responses to racist practices. For within an often clearly circumscribed area of poor housing, with its rodent infestation, vacant lots strewn with debris, and empty, boarded-up buildings, live people with clearly middle-class values. These individuals value friendships, honesty, religion, family, and the interconnectedness of these attributes as they strive for success. Another belief shared by this subgroup is the universality of the "American Dream," which includes African Americans, one group on whose backs this nation was built. For many African Americans, the royal heritage of their West African forebears is as significant to the story of America's origins and achievements as is the coming of the *Mayflower.*

Separations in Relation to Historic Periods

Historically, the earliest separations for African Americans as a people came as they were forcibly moved from Africa. The institution of slavery was constructed to contain these people permanently within and beneath American society. There was no attempt by most white slave masters to keep families of slaves together, except when there was an economic incentive to do so. The slave masters repressed the languages, cultures, and religious practices of slaves in an effort to forcibly acculturate them to their new subservient state. Many slave mothers were separated from their children and forced to nurture and suckle the children of the slave masters. The children of these slaves were then left to be cared for by the greater slave group.

Almost 130 years after its official abolition, vestiges of slavery can still be seen in this society. It affects the lives of black people through institutional racism, with its varied resultant psychological repercussions (Spurlock and Lawrence 1979).

Into the 20th century, African American women were allowed into the work force primarily as domestic or service workers, while African American men were employed as unskilled or semiskilled laborers. Many of these women have continued to work as domestics, providing care for children of the majority culture, while many of their own children experience their mothers' unavailability as a major loss. Writer Toni Morrison (1970) provides a vivid illustration of this pattern in her novel *The Bluest Eye.*

The novel's protagonist, Pecola, and two of her friends arrive at the residence of her mother's employer. They wait in the kitchen while Pecola's mother goes to fetch the wash she had done. The employer's daughter enters the room and appears to be afraid upon seeing these "strange" children and calls out for Pecola's mother, Polly. At the same time, Pecola and her friends move toward a berry cobbler that was cooling on a counter.

It may have been nervousness, awkwardness, but the pan tilted under Pecola's fingers and fell to the floor, splattering blackish blueberries everywhere. Most of the juice splashed on Pecola's legs, and the burn must have been painful, for she cried out and began hopping about just as Mrs. Breedlove (the name that Pecola used to address her mother) entered. . . . In one gallop she was on Pecola, and with the back of her hand knocked her to the floor. . . . The little girl in pink started to cry. Mrs. Breedlove turned to her. "Hush, baby hush. Come here. Oh, Lord, look at your dress. Polly will change it." (p. 86)

The mother yells at Pecola and her friends to leave. As they scurry out, they hear Mrs. Breedlove comforting her employer's child.

"Who were they, Polly?"
"Don't worry none, baby."
"You gonna make another pie?"
"Course I will."
"Who were they, Polly?"
"Hush. Don't worry none," she whispered, and the honey in her words complemented the sundown spilling on the lake. (p. 87)

This excerpt illustrates the black mother's attentiveness, concern, and compassion for the child of her employer, whereas her feelings for her own child demonstrate anger and lack of empathy. While ignoring the real pain and distress of her own child, the mother fails to even legitimize the very real trauma that Pecola has experienced and, furthermore, gives her "the back of her hand."

Migration

At the turn of this century, the majority of African American people lived in the South. By the early 1930s and 1940s, many had migrated to the North, usually driven by the motivation for greater economic stability (Haynes 1922, 1923). Many of these immigrants, who had lifelong farming experience, were unable to find work as the country became more industrialized. Often, many left their children as well as important extended family members and social connections as they journeyed alone into new areas. Many times, the children were left abruptly with little preparation or attention to their perception of the separation. The parents migrated into new environments and subcultures, each with their own demands. Regardless of the socioeconomic improvements, there were, for many of these families, psychological costs in their attempts toward acculturation. When the children did join their parents, often years later, they were expected to accommodate themselves to the current family situation and to be unaffected by the hiatus in the parent-child relationship. The following case, known to one of the authors of this chapter, provides a dramatic illustration of the severe costs of such separations.

Case Study

A 23-year-old African American woman had left her 5-year-old son in South Carolina and, following older siblings, moved north to find employment. She had difficulty establishing herself financially and felt thwarted in her attempts to save enough money for a permanent reunion with her son. Through the years, however, she did maintain visits with the family during the Christmas holidays.

Approximately 6 years following the initial separation, the woman sent for her son. By this time, she was married and had a 2-year-old daughter. The son, now 10 years old, had always lived with his maternal grandmother in the rural South. He was intelligent, had done well in school, had friends, and had no behavioral problems. He arrived in the summer before the start of school and recalled that this was the first time he had ever lived in a city. He felt confined, as he was not able to play outside because of the roughness of the neighborhood and its unfamiliarity.

Initially, the boy did well in the new school, but his performance soon began to deteriorate. One day, he reported to his teacher that while he was taking a bath, his mother threatened to shoot him in the head. As a result of the school's report of this incident, the State Social Services and the courts became involved. In a subsequent diagnostic evaluation of the boy, he spoke of his sadness about leaving his grandmother, his fear of a mother whom he did not know, his sense of estrangement from his new environment, and his worry about the future.

The feelings expressed in this story are not unusual. For many children, the reunifications of these long-separated families are experienced as major losses and may be expressed by failure in school or dropping-out, embattled relations with parents, substance abuse, and in some cases, delinquent behavior. Frequently, these behaviors have prompted referrals by the schools or courts for mental health services for these children. For some children, the response is a precipitous return to the extended family, often without adequate preparation.

A similar phenomenon has been noted among people of African descent who have migrated from Caribbean countries to the United States and Canada. Many of the immigrants from these Caribbean nations traced their roots to Africa and slavery, but the inhabitants of these lands were able to obtain independence through war (e.g., Haiti) or through negotiations (e.g., Barbados). Therefore, many of these immigrants have maintained a strong sense of connectedness with and pride in their native countries. They have viewed themselves and their histories as distinctly separate from that of African Americans. Afro-Caribbean immigrants may continue their customs, languages, and/or dialects, while maintaining old family ties and interpersonal relationships through frequent visits to the homeland. Notably, many of these immigrants have a keen sense of the American Dream's potential for them. Moving to the United States in search of jobs has often meant that they have doubled or tripled their earning capacity. They frequently maintain two full-time jobs to achieve greater financial success. In many instances, money has been sent to help support relatives in the Caribbean nations.

Once immigrant parents are established in the United States, their children are brought to their new homes, but often without planning for their psychological needs. As with African American children who moved from the South, these children are expected to move into a new system with only minimal conflict and to achieve success in this unfamiliar environment.

Often, because Afro-Caribbean immigrants have insisted on maintaining old cultural connections, a separateness may result in their relationships with

African Americans. Thus, the Caribbean-born children may find themselves a minority in a larger minority community in a foreign land. The attempts by these Afro-Caribbean immigrants at self-sustenance may be viewed suspiciously by African Americans as efforts toward superiority and the need to be differentiated from other blacks. And, indeed, many foreign-born blacks may be reluctant to give up their own cultures and to completely merge their identities with those of African Americans.

In the late 1970s and 1980s, we witnessed a new migration of African Americans from North to South. In part, this migration has been a move toward better jobs, as many corporations have relocated to the less costly South. There appears to be, however, another motive for these changes. Many African American families have viewed the disintegration of the large Northern cities where they have concentrated as a cause for great concern. This is more than an economic disquietude; it is now viewed as a question of life or death.

Upward Mobility and Losses

The move up the socioeconomic ladder does not provide immunity from losses and painful separations. Many African American families come to suburbia prompted by greater economic stability and the ever-present desire to provide better housing conditions and educational opportunities for their children. Often, there is a downside to such moves. Not only are the children separated from their friends, but in many instances there is a loosening of the close relationship with grandparents and other relatives who remained in the old neighborhood.

Many children also lose a sense of independence. Previously, they had been able to get to after-school events and weekend activities on their own by using public transportation. The painful sequelae of the separation and losses, coupled with the untoward experiences of the hostile environment of some suburban communities, can lead to impairment of family relationships, as well as to inner turmoil for children and parents. The problems are usually compounded when both parents are working outside the home, as most are, and the work is studded with stresses that are "colored" racist. The following vignette is illustrative.

> The psychological distress provoked by such experiences (related to the racist atmosphere of the workplace) is not dissipated when an individual leaves the office. The sequelae are likely to be especially troublesome for parents who

have legitimate demands made of them when they arrive home. The conflicts engendered by the apparent racist atmosphere of the work environment are compounded when 8-year-old Jamal reports, "My teacher says black people can't follow instructions. That's why I didn't do the right assignment," or 16-year-old Judy pleads for permission to live with an aunt and go to school in the city. Her voice escalates as she complains that the black boys aren't interested in dating the black girls in her school. Judy's anger is redirected toward her parents; she suggests that they made a bad decision; their move to suburbia so that she and her brother could have a better education had backfired—at least for her. She was so miserable that she was unable to direct full attention to her studies. (Spurlock and Booth 1988, p. 82)

Self-Concept

It is true that some African Americans have been able to move into America's mainstream by achieving academic, vocational, and/or financial success. From the outsider's perspective, these individuals appear to have "made it." African Americans who are successful are sometimes seen as exceptions who are "not really black." These comments are often presented as "compliments," with no recognition by the dominant group of their denigrating effect. How can it be anything but a put-down when African Americans know that they are perceived to be apart from their people because of their successes (Norris and Bell 1985)? Pierce (1988) has noted that in almost all black and white interactions, "operationally, Whites act to keep Blacks in the inferior, dependent, and helpless role" (p. 33). He characterized these "microaggressions" as pervading African Americans' daily life experiences and as being especially prevalent in the media.

Some studies (Greenberg and Dervin 1972; Greenberg and Dominick 1969) have indicated that African American and other minority children spend more time watching television than do nonminority children. The importance here is that many minority children will, from the cradle, come to learn much of their value system and potential for the future from a medium rife with negative stereotypes of African Americans. Television often presents African Americans as ragingly violent and out of control, as well as undependable, unintelligent, and incapable of holding leadership positions. Therefore, many African American children are "acculturated" by the media in a way that separates them from the possibility of achieving the same future open to nonminority children.

On the other hand, many African American children appear not to be affected adversely by the negative portrayal of black people on television. Although aware of the broader society's devaluation of African Americans, some children from this group have been able to make a distinction between the view held by the broader society and their perception of themselves (Norton 1983; Powell 1974; Rosenberg and Simmons 1972; Spurlock 1986). The positive role models that exist in African American communities serve to reinforce a positive concept of blackness. Unfortunately, these positive role models are often overlooked by mental health service providers, teachers, and others who provide services for children, because they do not meet middle-class criteria (Taylor 1976).

Absence of Fathers

The absence of the child's biological father need not yield disastrous consequences, as many have been led to believe. In a study that was conducted in the 1970s (Wilkinson and O'Connor 1977), the investigators observed adolescent males, who were reared in single-parent, female-headed families, to be achievement oriented; the amount of antisocial activity was minimal. Herzog and Lewis (1970) posited that

> Father absence is only one among an interacting complex of factors which mediate and condition its impact on a growing child . . . even if eventually a significant association can be demonstrated between father absence and one of the adverse affects attributed to it, that impact is dwarfed by other factors of interacting couples. (pp. 381–382)

In a study of family structure of inner-city African American residents and the mental health of their children (Kellam et al. 1977), the investigators determined that "the absence of the father was less important than the aloneness of the mother in relation to risk [of emotional disturbance in her children]" (p. 1012). A parallel finding pertained to the importance of other adults in the household or community, and the supportive role undertaken by that person (or persons)—often the maternal grandmother. The following story illustrates these findings.

> A teenage girl and her younger brother were separated from their father when they were 6 and 4 years of age, respectively. The initial separation came about with the dissolution of the parents' marriage and the father's move to another city. Early on, the emotional ties between the father and his children were regularly maintained by summer visits, letters, and telephone communications.

However, some 3 years later, contact became erratic when the father was hospitalized following a psychotic break.

The children responded with heightened depressive behaviors and brief episodes of regressive behavior. The support provided by the extended family, which had been helpful throughout the life of these youngsters, was especially helpful at the time of this crisis. Their maternal uncles who had served as significant father surrogates from time to time made themselves more available to the children. Other relatives were supportive to the family in a variety of ways.

The church must be included in the support system that benefited this family. Various church programs provided the mother and her children the opportunity to be benefactors; for example, they participated in the preparation and serving of Thanksgiving dinners for the elderly in the community in which the church is located. Such efforts are commonplace in many pockets of African American communities. Several staff members of a community mental health center had been another source of support for this family. Although contact had been brief, the mother had received guidance as to how to discuss their father's illness with the children.

The reader may ask, of what significance is the racial identity of the aforementioned family? Are there specific cultural factors that played a role in their being able to overcome adverse circumstances? We learned that both parents had been involved in African American activities since their college days and that they had instilled a positive sense of their African heritage in their children. The children had been brought up to be knowledgeable about racial discrimination and to be achievement-oriented and mindful of the roles they might play in the determination of their future. The children had been taught about the importance of the extended family, which they came to know as a common characteristic of their culture. The culture of "broken families" was reflected in the decline of their financial standing, which took another dip with the onset of the father's illness. For the most part, the "blackness" of this family had been "colored" positive.

Other African American children who have "lost" a father have not fared so well. Sometimes their misfortunes have been compounded by negative self-image, which has become associated with their racial identity and the particular culture of their immediate family and neighborhood. The frequent comings and goings of the men in a mother's life can be accounted for, in part, by a negative sense of self, coupled with a need for male companionship. The development of a relationship between her child or children and her companion is often thwarted in its beginning by the departure of this hoped-for father figure. The repetition of such an experience reinforces distrust and difficulties in establishing meaningful relationships. For example, a child may hide the pain of disappointment generated by a series of separations from father surrogates with antisocial behavior. Many of the youngsters we have evaluated because of their disruptive behavior in the classroom, on the school playgrounds, and at home have such a history.

Poverty, Violence, and Losses

According to a report of the U.S. Department of Justice (1983), blacks are victims of violent crimes more often than any other ethnic or racial group. Within many inner-city communities, deaths of African Americans have become a crisis of emergency proportions. African Americans have a higher mortality rate in every age group, beginning in infancy. The rate of white infant mortality in the United States in 1987 was 8.6 infant deaths per 1,000 live births; for blacks, it was 18.0 infant deaths per 1,000 live births ("Black and white death rates continue to differ" 1989). There are a number of factors that impede the delivery of healthy African American children, foremost among them poor prenatal care, early adolescent pregnancies, inadequate prenatal diets, and substance abuse during pregnancy.

Many of these factors are directly related to poverty. As Lawrence (1975) noted:

> An infant born in poverty in the Harlem community has a strong chance of being born prematurely, or, even if he achieves full term birth, he may be so small that the physical component of his ego is impaired. His mother may have been malnourished during her pregnancy, or ill without medical care, or an addict, and her child can be born small, weak, and addicted to a habit-forming drug. These are some of the reasons for the high incidence of minimal brain dysfunction or development lags, diagnoses which we often used in describing impaired "nature" in Harlem children. (pp. 33–34)

This analysis of issues affecting Harlem-born children can be extended to include minority communities throughout the United States.

According to a 1989 report ("Fatal shootings among youth are studied" 1989), 1 in 10 people in the United States who die before age 20 are killed by a gun. This weapon is associated with more than 40% of the deaths of young African American males, compared with 16% of the deaths of young white males. Homicide committed by peers of like culture is a leading cause of death of African American men between the ages of 15 and 44. These deaths represent fathers, husbands, sons, brothers, and friends, and the impact of these losses is felt beyond the immediate family and the local inner-city community. These deaths represent assaults on the psychological stability of the community, on its residents' sense of comfort and safety, and on the potential aspirations and development of the community's children.

In recent years, we have noted a difference in the manner in which young African American people are experiencing these deaths. In some individuals, there appears to be a dampening of affect with respect to loss, while others seem to minimize the value of life and danger through provocative behaviors. These attitudes were verbalized by a 15-year-old youth, who had been referred to one of us for a psychiatric evaluation. He had been arrested for seriously assaulting another boy who had bumped into him. This young man had been arrested on several other occasions, all for assaults. When questioned by the examiner about the nature of his response to the incident, he replied that his actions were justified. When pressed further, he noted that the potential danger of his action was never a concern. He related his knowledge of others who had been sent to jail or who had been killed; he fully expected to be sent to jail and said, "If I die, I die."

Clearly, this young man evidenced a hopelessness about his future—a hopelessness that constantly affected his relationships with other people. Although he did not outwardly show anxiety, it appeared that he may have, at all times, been at a resting level of panic.

Bowlby (1982) has defined defensive exclusion "as a defense against being aware of signals, arising from both inside and outside the [people themselves], that would activate their attachment behavior and that could enable them both to love and to experience being loved" (p. 674). We question whether or not this is happening with youngsters who now find themselves and their communities in a constant siege of terror. A reaction-formation defense mechanism becomes evident as these children take greater and greater risks.

Children who have been exposed to violence, especially when they themselves have been abused, are likely to be at increased risk for suicide (Green 1978). Heacock (1990) refers to a study (Kirk and Zuckor 1979) that tested the hypothesis that there is a high incidence of depression and diminished black consciousness and group cohesiveness in the suicidal African American population. Findings supported only that part of the hypothesis that pertained to a low level of black consciousness. Bell (1986) noted that there is a high incidence of head and brain injuries in segments of the African American community and called for investigative studies to determine the relationship between central nervous system injury and violence in these communities.

Conclusion

Separations and losses for African American children are intertwined with this country's history. The untoward effects of these losses were noted in reports from the literature, as well as in the reported findings of mental health practitioners. More frequently than not, separation from and loss of parents appear to be rooted, directly or indirectly, in the prejudicial attitudes of the broader society (e.g., the practices of slavery; unemployment and underemployment of African American men; and destructive behavior stemming from despair, which often is the result of society's efforts to forestall upward mobility of African American people). Attention was also directed to the losses that accompany poverty as well as upward mobility.

It was recognized that African American children, like children of other racial and cultural backgrounds, may differ significantly in their response to trauma, and that factors other than racial and cultural background must be considered in an assessment of any child. On the other hand, a clinician should not disregard specific cultural factors that may have had an impact on the child and her or his family.

Although there was discussion of children who have coped with adverse circumstances reasonably well, it was recognized that more intensive and extensive studies of resilient children are warranted. Separations and losses are inherent in living; knowledge of the development of self-confidence and mastery will allow for the promotion of resilience in all children who are under stress.

References

Bell CC: Coma and the etiology of violence, part I. J Natl Med Assoc 78(12):1167–1176, 1986

Black and white deaths continue to differ. The New York Times, September 27, 1989, p A20

Bowlby J: Attachment and loss: retrospect and prospect. Am J Orthopsychiatry 52(4):664–678, 1982

Burlingham D, Freud A: Infants Without Families. New York, International University Press, 1944

Fatal shootings among youth are studied. The New York Times, October 29, 1989

Furman E: Studies in childhood bereavement. Can J Psychiatry 28(4);241–247, 1983

Green AH: Self destructive behavior in battered children. Am J Psychiatry 135(5):579–582, 1978

Greenberg BS, Dervin B: Use of the Mass Media by the Urban Poor. New York, Praeger, 1972

Greenberg BS, Dominick JR: Racial and social class differences in teenagers' use of television. Journal of Broadcasting 13:331–334, 1969

Haynes E: Two million Negro Americans at work. The Southern Workman 51:64–72, 1922

Haynes E: Negroes in domestic service in the United States. Journal of Negro History 8:384–442, 1923

Heacock DR: Suicidal behavior in Black and Hispanic youth. Psychiatric Annals 20(3):134–142, 1990

Herzog E, Lewis H: Children in poor families: myths and realities. Am J Orthopsychiatry 40(3):375–387, 1970

Kellam SG, Ensminger ME, Turner RJ: Family structure and the mental health of children: concurrent and longitudinal community-wide studies. Arch Gen Psychiatry 34(a):1012–1022, 1977

Kirk AR, Zuckor RA: Some sociological factors in attempted suicide among urban black males. Suicide Life Threat Behav 9:76–86, 1979

Lawrence MM: Young Inner City Families: Development of Ego Strength Under Stress. New York, Behavioral Publications, 1975

Looff D: Sociocultural factors in etiology, in Basic Handbook of Child Psychiatry, Vol II. Edited by Noshpitz JD. New York, Basic Books, 1979, pp 87–99

Morrison T: The Bluest Eye. New York, Pocket Books, 1970

Norris D, Bell A: Success: psychological conflict for black Americans. Paper presented at the annual meeting of the American Psychiatric Association, Dallas, TX, May 1985

Norton DG: Black family life patterns, the development of self, and cognitive development of black children, in The Psychosocial Development of Minority Group Children. Edited by Powell GJ. New York, Brunner/Mazel, 1983, pp 181–193

Pierce CM: Stress in the workplace, in Black Families in Crisis: The Middle Class. Edited by Coner-Edwards AF, Spurlock J. New York, Brunner/Mazel, 1988, pp 27–34

Powell GJ: Self-concept in white and black children, in Racism and Mental Health: Essays. Edited by Willie CV, Kramer BM, Brown BS. Pittsburgh, PA, University of Pittsburgh Press, 1974

Rainwater L: Behind Ghetto Walls. Chicago, IL, Aldine Publications, 1970

Robertson J: A two-year old goes to the hospital (film). New York, New York University Film Library, 1952

Rosenberg M, Simmons RG: Black and White Self-Esteem: The Urban School Child. Washington, DC, American Sociological Association, 1972

Sekaer C: Toward a definition of childhood mourning. Am J Psychother 41(2):201–219, 1987

Spitz R: Hospitalism: an inquiry into the genesis of psychiatric conditions in early childhood. Psychoanal Study Child 1:53–74, 1945

Spitz R: Anaclitic depression. Psychoanal Study Child 2:313–342, 1946

Spurlock J: Assessment and therapeutic intervention of black children. Journal of the American Academy of Child Psychiatry 24(2):168–174, 1985

Spurlock J: Development of self-concept in Afro-American children. Hosp Community Psychiatry 37(1):66–70, 1986

Spurlock J, Booth MB: Stresses in parenting, in Black Families in Crisis: The Middle Class. Edited by Coner-Edwards AF, Spurlock J. New York, Brunner/Mazel, 1988, pp 79–89

Spurlock J, Lawrence LE: The black child, in Basic Handbook of Child Psychiatry, Vol I. Edited by Noshpitz JD. New York, Basic Books, 1979, pp 248–257

Taylor RL: Psychosocial development among black children and youth: a reexamination. Am J Orthopsychiatry 46:4–19, 1976

U.S. Department of Justice: Report to the Nation on Crime and Justice. Washington, DC, U.S. Government Printing Office, 1983

Wilkinson CB, O'Connor WA: Growing up male in a black single-parent family. Psychiatric Annals 7(7):50–59, 1977

8 Psychiatric Care of American Indians and Alaska Natives

James W. Thompson, M.D., M.P.H.
R. Dale Walker, M.D.
Patricia Silk-Walker, R.N., Ph.C.

Background Information

American Indian and Alaska Native People

This chapter deals with mental illness and its treatment in people who are descendants of the pre-Columbian inhabitants of North America, including Alaska. Native Hawaiians are not included, although this population is equally deserving of the title "Native American." Census reports have revealed that there are 1.4 million American Indian, Eskimo, and Aleut people in the United States (U.S. Bureau of the Census 1983), 312,765 native Indians and Inuit in Canada (Statistics Canada 1981), and an estimated 4 million Indians in Mexico (Weil 1975). Although these groups are enormously diverse, we will use the designation "Indian" to refer to all American Indian, Alaska Native, and Canadian and Mexican Indian people. "Pre-Columbian" and "precontact" refer to the time before Europeans "discovered" the North American continent, usually dated as 1492, although it had clearly been "discovered" long before (Gaddis 1977; Snow 1979). (An outline of significant dates and periods in the recent history of American Indians and Alaska Natives is presented in Table 18–6.)

Although it is not known exactly how many precontact tribal groups existed in the United States, the usual number cited is approximately 300

To be consistent with terminology used throughout this book, the term "white" is substituted in this chapter for "Caucasian." However, "Caucasian" is considered a less value-laden term by the authors of this chapter, who recommend using this term in the clinical setting.

(Walker and LaDue 1986), with many subdivisions within tribal groups. However, the modern notion of a "tribe" as a centralized political system, with firm geographic boundaries and a common culture and language, is a European conception (Berkhofer 1978). Indian peoples of the Americas spoke more than 1,000 distinct languages (McNickle 1975), derived from 56 language families (Powell 1966). Some of these languages were written, but many were not. Most were destroyed by European conquerors in the name of "civilization" (Walker and LaDue 1986).

The diversity among Indians is enormous (Sturtevant 1978ff; Wauchope 1964–1969). Levine and Lurie (1970) pointed out that the differences in the backgrounds of two Indian people might be greater than the differences between two Europeans from different countries. Tribes that were geographically separated had little in common, and tribes that were geographically close often had quite different cultures and traditions. Deculturation (the loss of traditional ways) and reculturation (the assumption of the ways of the majority), as well as intermingling among tribes, has today blurred some of the differences, but it would be a great mistake to assume that either the cultures or the psychopathologies of Indian people are all the same.

Countries of Origin

It is believed that Indian people migrated from Asia over a land bridge at the Bering Strait during a recent ice age. The time of the westward migration is usually accepted as 20,000 to 27,000 years ago (Snow 1979; Walker and LaDue 1986), although much earlier dates have been proposed (Gaddis 1977). There is other evidence to indicate a migration from the east, over the Atlantic Ocean. The creation myths of many tribes (including the Sioux, the Delaware, and the pre-Inca Chimus) speak of a sea arrival from the direction of the rising sun (Gaddis 1977). Still other evidence has been advanced to support the theory that modern *homo sapiens* originated in the Americas, with the migration being from the New World to the Old (Goodman 1981). In guiding study in this area, Snow (1979) cautioned that works on the prehistory of Indians published prior to 1970 should be avoided as inaccurate and recommended books by Forbis (1975) and Jennings (1978) for historic reference.

The Precontact Period

Before the coming of the Europeans, there were two large geographic areas that were largely occupied by Indians who practiced farming (Dobyns

1983; McNickle 1975). One of these areas followed the Rocky Mountains. The other area occupied the eastern half of the United States from the Gulf of Mexico to Canada. In most other sections, hunting and gathering was the predominant subsistence activity. Southern Mexico was dominated by empire builders and city-states. In addition, before Europeans arrived, groups of Indian people were on the move. The Apache, for example, historically traveled from Alaska and Canada to Arizona. Only during the last several thousand years did Indian people become distributed as they were when the first Europeans stepped on shore.

Walker and LaDue (1986) reviewed the precontact period with regard to medical treatment. They pointed out that there are commonalities in the beliefs and traditions of many Indian peoples, but their differences are also profound. For example, the language, appearance, and beliefs of the Eskimo are very much like those of their Siberian ancestors; the people of the Eastern Seaboard have an appearance closer to that of their European conquerors, but have a culture that is different from either that of Europeans or other Indian peoples. The clinician who seeks to understand Indian history and traditional beliefs faces a task as awesome as learning what is usually referred to in American schools as "world history." The most the clinician can hope for is to understand some of the history and beliefs of the tribes with whose members he or she is working. Having done this, however, he or she will be much better prepared to relate to Indian patients, understand their problems, and deal effectively with their psychopathology.

The Postcontact Period

Although some of the early contacts between Indians and Europeans were quite positive (Penn 1683/1970), they were, by far, the exception. As Berkhofer (1978) stated, "White hopes for the exploitation of Indians and their lands certainly shaped their perceptions of Native Americans from the very beginning of contact. . . . Images of the good Indian suggested the ease of exploitation . . . " (p. 118). Simultaneously, the image of the "savage" Indian rationalized European conquest. Berkhofer discusses the functions of these contradictory images at length and points out that the images still exist today.

At contact, there were several million Indian people. However, during the holocaust period for Indians (from about 1500 A.D. to 1900 A.D.), several factors led to their near-extermination. One was disease. Europeans brought with them infectious diseases for which Indian people were not prepared immunologically (Dobyns 1983). Lawson (1986) estimates that five-sixths of some Indian populations were killed by early epidemics. Walker and LaDue (1986) pointed out that leaders and other elders also died, leaving many communities without leadership. The power and leadership of the medicine men and women were also greatly reduced, because they could do little to effect cures for diseases about which they had no knowledge. Later epidemics were equally devastating. It has been argued that disease, rather than the superiority of European military power, resulted in the near-annihilation of Indian people (Dobyns 1983). Disease and military conquest were not totally separate threats, however; some of the epidemics resulted from deliberately providing Indians with infected blankets as "gifts," an early form of germ warfare (Vogel 1972).

Another factor leading to the near-extermination of Indian groups in the United States was the federal government's policy to move Indians out of areas desired by white settlers. These forced relocations, which still occur for Indians (O'Sullivan and Handal 1988), resulted in many Indian deaths (Berkhofer 1978; Brown 1971; de Tocqueville 1835/1975; Vogel 1972). Another mechanism of removal was simply to send in the cavalry to destroy a community (Brown 1971).

Alcohol was another factor in the Indian holocaust. Very early, it became clear that Indian people were susceptible to the effects of ethanol. The provision of whiskey to Indians thus became an easy way to "buy" land and otherwise take advantage of Indian people (Berkhofer 1978). In addition, alcohol led to disability and death for many.

The introduction of Christian religion and a forced removal of Indian children from their families in the name of education were central to the near-annihilation of Indian people, not in body, but in spirit. From earliest contact, Europeans were totally unwilling to accept Indian religious beliefs and were determined to stamp out "pagan" thought and practices and to Christianize the "heathen" Indians (Vogel 1972). This was not too difficult a task once the leadership, the culture, and the medicine people were destroyed or discredited (Walker and LaDue 1986). Many Indian people were comforted to have something to fill the spiritual void. In so doing, however, they were often forced to drop the last vestiges of their traditional culture and adopt European history and custom as their own.

Just as devastating as the introduction of Christian religion was the insistence by the conquerors that Indian children be schooled in European traditions. Children were taken from their families and placed in residential boarding schools intended to teach Indian children to be "white" (Coolidge 1977; Meriam 1977). They were severely punished for speaking their native languages or doing anything remotely "Indian." (Driver 1969, p. 492; Goldstein 1974) The psychological sequelae were profoundly negative for generations of Indian children (Kleinfeld and Bloom 1977).

The last 100 years have been referred to as the "assimilation era" (Walker and LaDue 1986). Primarily during this century, the overt policy of extermination of Indian people was changed into a more subtle one of absorbing the Indian into mainstream society. The Dawes Act of 1887 stipulated that communally owned (Indian) lands be divided into individual "allotments" of land to own and farm (Debo 1970). As was the case many times before, much of this land found its way into the hands of non-Indians, often by fraud (Berkhofer 1978; Brown 1971; Debo 1984). On reservations—often remote areas to which the remnants of many tribes had been relocated—disease and starvation were common. In effect, the official policy of the federal government during this era was "become assimilated, or die" (Neihardt 1961).

The history just presented remains very much in the minds of contemporary Indian people and has profoundly shaped their worldview. However, present day non-Indians know little of this history. Vogel (1972) recounted the ways in which American history textbooks have created or perpetuated false impressions about Indian people and their history. He remarked that although the genocidal aims of non-Indian America toward the Indian fell short of complete accomplishment, "the historical obliteration of the Indian was more nearly successful"; American history textbooks "obliterate, defame, disembody, or disparage" Indian people (Vogel 1972, pp. 284–285). To most Americans, Indians no longer exist. When non-Indians meet an Indian, often the first question is, "How much Indian are you?" Any answer of less than 100% (blood quantum) is met with an expression of satisfaction that, indeed, "real" Indians no longer exist. This "nonperson" status profoundly affects the Indian person's self-perception.

The Indian Health Service

One of the few federal government policies in the United States that has benefited Indian people was the development of the Indian Health Service (IHS). The government's responsibility for providing health care for Indians is a principle derived from many treaties with the tribes—possibly the only treaty obligation that has been kept.

The provision of health care to Indians is considered by many to be the oldest prepaid health care system in the United States. From the early 1800s until 1849, the Bureau of Indian Affairs (BIA), which included Indian health care in its purview, was under the auspices of the U.S. War Department. In

1849, the BIA was transferred to the U.S. Department of Interior. Within 25 years, health care was made much more available, with half of Indian Agencies having a physician (Public Health Service 1957). In the 1880s, formal health care was made available to children in boarding schools and became more generally available by 1900. In 1903, the BIA opened a psychiatric hospital, but it was closed in 1933. Patients were then transferred to state hospitals and to St. Elizabeth's in Washington, DC (Public Health Service 1957).

The IHS was formed in 1955 as a component of the U.S. Public Health Service, partially because the health status of Indians had remained poor. All responsibility for Indian health care was transferred from the BIA to the IHS. The IHS has had considerable success in reducing infant and perinatal mortality and the incidence and prevalence of infectious disease (Indian Health Service 1989a). As these acute general medical conditions have improved, however, it has become apparent that psychiatric conditions are a major problem in many Indian populations.

The IHS has done much less well in combating psychiatric illnesses and their sequelae. Treatment of these illnesses is split between a "mental health" program and an "alcoholism" program, which are often competitive rather than coordinated. Further, neither program is well coordinated with the general health care system, although the IHS has been making efforts in this direction (C. Vanderwagen, Indian Health Service, Rockville, MD, personal communication, May 1989). Both the mental health and alcohol programs are sparsely staffed and are so decentralized that effective planning, evaluation, and quality control are difficult to maintain at best. The programs are chronically underfunded and in many cases are run by minimally trained personnel. Bettering these programs so that they can help to improve the psychiatric status of Indian people is among the greatest challenges for the IHS.

Compared with the United States or Mexico, Canada historically has had better success in providing health and mental health services to its Indian population, although some would disagree with this assertion (Cardinal 1969). As residents of a province or territory, Indians are entitled to benefits of medical care and hospital insurance. These benefits are supplemented by the Native Health and Welfare Department, which provides transportation, medication, and comprehensive public health services. In addition, a network of 200 health facilities provides services to Indians, and a native alcohol abuse program funds locally run services (Statistics Canada 1981). Some authors maintain that health services provided to Canadian Indians are far superior to those provided to Indians in the United States (Driver 1969).

In Mexico, there is a complex system of private and public health care, which is theoretically available to all. However, in rural areas, where most Indians live, there is a serious problem with availability of health care. There is heavy reliance by Indians on native healers (*curanderos*) and herb dealers (*yerberos*), as there is throughout Mexico, but many Indians use these practitioners to the near-exclusion of Western medical care (Weil 1975).

Current Distribution and Demographics

Although most states have substantial Indian communities, the majority of the Indian population in the United States presently lives in California, Oklahoma, New Mexico, Arizona, Alaska, North Carolina, and Washington (U.S. Bureau of the Census 1983). In 1980, 52% of American Indians lived in urban areas and 48% in rural areas. A total of 643,000 Indian people lived on 277 U.S. reservations, most of which are rural, and 50,000 Alaska Natives lived in 209 native villages (U.S. Bureau of the Census 1983).

In Canada, the Indian population is much more evenly distributed, with Ontario and British Columbia having the largest Indian populations. Sixty-four percent of Canadian Indians live on reserves, 28% are off reserves, and the remainder are on "crown land" (Statistics Canada 1981).

About one-half of Mexicans are of predominantly Indian extraction, but few identify themselves as Indian. Most Indians who identify themselves as such live in one of three regions: the central plateau, the south Pacific coastal area, and the Gulf Coast (Weil 1975).

It is important to distinguish population distribution per se from tribal distribution. In some states or provinces in North America, a tribe or a group of unrelated tribes, such as the Navajo, Hopi, and Pueblo peoples, may live in the same geographic area because of the presence of reservations or reserves. In other states or provinces, there are rural Indian communities but no reservations. These communities, such as many in Alaska, may be made up of single tribes or may consist of members of diverse tribes, such as many communities in Oklahoma. In urban areas, Indian people may be from a great variety of tribal backgrounds living in loosely defined communities; or they may be largely homogeneous, such as the Lumbee in Baltimore, Maryland, and the Chippewa in cities in Minnesota.

These geographic patterns can contribute greatly to the differences in the already diverse Indian population. For example, in urban areas in the United States, there tends to be more deculturation and assimilation into majority society then on reservations. Such factors may result in a very different character and distribution of mental disorders among Indians.

The 1980 census profiled the Indian population of the United States as shown in Table 8–1.

Epidemiology and Other Studies

Epidemiology is concerned with the character and distribution of disease in a population and the etiology of illness (Kleinbaum et al. 1982). Therefore, it is appropriate in this section to discuss both the distribution and the etiology of mental disorders in Indian people. It is tempting, given the history of Indian people over the last 500 years, to attribute much of the psychopathology in the group to this historical experience. Many have in fact used this reasoning to explain high rates of alcoholism, depression, and suicide in some Indian groups. However, although cultural factors are important in the expression of illness, some scholars question whether cul-

Table 8–1. Population characteristics of American Indian and white people in the United States, 1980

Population characteristic	American Indians[d]	Whites
Percent under 20 years of age[a]	43.8%	30.3%
Percent age 65 and over[a]	5.3%	12.2%
Median age in years[a]	22.8	31.3
Percent of men 15 and older presently married[a]	49.6%	62.5%
Percent of women 15 and older presently married[a]	48.0%	57.4%
Median household income in dollars[b]	$12,256.00	$17,680.00
Mean years of formal education (age 25 and older)[c]	9.6	10.9
Percent of families below poverty line[b]	23.7%	7.0%
Percent of households that are family households[b]	82.0%	73.0%
Percent of family households consisting of a married couple with children[b]	43.0%	30.0%
Mean household size[b]	3.28	2.60

[a] U.S. Bureau of the Census 1983.
[b] Sandefur and Sakamoto 1988.
[c] Manson et al. 1987.
[d] Census data on American Indians has long been considered suspect. Passel and Berman (1986) in general note underreporting of American Indians, but with some selective over-reporting.

ture-related factors should ever be regarded as causative of mental disorders (Graves 1970; Levy and Kunitz 1974). It is important to continue to search for more basic underlying processes rather than to rely on "cultural" explanations.

Other etiologic explanations of mental disorders are the stress of reservation or urban ghetto living, being caught between two cultures, and the removal of traditional culture per se. We believe, however, that the most parsimonious explanation of the etiology mental disorder in Indian groups is that mental disorder in Indian people is caused by the same factors as in non-Indians. This is not to minimize the importance of cultural factors in determining the expression of illness; rather, we propose that the causes of psychopathology in Indian people are more similar to the majority culture than they are dissimilar. In the absence of empiric evidence to the contrary, we will assume that this is the case.

Definition of Mental Disorder

We define mental disorder as a group of diseases, using the dictionary definition of disease as "a condition in which bodily health is impaired." Implicit here is the assumption that the mind and spirit are an integral part of the body. The origin of the mental disorder may be in the brain, in another part of the body, in the external environment, or in a combination of these (such as in alcoholism).

Mental disorder leads to problems in the way the mind experiences or reacts to the person's internal milieu or to the environment. These difficulties can be entirely internal, or between the person and others, or in relationship to societal norms. The problems must be severe enough to warrant intervention or treatment by a healer. For example, a simple problem in living with little resulting disability would not qualify as a mental disorder. Nor would a problem between the person and society (e.g., crime) be a mental disorder, unless it resulted from a difficulty within the mind in experiencing or reacting either to the person's environment or internal milieu (e.g., a psychosis).

Services Utilization Data

Much of the literature about mental disorder in Indian people consists of reports on service utilization, a poor substitute for true prevalence data. Rhoades and colleagues (1980) collected data on visits during 1975 to outpatient general medical facilities run by the IHS. They did not include data from mental health or alcoholism programs. The data were analyzed by age group, an important factor to consider in any study of Indians, because the individual Indian population is young compared with the majority population. Unfortunately, Rhoades and colleagues calculated rates using the IHS service population rather than total outpatient visits to the IHS. Comparing visits with population tends to overstate rates, because many visits may be made by the same patient. It should also be noted that the IHS service population includes few urban Indians and no members of federally "unrecognized" tribes.

Rhoades and colleagues (1980) found that the highest visit rates were in the 20-to-54 age group, for alcoholism and neurosis (largely depression). The 40-to-44 age group had the highest rates for both of these conditions, with 10% having had a visit for alcoholism and 11% for neurosis. All ages taken together had visit rates of 3% for alcoholism, 0.1% for organic brain syndromes, 0.8% for schizophrenia, 4% for neurosis, 0.2% for personality disorder, and 0.3% for drug abuse.

May (1988) did a 10-year chart review in the Albuquerque Area of the IHS. This study is perhaps the only trend analysis of both inpatient and outpatient visits for psychiatric disorder by Indian people. Both the IHS general medical records and the records of the IHS mental health programs were reviewed. In the general medical charts, alcohol abuse headed the list of episodes, followed by drug overdose, conversion reaction, adjustment disorder in adolescence, and anxiety. The most common disorders in mental health program charts were marital problems, alcohol abuse, adjustment disorder in adolescence, depression, and parent-child problems.

Neligh (1988b) reviewed data on 17,044 visits to the Billings Area IHS mental health program, and noted that more than half of the visits were coded with V codes (i.e., conditions not attributable to a mental disorder that are the focus of attention or treatment). Neligh suggested that the staff used the V codes so often because they were reluctant to stigmatize patients. We surmise that this coding was probably also a reflection of personnel who are not educated in making a DSM-III-R (American Psychiatric Association 1987) diagnosis. In the 6,802 visits for which a DSM-III-R diagnosis, rather than a V code, was reported, 18% were for alcohol dependence, 14% for major depressive disorder, 12% for adjustment disorder, and 10% for personality disorder. These were followed by anxiety/hysteria (8%), nondependent use of drugs (6%), and schizophrenia (6%). All depressive disorders and suicide-related visits taken together accounted for 20% of visits, and all alcohol- and drug-related visits accounted for 26% of visits. (The latter figure is impressive in that it does not include visits to the alcohol programs per se.) Bipolar disorder accounted for 2% of visits. As Neligh has cautioned, service usage data should not be viewed as indicative of community prevalence.

Epidemiologic Data

There have been only three published community epidemiologic studies of Indians. Roy and colleagues (1970) reported on disorders among the Indians of Saskatchewan, whereas Shore and colleagues (1973) studied a U.S. Indian village and Sampath (1974) an Eskimo community. These relatively small studies do not paint a comprehensive or representative picture of mental disorder in Indian people, although they have been helpful in obtaining an overall view of one community. More recently, epidemiologic studies have focused on a particular disorder, across several tribal groups or communities. This more recent epidemiologic literature is covered in a later section on psychopathology in this chapter.

Evaluation of Existing Data

Some of the continuing stereotypes about Indian people (e.g., that all Indian groups have high alcoholism and suicide rates) are fostered in part by the scientific literature. Studies are still published that make much of very few cases (e.g., Spaulding 1985–1986). The IHS continues to report national Indian data from the National Center for Health Statistics (Indian Health Service 1989a) that are then widely quoted as being representative of all Indians.

There is a very real problem in assembling meaningful data on any Indian health condition. Collecting data from many tribes means that several diverse groups are being combined into one questionably meaningful group. Collection of data from a smaller but culturally homogeneous group, however, means that the incidence and prevalence rates for most conditions will be derived from only a few cases, yielding data of questionable statistical significance or epidemiologic utility.

Another problem in interpreting data is in the operational definition of who is an Indian. For the IHS, Indians are only those who live in the 32 "reservation states" where the IHS provides services (Indian Health Service 1989a). Only these groups are reported in IHS statistics. Some tribes are not "recognized" by the federal government and, therefore, are not included in most statistics. Another complicating factor is that some tribes impose a blood quantum on their membership, while others do not, meaning that tribal membership is subject to great variability. Blood quantum is by itself an insufficient measure of "Indianness." It should be noted, however, that there may be genetic and age-cohort effects of high blood quantum, and there is a tendency for high–blood quantum individuals to be more traditional in their beliefs.

There are other biases in the collection of data on Indians. For example, selective underreporting for Indians may occur in urban areas, where Indians may be mistaken for other racial groups. On the other hand, in rural areas there may be a *relative* overreporting of some health-related events for Indians compared with whites. There is no other population more counted and scrutinized then rural Indians, especially with regard to such events as suicide—perhaps leading to accurate reporting for Indians, whereas there is underreporting for whites (Harras 1987).

There also is clearly a bias in the reporting of census data on Indians. There was an undercount of Indians in the 1970 census, and a more accurate count in the 1980 census (Indian Health Service 1989a; Passel and Berman 1986). In fact, there may have been an overreporting of Indian people in the 1980 census, although this seems to have been confined to "non-Indian" states (Passel and Berman 1986). To the extent that there was a 1970 undercount, rates for disorders would be inflated when the denominators are from 1970 census data. Similarly, a 1980 census overcount would decrease rates.

Another problem in assessing data on Indians is that little of it deals with the level of acculturation (i.e., deculturation from native culture and reculturation into majority culture). It is not clear whether acculturation increases or decreases rates of particular psychiatric disorders, changes their presentation, or has other effects. Also, the assumption may not be valid that all members of a family, community, tribe, or reservation are similarly acculturated.

The clinician should be wary of approaching diagnosis and treatment of Indian people based on currently available statistics. Prospective, longitudinal studies are needed, with sound methodology and thoughtfully chosen comparison groups. Until such literature is available, caution in the use of currently available data is advised.

Need for Psychiatric Care

Determining the need for psychiatric care among Indian people has been hampered by differences concerning what the focus of care should be. Competing camps may define the "basic problem" as mental illness, substance abuse, problems in living (e.g., stress, grief, adjustment reactions), or social and economic difficulties. Undoubtedly, all of these problems are worthy of attention, but, as we noted earlier, Indian health programs have never been adequately funded, making the setting of priorities necessary. Congress, through its funding mechanisms, has de facto set the priority as alcoholism treatment programs, which have a much larger budget than that for non-substance abuse mental health care. Little of the care given in the alcohol programs could be accurately described as "psychiatric," because service is largely provided by people who are themselves recovering from alcoholism and who have no formal health education or special psychiatric training. One well-informed commentator (Levy 1988) has, in fact, expressed the opinion that the IHS alcohol programs are not treatment programs but are, rather, tribal employment programs. The IHS is quite aware of the need to increase the quality and training of its alcoholism treatment staff and to increase its salary levels to attract such personnel (C. Vanderwagen, Indian Health Service, Rockville, MD, personal communication, May 1989).

The IHS mental health program (which excludes substance abuse) is much smaller than the alcohol program. Within local mental health services, problems in living have often been the focus. There is no doubt that major efforts are made by nonprofessionals to provide care. But because these staff persons have little or no formal professional preparation, they simply do not know how to deal with complex psychiatric issues, meaning that problems in living receive most clinical attention.

In the setting of priorities for Indian psychiatric care, we put our vote firmly in favor of active clinical treatment of serious mental illness (including substance abuse), delivered by highly trained professionals who can apply the best psychiatric technology available. Clinical treatment services have been successful in reducing morbidity and mortality in the majority culture, and there is every reason to believe that these services would be successful in Indian communities. The often stated belief that clinical services delivered by highly trained professionals "don't work" with Indian people is vacuous. Such services have seldom been tried, or when tried have been underfunded, understaffed, and/or delivered with little cultural sensitivity. Neither has there been any follow-up of these or any other services delivered to Indian people to judge the efficacy of such services. It is important that the professional who works with Indian people or helps plan their care not accept such myths as fact but instead insist on the provision of quality psychiatric care by psychiatrists and other highly trained mental health professionals.

Prevention

Although prevention programs are currently the vogue in Indian country, most have never proven successful (Neligh 1988a; Silk-Walker et al. 1988). This is especially true of primary prevention (which often travels under the name of "health promotion" or "promoting positive mental health"). Simply stated, there is no evidence that improving the overall quality of life in an Indian community, making people happier, or improving their self-concept prevents mental disorder. There are severely limited resources available for psychiatric care for Indians. These limited resources can be spent on unfocused primary prevention programs, for which there is no evidence of effectiveness; or they can be used to buy treatment and rehabilitation personnel and services that we know *do* work. The only potentially effective strategy for primary prevention is the identification of risk factors for specific mental disorders, leading to focused interventions to reduce such risk factors. Even such focused strategies, however, have shown few positive results in psychiatry.

Although primary prevention is not currently useful in Indian psychiatric care, many of the principles of public health are highly useful. These include the identification of individuals with early symptoms of particular disorders, clinical intervention with these persons (secondary prevention), and aftercare services to decrease the reoccurrence of illness (tertiary prevention).

With regard to the public health approach, the clinician should not make the mistake of equating the Public Health Service (the agency containing the IHS) with a such an approach. The IHS, for all its good work, is oriented toward acute primary care of nonpsychiatric medical illness, not toward chronic illnesses or psychiatric illnesses. Because chronic illnesses and psychiatric illnesses are major problems for Indian people, the IHS will have to move toward a redefinition of its mission if it is to deal with such conditions successfully.

Myths and Realities

There are many myths and stereotypes about Indian people. Some of these are directly or indirectly related to psychiatric illness in Indians. They are discussed elsewhere in this chapter and are only mentioned here.

Traditional Culture

It is true that some tribal cultures have been largely destroyed, but traditional culture is alive and well in many Indian tribes. Traditional cultural practices may appear strange to non-Indians, but these are not pathological. For example, Beiser (1974) pointed out that ceremonials are positive and reinforcing, and Jelik (1974) suggested that indigenous therapeutic practices are not only helpful to individuals but also maintain the culture in which such practices occur.

Psychiatric Disorder and Services

There is little empirical evidence that the rates for most psychiatric illnesses are higher in Indian people than in whites. An exception is that in some Indian groups, but not all, alcoholism rates are high. Even in groups with high rates, it is not the case that all Indian people are alcoholic. Neither is it the case that a large number of suicides occur among Indian people. There are about 200 Indian suicides per year in the United States compared with 30,000 non-Indian suicides (Indian Health Service 1989a).

Also, there is little evidence concerning the differences between Indian and white presentations of psychiatric illness or its treatment. There is every reason to think that there are more similarities than differences, as has been shown to be the case for depression (Manson et al. 1985). When diagnoses are made or treatment is delivered without respect for culture's role, this may present problems, but this is a issue separate from the validity of the diagnostic system or the efficacy of specific treatment modalities.

With regard to psychiatric services, Indian people do have access to mental health care, although much of it is substandard and underfunded. Mental health programs are often separated from and poorly coordinated with the general medical health and substance abuse programs.

Images of Indians

As we have previously discussed, Indian people are not homogeneous but are instead quite diverse. Indians are not disappearing; in fact, the population is growing. Also, as we have discussed, the stereotype of the "good" Indian served the purpose of suggesting the ease of exploitation, whereas the stereotype of the "heathen" rationalized European conquest. These dichotomous stereotypes still exist in the image of the romanticized Indian who loves the environment and that of the "drunken Indian" who cares for naught.

The Stigma of Mental Illness Among Indian Peoples

Because of the diversity of Indian peoples, it is very difficult to make generalizations about stigma. Moreover, the degree of stigma is not the same for all psychiatric disorders. Some tribal groups attach very little stigma to any mental disorder, because they make little distinction between mental and physical symptoms. Others attach a great deal of stigma to mental disorder, but not to alcoholism. Still others attach stigma to particular events, such as suicide, in part because of the enormous amount of media attention that has been directed toward suicide among Indian youth. Finally, some tribal groups attach stigma to any and all mental disorders, including alcohol and other substance abuse.

Another factor that affects the degree of stigma attached to mental disorder is the degree of deculturation from traditional belief systems and reculturation into the belief systems of the majority culture. Generally, the greater the deculturation, the more similar the perception of stigma to that of the majority culture. There also appear to be urban-rural differences, which cloud the picture. The clinician can learn about the degree and character of stigma in a particular Indian community by asking patients and Indian health personnel how they understand mental illness symptoms and disorders and how they perceive theories of causality.

The origins of stigma concerning mental illness vary among Indians. For example, some traditional belief systems view mental illness as a form of supernatural possession, whereas others see it as a sign of imbalance with the rest of the natural world. Still others see persons with such symptoms as possessing a special gift. Different attitudes about mental disorder arise from each of these belief systems. Some tribal groups see mental disorder as a hopeless state—that is, as the terminal event in any illness (Kunitz 1983).

There are several manifestations of stigma in the treatment setting. One is that the common problem of sharing one's innermost thoughts with a psychiatrist is compounded by the general distrust of federal medicine and doctors (Lockart 1981). This may be articulated as a mistrust of white doctors, but it is more likely to be a result of the way federal institutions per se interact, and have always interacted, with Indian people. This mode of interaction may be summarized as one of "forced control." Some of the stigma attached by Indian people to the treatment of mental disorder derives from their mistrust of these federal institutions. For example, in the early 1970s, physicians in the IHS stopped wearing military-style uniforms for several years. When this happened, many Indian people expressed relief that they were no longer being treated by "army doctors." (The U.S. Army evokes visions of the U.S. Cavalry, which had as a major mission the elimination of Indian people.) Unfortunately, in the 1980s IHS physicians again began wearing uniforms. This makes going to see any doctor, especially a psychiatrist, difficult for some Indians.

Another problem in the clinical setting is confidentiality. In small, close-knit Indian communities, there are realistic concerns about confidentiality. Indeed, relatives and acquaintances may work in the medical records room of the hospital or clinic. The patient may not want to tell his or her "secrets," for fear that such utterances will be recorded in a medical record that is for all practical purposes a public document.

Still another difficulty the clinician may encounter is a negative reaction to the non-Indian health worker's knowledge of the Indian patient's culture. As we have stated elsewhere, such knowledge is usually quite helpful in the clinical setting. Some patients, however, may not know their own culture well, and react with anxiety and shame as the health professional shares his or her knowledge with the patient. The advantages of learning about the culture far outweigh this occasional reaction, but the clinician should be aware of this as a possible source of difficulty in relating to some patients.

An additional type of stigma has to do with tribal competition for shrinking mental health dollars. This competition becomes tribal-specific, recalling old wounds and competitions between tribes. Tribal members may be quite conscious of these old wounds, or they may be unaware that they are refighting old wars.

There is no simple answer to the dilemma of stigma. However, as in any clinical setting, the clinician must be open to learning about the Indian patient's culture and the individual patient's attitudes toward mental illness and IHS physicians. Being empathetic with the patient's difficulties in sharing their secrets with "the enemy" is helpful. This empathy is often best not spoken but may be offered by quiet acceptance of the patient's veiled or not-so-veiled criticisms. Taking clear steps toward the assurance of confidentiality and explaining these steps to the patient are also important.

Folk, Traditional, and Mainstream Psychiatric Care

Folk Medicine

"Folk medicine" and "folk remedy" are terms often used pejoratively in the majority culture to refer to an understanding of disease and treatments that

is based on hearsay, superstition, or outright fakery. Western medical practitioners may believe that "folk treatments" are totally ineffective, in part
because they see value only in medicine based on the scientific method—a
viewpoint that disapproves of even the majority culture's folk medicine.
This attitude is also in part due to the ethnocentrism of majority culture,
which brands everything not part of that culture's approach to medicine as
"folk." In the service of this ethnocentrism is an understanding of Western
(i.e., European) medicine as cognitively oriented and based completely on
the scientific method. In short, if the understanding or method did not
come from "our" culture, if it is not completely understandable in Aristote-
lian terms, and if it has not been shown to be effective in controlled clinical
trials, it must be worthless.

This is an unfortunate position for physicians to take, even if they never
deal with someone from another cultural background. The history of Western medicine is replete with examples of treatments and rationales that were
(and are) not in the least "scientific" or "proven," in the Western sense. Such
practices are still very much a part of Western medicine. As examples, every
physician learns the importance of the "placebo effect" and the "laying on of
hands"; savvy physicians also recognize that the patient who believes in the
doctor and his or her treatment does better in surgery or on medication.

The plea of La Barre (1942/1970) is still relevant today:

> As scientists we cannot afford the luxury of an ethnocentric snobbery which
> assumes *a priori* that primitive cultures have nothing whatsoever to contribute
> to civilization. Our civilization is in fact a compendium of such borrowings,
> and it is a demonstrable error to believe that contacts of "higher" and "lower"
> cultures show benefits flowing exclusively in one direction. (pp. 199–200)

Indian Medicine

At the time of the first contact between Indians and Europeans, Indian
medicine was highly developed, and the Indians' health in general was described by European historians as being better than their own (Walker and
LaDue 1986). Indians north of Mexico used 150 medications that were
later included in the *U.S. Pharmacopoeia*, and Mexican Indians contributed
50 more (Vogel 1972). The Spanish considered Aztec medicine to be superior in some ways to their own (Driver 1969).

The medicine of Indian people takes many forms. These include herbal
medicine, sweats and other ceremonials, feasts, and the use of natural phenomena, such as mineral springs (Weslager 1973). The effects of ceremonials

are akin to psychotherapy, because they persuade the patient or give permission to the patient to be renewed. The use of herbs and other plants to affect thought and feeling is, of course, psychopharmacology.

Herbal medicine was and is used extensively by Indian healers, who are called by various names, although "medicine man [or woman]" is the most familiar. There is ample evidence that Indian people have long known of the uses of plants for laxative, diuretic, emetic, and fever-reducing purposes, as well as for many other specialized uses. For example, foxglove was used for its cardiac stimulant properties for hundreds of years before Withering discovered digitalis in England (Vogel 1970).

A "sweat" is a ceremony held in a small space, such as a tepee, with steam provided by pouring water over hot rocks. Sweats are held for purposes of cleansing, prayer, and healing. The healing is often in the form of psychological catharsis and relaxation, and it can have effects similar to group therapy and relaxation therapy. It is also a way in which part of the community is mobilized for the benefit of an individual or the community as a whole.

Healing ceremonies take many forms, and are used to prevent as well as cure illness. There are various charms, amulets, and instruments used in ceremonies, which may represent the healing power, the illness itself, or may serve a purpose recognizable to Western medical personnel (e.g., a syringe made of an animal bladder and a hollow bone [Vogel 1970]). Prayers, songs, and dances are also used.

Feasts also serve both preventive and curative purposes. Weslager (1973) gives the example of a young girl who became ill and was diagnosed by the medicine man as having a spiritual infection caused by setting a pet otter free some years earlier. The medicine man indicated that the otter was now wandering around hungry with no one to feed it. A feast was held in honor of the otter to give the girl immunity from the illness this was causing, and she improved. This anecdote demonstrates the working-through of guilt in a community setting with a sharing of food or "breaking of bread."

The physician who treats Indian patients cannot ignore traditional beliefs about health and disease, traditional therapies, and traditional healers without the risk of being ineffective in his or her own work. This is because the success of any therapy is in part dependent on the *patient's* understanding and acceptance of that therapy. The difficulty is that there is little written material on Indian beliefs and medicine, and the small amount available represents few tribes. Most learning must therefore take place on site from Indian people themselves.

In this context, although the clinician should work to understand traditional beliefs about health, disease, and healing, such understanding will seldom include knowledge of how a particular healing ceremony is performed. One must be very careful about questioning Indian people, particularly Indian healers, about such details. They may feel that to give away secrets of healing is to give away the power of those secrets or to hand them to someone who could use them to do harm. If these secrets are to be revealed at all to non-Indians, or even to someone from another tribe, it is only after a long and trusting relationship has been established. Even if details about healing methods are never shared, this in itself is not a negative reflection on the non-Indian physician and does not preclude the physician's learning about the Indian approach to health and illness.

To conclude this discussion, we offer a few broad guidelines concerning Indian traditional medicine:

1. Indian patients may use both traditional and Western medicine. This may depend in part on how much the person is deculturated from his or her native culture and recultured into the majority culture. For example, a 21-year-old woman who was university trained and working in a health clinic approached the IHS doctor and told him that she had suffered from a skin condition for a number of weeks. Her "Indian doctor" had been treating it, and though she planned to continue these treatments, she wondered whether the IHS doctor might also be able to contribute.

2. Many Indian people subscribe to the idea that illness is a state of imbalance with the world. They may express this idea in physical, psychological, and/or spiritual terms. When in Western medicine we speak of "homeostasis," we are speaking only of an individual's physiology. This Western notion must be expanded to capture the Indian concept of "balance."

3. Indian people often do not tend to see mental illness as separate from physical or spiritual illness. The mental, physical, and spiritual are all seen as influencing the health of an individual, and all must be considered when treatment is planned.

4. Many Indian people are extremely pragmatic. They want to do what will work and see no problem in combining Western and traditional treatments.

5. Traditional treatments are perceived to work just as well as Western treatments: herbal preparations have pharmacologic properties; ceremonies have therapeutic value to the patient; and "grandmothers" may be marvelous auxiliary psychotherapists.

Mainstream Psychiatric Care

The main source of psychiatric care for Indian people on reservations and in rural areas in the United States is the IHS (Indian Health Service 1989b). It was not until 1965 that there was an organized mental health program. In 1989, the mental health program had a budget of $13 million, which was 1.3% of the IHS budget for that year. Eighty percent of the 127 local Service Units in the IHS have formal mental health service programs. The authority for spending the budget rests with the 12 regional IHS offices (Area Offices), which spend from $6.00 to $20.50 annually per person (1988 figures), depending on the area. The actual administration of the programs is under either IHS Area Office or tribal control. The IHS central offices in Rockville, Maryland, and Albuquerque, New Mexico, have responsibility for policy-making, planning, budget allocations, and other systemwide administrative functions.

The IHS mental health budget supports 236 IHS and tribal staff. Eighty-one percent are employed by the IHS. One hundred and ninety-eight of the 236 staff are direct service staff, of which 41 are Indian people. Table 8–2 lists staff by discipline, Indian status, and whether or not they have additional training in working with children.

Of psychiatrists, 10 of the 22 (46%) are located in one Area (Navajo), and 4 of 12 Areas (33%) have no psychiatrist. Forty percent of the total staff and 62% of the Indian staff are paraprofessionals. The IHS estimates that at least 550 direct treatment staff would be needed to deliver adequate ambulatory mental health care (Indian Health Service 1989b). Therefore, by their own estimates, the IHS is functioning with only 43% of the necessary staff. To provide state-of-the-art psychiatric care, it is probable that still more staff are needed; certainly, more formally trained staff are needed.

The IHS runs two short-term psychiatric inpatient units: a 14-bed unit in Gallup, New Mexico, and a 9-bed unit in Rapid City, South Dakota. Inpatient services are also provided under contract to local general hospital psychiatric units or private psychiatric hospitals. State hospitals are also used at times, with the bill often paid by the IHS with "contract" monies. Using a model derived from national majority culture figures, the IHS estimates that 7,127 inpatient admissions would have been expected in 1985, but there were only 4,515 (Indian Health Service 1989b). That is, almost 37% of those estimated to be in need of inpatient treatment do not receive it. Also, the IHS indicates that a mentally ill Indian person may be placed inappropriately in jail.

Public outpatient mental health facilities may be utilized by Indians in most areas, but these are often geographically distant, have fee requirements, or lack sensitivity toward and relevance to Indian people. There are no Indian programs for partial hospitalization, transitional living, or children's residential treatment, except through non-Indian public facilities. The caveat is that state and local governments will often not provide services to Indians, stating that they receive their care from the IHS. Thus, Indians often are effectively denied access to care.

Alcoholism and other substance abuse programs are largely run by the tribes themselves, using IHS funding. There are between 275 and 300 such programs, and as noted previously, quality and training of staff is a major problem. There is often no staff person who specializes in treatment of substance abuse other than alcohol. Nor does an Indian diagnosed with both substance abuse and another mental illness have services designed specifically for him or her (C. Vanderwagen, Indian Health Service, Rockville, Maryland, personal communication, May 1989).

Psychiatric care is also delivered through the general medical clinics of the IHS. Unfortunately, there is little coordination among the general health, mental health, and alcohol programs at the administrative or program level, although there are ongoing efforts to improve this state of affairs. Psychiatric care for Indian people is fragmented and incomplete, and there is little specialized care for children, elders, victims of domestic violence, patients who are severely and persistently mentally ill, or veterans.

A very large group that receives even fewer services than reservation and rural Indians is the urban Indian population. This group, which makes up 52% of the Indian population in the United States, is served in some cities by urban clinics supported by the IHS. Even in these cities, there is little ability to serve the great need. The total federal budget for all urban health programs (*not* just mental health programs) ranges between $8 million and $10 million, and even that is annually threatened by federal budget cuts.

Concepts of Mental Health and Mental Illness

There is much in the literature about the belief systems of Indian people, including much about health and illness. A great deal of this material, however, is about a relatively few tribes. Even within a single tribe, there are many beliefs. For example, Luckert (1972), a historian, describes four theories of disease and healing in the Navajo, which he derived from conversations with a medicine man. Although a complete discussion of this topic is not possible here, we have covered several important concepts.

Walker and LaDue (1986) indicated that in spite of the diversity of the many tribal groups in North America, before contact with Europeans there was some consistency in the guidelines for living developed by Indian people. They further described these acquired roles and rules as a "survival pact" between the individual, the group, and the earth, including all living things. When the laws of the pact are followed, all goes well. When the laws are not followed, all of the actors in the symbiosis are at risk. Walker and LaDue also noted that prior to contact, there was no theory of mental illness per se. Rather, physical illness (e.g., object intrusion or soul loss) was seen as the cause of mental illness. Deviant behavior was seen as misbehavior (i.e., breaking the rules of the survival pact) and was treated as such, rather than as illness.

Vogel (1970) briefly reviewed Indian theories of disease. He pointed out that humans in general attribute diseases to one of three causes: human agency, supernatural agency, and natural causes. Human agency is the same in Indian people as in the majority culture and includes wounds inflicted by self and others, poisoning, emotional reactions to loss, and so on. Natural causes include water accidents, fire, and wind. Indian treatment of illnesses resulting from human agency and natural causes is in part similar to that of Western medicine; these include surgery, ointments and other herbal medicines, and nursing care. Treatment may also involve ceremonials, feasts, songs, and other interventions.

Supernatural causes listed by Corlett (1970) include the spirits of animals (who gain revenge for slights and abuses, such as a fisherman wasting his catch); disrespect toward fire, a river, or the sea; human ghosts or witches; dreams, omens, or neglected taboos; and the influence of a woman during her menstrual period. Common themes are respect for life and that which sustains life (fire and water) and being in balance with nature and society.

In object intrusion, a small animal, a worm, a snake, or an insect has entered the body and caused disease. (Western physicians will recognize this as an analogy to germ theory and the role of parasites in causing illness.) Sucking, using a hollow bone, is often used to remove such objects, which often represent evil spirits. The venom of snakes and the pus from wounds may also be removed by this means (Vogel 1970).

Spirit intrusion is a concept related to object intrusion and refers to disease-causing spirits. They may be the result of a charm or a spell, a poisonous plant, or the souls of the dead. The medicine man or woman decides which spirit is causing the problem and prescribes an appropriate treatment. Soul loss occurs when the body leaves during a dream and travels about; the soul must be brought back, or the person will die (Vogel 1970).

Especially interesting to Western psychiatrists is the Indian conception of disease being caused by unfulfilled dreams or desires. This belief includes the concept of the unconscious, in the sense that the person may be unaware of these libidinal drives (Jouvency 1970). Part of the Indian therapy for such disease is often the interpretation of dreams.

Some Mexican Indians believe that air and wind can invade the body and cause disease. They also associate illness with disturbed emotional states and periods of delicacy (e.g., in childhood). Maintaining a balance between polarities of heat and cold, or strength and weakness, is used in diagnosis and in curing illness (Weil 1975).

Of course, Indian people also have to a lesser or greater degree adopted the belief systems of the majority culture concerning health and illness, although the degree of reculturation cannot be easily predicted from the patient's tribal origin or urban or rural status. To some extent it may be predicted by age. Older Indian people tend to have a more traditional view, but there is still a wide range of beliefs. Some highly deculturated Indians may have adopted Western beliefs almost entirely, at the expense of more traditional ones. Others have adopted very few majority beliefs, although, as noted previously, some Indian concepts are quite similar to those of the majority. Others have melded the two systems. Often, the melding is subtle and may not be a conscious effort on the part of the patient. For example, a patient may refer to an illness by saying "he," rather than "it." For native language speakers, this may be a translation phenomenon, but it may also be a personalization of the illness as an intruder into the body or mind. The clinician should not use this grammatical form, however, because patients may consider it affected or as poking fun.

Table 8–2.   Direct service staff supported by the Indian Health Service, 1989

Discipline	American Indian	Child/Adolescent[*]	Total #
Psychiatrists	0	5	22
Psychologists	4	3	37
Nurses	1	2	7
Social workers	37	5	52
Social work associates	2	0	3
Mental health technicians	41	0	45
Other	24	2	32
Total	109	17	198

* Formally trained to do subspecialty clinical work with children and/or adolescents.

The key to understanding and utilizing the patient's belief system in treatment is to find explanations of diagnostic terms and treatment strategies to which the patient can relate. A balance must be struck between explanations and treatment modalities with which the physician and the patient feel comfortable. Diagnosis and treatment that do violence to a patient's beliefs leads to noncompliance and ineffectiveness. Even if the clinician and patient start far apart in their understandings, if both are able to discuss how each sees particular terms and treatments, over time they can move closer together in their understandings and join forces to deal effectively with the patient's illness.

Psychopathology

Expressions of Mental Illness

Discussion of mental disorders in Indian people is difficult, in part because of the diversity of Indian people, but also because there is little scientific literature reviewing their psychopathology. Most of the literature has focused on sociocultural aspects of dysfunctional and destructive behavior in Indian people, and almost never on the diagnosis of mental disorder per se. The result is that the clinician must operate to some extent in the dark and may be forced to make difficult choices. He or she can assume that Indian mental disorders are very much *unlike* mental disorders in whites, leading to an idiosyncratic approach to diagnosis, which is geared only toward the social and cultural aspects of problems that are brought to her or his attention. Or he or she can assume that Indian mental disorders are very much *like* majority culture mental disorders, using diagnostic methods straight out of the major textbooks of psychiatry. However, a third possibility, which we espouse, strikes a middle ground. We propose that psychopathology in Indian people is indeed very much like that found in whites, but that social and cultural influences alter the presentation of these disorders (see Shore et al. 1987; Sue 1988; Sue and Zane 1987).

To strike such a balance in assessing psychopathology, the distinction that Kleinman and colleagues (1978) make between disease and illness is also instructive. It is important to assess both the *disease* (a malfunctioning or maladaptation of biologic and psychophysiologic processes) and the patient's *illness* (the personal, interpersonal, and cultural reactions to the disease or discomfort). As these writers state, the "systematic inattention to illness is in part responsible for patient noncompliance, patient and family dissatisfaction with professional health care, and inadequate clinical treatment" (Kleinman et al. 1978, p. 252). We add that inattention to the disease (i.e., mental disorder per se) in Indian people is equally problematic. Disease, illness, and their interaction are key factors in diagnosis and treatment.

Affective Disorders

Apart from substance abuse, affective disorders in Indians have been written about more than any other group of mental disorders. Shore and colleagues (1987) reviewed the literature on rates of depression in Indian people. They report high rates of depression relative to the majority (Shore and Manson 1981). The work of Shore and colleagues (1987) and Manson and colleagues (1985) is perhaps the best work in affective psychopathology in Indians. These investigators administered a standard psychodiagnostic instrument to Indian people in three different tribal cultures. The results were very similar among tribes and similar to the picture of depression in the majority culture. The three major depression subgroups were 1) an uncomplicated pattern, 2) secondary depression with a history of alcoholism, and 3) complicated depression superimposed on an underlying chronic depression or personality disorder. They pointed out that treatment of each may be different and influenced by cultural factors. Their study design is well worth repeating for other Indian groups and for other diagnostic categories.

A condition related to affective disorder in Indians is alcoholism and abuse of other substances. The clinician may see a patient's depression, with substance abuse representing an effort at self-treatment, or may see the substance abuse as primary with a secondary affective disorder. In either case, both of the patient's conditions should be vigorously treated.

Another behavior related to depression is suicide. Much has been written on Indian suicide, and this represents another set of myths surrounding Indian people (i.e., that they are all suicidal and that large numbers commit suicide; Shore 1975; Shore and Manson 1981; Thompson and Walker 1990). In fact, there are about 200 Indian suicides per year, and these are highly clustered by age and sex (Indian Health Service 1989a), with young males accounting for a large percentage of cases. Older Indian people have very low rates, and rates among women are equal to or lower than those in the majority culture.

Suicide is related to alcohol and substance abuse, and clinicians should encourage the use of Breathalyzer data and serum toxicology when a patient presents with suicidal behavior. Other destructive behaviors may also be related to suicide. These include auto accidents (Holinger 1980) and homicide

(Shore 1975). Suicide and other self-destructive behaviors are discussed in greater depth in a later section.

There has been little study of bipolar illness in Indians. It was once thought that bipolar illness almost never occurred in Indians (Association of American Indian Physicians 1978; Rhoades et al. 1980), but our clinical experience contradicts this assertion, as does recent mental health utilization data (Neligh 1988b).

Alcoholism

Although high alcoholism rates are widely reported in the literature, the stereotype of the "drunken Indian" is just as inaccurate as the stereotype of the "suicidal Indian," although Indians themselves may believe these myths (May and Smith 1988). Alcoholism rates are high in some communities, but prevalence rates vary by tribe and location (Stratton et al. 1978; Westermeyer 1974; Westermeyer et al. 1981). In Oklahoma, for example, Indian people in the western part of the state have higher alcoholism rates than those in the eastern part of the state. Within a given community, some researchers have found that many of the alcoholism cases are concentrated in a small part of the population (Levy and Kunitz 1974).

The patterns of use of alcoholism between tribes are as varied as the prevalence rates of alcoholism. The factors in this variation are far from clear. Westermeyer (1972) demonstrated that the Chippewa were no different from whites in percentage of the population addicted to alcohol, although the Indian group showed more severe withdrawal, possibly the result of having delayed treatment. There is, however, no syndrome of "Indian alcoholism" that differs from that found in the majority population.

There may also be more severe withdrawal in groups with a history of binge drinking, head trauma, intercurrent infection, low access to treatment facilities, and delay in seeking treatment. These are important factors, of course, for all populations. Laboratory tests appropriate for assessing the Indian alcoholic patient, especially in withdrawal, include serum protein, iron, vitamins A and C, and hemoglobin (Westermeyer 1972). Physical examination should include a neurological exam, a cranial exam, and an evaluation for signs of infection. If head trauma is suspected, imaging studies may be indicated.

The long-term course of alcoholism in Indian peoples has not been studied, but one important observation is that alcoholism appears to diminish with age (Association of American Indian Physicians 1978). Also, in some tribes, severe alcohol use and its sequelae are seen in adolescents. Therefore, alcoholism may start earlier and end earlier in some Indian groups than in the majority culture. As in similar studies in the majority culture, the few follow-up studies of alcohol treatment in Indians have not been encouraging (Kivlahan et al. 1985; Walker et al., in press; Westermeyer and Peake 1983). There are, however, many factors in addition to treatment that may contribute to successful outcome. These include aftercare, removal from the environment where substance abuse occurred, and treatment of concomitant depression. One research group also suggested the need for simultaneous treatment and follow-up of the entire drinking network (Silk-Walker et al. 1988). Community commitment to abstinence among its members is also an important factor (Alhali Lake Indian Band, undated).

The etiology of alcoholism in Indians has been written about extensively, but no convincing conclusions have been reached. Westermeyer and co-workers (1981) discuss factors possibly contributing to substance abuse among Indian people. High unemployment is one possible factor, but it is not clear whether this is the cause or the result of alcoholism. Suggested cultural influences include a reliance in pre-Columbian times on magical power, which might be replaced by alcohol (to explain high current rates in some groups; Kunitz and Levy 1974) and reculturation into white culture (to explain low rates in some groups; Stratton et al. 1978). Biological theories have also been suggested, but Westermeyer and co-workers (1981) cite multiple methodological problems in this research, which place the findings in doubt. May and Smith (1988) indicate that there is no proof of genetic, metabolic, or other differences in Indians that would negatively affect the processing of alcohol or that would differentially affect the functioning of Indians while they are under the influence of alcohol.

What is clear, however, is that many Indian people are adversely affected by the medical (psychiatric and nonpsychiatric) and social sequelae of alcohol abuse. Where there are high rates of cirrhosis, automobile accidents, suicide, and homicide in Indians, alcohol is often an important factor. However, it is not clear whether alcohol use is the primary pathology or is secondary to other mental disorders, social problems, or other factors.

A condition related to alcoholism and of great importance in Indian people is fetal alcohol syndrome (May et al. 1983). The clinical approach to this condition should include prevention (i.e., discontinuing drinking in the pregnant mother), family and individual therapy with the parents of an affected child, and careful evaluation of the child by a pediatrician and a psychiatrist specializing in infants.

In terms of the perception of alcoholism by Indian people, there has been a theoretical perspective promulgated in the literature that alcoholism in some Indian communities is not seen as deviant, and, therefore, is neither maladaptive nor an illness (Kunitz and Levy 1974). An alternate conceptual perspective is the symbolic interactionist model (Heath 1988), which views drinking by Indian people as a "protest demonstration" (Robbins and Lurien 1971). It is true that alcohol abuse is so common in some Indian communities that it may be accepted as the norm. Increasingly, however, Indian people and communities have been speaking out against this point of view, in an attempt to redefine alcoholism as clearly deviant and maladaptive. Many communities have declared themselves to be "alcohol free" and have accomplished much in terms of ridding their people of this disorder (Alhali Lake Indian Band, undated). Health personnel will serve their Indian patients best by seeing alcohol abuse, alcohol dependence, and heavy drinking as abnormal, and never as adaptive or healthy, despite the fact that they might be common.

Other Substance Abuse
Given the large body of literature on alcoholism in Indian people, there is surprisingly little information on the abuse of other substances. Inhalants have been studied to some extent, with at least one author labeling adult inhalant abuse as "prealcoholic behavior" (Albaugh and Albaugh 1979), but little else is available in the literature about the use of nonalcohol substances by adult Indians.

With regard to Indian youth, it has been noted that there is evidence of the use of marijuana, inhalants, and stimulants (Westermeyer et al. 1981) but little use of cocaine, heroin, or sedatives. Other authors, who surveyed 35,000 Indian youth over the age of 12, indicated that there was evidence of heavy use of marijuana but also of cocaine, phencyclidine (PCP), and other substances (Beauvais et al. 1985). Loretto and colleagues (1988) suggested that although drug use by Indian youth is high, the rates are leveling off. They also pointed out that use among Indian youth tends to follow national trends. Unfortunately, the data of Loretto and colleagues were derived from only one reservation and generalized to all other reservations in the United States, and the validity of such generalization is highly improbable.

Hydrocarbon abuse among Indian youth has also been studied (Kaufman 1973; Schottstaedt and Bjork 1977; Westermeyer et al. 1981). This abuse is especially profound, because it carries with it serious permanent sequelae, such as brain damage and/or asphyxiation. In addition, children who use these substances develop habit patterns and ways of coping that foster dependence on external agents and may move on to alcoholism in adult life (Schottstaedt and Bjork 1977). These authors believe that the substance abuse among subjects in their sample is a symptom of emotional distress, and they suggest ways to meet basic emotional needs more adequately. Hydrocarbon sniffing has been considered a gateway drug for other substance abuse in Indian adolescents, and such abuse continues to exist (Strimba and Sims 1974). Diagnostically, serum lead levels have been used to screen for gasoline sniffing among youth (Westermeyer et al. 1981), although the advent of unleaded gasoline has lessened the usefulness of this technique.

Disorders Usually First Evident in Childhood

Beiser and Attneave (1982) compared national data on use of outpatient mental health services by white and Indian children and found that except for those ages 5 through 9, Indian children were at a higher risk for entering the treatment system. They proposed that these findings represented in part methodological artifact and in part a higher prevalence of mental disorder. By adolescence, more than one-third of Indian children had left school. These children entered the mental health system at a high rate, largely because of antisocial behavior. Alcoholism rates were also estimated to be high among Indian adolescents. Finally, Beiser and Attneave reported a high rate of suicide in Indian adolescents.

Green and colleagues (1981) reviewed the psychiatric epidemiology literature on Indian children and noted that there was little careful work in this area. Articles quoting prevalence figures often provide little more than guesses about the extent of "mental health problems" in Indian youth; figures range from very low "rates" to one-third of Indian youth. Green and colleagues (1981) noted another problem in the psychiatric epidemiological literature on Indian children: it seldom uses the conventional categories of psychopathology, relying instead on classification of social conditions, such as child abuse, delinquency, and school problems. Work is needed to make the connection between these factors and psychiatric illness. Berlin (1986) has made such an attempt, discussing in brief such topics as the effects on infants of having a mother who is both depressed and alcoholic, the relationship of developmental problems to depression and hyperactive aggressive behavior, and adolescent pregnancy as a symptom of depression.

Berlin (1986) notes that psychopathology among Indian adolescents appears qualitatively similar to that found in the rest of the United States adolescent population but that there are substantial quantitative differences among tribes in comparison to non-Indian adolescents. We believe this to be true of childhood disorders in general. Some of the quantitative differences are related to fetal alcohol syndrome, substance abuse, and the dual diagnosis of depression and substance abuse.

When parents are themselves depressed and abusing substances, child abuse and neglect may occur, which may contribute to any psychopathology the child may exhibit. As noted previously, teenage pregnancy may represent a "symptom" of depression (Berlin 1986), and infants born to these teenage mothers may themselves be at high risk for mental disorder. It is perhaps in the youth that the effect of extreme levels of unemployment in some Indian communities is most obvious (Berlin 1986). In some communities, there is no progression from adolescence into self-sufficiency (i.e., getting a job and supporting himself or herself and a family). Substance abuse and mental disorder are possible outcomes for someone trapped in such a powerless state.

It is also well for clinicians to remember that developmental processes for Indians may not fit majority norms (Berlin 1986). Consultation with those familiar with "normal" childhood development in a particular tribe is always advisable.

Foster Care and Adoption

Although they are, of course, not mental disorders, it has been suggested that foster care and adoption are linked to mental disorder in Indians. However, the literature on foster care and adoption is aimed entirely at advocacy and legislative action, rather than at examining this possible link scientifically. There are persuasive arguments for the placement of Indian children with Indian foster and adoptive parents, as opposed to placement with white families (Shore 1978; Unger 1977). Placement of Indian children with whites has indeed been a problem. For many years the non-Indian social welfare system removed Indian children from their families in order to place them with white adoptive families, with little or no justification. Where the social welfare worker perceived problems in an Indian family, there were seldom attempts to work with the family or community to resolve these problems (Mindell and Gurwitt 1977). Work on this issue led to the passage of the Indian Child Welfare Act in 1978 (U.S. Congress 1978). The Act provides that Indian families be given preference in adoption of Indian children.

It must be recognized, however, that in spite of strongly held convictions by advocates of Indian family placement and clear implications for the integrity of Indian communities and culture, there is no research supporting the idea that Indian children brought up by white families develop mental disorders more frequently than children brought up in their native cultures. It should also be pointed out that there is no such research in the majority culture on the effects of adoption. The fact of having been adopted into a non-Indian family may well be expressed in the dynamics of the illness of those Indian people who do develop mental disorders. These dynamics may include the usual ones associated with adoption (e.g., being wanted or un-wanted and being uncertain of one's identity), and they may also include issues of anger at having been denied one's cultural heritage. However, in the absence of scientific evidence, it should not be assumed that the adoptive experience is causal of mental disorder.

The Psychoses

There is little written on psychosis in Indian people. The presence of psy-chotic-like signs (e.g., hallucinations) may or may not be symptoms of mental disorder, because there are situations in which some symptoms of psychosis are culturally acceptable. This observation also holds true for the majority culture. For example, some hallucinations occurring in an un-complicated grief reaction are not considered pathologic. In evaluating psychotic symptoms in an Indian person, it is important not to apply exclu-sively the majority culture's standard of what is "normal" or "abnormal."

Presentation of the psychoses in Indians appears to be very much as in the majority culture, although the content of delusions and hallucinations may be culturally influenced. Especially with nonbizarre delusional material, the psychiatrist may have difficulty in determining whether such material is par-tially or completely based in reality. Discussions with health care personnel familiar with the patient's culture and with members of the patient's family may be necessary in order to make the distinction between normality and pathology. It should also be remembered that some Indian people have learned to be quite suspicious of "white people" and "white medicine." But suspiciousness alone should not lead to a diagnosis of paranoid psychosis or paranoid personality.

In studies of a single tribe, Kunitz (1983) indicated that "mind loss" (faints, dissociative reactions, and seizures) are thought to be the final stage of all diseases. This may lead the mentally ill patient or the family to go to a general practitioner rather than a psychiatrist or other mental health profes-sional. It may also lead to resistance to psychiatric treatment, because this is seen as an "end-stage" phenomenon. Intervention may therefore seem use-less to the patient and his or her family.

Kaplan and Johnson (1964) pointed out that extremes of behavior often appear to signal the need for treatment in the Navajo. Levy (1983), in a study of 16 Indian patients in an IHS treatment facility who were diagnosed as having schizophrenia, indicated that males with schizophrenia were hospi-talized when there was increased potential for violence, and females with schizophrenia were brought to the hospital when they became withdrawn and were no longer caring for their family (e.g., cooking and weaving).

Destructive Behaviors

Although not a mental disorder, self-destructive behavior in Indians has been written about widely in the psychiatric literature, and strong inferences have been drawn concerning causality between such behavior and mental disorders. As we have discussed previously, although there are a number of studies showing high rates of suicide (Conrad and Kahn 1974; Ogden et al. 1970), the stereotype of the "the suicidal Indian" is a myth (Shore 1975). In fact, the suicide rate for Indian tribes varies widely, from higher to lower than that of the general population. Unfortunately, the stereotype of the "suicidal Indian" remains, and a cluster of adolescent Indian suicides still sends the news media scrambling for data and commentary on "the Indian suicide problem" ("Body of 8th Indian suicide victim found" 1985; National Public Radio 1985). In practice, the clinician must strike a balance between overreacting to a rash of suicides and dealing forthrightly with the serious difficulties periodically posed by suicide in some communities.

Other forms of self-destructiveness are also problems in some Indian communities (May 1987). The rates of automobile accidents and other accidents (some of which may not be "accidents"), unprotected sexual contact, and unwanted and teenage pregnancy are high in some areas. Although the same cautions to clinicians not to overreact also apply, such problems do indeed pose difficulties for some communities. Psychiatrists can be of help in analyzing and helping the community to deal with these problems.

The link between some forms of self-destructiveness and mental disorder per se is quite clear. There is much in the literature linking suicide with depression, substance abuse, psychosis, and other mental disorders. Holinger (1980) indicated that many other self-destructive acts may be related to these disorders. It is clear that auto accidents are linked to alcohol use. Single-car accidents (May 1987) and some homicides (Shore 1975) may be forms of suicide. Unwanted or teenage pregnancy may be an attempt to "cure" loneliness and depression. As with any population, the clinician must pay attention to the possible links between such behaviors and mental disorders.

The clinician's first tasks must be to provide quality diagnosis and treatment of mental disorders. There may be a temptation to regard these tasks as unimportant in view of the great social and economic problems in some Indian communities—a perspective that may be reinforced by those who believe that mental disorder is simply a response to a "sick society." To avoid this temptation and yet be responsive to community needs, we favor an approach that recognizes different levels of intervention. The clinical level is the clinician's primary and most important area of intervention. Indian people have long been deprived of clinical services. Another valid level is the community level, which may include service on community boards, volunteer work in schools and social agencies, and other community activities. The advocacy level can also be a valid one for the clinician, whether this be in national organizations, in the legislative arena, or within the IHS itself. Some clinicians may choose to be active on only the clinical level, whereas others may be active on all levels.

Other Mental Disorders

The existence of organic mental disorder (OMD) in Indian elders has been studied systematically only in nursing homes, where one author found a lower rate of cognitive impairment than in the majority population (Mick 1983). It is not clear whether this is a "survivor effect" or evidence of a lower rate for Indian elders. Neligh (1988b) anecdotally reported a high count of OMD in all age groups in one IHS Area, with the presumed etiologies being alcohol use and head trauma. The presentation of organic mental disorders in Indian people is similar to that in the majority population, but again, this has not been systematically studied.

There is little available in the literature on the presentation of other mental disorders in Indian people. Neligh (1988b) anecdotally reported that in one IHS Area, patients appear to present with anxiety, somatization, and eating disorders much as they do in the majority population. He also questioned the validity of personality disorder diagnoses made in Indian people, although the problem may be based on difficulties with instrumentation rather than with basic constructs.

Assessment

Perhaps the greatest value of culture-sensitive psychiatry is in making assessments. With regard to psychological testing, Goldstine and Gutmann (1972) used the Thematic Apperception Test (TAT; Murray 1943) in a study of Navajo males, with findings similar to those with subjects in other cultures. Some differences, however, have been found in the use of the Wechsler Intelligence Scale for Children, Revised (WISC-R; Wechsler 1974 [Browne 1984; McShane and Plas 1982]). Dana and colleagues (1984) developed limited local, culturally relevant, nondiscriminatory norms for measures of life stress, locus of control, worldview, and values in the Rosebud Sioux. Pollack and Shore (1980) studied the validity of the Minnesota Multiphasic Personality Inventory (MMPI; Hathaway and McKinley 1970) with Indians, and found that it had limited usefulness in determining mental normalcy from mental illness or in distinguishing among various types of mental illness. In the validation and use of psychological tests, it is important not only to compare responses among cultures, but to assure that "psychological tasks . . . evoke the same kinds of behaviors in subjects from different cultures" (Cole et al. 1971, pp. xii–xiii). It must be determined that Indians are applying the same cognitive processes as those people in whom the test was originally validated.

Baron and colleagues (in press) studied whether the National Institute of Mental Health (NIMH) Center for Epidemiologic Studies Depression Scale (CES-D; Radloff 1977) was a useful screening tool in Indians. They argue for its use in targeting preventive intervention strategies but note that its use as a diagnostic instrument is suspect. Manson and colleagues (1985) studied how a particular tribe (the Hopi) conceptualizes depression. The goal of the study was to construct a culturally appropriate diagnostic instrument. At the time the article was published, the instrument, the American Indian Depression Scale, was being administered to a sample of Hopi subjects.

Diagnostic instruments can be useful with Indian people, but standardization, reliability, and validity must be determined in the group for which the instrument is to be used. Little of that research work has been done. Standardization with one tribe does not necessarily translate into standardization with another. However, clinicians should not therefore adopt a nihilistic view of existing instruments. As Manson and colleagues (1987) point out, many instruments can accurately assess mental illness among Indians, provided they are modified to reflect Indian cultural heritage and experience.

Case Study

A 12-year-old Indian girl is admitted to the hospital with a history of school difficulties and seeing "spirits." The elders in her tribe feel that she is a gifted individual because of her visions. Her family is quite traditional and appreciates the special nature of her gift, but nevertheless her relatives are troubled because she becomes so engrossed in the visions that she neglects friends, family, and schoolwork. She has no history of substance abuse, and there is no history of substance abuse or mental disorder in her family. On being given a mental status exam, she is revealed to be a friendly and happy child, of average intelligence, who easily relates the above history. She is not disturbed by her visions, which she describes as elders appearing before her to give advice about her daily activities. She exhibits no other signs of psychosis, except that some of her explanations seem verbose and do not closely hang together.

Discussion of Case: Although seeing visions may well be viewed as normal in this patient's culture, and, indeed, may receive support from her tribal members, nevertheless, her schoolwork is impaired. It is not clear whether she is in fact dissociating while having the visions and therefore cannot concentrate on schoolwork, or whether she is not confident about her academic abilities and uses a culturally acceptable method of avoiding the work. This distinction would be important diagnostically. If possible, treatment would be aimed at dealing with the school problem, rather than removing the hallucinations per se, because the hallucinations may well serve an important function for her in her society. It would also be important to encourage her parents to seek out the traditional healers in their community and for them to discuss the problem as they see it with both the Western and traditional healers.

Alternate Presentations of Mental Disorder

The concept of "culture-bound syndromes" has a long history in cross-cultural psychiatry. This concept has never been well defined, however, and has led to the unfortunate sequestering of nonmajority psychopathology into what one writer has called the "twilight zone" (Hughes 1985). Such researchers question the utility of such a concept. "Culture-bound" implies that some psychopathology is found only within a single culture, and at times, there is the implication that the culture must in some way have caused the psychopathology. Neither may be the case, however. As has been demonstrated by Manson and colleagues (1985), in at least one psychiatric illness in Indian people (depression), DSM-III (American Psychiatric Association 1980) criteria are quite valid, but the presentation of illness may be different from that of the mainstream culture. Likewise, Kunitz (1983) quoted Levy's work showing that in Indian patients with schizophrenia, the usual psychiatric symptoms were present, but the Indian families he studied often responded to other stimuli to lead their schizophrenic family member to treatment.

The danger of accepting syndromes as culturally bound is that the clinician will feel that he or she cannot understand or deal with the condition because it seems so foreign and may miss psychopathology with which he or she *can* deal (e.g., S. M. Manson, unpublished data [Physicians and American Indian healers: issues and constraints in collaborative health care], June 1992). The psychiatrist can avoid this temptation by attempting to interpret what he or she is seeing and hearing in the context of both Western and traditional cultures. The assumption should be that part or all of the patient's condition can be understood with a culturally sensitive application of Western psychopathology until proven otherwise. This having been said, several culture-bound conditions are mentioned in the following paragraphs. None of these has been empirically studied from the dual contexts of Western and traditional medicine, and we would discourage their use in the clinical practice of psychiatry with Indians.

Simons and Hughes (1985) provided a useful categorization of culture-bound syndromes, which they apply to all peoples, including the majority cultures of the United States and Canada. These categories (or "taxons") are "startle matching," "sleep paralysis," "genital retraction," "sudden mass assault," "running," "fright illness," and "cannibal compulsion." Several of the Indian syndromes fit into these categories. Many of those covered in detail by Simons and Hughes have been observed in the Eskimo: sleep paralysis, *pibloktoq* (a sudden mass assault syndrome), and "Arctic hysteria" (a running syndrome). Another sudden mass assault syndrome mentioned is *wihtiko* (in the Cree people). The chapter by Marano (1985) covers *windigo* (a delusional cannibal compulsion, or fear of it, in the Algonkian people) and discusses the misunderstandings that have long surrounded this condition. Simons and Hughes end each section of their book with a discussion of DSM-III diagnoses in light of the group of culture-bound syndromes. (See also Chapter 3.)

There are several scholarly reviews that speak specifically to Indian depressive syndromes, including those of Trimble and colleagues (1984) and Shore and Manson (1981). The latter authors discuss "*windigo* psychosis," noting that it is seen in several tribes, as well as several depression-related syndromes, *hiwa-itck* (Mohave), *wacinko* (Oglala Sioux), "self-destructive syndrome" (Nez Percé), *tawatl ye kni* or "totally discouraged" (Dakota Sioux and other tribes), and "excessive Navajo mourning." They conclude that depression results from a variety of responses with multiple etiologies.

Knowledge of so-called culture-bound syndromes is useful in understanding a particular Indian culture, but it may be of limited usefulness in diagnosis and treatment of mental disorders. Perhaps the best approach is to temper Western understandings and approaches with those of particular Indian cultures, including potential culture-bound syndromes. Such syndromes, although questionable diagnostic entities in themselves, may be alternate presentations of mental disorders and may say a great deal about the cultural function of the syndrome for the individual.

Other Folk or Traditional Categories of Mental Illness

Although Indian people traditionally had ways of grouping illnesses that helped them in their conceptualizations of pathology and its treatment, there is little if any written information about such "nosologies." In this chapter's section "Concepts of Mental Health and Mental Illness," limited information about categorization systems is provided. A key point is that these traditional systems did not separate "mental" disorders from disorders of general health or of the spirit. It is clear from writing done at the time of European contact that the health status of Indian people was relatively high (Walker and LaDue 1986) and that medical care was quite advanced (Vogel 1970). It would follow that Indian conceptualizations of mental illness were also advanced and functional.

Medicine men and women still rely on traditional conceptualizations of illness in their diagnosis and treatment activities, but as we noted previously, little of their beliefs and practices is known outside of their communities. Therefore, the Western physician must, and should, rely on Western nosology, tempered with knowledge of the culture at hand.

Traditional Healers

Indian people have their own healers, called by a variety of names, including "medicine man [or woman]." These healers serve a wide variety of functions, including physician, counselor, priest, and historian (Fields 1976). Bergman (1974) added the profession of law to those of theologian and physician in explaining the roles of medicine men. To many Indian people, there is no difference between a healing ceremony and worship (Beiser and DeGroat 1974). The medicine man traditionally was the agent of both, and before European contact, was also the "judge" in settling disputes. Bergman (1974) pointed out that medicine men have largely turned over the technical and pharmaceutical role to Western medicine and have focused "on what they always considered most important—roughly what we would call psychotherapy or . . . pastoral counseling" (p. 133). This is an oversimplification of the role of medicine men and women, because many still concern themselves very much with "physical" illness. Nevertheless, it is true that these healers play a large part in assuring the emotional and spiritual health of Indian people.

A few descriptions of the philosophy of Indian healers do exist (Beiser and DeGroat 1974; Lake 1983). In this regard, it is important to dispel the myth that medicine men and women practice witchcraft. They practice healing, although in some cases it may be for the purpose of undoing the evil that some people do to others (Fields 1976). But they do not practice black magic or sorcery. Jelik and Todd (1974) described how native healers in one tribe moved from being seen as crazy witch doctors to auxiliary psychotherapists. (Exceptions to this general principle are some Mexican healers who can do harm as well as good and may practice witchcraft. However, witchcraft is used by these curers [and others in the society] largely against people who have broken social rules, rather than against the sick [Weil 1975]).

There have been several attempts to have Western medicine and traditional medicine collaborate, some successful and others unsuccessful. Attneave (1974) described two types of Western health professionals who are unsuccessful in relating to traditional medicine. These are 1) those who, when offered a glimpse into the traditional life of the tribe, "lack the sensitivity to perceive when the curtains are pulled aside" (p. 53), and 2) the politically liberal professional who is determined not to interfere with Indian culture and so never cultivates relationships among Indian people. She also describes a third and preferable interface between Western and traditional medicine, which "recognizes the mutuality of interests, the shared techniques, and the selective appropriateness of psychiatric and traditional practices" (p. 55). Attneave gives several examples of such a relationship, although these are widely scattered. They include a training program for medicine men that existed in Rough Rock, Arizona, throughout the 1970s (Fields 1976) and a traditional healing room within the IHS hospital in Chinle, Arizona (S. M. Manson, unpublished data [Physicians and American Indian healers: issues and constraints in collaborative health care], June 1992). During the 1970s, the University of North Carolina School of Medicine at Chapel Hill had a medicine man on staff who taught medical students and consulted on patient care.

Manson (S. M. Manson, unpublished data [Physicians and American Indian healers: issues and constraints in collaborative health care], June 1992) studied 60 cases of attempted collaboration between traditional and Western medical practitioners. He identified the following problems:

1. Problems of definition (of abnormality and of "legitimate" traditional healing);
2. Problems of explanation (for why certain techniques are used by medicine men);
3. Problems of credibility (for both traditional and Western healers);
4. Problems of reimbursement for traditional healers;
5. Problems of patient expectations (the patient does not agree with the collaboration); and
6. Problems of professional integrity (the biases of both Western and traditional healers toward each other).

Manson concluded that locally relevant mechanisms for collaboration must be developed, ranging from formal inclusion of traditional healing in Western health facilities, to separate, coordinated services. The clinician working with Indian people cannot automatically use the model of collaboration he or she uses to relate to other Western physicians.

The Family and Mental Illness

Family support issues are important in psychiatric practice with Indian people and should be attended to in any treatment plan. Care must be taken, however, to avoid the notion that such interventions are the *only* ones necessary, as has often been implied (National Indian Council on Aging 1982).

Much of the literature on families has focused on social support for the Indian elderly or on the interaction between the elderly and younger generations. Shomaker (1989) discussed the problem found in some Indian families wherein parents did not meet the needs of their children, leaving informal "grandmothers" to care for these children. The stress on these older women was discussed, as was the mechanism of intergenerational relationships. John (1985) and Manson and Callaway (1984) examined social support for the elderly, with some attention to mental health. Porter (1982) made recommendations that the Indian elderly need the availability of safe and comfortable housing; delivery of health support services (e.g., homemaker and chore services, community health representative programs, and nutrition programs); community programs on aging; special health and mental health care programs; a community support system; legal services; and long-term care (preferably not in nursing homes away from their reservations).

Although Robert Coles' (1977) work is not specifically about psychiatry or family support, he provides an empathetic and instructive account of Eskimo and Indian families using the words of children from these groups. Other relevant issues involving children in the Indian family are child abuse (Berlin 1986; May 1988), children of alcoholics, and fetal alcohol syndrome. Issues of general concern for families are elder and spouse abuse, survivors of suicide and homicide, and dealing with family members who are severely mentally ill. However, there is little psychiatric literature available on these topics regarding Indians.

Finally, there have been movements in the past to reestablish the community social network for the benefit of a distressed individual or family (Speck and Attneave 1973). Today, there are a growing number of community activities among Indian people that seek to revitalize the community as a functioning unit and to strengthen valued traditional practices. Among these efforts are the Alaskan "spirit camps," where the community comes together for the benefit of its members, sharing traditional practices and fostering communication among generations (W. Richards, Native Health Service, Anchorage, Alaska, personal communication, June 1989).

Clinical Treatment Issues

The treatment of mental disorders is too extensive an area to cover in detail here. General issues surrounding treatment of Indians are discussed, as well as the use of specific treatment modalities with Indian people.

General Issues

Often there is the assumption by those in practice that Western treatments are not effective in the Indian setting, but evidence for that position is lacking. There is every reason to believe that treatments for mental disorders that are effective for non-Indians are indeed effective for Indians. However, the latter assumption has likewise not been studied. Given the absence of scientifically derived outcome data and positive anecdotal reports of effectiveness of Western treatment with Indians, we believe that it is improper to withhold state-of-the-art treatment from Indian people on the basis that Indians are different, or that Western treatment "doesn't work" for Indians. However, it is equally improper to approach diagnosis and treatment without considering social and cultural influences.

It is important to appreciate the complexity of "the system" with regard to the treatment of Indian people. In fact, multiple systems are involved, not just the formal health care system. Although this is true of all populations, Indian people are affected by several entities not found in the majority society. Specifically with regard to Indians, the Western health system may have several forms. To name a few, these include the IHS, tribally run programs, and private and public practices of Western medicine that Indians also use. One must consider the influence on the patient of the tribe, the BIA, and the social service system (both of the majority culture and of the tribe). In addition, the medicine man or woman is important for many Indians, and the religious portions of the person's belief system, both traditional and Christian, must be considered.

Another issue is that within the formal (Western) health care system, there are not now and have never been enough resources for the treatment of Indians (with "enough" defined as parity with the majority health care system). Because of the lack of resources, many Indian people with mental disorders go untreated. A striking example is found in the care of chronically mentally ill Indian people. Many have never been on neuroleptic medication, a keystone of treatment of chronic psychosis. However, the situation is not hopeless. Advances made in general Indian health (e.g., in maternal and child health and in infectious diseases) were also made with limited resources. The IHS believes that doubling the mental health budget would allow for large advances, and work is also under way to improve the staffing in the mental health and substance abuse programs. These and similar actions are quite within the realm of possibility and could lead to successes in the psychiatric care of Indians similar to successes in nonpsychiatric medicine.

Though the basic treatment of mental disorders in Indians is similar to that for the majority population, there are important cultural considerations. This may not mean, however, that specifically "Indian" programs are uniquely effective. Because of inadequate opportunities for research on specifically Indian treatment programs, there is no scientific evidence for or against such programs. Walker (1990) discusses this point with regard to treatment of alcohol dependence. There are cultural influences that are important to consider, however. Westermeyer and Walker (1982) indicated that cultural sensitivity includes giving ample time for the development of rapport; prolonged facilitation and clarification to allow patients time to tell their story and express their feelings; probing with discretion across cultural boundaries; and gentle confrontation, lest the patient interpret this as the same rejection that he or she has experienced with non-Indians in other majority institutions. They also indicated that the use of network or systems therapy (i.e., bringing in all of the people important in the treatment process) may be more effective than individual therapy. Finally, they pointed out that there are data supporting the beneficial effects of traditional folk healing practices.

Some of the most practical advice for clinicians comes from a Sioux physician, who wrote about the delivery of general health care (Schmidt 1988). She stated that in medicine, we are taught to look for certain responses or signs, and when we do not receive them we begin to draw conclusions about the patient. That can be a dangerous practice, however. She gave the example of eye contact, which is valued in the majority society as a sign of respect and attentiveness. For some Indian people, however, it is a sign of *disrespect* to look someone in the eye, and to try to do so may make the patient quite uncomfortable.

Schmidt (1988) also wrote about the concept of time. For some Indian people, time is "flowing" or "flexible." They may miss an appointment or may be late because they have been taught that it is not important to be precisely "on time." The physician may interpret this as not caring about their health, "acting out," or in other psychodynamic ways. These may also be correct, but the cultural interpretation should also be considered. Similarly, some Indian people may look only at the present, rather than the future, and therapies must therefore be present-oriented. (Non-Sioux Indian people may or may not share these beliefs and perceptions.)

Another issue that is difficult for the non-Indian clinician to understand is the Indian concept of ownership. Ownership is often not focused on material goods but rather on caretaking and sharing. An example of this is "giving away," in which a person who is being honored *gives* gifts to others rather than *receiving* gifts as he or she might in the majority culture. Schmidt also cited this as a reason why some Indian people prefer to care for patients at home rather than placing them in a nursing home.

Finally, Schmidt (1988) discussed her experience that Indian patients frequently do not ask a lot of questions, because it is considered disrespectful. Therefore, reviewing or demonstrating instructions may be important. On the other hand, one family member may be in charge of health care in the family and may question the physician about treatment. It is important to understand this family role and to take such questioning as clarification of instructions. A successful interaction with the family health care overseer can lead to greater compliance with the treatment plan.

Geography may also greatly affect how a clinician should approach treatment. Richards and Oxereok (1978) described some of the problems in treating Alaska Natives across great distances. They stressed the importance of flexibility, because the clinician on hand may be the only trained person within many miles. Richards and Oxereok gave the negative example of a counselor called upon in a crisis situation, who exclaimed, "But I only do Gestalt therapy." They also indicate that because of the great distances involved, it may be possible to see a patient only sporadically and for only a few sessions. The use of self-help groups and identification of the healthiest member of the family in order to recruit him or her as a "co-therapist" were also recommended. Brief therapy and crisis treatment was also suggested as a major part of treatment planning, with a short-term contract and limited objectives. (Similar approaches may be useful in remote areas in the southwestern United States, Mexico, and Canada.)

Specific Treatment Modalities

There are few research studies on the use of specific treatment modalities in Indian people, but at least two authors reviewed literature on treatment of Indians (Manson et al. 1987; Neligh 1988b). Neligh reported the wide use of all classes of psychotropic medication with Indians with apparent success, although none has not been systematically reviewed or studied. He also noted the controversy within the IHS with regard to the use of benzodiazepines for the treatment of anxiety and sleep disorders. Manson and colleagues (1987) focused on psychoanalysis and psychotherapy but made no evaluative comments as to their effectiveness or ineffectiveness. Neligh (1988b) indicated that although informal "counseling" (i.e., general supportive psychotherapy) is widely practiced by nonphysician mental health workers, largely in response to a perceived cultural resistance to more structured and directive styles of therapy, the effectiveness of this style of therapy has not been shown.

One viewpoint, which Manson and colleagues (1987), Neligh (1988b), and we ourselves share, is that group therapy with Indians is useful, an assertion that contradicts the commonly held belief that it was not an appropriate modality for Indians (Neligh 1988b). This modality, combined with traditional activities, has also proven very useful in Alaskan "spirit camps" (W. Richards, Native Health Service, Anchorage, AK, personal communication, June 1989). A related modality, family network therapy (Manson et al. 1987; Speck and Attneave 1973), is also promising. The treatment of severely mentally ill people is persistently neglected in Indian country. There are definitional problems in the identification of psychosis in Indians (Neligh 1988b), but there is little doubt that such psychosis exists. The neglect of this group of patients is especially unfortunate in light of the rapid progress that has been made in the treatment and rehabilitation of people with severe mental illness in the majority culture. Neligh (1988b) called for the creation in Indian country of modalities that are used in Anglo medicine, such as partial hospitalization, skills training, and case management. As in the majority culture, neuroleptics should be the cornerstone of the care of this patient group.

Traditional methods of treatment are covered elsewhere in this chapter but are equally important modalities in the psychiatric treatment of Indian people.

Non-Indian Therapists

The use of non-Indian therapists clearly carries with it some difficulties (Lockart 1981). Nevertheless, we maintain that a skilled and culturally sensitive non-Indian therapist, who is willing to learn from the patient as therapy progresses, can be of great help to the Indian patient. Although the ideal arrangement might be a well-trained, culturally sensitive therapist from the patient's own tribal group, that will seldom be possible because of the limited number of Indian health care professionals. In many cases, the decision as to which therapist will treat the patient will be made on the basis of who is available, rather than what is the best fit for the patient. Important factors in the decision regarding formal training and skill versus "Indianness" are the severity and chronicity of the condition being treated, the need to use the formal psychotherapies and pharmacotherapy, and the existence of general medical comorbidity. In no case should an Indian patient be denied state-of-the-art treatment with the rationalization that treatment by a fellow Indian is of overriding importance.

Use of a Translator

There are large numbers of Indians who do not speak English at all or who speak it as a second or third language. The use of a translator in relating to an Indian person is much the same as with any other person who speaks another language. The clinician should be aware, however, that translation is often not so much an exercise in finding equivalent words but rather in finding equivalent concepts. Related to this is the problem of *cultural* translation, which can only be accomplished by someone who is very familiar with both cultures. The clinician who works with a particular Indian group will do well to learn as much about that group as possible and to regularly consult with Indian people, so he or she can make the cultural translation. Use of a translator for psychiatric practice requires practice and patience. Also required is sensitivity to the translator's perceived role in the community and the potential for countertransference between translator and patient.

Conclusion

We have reviewed many unmet needs in the psychiatric treatment of Indian people. These include the need for more funding of services, the need to focus on illness, the need to coordinate services, and the need for more research—epidemiological and clinical. But no need is more critical than the need for well-trained personnel, both Indian and non-Indian.

The psychiatric treatment of Indian people can be challenging and rewarding. Unfortunately, inadequate understanding has too often led to frustration in both patient and psychiatrist, and thus to a less than pleasant (and a less than therapeutic) encounter. We hope that this chapter will assist in alleviating that lack of preparation. However, what we have written here cannot take the place of talking with Indian people and to others who have worked with Indian people. Nor can it take the place of gaining the trust of Indian people in the clinical setting, learning about them slowly, and allowing them to learn about oneself. With patience on both sides, the Indian community and the psychiatrist can each learn that the other has knowledge and skills that can help troubled patients. With time and effort, the community will incorporate the Western healer and allow him or her to participate in a common task—the curing of disease and the healing of illness in Indian people.

References

Albaugh B, Albaugh P: Alcoholism and substance sniffing among the Cheyenne and Arapaho Indians of Oklahoma. Int J Addict 14:1001–1007, 1979

Alhali Lake Indian Band: The Honour of All, Part I and Part II (videotape). Available from Alhali Lake Indian Band, P.O. Box 4479, Williams Lake, British Columbia, Canada V2G 2V5. Undated

American Psychiatric Association: Diagnostic and Statistical Manual of Mental Disorders, 3rd Edition. Washington, DC, American Psychiatric Association, 1980

American Psychiatric Association: Diagnostic and Statistical Manual of Mental Disorders, 3rd Edition, Revised. Washington, DC, American Psychiatric Association, 1987

Association of American Indian Physicians: Report on Physical and Mental Health of Elderly Indians. Final report of a contract with the Indian Health Service. Rockville, MD, Indian Health Service, U.S. Public Health Service, U.S. Department of Health, Education and Welfare, 1978

Attneave CL: Medicine men and psychiatrists in the Indian Health Service. Psychiatric Annals 4(9):49–55, 1974

Baron AE, Manson SM, Ackerson LM, et al: Depressive symptomatology in older American Indians with chronic disease: some psychometric considerations, in Depression in Primary Care: Screening and Detection. Edited by Atkinsson C, Zich JM. New York, Routledge, 1990, pp 217–231

Beauvais F, Oetting ER, Edwards RW: Trends in drug use of Indian adolescents living on reservations: 1975–1983. Am J Drug Alcohol Abuse 11(3 & 4):209–230, 1985

Beiser M: Indian mental health. Psychiatric Annals 4:6–8, 1974

Beiser M, Attneave CL: Mental disorders among Native American children: rates and risk periods for entering treatment. Am J Psychiatry 139:193–198, 1982

Beiser M, DeGroat E: Body and spirit medicine: conversations with a Navajo singer.

Psychiatric Annals 4(9):9–12, 1974

Berkhofer RF: White Man's Indian. New York, Alfred A Knopf, 1978

Bergman RL: The medicine man of the future—reuniting the learned professions, in Beyond Clinic Walls. Edited by Tulipan AB, Attneave CL, Kingstone E. University, AL, University of Alabama Press, 1974, pp 131–143

Berlin IN: Psychopathology and its antecedents among American Indian adolescents, in Advances in Clinical Child Psychology, Vol 9. Edited by Lahey BB, Kazdin AE. New York, Plenum, 1986

Body of 8th Indian suicide victim found. Tulsa Daily World, September 29, 1985

Brown D: Bury My Heart at Wounded Knee. New York, Holt, Reinhart & Winston, 1971

Browne DB: WISC-R scoring patterns among Native Americans of the northern plains. White Cloud Journal 3(2):3–16, 1984

Cardinal H: The Unjust Society: The Tragedy of Canada's Indians. Edmonton, Alberta, MG Hurtig, 1969

Cole M, Gay J, Glick JA, et al: The Cultural Context of Learning and Thinking: An Exploration in Experimental Anthropology. New York, Basic Books, 1971

Coles R: Eskimos, Chicanos, Indians: Vol IV, Children of Crisis. Boston, MA, Little, Brown, 1977

Conrad RD, Kahn M: An epidemiological study of suicide among the Papago Indians. Am J Psychiatry 131:69–72, 1974

Coolidge D: "Kid catching" on the Navajo reservation: 1930, in The Destruction of American Indian Families. Edited by Unger S. New York, Association on American Indian Affairs, 1977

Corlett WT: The Medicine Man of the American Indian and His Cultural Background. Springfield, IL, Charles C Thomas, 1935. Quoted in Vogel VJ (ed): American Indian Medicine. Norman, OK, University of Oklahoma Press, 1970

Dana RH, Hornby R, Hoffmann T: Local norms of personality assessment for Rosebud Sioux. White Cloud Journal 3(2):17–25, 1984

Debo A: A History of the Indians of the United States. Norman, OK, University of Oklahoma Press, 1970

Debo A: And Still the Waters Run: The Betrayal of the Five Civilized Tribes. Norman, OK, University of Oklahoma Press, 1984

de Tocqueville A: Democracy in America, Vol 1 (1835). Translated by Reeves H. New York, Appleton-Century-Crofts, 1898. Quoted in McNickle D: They Came Here First. New York, Perennial Library, 1975

Dobyns HF: Their Number Become Thinned. Knoxville, TN, University of Tennessee Press, 1983

Driver HE: Indians of North America, 2nd Edition, Revised. Chicago, IL, University of Chicago Press, 1969

Fields S: Folk Healing for the wounded spirit, I: Medicine Men: purveyors of an ancient art. Innovations 3(1):12–18, 1976

Forbis RG: Eastern North America, in North America. Edited by Gorenstein S. New

York, St. Martin's Press, 1975

Gaddis VH; American Indian Myths and Mysteries. Radnor, PA, Chilton Book Company, 1977

Goldstein GS: The model dormitory. Psychiatric Annals 4:85–92, 1974

Goldstine T, Gutmann D: A TAT study of Navajo aging. Psychiatry 35:373–384, 1972

Goodman J: American Genesis. New York, Summit Books, 1981

Graves TD: The personal adjustment of Navajo Indian migrants to Denver, Colorado. American Anthropologist 72:35–54, 1970

Green BE, Sack WH, Pambrun A: A review of child psychiatric epidemiology with special reference to American Indian and Alaska Native children. White Cloud Journal 2(2):22–36, 1981

Harras A: Issues in adolescent Indian health: suicide. Tucson, AZ, U.S. Department of Health and Human Service, Health Resources Services Administration, Indian Health Service, Office of Health Program Development, 1987

Hathaway SR, McKinley JC: Minnesota Multiphasic Personality Inventory, Revised. Minneapolis, MN, University of Minnesota, 1970

Heath DB: Emerging anthropological theory and models of alcohol use and alcoholism, in Theories on Alcoholism. Edited by Chaudron CD, Wilkinson DA. Toronto, Ontario, Addiction Research Foundation, 1988

Holinger PC: Violent deaths as a leading cause of mortality: an epidemiologic study of suicide, homicide, and accidents. Am J Psychiatry 137:472–476, 1980

Hughes CC: Culture-bound or construct-bound?: the syndromes of DSM-III, in The Culture-Bound Syndromes: Folk Illnesses of Psychiatric and Anthropological Interest. Edited by Simons RC, Hughes CC. Dordrecht, Netherlands, D Reidel, 1985

Indian Health Service: Trends in Indian health, 1989. Rockville, MD, U.S. Department of Health and Human Services, Program Statistics Branch, Indian Health Service, 1989a

Indian Health Service: National plan for Native American mental health services. Rockville, MD, U.S. Department of Health and Human Services, Mental Health Programs, Indian Health Service, 1989b

Jelik WG: Indian healing power: indigenous therapeutic practices in the Pacific Northwest. Psychiatric Annals 4(9):13–21, 1974

Jelik WG, Todd N: Witchdoctors succeed where doctors fail: psychotherapy among the Coast Salish Indians. Canadian Psychiatric Association Journal 19:351–356, 1974

Jennings JD: Ancient Native Americans. San Francisco, CA, Freeman, 1978

John R: Service needs and support networks of elderly Native Americans: family, friends, and social service agencies, in Social Bonds in Later Life: Aging and Interdependence. Edited by Peterson WA, Quadagno J. Beverly Hills, CA, Sage, 1985

Jouvency J: untitled, quoted in Vogel VJ: American Indian Medicine. Norman, OK, University of Oklahoma Press, 1970, p 20

Kaufman A: Gasoline sniffing among children in a Pueblo Indian village. Pediatrics 51:1060–1064, 1973

Kaplan B, Johnson D: The social meaning of Navajo psychopathology, in Magic, Faith, and Healing. Edited by Kiev A. New York, Free Press, 1964

Kivlahan DR, Walker RD, Donovan DM, et al: Detoxification recidivism among urban American Indian alcoholics. Am J Psychiatry 142:1467–1470, 1985

Kleinbaum DG, Kuper LL, Morgenstern H: Epidemiologic Research. Belmont, CA, Lifetime Learning Publications (Wadsworth), 1982

Kleinfeld J, Bloom J: Boarding schools: effects on the mental health of Eskimo adolescents. Am J Psychiatry 134:411–417, 1977

Kleinman A, Eisenberg L, Good B: Culture, illness, and care: clinical lessons from anthropologic and cross-cultural research. Ann Intern Med 88:251–258, 1978

Kunitz SJ: Disease Change and the Role of Medicine: The Navajo Experience. Berkeley, CA, University of California Press, 1983

Kunitz SJ, Levy JE: Changing ideas of alcohol use among Navajo Indians. Quarterly Journal of Studies on Alcohol 35:243–259, 1974

La Barre W: Folk medicine and folk science. Journal of American Folk-Lore 1942; 55:199–200, quoted in Vogel VJ (ed): American Indian Medicine. Norman, OK, University of Oklahoma Press, 1970

Lake RG (Medicine Grizzly Bear): Shamanism in Northwestern California: a female perspective on sickness, healing and health. White Cloud Journal 3(1):31–42, 1983

Lawson J: History of North Carolina (1714). Durham, NC, Richmond, Garrett and Massie, 1937, cited in Walker RD, LaDue R: An integrative approach to American Indian mental health, in Ethnic Psychiatry. Edited by Wilkinson CB. New York, Plenum, 1986

Levine S, Lurie NO (eds): The American Indian Today. Baltimore, MD, Penguin, 1970

Levy J: Untitled, quoted in Kunitz SJ: Disease Change and the Role of Medicine: The Navajo Experience. Berkeley, CA, University of California Press, 1983

Levy JE: Discussion following alcoholism, alcohol abuse, and health in American Indians and Alaska Natives, quoted in Silk-Walker P, Walker D, Kivlahan D: Behavioral Health Issues Among American Indians and Alaska Natives (Monograph No 1). Edited by Manson SM, Dinges NG. Denver, CO, American Indian and Alaska Native Mental Health Research, 1988, p 86

Levy JE, Kunitz SJ: Indian Drinking: Navajo Practices and Anglo-American Theories. New York, Wiley, 1974

Lockart B: Historic distrust and the counseling of American Indians and Alaska Natives. White Cloud Journal 2(2):31–34, 1981

Loretto G, Beauvais F, Oetting E: The primary cost of drug abuse: What Indian youth pay for drugs. American Indian and Alaska Native Mental Health Research 2(1):21–32, 1988

Luckert KW: Traditional Navaho theories of disease and healing. Arizona Medicine 29:571–3, 1972

Manson SM, Callaway DG: Problematic life situations: cross-cultural variation in support mobilization among the elderly (Final Report on Grant No. 0090-AR-0037).

Washington, DC, Administration on Aging, 1984

Manson SM, Shore JH, Bloom JD: The depressive experience in American Indian communities: a challenge for psychiatric theory and diagnosis, in Culture and Depression. Edited by Kleinman A, Good B. Berkeley, CA, University of California Press, 1985

Manson SM, Walker RD, Kivlahan DR: Psychiatric assessment and treatment of American Indians and Alaska Natives. Hosp Community Psychiatry 38:165–173, 1987

Marano L: Windigo psychosis: the anatomy of an emic-etic confusion, in The Culture-Bound Syndromes: Folk Illnesses of Psychiatric and Anthropological Interest. Edited by Simons RC, Hughes CC. Dordrecht, Netherlands, D Reidel, 1985

May PA: Suicide and self-destruction among American Indian youths. American Indian and Alaska Native Mental Health Research 1(1):52–69, 1987

May PA: Mental health and alcohol abuse indicators in the Albuquerque Area of Indian Health Service: an exploratory chart review. American Indian and Alaska Native Mental Health Research 2(1):33–46, 1988

May PA, Smith MB: Some Navajo Indian opinions about alcohol abuse and prohibition: a survey and recommendations for policy. J Stud Alcohol 49:324–334, 1988

May PA, Hymbaugh KJ, Aase JM, et al: Epidemiology of fetal alcohol syndrome among American Indians of the southwest. Soc Biol 30:374–387, 1983

McNickle D: They Came Here First. New York, Perennial Library, 1975

McShane DA, Plas JM: WISC-R factor structures for Ojibwa Indian children. White Cloud Journal 2(4):18–22, 1982

Meriam L: The effects of boarding schools on Indian family life (1928), in The Destruction of American Indian Families. Edited by Unger S. New York, Association on American Indian Affairs, 1977

Mick C: A profile of American Indian nursing homes (Working Paper and Reprint Series, Long-Term Care Gerontology Center). Tucson, AZ, University of Arizona, 1983

Mindell C, Gurwitt AL: The placement of American Indian children—the need for change, in The Destruction of American Indian Families (Official Position Paper of the American Academy of Child Psychiatry, January 25, 1975). Edited by Unger S. New York, Association on American Indian Affairs, 1977, pp 61–66

Murray HA: Thematic Apperception Test Manual. Cambridge, MA, Harvard College, 1943

National Indian Council on Aging: Indian elders: a tribute: final report on the Fourth National Indian Conference on Aging. Washington, DC, National Indian Council on Aging, 1982

National Public Radio: Adolescent Indian Suicide. News feature on All Things Considered, Washington, DC, National Public Radio, October 5, 1985

Neihardt JG: Black Elk Speaks. Lincoln, NE, University of Nebraska Press, 1961

Neligh G: Secondary and tertiary prevention applied to suicide in American Indians. American Indian and Alaska Native Mental Health Research 1(3):4–18, 1988a

Neligh G: Major mental disorders and behavior among American Indians and Alaska

Natives, in Behavioral Health Issues Among American Indians and Alaska Natives (Monograph No 1). Edited by Manson SM, Dinges NG. Denver, CO, American Indian and Alaska Native Mental Health Research, 1988b

Ogden M, Spector MI, Hill CA: Suicides and homicides among Indians. Public Health Rep 85:75–80, 1970

O'Sullivan MH, Handal PJ: Medical and psychological effects of the threat of compulsory relocation for an American Indian tribe. American Indian and Alaska Native Mental Health Research 2(1):3–20, 1988

Passel JS, Berman PA: Quality of 1980 Census data for American Indians. Soc Biol 33:163–182, 1986

Penn W: The Indians (1683), in William Penn's Own Account of the Lenni Lenape or Delaware Indians, Revised Edition. Edited by Myers AC. Somerset, NJ, Middle Atlantic Press, 1970

Pollack D, Shore JH: Validity of the MMPI with Native Americans. Am J Psychiatry 137:946–950, 1980

Porter D: Mental health treatment and prevention: focus on elders, in American Indian Families: Developmental Strategies and Community Health. Edited by Mitchell W, Red Horse J. Phoenix, AZ, Arizona State University School of Social Work, 1982

Powell JW: Indian linguistic families of American north of Mexico, in American Indian Languages. Edited by Holder P. Lincoln, NE, University of Nebraska Press, 1966

Public Health Service: Health Services for American Indians (PHS Publ No 531). Washington, DC, U.S. Government Printing Office, 1957

Radloff LS: THe CES-D Scale: a self report depression scale for research in the general population. Journal of Applied Psychological Measurement 1:385–401, 1977

Rhoades ER, Marshall M, Attneave C, et al: Mental health problems of American Indians seen in outpatient facilities of the Indian Health Service, 1975. Public Health Rep 95:329–335, 1980

Richards B, Oxereok C: Counseling Alaskan Natives, in Transcultural Counseling: Needs, Programs, and Techniques. Edited by Walz GR, Benjamin L. New York, Human Sciences Press, 1978

Robbins RM, Lurien NO: The world's oldest ongoing protest demonstration: North American Indian drinking patterns. Pacific Historical Review 40:311–332, 1971

Roy C, Chaudry A, Ivine D: Prevalence of mental disorders among Saskatchewan Indians. Journal of Cross-cultural Psychology 4:383–392, 1970

Sampath HM: Prevalence of psychiatric disorders in a southern Baffin Island Eskimo community. Canadian Psychiatric Association Journal 19:363–367, 1974

Sandefur GD, Sakamoto A: American Indian household structure and income. Demography 25(1):71–80, 1988

Schmidt SM: American Indian health care: An Indian physician's perspective. S D J Med 41(2):13–16, 1988

Schottstaedt MF, Bjork JW: Inhalant Abuse in an Indian Boarding School. Am J Psychiatry 134:1290–1293, 1977

Shomaker DJ: Transfer of children and the importance of grandmothers among the Navajo Indians. Journal of Cross Cultural Gerontology 4:1–18, 1989

Shore JH: American Indian suicide—fact and fantasy. Psychiatry 38:86–91, 1975

Shore JH: Destruction of Indian families—beyond the best interests of Indian children. White Cloud Journal 1(2):13–16, 1978

Shore JH, Manson SM: Cross-cultural studies of depression among American Indians and Alaska Natives. White Cloud Journal 2(2):5–12, 1981

Shore JH, Kinzie JD, Hampson JL, et al: Psychiatric epidemiology of an Indian village. Psychiatry 36:70–81, 1973

Shore JH, Manson SM, Bloom JD, et al: A pilot study of depression among American Indian patients with Research Diagnostic Criteria. American Indian and Alaska Native Mental Health Research 1:4–15, 1987

Silk-Walker P, Walker D, Kivlahan D: Alcoholism, alcohol abuse, and health in American Indians and Alaska Natives, in Behavioral Health Issues Among American Indians and Alaska Natives (Monograph No 1). Edited by Manson SM, Dinges NG. Denver, CO, American Indian and Alaska Native Mental Health Research, 1988

Simons RC, Hughes CC (eds): The Culture-Bound Syndromes: Folk Illnesses of Psychiatric and Anthropological Interest. Dordrecht, Netherlands, D Reidel, 1985

Snow DR: Native American Prehistory: A Critical Bibliography. Bloomington, IN, Indiana University Press, 1979

Spaulding JM: Recent suicide rates among ten Ojibwa Indian bands in Northwestern Ontario. Omega 16:347–354, 1985–1986

Speck RV, Attneave CL: Family Networks. New York, Pantheon, 1973

Statistics Canada: Canada Year Book, 1980–81: A review of Economic, Social, and Political Developments in Canada. Ottawa, Ontario, Minister of Supply and Services, 1981

Stratton R, Zeiner A, Paredes A: Tribal affiliation and prevalence of alcohol problems. J Stud Alcohol 39:1166–1177, 1978

Strimba JL, Sims PS: A university system drug profile. Int J Addict 9:569–583, 1974

Sturtevant WC (ed): Handbook of North American Indians, Vols 1–20. Washington, DC, Smithsonian Institution, 1978ff

Sue S: Psychotherapeutic services for ethnic minorities: Two decades of research findings. Am Psychol 43:301–308, 1988

Sue S, Zane N: The role of culture and cultural techniques in psychotherapy: a critique and reformulation. Am Psychol 42:37–45, 1987

Thompson JW, Walker RD: Adolescent suicide among American Indians and Alaska Natives. Psychiatric Annals 20:128–133, 1990

Trimble JE, Manson SM, Dinges NG, et al: Towards an understanding of American Indian concepts of mental health: some reflections and directions, in Intercultural Applications of Counseling and Therapies. Edited by Marsella A, Pederson P. Beverly Hills, CA, Sage Publications, 1983

Unger S (ed): The Destruction of American Indian Families. New York, Association on American Indian Affairs, 1977

U.S. Bureau of the Census: 1980 Census of Population, Vol 1: Characteristics of the Population, Chapter B, General Population Characteristics, Part 1, United States Summary, PC80-1-B1. Washington, DC, U.S. Department of Commerce, 1983

U.S. Congress: Public Law 95–608. Indian Child Welfare Act of 1978. Congressional Record, 92 Stat. 3069, November 8, 1978

Vogel VJ: American Indian Medicine. Norman, OK, University of Oklahoma Press, 1970

Vogel VJ: This Country Was Ours: A Documentary History of the American Indian. New York, Harper & Row, 1972

Walker RD: Special populations, in Broadening the Base of Treatment for Alcohol Problems. Edited by Glazer F, Deisenhaus H. National Academy Press, 1990

Walker RD, LaDue R: An integrative approach to American Indian mental health, in Ethnic Psychiatry. Edited by Wilkinson CB. New York, Plenum, 1986

Walker RD, Benjamin GA, Kivlahan DR, et al: American Indian alcohol misuse and treatment outcome, in Alcohol Use Among Ethnic Minorities: National Institute on Alcohol Abuse and Alcoholism Research Monograph 18 (DHHS Publ No ADM-87-143). Edited by Westermeyer J. Washington, DC, U.S. Government Printing Office, 1989, pp 301–314

Wauchope R (ed): Handbook of Middle American Indians, Vols I–VIII. Austin, TX, University of Texas Press, 1964–1969

Wechsler D: Manual for the Wechsler Intelligence Scale for Children—Revised. New York, Psychological Corporation, 1974

Weil TE: Area Handbook for Mexico, 2nd Edition. Foreign Area Studies of the American University (DA Pam 550–579). Washington, DC, U.S. Government Printing Office, 1975

Weslager CA: Magic Medicines of the Indians. Wallingford, PA, Middle Atlantic Press, 1973

Westermeyer J: Chippewa and majority alcoholism in the Twin Cities: a comparison. J Nerv Ment Dis 155:322–327, 1972

Westermeyer J: "The drunken Indian": myths and realities. Psychiatric Annals 4(9):29–36, 1974

Westermeyer J, Peake E: A ten-year follow-up of alcoholic Native Americans in Minnesota. Am J Psychiatry 140:189–194, 1983

Westermeyer J, Walker D: Approaches to treatment of alcoholism across cultural boundaries. Psychiatric Annals 12:434–439, 1982

Westermeyer J, Walker D, Benton E: A review of some methods for investigating substance abuse among American Indians and Alaska Natives. White Cloud Journal 2(2):13–21, 1981

Glossary of Related Terms

Alaska Native
Descendants of the pre-Columbian inhabitants of what is now Alaska. This designation includes a diverse group of American Indian, Eskimo, and Aleut people. (The term "Alaskan Native" refers to someone born in the state of Alaska.)

American Indian
Descendants of the pre-Columbian inhabitants of North America. The term "Native American" is not preferred, because many believe this to mean "born in America." In Canada, Indian people are referred to as "Native Indian."

Giveaway
A ceremony during which a person who is being honored *gives* gifts to others, rather than *receiving* gifts as he or she might in the majority culture. This is an example of the Indian concept of ownership, which is often not focused on material goods, but rather on caretaking and sharing. Also called a *potlatch* (pronounced "pot-latch") in some communities in the Pacific Northwest. (*Potlatch* is from the Chinook word *patshatl*, meaning "giving" or "a gift.")

Indian Health Service (IHS)
Founded in 1955 as a component of the U.S. Public Health Service (PHS), the IHS is the sole source of medical care for many Indian people. It consists of both civilian employees and members of the PHS Commissioned Corps, a nonmilitary uniformed service. As a federal agency, the IHS reports directly to the Assistant Secretary for Health, Department of Health and Human Services.

Pow Wow
An American Indian social gathering, held in the summer, featuring dancing, singing, contests, food, giveaways, and handicrafts. Many of these are open to all (Indian and non-Indian), although some are only open to a particular tribe or tribes.

Reservation
A parcel of land set aside for exclusive use of a particular Indian tribe or tribes. There are reservations throughout the United States, from New York to California. Less than half of the U.S. Indian population lives on reservations. In Canada, these areas are referred to as "reserves."

Spirit Camp
A gathering in Alaska, wherein traditional activities are combined with small group discussions. These meetings are intended to pass along traditional ways to younger people and to give them a sense of their place in the community.

Sweat Lodge
A small space in which a "sweat" ceremony is held. It is specially prepared for each sweat. A medicine man presides over the ceremony, and individuals can participate only by invitation. Sweats are held for purposes of cleansing, prayer, and healing.

Traditional Medicine
Medicine as practiced by medicine men and women. It includes pharmaceutical, psychological, and spiritual interventions. Medicine practiced by physicians trained in the Western medical tradition is referred to as "Western medicine," or more colloquially as "white medicine." There is no inherent conflict between traditional and Western medicine.

9 Psychiatric Care of Chinese Americans

Albert C. Gaw, M.D.

I n this chapter, the term "Chinese American" refers to both United States citizens of Chinese ancestry and Chinese citizens who reside permanently in the continental United States, Hawaii, and U.S. Pacific Territory islands. The 1990 census registered 1,645,472 Chinese Americans, making them the largest Asian group among the various Asian immigrant communities in the United States.

Chinese Americans are a heterogeneous group. To understand them and effectively treat their mental illnesses, it is important to appreciate their varied cultural and ethnic background, their beliefs and cultural values, and their immigration experience in the United States. It is also essential to understand how psychiatric symptoms are manifested among Chinese Americans in ways similar to or different from other ethnic groups, how they view mental illness, what role the family plays in the care of mentally ill relatives, and why it is necessary to prescribe treatments that are acceptable in the context of Chinese American cultural experience.

China: The Land, Its People, Religion, and Values

China is located in the central portion of the Asiatic continent. It is the second largest sovereign area in the world, next to the Russian Republic of the Commonwealth of Independent States. It has a land mass of 3 1/3 million square miles, which is more than 300,000 square miles larger than the United States. However, because of its rugged interior terrain, most of the

In general, the Wade-Giles system of romanization has been used for Chinese words throughout this book. In some cases, Pinyin romanization has been substituted or provided as an alternative for certain geographic names and common terms. The glossary in the back of this book provides a more detailed discussion of Wade-Giles romanization and of the tonality of the spoken Chinese language, as well as a complete listing of Chinese characters for each term used.

Chinese people live in 1 million square miles south of the Great Wall, a region that is only about 30% of the entire land area and about 43% the size of the continental United States. All the major population centers and the major centers of national economic enterprise are located within 1,000 miles of the eastern coast of China (Winfield 1948, pp. 18–22).

The Chinese population, currently estimated to be 1 billion, constitutes about one-fifth of all the people on earth. China is primarily an agricultural country. The Chinese language is formed by more than 40,000 characters or ideographs that were developed from picture writing. Although several distinct dialects are spoken in different regions of the country, Mandarin or *kuo-yü* is the national language. In addition to Mandarin, other dialects commonly spoken by American expatriates from China are:

1. Cantonese and Taishanese from the Kwangtung (Guangdong) province in southern China and Hong Kong;
2. Fukienese, Amoy, and Taiwanese, from the province of Fukien (Fujian) along the southeastern coast and Taiwan;
3. Shanghainese, from the Shanghai region;
4. Hakka, from a region extending along an east-west axis from Fukien to Kwangsi (Guangxi); and
5. Szechwanese, from the Szechwan (Sichuan) province of western China.

China has one of the world's oldest continuous civilizations. Yang (1961) pointed out that religion assumes a key role in traditional Chinese social life and organizations and thus provides a basis for its existence and development. Because religious beliefs strongly shape traditional Chinese values and behavior, key religious beliefs that molded traditional Chinese values are briefly described here.

Two major cultural elements in the religious traditions of China are generally recognized: 1) a complex of varying but related local beliefs and practices of the common people, and 2) the three great literate religious traditions of the educated class—Confucianism, Taoism, and Buddhism (Hu 1960).

Chinese Folk Religious Beliefs

Ancestral Cult

Hu (1960) pointed out that ancestral cult is the oldest and most pervasive of all Chinese religions (p. 111). It is based on the belief that the living can directly communicate with the dead; the dead, though now living in a different world, can still influence and be influenced by events in this world. This belief forms the basis for the veneration of ancestral spirits.

The rituals of ancestral worship were primarily personal and familial ones. Most homes had a shelf containing ancestral tablets where incense was burned and ceremonies and offerings to ancestors were made. Complete meals were offered during special festivals, such as the Chinese New Year or during the death anniversaries of ancestors. For All Saints Day (*Ch'ing-ming*), the family graveyard was cleaned, and yellow paper currency and foods were offered to the departed. Thus, ancestor worship served to perpetuate strong family ties, a hallmark of Chinese culture, and it provided the matrix in which certain folk religious beliefs thrived.

Folk Religion

Folk religion consisted of a curious mixture of popular beliefs derived from ancestor worship and the world of spirits and from the three literate religious traditions of Confucianism, Taoism, and Buddhism (Hu 1960, p. 112). The conceptual basis for folk religion is a belief in a direct and reciprocal relationship between the terrestrial and the spiritual world, and between and among human beings, gods, and spirits.

The celestial world is believed to be populated by departed ancestors, gods, ghosts, demons, animal spirits and deified heroes of the Chinese history. Divinities were thought to be organized in a celestial bureaucracy superintended by the Jade Emperor—a hierarchy quite akin to the traditional Chinese imperial order. As I discuss later in this chapter, in the mind of the peasants, these celestial beings played a key role in the affairs of the common people. For example, Hu (1960) mentioned that there is a kitchen god who kept account of all the good and bad deeds of the family. Each village has a tutelary god, *T'u-ti*, who had charge of the local census and received reports of death. *Ts'ai-shen*, the god of wealth, is particularly welcomed by merchants during the Chinese New Year.

Some malevolent spirits, called *kuei*, were also believed to inhabit the celestial world. Certain animals like foxes and snakes were thought to possess supernatural powers and could assume charming forms to seduce young men.

The expert in dealing with the spiritual world is the shaman, or *wu*. The shaman is called upon to intercede on a sick person's behalf, particularly when the patient was thought to be possessed by a malevolent spirit.

The Literate Traditions

Confucianism

Strictly speaking, as Yang (1961, p. 244) had pointed out, Confucianism is not a full-fledged theistic religion, because it poses no gods or supernatural dogma as symbols of its teachings. Yang reiterated that Confucianism is concerned with the elaboration of *Tao* or the Way in the social sphere. It deals with visible facts, is formal, values self-restraint, order, and ceremonious correlates of deportment, and cultivates deportment.

Confucianism stressed family solidarity, friendship, social relations, and imperial allegiance. The Confucian ethic included the concept of filial piety, principles of moral cultivation, and rules for detailed application of the virtues to human relationships and problems (Hu 1960, p. 474). Chinese values such as *jen* (goodness in interpersonal relationships), *li* (propriety in interpersonal relationships), and the emphasis on morality and on conformity of prescribed role behavior are Confucian in origin.

Taoism

Taoism, like Confucianism, was both a philosophy and a religion (Hu 1960, p. 118). Hu has pointed out that as a religion, Taoism was eclectic, borrowing many important features (especially its organizational and ritualistic aspects) from Buddhism and incorporating many practices and beliefs from folk religion. Unlike Buddhist monks, Taoist priests, called *tao-shih,* kept their family names and were not expected to shave the hair on their heads. Taoism is closely identified with alchemy, geomancy, divination, witchcraft, fortune-telling, astrology, communication with the dead, as well as breathing control and a special diet designed to prolonged life. Thus, Taoism appealed to the mystical side of human nature; it evolved into a warm, personal religion and fulfilled a human need that Confucianism had not (Hu 1960, p. 118).

Buddhism

Buddhism, based on the teachings of Siddhārtha Gautama, originated in India and was introduced into China around the first century A.D. (late Han Dynasty). Its chief appeal lay in its promise of salvation (Hu 1960, p. 120). The Goddess of Mercy is *Kuan-yin.* Amida Buddha (Amitabha) is the ruler of Western Heaven. Buddhism seeks enlightenment and avoidance of earthly or blind desires of ignorance. Buddhism teaches the eternity of life and the idea of rebirth—that one's conduct and deportment in this world can influence the eventual form of existence in the next world.

Buddhism became adapted to suit the prevailing Chinese culture. Buddhist gods, like Taoist gods, lived in palaces as the emperors did. Ceremonies of penitence and of the sacrifices to dead ancestors won the favor of the masses. The Buddhist Dhyana meditative school grew into the prominent Ch'an contemplative school and, in turn, was introduced to Japan under the name Zen.

As I discuss later, traditional Chinese religious beliefs became incorporated into traditional Chinese medical thinking and served as the underpinning for the conceptual basis of health and disease, healing practices, and guidelines for deportment and interpersonal relationships.

Chinese Immigration to the United States

Chinese were living on the American continent soon after the arrival of European settlers. Chinese were reported among the servants of the early Spanish galleon traders, and were aboard the ships of nations engaged in the China Trade (Lai 1980). However, the impetus for large-scale immigration to the United States did not take place until the mid-19th century. (See Table 18–7 for an outline of significant dates and events in the history of Chinese immigration to the United States.)

Prompted by the discovery of gold in California in 1848 and the need for manual labor for the construction of railroads and industrial development, and coupled with the presence of political unrest and natural disasters in China, large numbers of Chinese, especially from the coastal province of Guangdong, settled on the West Coast of the United States. Within 2 years of their first arrival, the Chinese population had swelled to 25,000 (Sung 1975). Most of the early settlers were peasants and unskilled laborers who spoke the Taishanese and Cantonese dialects. As aliens who staunchly maintained their habits and customs, they formed close-knit communities that evolved into present-day Chinatowns.

Competition with white laborers in a period of economic depression in the 1870s led to the emergence of anti-Chinese sentiments. These sentiments eventually were enacted into a series of Exclusion Laws. Beginning with the Exclusion Act of 1882, at least 14 pieces of discriminatory legislation were enacted by the U.S. Congress over the years. These laws prevented Chinese from bringing over their wives from abroad and denied them the right to citizenship and to due process of law (Kim 1973). In certain states, they were segregated in schools and theaters; refused services in barber shops, hotels, restaurants, and at public places; denied the right to purchase land; and not permitted to marry whites (Lai 1980). Furthermore, immigration quotas were imposed creating a barrier that virtually halted the immigration of Chinese into the United States. By 1920, the total Chinese population had declined from a high of 107,488 in 1880 to 61,639. Denied the opportunity to be reunited with their wives and families, early Chinese American communities were predominantly male.

Many of the early Chinese laborers were sojourners who had intended to return to China when they retired. But World War II and the Communist takeover of mainland China prevented these sojourners from returning. As a result, many were stranded in the United States, and they were forced to retire in America without the benefit of traditional family support.

Japanese military imperialism during World War II changed the landscape of political alliances. China became an ally of the United States. This new political alliance mitigated anti-Chinese feeling. Former restrictive immigration policy toward Asians became liberalized. The War Bride Act of 1946 allowed Chinese wives of American soldiers to join their husbands in the United States. Congress finally repealed the Exclusion Laws in 1965.

With changes in the national immigration quota system, the number of Chinese immigrants in the United States increased dramatically. From a low of 77,504 in 1940, the Chinese population rose to 1,645,472 in 1990.

The wave of immigrants following World War II consisted of wives, children, and family members of resident Chinese Americans, overseas students, semiskilled and skilled laborers, and merchants, as well as professionals from various East Asian countries. The reunion of Chinese family members offered the opportunity to restabilize the Chinese American family system, previously fragmented by the enactment of Exclusion Laws. (An outline of cohort experiences of Chinese American elders is presented in Table 18–8.) The influx of younger immigrants of diverse vocational backgrounds also provided a wider range of labor for Chinese American communities and the greater American society.

There were, of course, other sources of Chinese immigrants. After the Communist takeover of China and with the breakoff of diplomatic relations between the United States and the People's Republic of China (PRC), Chinese immigration drew exclusively from East Asian countries such as Taiwan, Hong Kong, Singapore, Malaysia, and the Philippines. The reestablishment of diplomatic relations between the United States and the PRC in 1978 provided an opportunity for students and professionals from mainland China to study at American universities. Some of these students eventually elected to stay in the United States.

The massacre at Tienanmen Square in Beijing in June 1989 and its political aftermath has further fueled the desire of a certain sector of Chinese students from the PRC and other Asian countries to seek permanent residency in the United States. In addition, the anticipated 1997 transfer of British sovereignty over Hong Kong to the PRC creates an impetus for many Hong Kong immigrants and businesspeople to resettle in North America. Many have settled on the West Coast and continue their business activities in East Asia. Another group includes expatriate Chinese refugees from Vietnam.

Thus, the influx of immigrants from different parts of China as well as other East Asian countries after World War II contributed to the complexity of the existing Chinese American communities. Each Chinese subcultural group has brought with it a unique dialect and system of values, beliefs, customs, food habits—and even, perhaps, a distinct illness-coping style.

Current Demography

The 1990 census figures for Asian American demography are not yet available. According to the 1980 figures (U.S. Bureau of the Census 1980), of the 812,000 Chinese Americans, 63% were foreign-born. The peak age distribution was in the 25-to-34 age group. Among people 25 years of age and older, the majority had completed 4 years of high school education or higher. The Chinese American civilian labor force numbered 415,000 with a 3.6% unemployment rate, ranking this group second only to Japanese Americans as the Asian American group with lowest level of unemployment. The prevalent family size and type was a married couple (average family size = 3.65 people). Median income was reported to be $22,559, which was above the national average of $19,917; 10.5% reported income below the poverty level.

Chinese American Communities

Chinatowns were formed by the early Chinese settlers from Guangdong, and the Cantonese dialect continues to be the predominant Chinese dialect spoken in this country. Chinatowns continue to be the entry point for many recent Chinese immigrants and refugees.

Non-Cantonese-speaking Chinese immigrants from Chinese provinces other than Guangdong tend to live in communities surrounding Chinatown and use Chinatown mainly as a place to shop, eat, socialize, and have cultural activities. In recent years, there has been more interaction between Chinatown residents and Chinese Americans from the suburbs, resulting in a positive interchange of talents that has benefited the entire Chinese American community. Substantial Chinatown communities in the United States are now found in major cities such as San Francisco, New York City, Los Angeles, Houston, Sacramento, Boston, Honolulu, and Chicago.

Although the various subcultural groups of the Chinese American community share Mandarin (Beijing dialect) as the common spoken Chinese national language, each subcultural group tends to maintain its spoken dialect as well. These dialects, including Cantonese, Taishanese, Shanghainese, Taiwanese, or Hakka, are phonetically different from one another; as such, they cannot serve as a medium for intergroup communication. The growing number of American-born Chinese Americans tend to speak primarily English, despite the tendency of the older generation to adhere to their native tongues. Thus, for purposes of intergroup communication among Chinese, either Mandarin or English is used.

Mental Health: Myths and Realities

Highly visible Chinatown communities tended to reinforce stereotypes about Chinese, and these stereotypes usually were reflective of the prevailing social, economic, and political events of the time. During the period of the enactment of the Exclusion Acts and the contemporaneous hard economic times and in order to justify discriminatory acts, Chinese were depicted as pigtailed, strange, exotic, filthy, unassimilable, immoral, treacherous, and cowardly (Kitano and Sue 1973). When China became an ally of the United States during World War II, these negative stereotypes gave way to more positive characterizations depicting Chinese as intelligent, law-abiding, quiet, loyal, hardworking model Americans.

Kitano and Sue (1973) regarded both types of stereotypes as potentially damaging, because in both cases individual and intragroup variation were being ignored. Furthermore, stereotypes provided an excuse for people to neglect the multiple mental health needs confronting Chinese American communities and prevent accurate assessment of their needs. For years, Chinese American communities were considered model communities that had low incidences of crime and mental illness. Many believe that the presence of a strong family system buttressed the Chinese against the emergence of mental illness. Glossed over were the realities of the various social forces such as poverty, overcrowding, poor working conditions, and a rising crime rate that tended in some cases to tear the contemporary Chinese American family apart.

When one examines the working conditions of the present-day Chinatown family, it is still common to find both parents working long hours in restaurants or other family businesses, leaving little time to attend to the care of their children. Cultural pride and community attitude of shunning public display of one's "dirty linen" used to prevent many Chinatown leaders from acknowledging the presence of mental health problems in the community and encouraging the establishment of mental health programs. This conservative attitude has now gradually given way to a more realistic appraisal of community mental health needs as more community-oriented individuals have taken the initiative to form community social and health agencies to address some of these needs (Gaw 1975).

The Stigma of Mental Illness

Concern about the stigma of mental illness may hinder many Chinese American patients and their families from seeking needed mental health care. This concern may be reflected in a range of behaviors, including a low rate of utilization of mental health services among Chinese Americans, the request from a patient or a family member asking for elaborate clarification of the qualifications of the treating psychiatrist, inordinate concern about confidentiality, reluctance to use insurance coverage, showing up late for or canceling appointments, lack of support from family members regarding the usefulness of treatment, insistence on having a white therapist, or even an outright refusal to seek psychiatric help even in the face of overt psychiatric symptomatologies.

The central role of the Chinese family in Chinese American culture also means that if one of its members is labeled "mentally ill," it will bring shame upon the entire family and raise concern about the marriageability of the patient, other family members, or their offspring. It is therefore not surprising that despite the availability of many modern psychotropic medications and various modalities of treatment, a clinician may still occasionally find a mentally ill Chinese American who has been kept for years in a Chinese household without receiving psychiatric help. These cases are brought to the attention of caregivers only when a crisis arises.

Lin and Lin (1981, pp. 388–391) cited several common popular Chinese views of mental illness that may contribute to the development of stigma:

1. It is viewed as "misconduct" requiring corrective thinking and rectification of behavior.
2. It is a sign of the wrath of the gods or ancestors caused by the transgression of family rituals in ancestor worship.
3. It is considered a result of an imbalance of yin and yang.
4. It is caused by a lack of hormones or vitamins or results from diminished brain function.
5. It is caused by hereditary defects.
6. It is a reaction to psychosocial stresses such as being jilted in love, failing in a business venture, or passing college entrance examinations.

The net result of these notions of mental illness is an acute feeling of shame, guilt, and embarrassment that, in extreme cases, may lead the person with mental illness to avoid all outside contacts. The stigma implies that misconduct and/or deficiency has occurred in the family and that family members have failed to guide, exhort, educate, manage, or provide for the patient—and, therefore, that they are deserving of shame.

Response of Chinese Families to Mental Illness

Lin and Lin (1981) studied the pattern of help-seeking behavior among Chinese Canadian families having a family member with a psychotic illness. The researchers tracked the families from onset of the family member's psychiatric problem to his or her admission to a mental health institution or agency. They described five phases in the pathway of family coping:

1. Confinement of coping exclusively within the family;
2. Inclusion of certain trusted outsiders;
3. Consultation with outside agencies and professionals;
4. Hospitalization after the patient has been diagnosed with a mental illness; and
5. Scapegoating and final rejection of the patient by the family.

The Lin and Lin (1981) study suggests that Chinese families would attempt prolonged management of the patient's deviant behavior within the family by mobilizing its own resources and remedies with minimal outside assistance, and without initially regarding the family member in question as "mentally ill." When these efforts failed, assistance from outside agencies and providers, including physicians and psychiatrists, would be sought while the patient was still kept at home. Hospitalization would be resisted until all other efforts had failed. The introduction of the label of mental illness seemed to hasten the transition from intrafamilial coping to hospitalization of the patient. Ultimately, the patient is rejected by family members and is scapegoated and blamed for things that went wrong within the family.

The cycle then repeats itself with each relapse. The period of intrafamilial coping is progressively shortened as the number of hospitalizations increases. When the family has reached a point of ceasing all contacts with the patient and is unwilling to take him or her back home, this is an indication that the patient is finally being rejected.

This pattern of intrafamilial coping is certainly not uniquely Chinese. Most families would try to take care of a mentally ill relative at home. What the Lin and Lin (1981) study does suggest is the degree to which a Chinese family would try to keep knowledge of such a problem from outsiders for fear of the shame, guilt, and stigma that such knowledge might bring upon the family should one of its members be labelled "mentally ill." Because of the centrality of the family in the lives of Chinese, Lin and Lin reminded providers not only to involve Chinese family members in the care of their relatives who are patients, but also to be keenly sensitive to the feelings and concerns of both patients and their families when treating Chinese Americans with mental illness.

Conception of Health and Disease in Traditional Chinese Medicine

"Chinese medicine" denotes a system of medical care that includes a broad category of traditional healing activities handed down through medical literati and folk practitioners in China (N. Sivin, unpublished data, July 1975). Such healing practices may range from diagnosis and treatment based on a traditional, highly abstract system of cosmology to treatment by exorcism and incantation. Chinese traditional medical practitioners, called *chung-i-shih,* encompassed the roles of herbalist, acupuncturist, bonesetter, diviner, shaman, and others. For heuristic purposes, the field of Chinese medicine can be broadly classified into two categories: classical and popular or folk.

Conception of Mental Illness in Classical Chinese Medicine

Classical Chinese medicine, best exemplified by the system of theory and prescribed medical practices expounded in *The Yellow Emperor's Classic of Medicine* (*Huang-ti nei-ching su-wen*), probably around the third or second century B.C., has evolved over millennia into a highly abstract system of Chinese metaphysics. The theory served as the basis of medical practice among the Chinese literati minority and the Imperial Court physicians. It was based on beliefs that defined health and illness according to a unitary worldview of cosmology. Humankind was conceived to be a microcosm of the macrocosmic universe, wherein the objective rhythm of the cosmos can intimately affect the workings of the human body. A state of health exists when there is a finely balanced and rhythmic working of the body, a well adjustment of the body to its physical environment, and a harmonious relation between bodily functions and emotion (N. Sivin, unpublished data, July 1975).

The opposite state, in which imbalance exists, constitutes illness. Because of the intimate relationship between the working of the body and the external environment, this conception of health, based on theories universal in natural philosophy, is emphatically ecological, dynamic, and holistic. It is unitary in that it treats somatic, psychologic, social, and ecological phenomena as an integrated system. "Emotions are expected not only to be appropriate in intensity and quality to specific situations, but also in harmony with the daily and seasonal cycles of nature" (N. Sivin, unpublished data, July 1975).

The key concepts are *yin-yang,* a bipolarity that is simultaneously both opposite and complementary; the Five Phases, which are also referred to as the Five Elements; and *ch'i* (energy or vitality). Table 9–1 illustrates the correspondences between the Five Phases, the external physical environment, and the internal milieu of the human body. *Ch'i* is believed to be an all-pervasive force that permeates the universe and the human body and is regulated by *yin-yang* and the Five Phases (Porkert 1974, p. 174).

Table 9–1.   Correspondences of the Five Phases

Phases	Season	Organ	Orifice	Emotion	Color
Wood	spring	liver	eyes	anger	green
Fire	summer	heart	ears	joy	red
Earth	late summer	spleen	nose	compassion	yellow
Metal	autumn	lungs	mouth	sorrow	white
Water	winter	kidney	genitals	fear	black

The human body is conceptualized to have different conduits or meridians that allow for the flow of *ch'i*. Impediments to the flow of *ch'i* result in illness. For example, the presence of pain in an inflamed joint is thought to result from excessive accumulation of *ch'i* in the affected joint. Treatment is then directed toward the restoration of the natural flow of *ch'i* through the use of acupuncture needles, massage, or other traditional methods. *Ch'i* is imbued with properties and is used in the present Chinese vernacular to denote many psychologic states (Table 9–2). The concept of *ch'i* also extends to the description of ancient theory of causation of mental illness (Liu 1981). At least two Chinese classical entities of behavioral disorder, *k'uang* and *tien*, are believed to be related to *ch'i*.

An ancient Chinese medical classic, *Nan Ching*, recognized a person afflicted with *k'uang* as having the following symptoms: feeling sad, eating and sleeping less, developing megalomania with an exaggerated opinion of his or her own intelligence, scolding day and night or stopping to talk, running about restlessly, singing, behaving strangely, and seeing and hearing things. This condition, much akin to a modern picture of a bipolar disorder, is attributed to excessive *yang* energy as well as *ch'i* disturbance. Treatment is accordingly directed to reducing food intake and the utilization of measures such as prescribing herbal medicines that would reduce *yang* to restore the *yin-yang* balance in the person's body.

On the other hand, a person who has *tien* manifests a more quiet and withdrawn form of mental illness. Such an individual will fall to the ground with eyes closed and appear to be asleep. From the perspective of modern nomenclature, this condition may appear to be either epilepsy or schizophrenia. Ancient Chinese medical theory attributes a person's development of *tien* to a preponderance of *yin*. It is speculated that a prenatal predisposition to *tien* can be caused by sudden fright during pregnancy, resulting in an insufficiency of *ch'i* and *ching* (i.e., "vital essence") in the fetus.

Table 9–2. Some dynamic meanings of *ch'i*

Chinese Term	Literal Chinese Meaning	English Meaning
Sheng-ch'i	To produce *ch'i*	To get angry
Ch'u-ch'i	To let *ch'i* out	To get rid of one's anger
Huo-ch'i	Fiery *ch'i*	To have a hot temper
Ch'en-ch'i	Sunken *ch'i*	To be sullen or to feel despair
Ch'i-se	Color of *ch'i*	To describe the facial color or vitality of a person

Conception of Mental Illness in Popular Chinese Medicine

Just as Imperial Court physicians had to develop a highly abstract theory of medicine known as the "classical tradition" as a rationale for dealing with daily stresses and ever-present illnesses, the Chinese peasantry also had to develop a cornucopia of folk therapies and notions of health and disease that gave meaning to the stresses and illnesses of their daily lives. This part of the medical tradition of the Chinese people, deeply rooted in a folk tradition traceable to ancient Taoist, Buddhist, and Confucian teachings, is known as popular medicine.

The folk healers in popular medicine were shamans, physiognomers, geomancers, bonesetters, and fortune-tellers, among others. They employed healing practices that Sivin has described as symbolic therapies ("verbal or non-verbal procedures directed at bringing about or preventing a specific change and usually having a religious significance"; N. Sivin, unpublished data, July 1975). Some of the ritualistic and magical cures they employed included charms, prayers, and exorcism.

In the realm of folk beliefs, the world of humans is surrounded by gods and demons. A hierarchy of gods exists that could invade the human body and feed upon its vital energy, causing illness, if proper rituals were not rendered. Because the daily lives and activities of the common man were thought ultimately to be involved with the celestial world, rituals and liturgies were performed to appease the gods.

The gods had their own arrangement of bureaucratic structure and rank. The Chinese would be intimately acquainted with these "gods." They would offer foods to the gods on special occasion, burn incense in front of their images at home, consult them regarding important business matters or before making key life decisions, and turn to them for guidance and succor during illness.

Like terrestrial officers, the gods could be appeased, pleased, angered, and sometimes even bribed. According to their functions, these gods could further be divided into two general categories. Those seen arising from *yang* are called *shen* and are responsible for all the good that befalls men, whereas those arising from *yin* are *kuei,* or demons.

In this rubric, the human body is thought to be infused with both *shen* and *kuei* at birth. At death, *shen* returns to the *yang* of heaven and *kuei* to the *yin* of the earth. *Kuei* can become a free-floating spirit called *hsieh-ch'i.* The presence of human transgressions such as family strife, failure to render filial obligations, interpersonal quarreling, and social immorality is thought to create a human anomaly that can invite the invasion of *hsieh-ch'i* into the human body and inflict illness. When *hsieh-ch'i* invades the body, a person is considered "possessed."

To treat the illness, a healer or shaman who professes to be possessed by the *yang* spirit and who can act as a medium can be called upon to perform a curing ritual that includes exorcisms, beatings, and ceremonies to call back lost souls. In the course of investigation, the healer attempts to "diagnose" by determining the culpable *kuei* in the family, in the community, or in the celestial bureaucracy. Once the cause of disorder is "diagnosed" and the offending spirit identified, the healer intercedes on the patient's behalf by appealing to the "superior" of the offending spirit in the spiritual hierarchy to drive out the *kuei* from the inflicted individual. In this manner, the healer tries to resolve interpersonal disputes among members of the family and relatives. When an anomaly is thought to exist in the community, the healer would prescribe ritualistic corrective measures.

This supernatural approach of healing also extends into the realm of morality and ethics, rehabilitation, and prevention. To prevent being infected by *kuei*, a person is taught to act in an upright, pure, and clean manner. Magical aids, such as charms containing the secret names of gods or certain drugs and incantations, were used to protect the individual from harm. Social order must be maintained to prevent anomalies from occurring.

Although the healing process in popular medicine is highly symbolic and ritualistic, this supernatural conception of illness and healing treats all aspects of illness—patient, healer, human relations, the social order, and the celestial hierarchy—as a holistic system. All parties who are involved (individual, family, healer, and gods) partake in the healing ritual in order to "cure" the afflicted individual.

The following case study illustrates how the traditional popular conception of illness manifested as a psychosomatic complaint in an elderly Chinese woman.

An elderly Cantonese woman presented with a chief complaint of morning belching. Examinations, including a physical and an upper gastrointestinal X ray, revealed no abnormal findings. She appeared depressed and teary-eyed when talking about her recently deceased husband. She was actively grieving.

When queried, the woman denied feeling depressed. Rather, she was preoccupied with the thought of having touched her dying husband when she last visited him at the hospital and feared that the touching had allowed the *ch'i* from her husband's body to enter her body. When she thought of him in the morning, she would begin to belch, a symptom indicating to her that she had excessive *ch'i*.

In accordance with traditional Chinese folk belief, the *ch'i* of a person leaves the body at death, roams the air, and can invade another human body. Believing that her husband's *ch'i* had infected her, the patient's belching was her symbolic way of expelling excessive *ch'i*.

Culture-Bound Syndromes

Yap (1969) regarded culture-bound syndromes as "certain systems of implicit values, social structure and obviously shared beliefs that produce unusual forms of psychopathology that are confined to special areas" (p. 38). Certain illnesses, known by their indigenous names, such as *koro* (*suk-yeong*), *latah, amok, hsieh-ping, shen-k'uei,* and *p'a-leng,* have been reported among overseas Chinese in East Asia (Tan 1981). With the ease of international travel and the increase in the Asian refugee population in the United States, some of these rather dramatic, confounding, and rarer forms of mental disorder may increasingly be found here and other industrialized countries.

Simons and Hughes (see Chapter 3) have reviewed the more common culture-specific disorders that may likely appear in Western countries, including the United States. Two of the more common categories of culture-specific disorders are described below.

Genital Retraction Disorder (*Koro* or *Suk-yeong*)

Koro is a condition characterized by a complaint about genital retraction with a fear of impending death, occurring where culturally sanctioned beliefs of folk disease or pathology are present. A male with this disorder may complain that his penis is shrinking into his abdomen and that this will kill him. A female with *koro* (a much rarer occurrence) may complain that her labia or breasts are shrinking and that this will kill her. During a state of acute panic, a person with *koro* may attempt to pull his penis or have others hold onto the penis, or he may use clamps or string tied to his penis to prevent it from retracting.

Although all age groups can be affected with *koro,* cases in children are rare, except in the course of an epidemic. The age at onset is early adulthood through the 30s. The disorder is usually self-limiting but may persist for days or weeks. Relapse is possible and recurrence does occur. Social, occupational, and psychologic functioning may be impaired and markedly disrupted. The condition is invariably accompanied by marked anxiety and/or panic, and insomnia is frequently present. The fear of death and the conviction of having a fatal illness may lead a person with *koro* to become depressed and suicidal.

Genitalia may be injured by the careless use of clamps or strings.

The disorder is uncommon except in the context of an epidemic. Although sporadic cases among Chinese immigrants in Western countries have been reported, *koro* occurs most frequently among Chinese in South China or Southeast Asia. Epidemics have also been reported among Thai, Asian Indian, and other Asian groups as well. The disorder usually affects individuals with little formal education, and male patients outnumber females. Individuals who have *koro* frequently have conflicting feelings about masturbation, sexual identity, and/or sexual intercourse.

The following sociocultural factors have been reported to be present in isolated cases and in different epidemic outbreaks of *koro*:

1. A belief in a folk disease called *koro* (among Malays), *suk-yeong* (among Cantonese Chinese), or *suo-yang* (among Mandarin-speaking Chinese);
2. A belief that the excessive loss of semen from too much intercourse may cause involution of the penis;
3. A belief in ghosts of the dead who are capable of stealing penises from the living;
4. A belief in the inducement of genital retraction by ingestion of contaminated foods; and
5. Other cultural beliefs.

Koro should be distinguished from delusional disorder, somatic subtype; body dysmorphic disorder; panic disorder; schizophrenia; organic delusional disorder; sexual disorder not otherwise specified; and from non-culture-specific complaints of genital retraction caused by primary genital diseases or other organic brain dysfunction, such as drug abuse, drug withdrawal state, brain tumor, epilepsy, and syphilis (Bernstein and Gaw 1990). Therapy is usually directed toward providing psychological and environmental support and relieving distressing symptoms through medication. Psychotherapy may be indicated for certain individuals.

Amok

Carr and Tan (1976) described *amok* as follows:

A furious assault commonly found in Malayan males, especially farmers and mountain dwellers, unrelated to suicide, drugs, or alcohol, but related to psychical stress in the form of fright, anger, grief, or nervous depression. The attacks are preceded by vertigo ("fever") and visions ("influences"), are directed against friend and foe alike, may last a few hours, and are followed by total amnesia and deep stuporous sleep for several days. (p. 1297)

Although originally described among Malays, this condition has also been reported to occur among Chinese (Carr and Tan 1976).

The psychosocial profile of people with *amok* is almost always of young or middle-aged men, usually living away from home, who have recently suffered a loss, an insult, or have otherwise "lost face." They are often in the military or recently discharged from it. They are usually poorly educated and from a low socioeconomic background. Often they are individuals who were known as quiet and withdrawn, even "schizoid." Although they may have a history of mental illness, most often these individuals are not exhibiting a concurrent Axis I disorder. Their past behavior patterns may have shown immaturity, impulsivity, poorly controlled emotionality, or social irresponsibility.

Amok needs to be differentiated from *amok*-like conditions that could be caused by epilepsy, infections (such as malaria or syphilis), schizophrenia, depression, psychosis, and dissociative reactions. Owing to the mass assault behavior characteristic of those with *amok*, most *amok* perpetrators are either incarcerated or killed. Treatment is directed toward preventing an individual from acting out mass assault behavior when a change in mental status such as brooding and preoccupation with murder is detected.

Epidemiologic Studies of Mental Disorders Among Chinese

Community survey of psychiatric epidemiologic data for Chinese Americans are lacking. Therefore, epidemiologic data for Chinese Americans have to be extrapolated from studies in other Chinese communities, particularly those done in Taiwan, Hong Kong, Singapore, and the PRC. The application of these data must therefore be limited; they are intended for general background information only.

Lin and colleagues (1981, p. 260) summarized some of these key epidemiologic and clinical findings among Taiwanese Chinese:

1. Prevalence rates of mental illness among Chinese, including rate for psychosis, are roughly similar to those reported from other cultures.
2. The rate for neurosis is lower in less economically developed and less modernized areas, but the rate for psychosis is higher.

3. Alcoholism is rare among Chinese.
4. Drug addiction, a major problem in the past, is currently not a prevalent problem in either Taiwan or the PRC.
5. Middle-aged Chinese show a greater predilection to develop mental disorders. In general, females have higher prevalence rates than males, except for suicide, where males and older people predominate.
6. Oldest sons and youngest daughters have higher rates of mental illness.
7. Neurosis, suicide, and psychophysiological reactions, but not psychosis, are correlated with urbanization and migration. Females and people of lower socioeconomic status are more adversely affected by migration.

In addition, in another study, Hwu and colleagues (1989) surveyed the lifetime prevalence of mental disorders among Taiwanese Chinese as defined by the Chinese Modified Diagnostic Interview Schedule (DIS-CM; Hwu et al. 1984a). Excluding tobacco dependence, the researchers found the prevalence rates for exhibiting any mental disorder were 16.3%, 28.0%, and 21.5% for subjects living in a metropolitan Taipei city sample, a small town sample, and a rural village sample, respectively. Generalized anxiety disorder, alcohol abuse, tobacco dependence, and cognitive impairment had higher prevalence rates in the small town and rural village samples than that of the metropolitan Taipei city sample. Females were found to have a higher prevalence rates for anxiety disorder, psychosexual disorders, depressive disorders, phobic disorder, somatoform disorder, and cognitive impairment. Males had higher prevalence rates for alcoholism, tobacco and drug dependence, and pathological gambling. People living in small towns had the highest prevalence rates for many disorders in the three study sites. Hwu and colleagues speculated that people living in nonmetropolitan areas in Taiwan, where traditional values are more prevalent, are more adversely affected by rapid socioeconomic change and experience more difficulties in adjusting to their new living situations.

Because the methodology in the Taiwan survey used the National Institute of Mental Health (NIMH) Diagnostic Interview Schedule (Robins et al. 1981) to ascertain cases, it was possible to compare the Taiwan results with those of the NIMH Epidemiologic Catchment Area (ECA) survey. Comparison of Taiwan survey data and ECA data revealed lifetime prevalent rates of psychiatric illness of 21.56% in Taiwan and 35.55% in the United States (Compton et al. 1991). The reason for this interesting variation is unclear.

Among Chinese Americans, studies on utilization of mental health facilities (Sue and McKinney 1975), hospitalization rates (Jew and Brody 1967), psychological testing performance of Chinese American students (Sue and Sue 1974), and comparative study of depression between Asian and white students (Marsella et al. 1973) indicate the following findings (Tsai et al. 1981, p. 292):

1. Chinese Americans underutilize mental health facilities.
2. Those Chinese Americans who get treatment tend to be patients who are more disturbed.
3. Somatization among Chinese American patients (expression of psychologic disturbance through bodily symptoms) is prominent.

Somatization and Depression

A number of investigators have reported the prevalence of somatization symptom among Chinese (Kleinman 1977; Marsella et al. 1973; Rin et al. 1966; Tseng 1975). Marsella and colleagues (1973) compared 196 depressed third-generation Chinese Americans and Japanese Americans with a comparable white population at the University of Hawaii and noted, "Chinese seemed to be the only group with rather definite patterns of depression associated with somatic functioning" (p. 447).

Furthermore, one study suggests that the degree of somatization may be class- and age-related. Lee and colleagues (1986) compared somatization symptoms between white outpatients in Rochester, New York, who were diagnosed as neurotic and Chinese patients in Taipei, Taiwan, who were diagnosed as neurotic using standardized protocols. They found that although both American and Chinese patients reported almost the same number of psychosomatic symptoms during structured interview, a significantly higher rate of somatic symptoms in the primary complaints was found in the Chinese subjects. In the absence of psychological symptoms, only 2.9% of the American subjects, in contrast to 37% of the Chinese subjects, reported somatic symptoms. They also indicated that the tendency to somatize emotional problems appears to be related to having less formal education and being older for the Chinese patients and possibly to lower socioeconomic status for the American patients. However, Kleinman (1977) finds somatization among Taiwanese Chinese in all socioeconomic groups and in those with varying levels of formal education.

These findings seemed to support Tseng's (1975) hypotheses that posit four reasons why Chinese tend to express dysphoric symptoms in somatic terms:

1. An organ-oriented conception of pathology that stems from traditional Chinese medicine. Chinese traditional medicine emphasizes close symbolic correspondences between human emotions and body organs (see Table 9–1 and the section in this chapter "Conception of Mental Illness in Classical Chinese Medicine"). With such cultural conception of health and diseases, Chinese may well be apt to express psychic distress through bodily organ symbols.
2. Chinese are reluctant to openly express sexual or aggressive feelings.
3. Expression of physical complaints is more socially acceptable to Chinese than expression of emotional complaints.
4. There is social reinforcement of concerns about bodily functions through the media.

Schizophrenia

Epidemiologic and clinical studies conducted since 1946 on incidence of schizophrenia among Taiwanese as well as among Taiwan's indigenous mountain people have yielded interesting data. Chen (1989) summarized these epidemiologic findings as follows:

1. The rate of schizophrenia is lower among Taiwan's indigenous mountain people than the rate for Taiwanese Chinese.
2. Those with schizophrenia among the indigenous mountain people of Taiwan tended to show acute onset with hyperkinetic excitement, incoherent speech, visual and auditory hallucinations, and occasional non-systematic persecutory delusions.
3. Notwithstanding socioeconomic changes that have occurred in Taiwan in the past 15 years, the rate of schizophrenia has remained stable.
4. Except for an overrepresentation in the 1961–1963 study of females with schizophrenia among those mainland Chinese who had migrated to Taiwan, there is no significant difference in the rate of schizophrenia among different Chinese populations.
5. The schizophrenia manifested by most of the females with the disorder was of the paranoid type.

For those living in metropolitan Taipei, Hwu and colleagues (1989) showed that the lifetime prevalence is 3.0 per 1,000 for schizophrenia and 4.8 per 1,000 for paranoid disorder.

Course and Outcome

Multinational studies from the International Pilot Study of Schizophrenia (Sartorius et al. 1977) has provided evidence of cross-cultural variability in the course and outcome of schizophrenia when the diagnosis was based on strict symptomatological criteria. The data further suggest that patients with schizophrenia who are from developing countries had considerably more favorable course and outcome than those living in developed countries (Lin and Kleinman 1988).

Lo and Lo's (1977) study of Chinese schizophrenic subjects is consistent with the above observation. They conducted a 10-year follow-up study (1965–1975) of a cohort of 133 Chinese patients with schizophrenia after their first admission to the Hong Kong Psychiatric Center. Eighty-two patients (62%) attended follow-up evaluation. Comparison of characteristics of the fully evaluated group and the group who did not attend showed no significant difference in demographic variables and clinical characteristics such as duration, onset of illness, and predominant symptom patterns. However, more patients in the fully evaluated group had a supportive relative as compared with the latter. The results showed that, despite some relapse, 65% of the fully evaluated group had full and lasting remission or showed no deterioration or only mild deterioration. Intragroup comparison showed that being female, having a shorter duration of illness, having an acute onset, having symptom-groups other than disturbances of emotion and volition, and having a supportive relative are factors associated with more favorable prognosis.

Cross-Cultural Comparison of Symptom Pattern

Rin and colleagues (1973) compared symptom patterns of 866 Japanese patients consecutively admitted to five mental hospitals in Tokyo, Japan, in 1963–1964, with 890 Chinese patients consecutively admitted to three hospitals in Taipei, Taiwan, in 1967–1969. Patients with the diagnosis of organic brain disorder were excluded from the analysis. The findings revealed that the Japanese patients showed symptoms of more *shinkeishitsu* (nervous temperament), depression, somatic gastrointestinal/sleep disturbance, hebephrenia, and apathy. The Taiwanese Chinese patients, on the other hand, showed more hostility, breaks with reality, and hypochondria/headache symptoms. Women in each cultural group were found to be more likely than men to show both more severe symptomatology and to have a higher incidence of the symptom patterns that reflect the particular symptomatology of their culture. Rin and colleagues concluded,

Japanese are likely to have disorders in arousal levels, to turn against themselves, and to see the major source of their problems as being within themselves, while the Taiwan Chinese are much more likely to direct their symptomatology outward, to act out against others, and to perceive the outside world in unreal ways. (p. 296)

Familial Genetic Studies

Tsuang (1972) conducted familial genetic study in Taiwan and reported that the risk of schizophrenia were 0.6% for the general population, 6.5% for full siblings of patients, and 4.7% for the parents of patients. Assuming a ratio of 1.0 for the general population, the risk of schizophrenia among full sibs of patients and parents of patients showed a ratio of 10.8 and 7.8, respectively. His study also suggests that "schizophrenias with heavy genetic loading are related to single dominant, major gene inheritance" (p. 225) and that "in Chinese families early-born subjects of both sexes might be more prone to schizophrenia and affective disorders than later-born subjects, perhaps because of psychological stresses due to familial overexpectation and because the early born are overburdened with family responsibilities" (p. 226).

Schizophrenia and Suicide

In a study assessing risks factors of suicide among people with schizophrenia in Hong Kong between 1981 and 1985, 74 Chinese subjects with schizophrenia who had committed suicide were age- and sex-matched with 74 Chinese subjects with schizophrenia who had not committed suicide (Cheng et al. 1990). Sociodemographic variables were found unrelated with suicide. Factors associated with suicide were:

1. Severity of illness (more frequent admissions, higher doses of medication, and earlier appointment);
2. A history of major depressive episodes and suicide attempts;
3. Last hospital admission for reasons other than schizophrenic symptoms alone; and
4. Suicidal ideation on mental status examination.

Affective Disorders

Lin's (1953) original study revealed that the prevalence rate for manic-depressive disorder among Taiwanese Chinese was 0.6%. This rate, repeated 15 years later, remained unchanged at 0.5% (Lin et al. 1969). In a recent survey (Table 9–3), Hwu and colleagues (1989) found that the lifetime prevalence rates of affective disorders in three different types of communities in Taiwan were as follows: for manic episodes, the rates were 1.6% for the metropolitan Taipei city sample, 0.7% for the small town sample, and 1.0% for the rural village sample. There were no significant differences in the rates between the sexes. For major depressive disorder, the lifetime prevalence rates were 8.8% for the metropolitan Taipei city sample, 16.8% for the small town sample, and 9.7% for the rural village sample. Higher prevalence rates for major depressive disorder were found in the small town samples and the females in all three samples. For dysthymic disorder, the lifetime prevalence rates were 9.2% for the metropolitan Taipei city sample, 15.1% for the small town sample, and 9.4% for the rural village sample. Females were found to have a higher prevalence rate than males for dysthymic disorder in the rural village sample only.

Symptom patterns of bipolar affective (manic-depressive) disorder were found not to be dissimilar to those commonly found among other ethnic groups, namely hyperenergy, decreased need of sleep, initial insomnia, early morning awakening, irritability, elation, lability, agitation, easy anxiety, hypertalkativeness, argumentativeness, shifting topics of speech, careless behavior, loud speech, overconfidence, grandiosity, overreligiousity, auditory hallucination, lack of insight, distractibility, and poor concentration.

Treatment

Yang (1985) studied 101 bipolar patients who had each had at least two manic episodes during 2 successive years prior to lithium treatment.

Table 9–3. Lifetime prevalence (per 1,000 residents) of affective disorders in metropolitan Taipei, small town, and rural village samples

Diagnosis	Metropolitan Taipei	Small Town	Rural Village
Manic-depressive disorders	8.8	16.8	9.7
Manic episode	1.6	0.7	1.0
Dysthymic disorders	9.2	15.1	9.4
Generalized anxiety disorders	37.4	104.9	77.8
Panic disorders	2.0	3.4	1.3
Phobic (total) disorders	42.3	56.6	34.5

Source. Hwu et al. 1989.

Lithium was given continuously to the subjects for at least 2 years. Most of the subjects who responded well to the medication showed mean individual plasma lithium levels from 0.5 mm/L to 0.79 mm/L.

Familial Genetic Studies

Tsuang's (1972) study of the risk of affective disorders in relatives of patients diagnosed with manic-depressive psychosis revealed findings of 0.2% among the general population, 6.6% among the full sibs of patients, and 3.9% among parents of patients, or a ratio of 1.0 for the general population, 33.0 for full sibs of patients, and 19.5 for parents of patients. Another familial genetic study by Hwu and colleagues (1987) using the Family History Schedule (Hwu et al. 1984b), key informants, and DSM-III criteria (American Psychiatric Association 1980) for bipolar affective disorder with inclusion of manic episode showed a ratio of 7.0 for full siblings of patients and 26.4 for parents of patients, as compared with the general population.

Suicide

Bourne (1973) reported a high suicide rate among Chinese in San Francisco's Chinatown. Between 1952 and 1968, the suicide rate among Chinese was 27.9 per 100,000 population per annum. Although this rate was not significantly different from that of the entire San Francisco population (27.5 per 100,000), it was nonetheless three times higher than the reported rate for the national average (10.0 per 100,000). Furthermore, Bourne found the frequency of Chinese men committing suicide was four to five times more than that of Chinese women. Especially suicide-prone were Chinese men despondent over physical ill-health. Barbiturate ingestion was the most common method of suicide. Because most Chinese immigrants earlier in the 20th century were men and the number of elderly men at the time of the study far outnumbered women (Li et al. 1972), this may partly explain why there were more elderly Chinese men committing suicide.

For Chinese women, Bourne's (1973) findings revealed that interpersonal conflict, coupled with a past history of psychiatric illness, was the most frequent cause of suicide. The most frequent method for suicide was by hanging. Bourne speculated that the subjugation of women by men in traditional Chinese society and the suppression of open expression of aggressive feelings, coupled with the traditional Chinese belief that the ghosts of those who died by hanging could return to torment the living, were all factors that made hanging seem like a means of achieving final and lasting vengeance.

Attempted Suicide

Characteristics of 307 cases of attempted suicide in Hong Kong in 1986 were studied by Chiu (1989). Chiu compared the demographics of people who attempted suicide with those of the general population and found that those who attempted suicide tended to be divorced female homemakers, aged 15 to 34, who lived alone.

The results of Chiu's (1989) Hong Kong study were also compared with Yap's (1954) study of people in Hong Kong who attempted suicide and with Morgan and colleagues' (1975) study of 368 patients who had been admitted to the Bristol, England, Royal Infirmary Accident and Emergency Department in 1972 following nonfatal acts of deliberate self-harm. The data revealed the following findings: for males, the peak incidence of attempted suicide in Chiu's sample was 57.9 per 100,000 among the 20-to-24 age group; in Yap's sample, 107.5 per 100,000 among the 30-to-34 age group; and in the Morgan and colleagues' sample, 334 per 100,000 among the 25-to-29 age group. The peak incidence of attempted suicide in Chiu's 1986 data sample was only one-half of that in Yap's 1954 sample and only one-sixth of that in the 1972 Bristol sample.

Among females, the peak incidence in Chiu's sample was 166.2 per 100,000 in the 20-to-24 age group; in Yap's sample, 170.9 per 100,000 among the 20-to-24 age group; and in the Bristol sample, 661 per 100,000 among the 25-to-29 age group. The peak incidence of attempted suicide for females in Hong Kong in the Chiu and Yap study samples remained almost the same and represented only one-quarter of the peak incidence in the 1972 Bristol sample.

Compared with the Yap study, the precipitating factors in Chiu's sample were found to be significantly related to interpersonal conflicts or psychiatric symptoms and significantly less related to economic stress. Methods of attempted suicide in 1986 were more likely to be through ingestion of hypnotics and sedatives and less likely to be by drowning. Alcohol consumption before attempting suicide was reported in 7% of Chiu's sample, whereas it was not mentioned in Yap's study.

Of the psychiatric diagnoses given to subjects in Chiu's sample, 59% were situational reaction, 14% were depressive illnesses, 9% were schizophrenia or paranoid disorder, 4% were personality disorder, 2% were alcohol or drug dependence, and 12% were without a psychiatric diagnosis. Chiu (1989) postulated that the dramatic fall in the peak incidence and peak age group of attempted suicide among men in the past 30 years may be related to the rapid economic growth and control of tuberculosis in Hong Kong. However, the disintegration of the traditional Chinese extended families and the establishment of nuclear families in public housing flats have caused increasing conflicts between spouses, and these factors are thought to lead to an increase in the incidence of suicide attempts by homemakers.

Nonpsychotic Disorders

Cheng (1988) conducted a community study of minor psychiatric morbidity (nonpsychotic disorder) on 1,050 subjects aged 15 years and older, randomly selected from a rural, a suburban, and an urban community in southern Taiwan. Samples were initially screened with a 12-item Chinese Health Questionnaire (Cheng and Williams 1986). Using the modified Chinese Version of the Clinical Interview Schedule protocol (Cheng et al. 1983), potential "cases" and one-third of the randomly selected "noncases" were then interviewed by a psychiatrist who was not informed of the subjects' screening scores. Cheng found an overall weighted prevalence rate of 18% for men and 33.3% for women. A higher risk for minor psychiatric morbidity was found to be associated with the following cohorts: 1) women aged 35 and over; 2) unemployed men; and 3) people of lower socioeconomic status. One-week prevalence rates for specific disorders from *The International Classification of Diseases, 9th Revision* (ICD-9; World Health Organization 1978) disorders were 15.7% for anxiety states, 7.4% for neurotic depression, 1.0% for adjustment reaction, and 0.2% for alcohol dependence syndrome. Cheng's results were consistent with Hwu and colleagues' (1989) lifetime prevalence study, which showed higher prevalence rates in anxiety disorders, depressive disorders, and somatoform disorders among women.

The higher prevalence of minor psychiatric morbidity among Taiwanese women in Cheng's survey was further investigated in 1989 in terms of demographic variables, socioenvironmental risk factors, and psychosocial stresses. The findings suggest that chronic psychosocial stressors accounted for the higher prevalence.

Sexual Disorders

Tsoi (1988) estimated the prevalence of transsexualism in Singapore by counting all who sought sex-reassignment surgery and were subsequently diagnosed as transsexuals by psychiatrists. There were a total of 458 Singapore-born transsexuals, of which 343 were males and 115 were females. A prevalence of 35.2 per 100,000 population for male transsexualism and 12.0 per 100,000 population for female transsexualism was estimated.

Chinese transsexuals were reported to be younger (mean age 24.1 years) than those reported in the United States, Sweden, England, and Australia (mean age 30 years). Intraethnic group comparison showed the Chinese (versus Singapore Malays and Indians) had the highest rate for female transsexualism (13.2 per 100,000). Tsoi attributed this high prevalence to the availability of sex-reassignment surgery in Singapore.

Alcoholism

Several studies in the United States and abroad have documented the low rate of alcoholism among Chinese (Cheng 1988; Chi et al. 1988; Hwu et al. 1989, 1990). Prevalence rates for DSM-III–defined alcohol abuse in Taiwan Chinese were 3.4% in the metropolitan Taipei sample, 8.0% for the small town sample, and 6.3% for the rural area sample (Hwu et al. 1988). For DSM-III–defined alcohol dependence, the prevalence rates were 1.5% for the metropolitan Taipei sample, 1.8% for the small town sample, and 1.2% for the rural area sample (Hwu et al. 1989). Although these rates were considerably higher than that reported in the initial survey findings by Lin (1953), the rates among ethnic Chinese were still low as compared with the rates for Taiwan's indigenous mountain people and other ethnic groups (Hwu et al. 1990). Both sociocultural and genetic reasons have been advanced to account for this low prevalence among Chinese. The interactive effect of these two factors on low prevalence rate have also been recently studied (Akutsu et al. 1989).

Chafetz (1964) has postulated the following sociocultural factors to account for the low prevalence rate of alcoholism among overseas Chinese in East Asia:

1. Alcoholic beverages are generally consumed only at parties and at mealtime as a means to promote social discourse and communication. Solitary drinking for whatever reason is frowned upon among Chinese.
2. There is a strong social sanction against drunkards and drunken behavior in Chinese culture.
3. The presence of a strong Confucian moral ethic that prescribes proper interpersonal conduct discourages the exhibition of deviant behavior, including drunken behavior.

A genetic hypothesis has focused on the possible role of a low mitochondrial isozyme of liver aldehyde dehydrogenase among Asians. Wolff's (1972) study has documented greater alcohol sensitivity among Asians as compared with whites. He found that Asian babies had marked facial flushing after consuming a small amount of alcohol that had no detectable effect on white babies. A number of studies have subsequently confirmed his finding (Ewing et al. 1974; Hanna 1978; Nagoshi et al. 1988; Wolff 1973). Goedde and colleagues (1979) had advanced a possible correlation between aldehyde dehydrogenase isozyme (ALDH I) deficiency and alcoholic sensitivity. In the process of metabolism in the body, alcohol is converted to acetaldehyde; ALDH is essential in the breakdown of acetaldehyde. Goedde and colleagues postulated that the deficiency of the faster migrating enzyme of ALDH (ALDH 1) to metabolize acetaldehyde quickly and effectively leads to a delayed oxidation of acetaldehyde, which in turn produces dysphoria, flushing, and tachycardia.

It is speculated that this probable greater autonomic reactivity on the part of Chinese and other Asians and the subsequent dysphoric effect induced by consumption of alcohol may discourage them from excessive alcohol intake (Akutsu et al. 1989). The fast-flushing response among Chinese may seem to deter them from excessive alcohol intake.

Using an epidemiologic approach, risk factors for alcohol abuse and alcohol dependence have been investigated by Hwu and colleagues (1990) in Taiwan. In a large community survey, alcohol abuse was found to be about five times more prevalent than alcohol dependence. Both cohorts of alcohol abuse and alcohol dependence were correlated with being male and having had behavioral problems in childhood or adulthood. Addition risk factors in the alcohol abuse group include being a jobholder, being born after World War II, and living in a nonmetropolitan area. The data of Hwu and colleagues further suggest a biological predisposition to alcoholism in both groups and that the higher prevalence rates of the alcohol abuse group may be linked to the culturally determined life-style associated with modernization in contemporary Taiwanese society.

Practical Guidelines in Psychiatric Care of Chinese Americans

In this section, I offer some practical guidelines for clinicians less familiar with the provision of mental health care for Chinese Americans. These guidelines were derived from major sociocultural themes expounded in earlier sections as well as from my own experience in providing psychiatric service to Chinese American patients in the Greater Boston area.

Paying attention to both individual and family crisis at referral, and acting decisively.   Given the inherent reluctance of many Chinese Americans to seek mental health care and the stigma in Chinese culture surrounding mental illness, Chinese American patients often delay seeking appropriate care. By the time someone finally does seek out psychiatric care, both the patient and the family may be in crisis. Thus, caregivers should respond quickly and act decisively. In addition to immediately focusing on the diagnosis and treatment of the patient's presenting problems, intervention also requires attention to the evaluation and relief of physical, familial, occupational, cultural, and even social problems.

Overcoming language barriers.   For non-English-speaking patients, interpreters are relied upon to obtain a history. Fortunately, most patients often bring their own interpreters when seeking mental health services. If the patient has no interpreter and one is needed, because of the variety of Chinese spoken dialects, it is imperative to ascertain first the patient's *dialect* instead of simply asking for an interpreter who speaks "Chinese."

Because the experience and skill of interpreters vary, the following pointers are offered to facilitate accurate translation. (See also Chapter 5.)

1. The clinician should instruct the interpreter to translate exactly what is said. The interpreter may inject his or her own notions into the questions; this should be avoided. Before the interview, both the interpreter and the patient should be encouraged to ask questions if the phrasing of a question is not clear.
2. Simple, short sentences should be used. A sentence-by-sentence translation avoids overwhelming the capacity of the translator to remember details.
3. Technical terms should be avoided. Words such as depression, psychosomatic, or conversion reaction may not be easily translated into Chinese. In such a case, it is best to ask the patient to describe the symptom-complex. The existence of depression, for example, can be ascertained by asking whether the patient feels sad, has been waking up very early in the morning, and has decreased appetite, crying spells, or suicidal ideation.
4. The clinician should avoid asking highly charged questions about emotional or sexual material in the first interview. Out of embarrassment, the patient may not acknowledge the presence of such highly guarded feelings. If the information is needed, an indirect line of inquiry, such as "How is the relationship between you and your father?" is preferable to "Are you angry with your father?"

5. Extra time should be allotted for the interview. Conducting an interview through an interpreter takes twice as long. The clinician needs to plan ahead by allotting this extra time.

Overcoming the language barrier requires institutional support. At mental health institutions, a pool of trained translators can be set up in advance.

Engaging the patient's family in diagnosis and treatment. Involving Chinese family members in the interview and treatment process comes naturally for most Chinese American patients. Lin (1982) has emphasized the importance of the role of the family in the care of Asians with mental illness. Family members often are called upon to make decisions for or with the patient, and their participation should be encouraged.

Engaging the Chinese American patient. Kim's suggestions on how to engage Korean American patients (see Chapter 12) are equally valid for Chinese American patients. From the outset, if the therapist maintains a attitude of wanting to learn more about the patient's culture and experience, not only can this foster a better working relationship, it can also promote a deeper appreciation of the therapist's own culture (Leighton 1982). The role of the psychiatrist and the use of psychotherapy may often not be understood by Chinese American patients who are more familiar with the hands-on practices of the traditional Chinese medical doctor. Psychiatrists should not hesitate to assume a traditional "medical" role and perform medical activities such as taking blood pressure, weight, and pulse; performing auscultation; ordering diagnostic tests; and writing prescriptions. This is especially pertinent if psychotropic medications are being considered as part of treatment. Once a rapport is established with a patient, the psychiatrist can gradually ask about more "intimate" matters.

Advice about food can be useful. Clinicians should familiarize themselves with the symbolic value of "hot and cold" properties of certain foods in balancing excesses of perceived *yin-yang* disturbances in the body (see Chapter 13). Such activities facilitate establishment of trust. In addition, mental illness can be better understood in the context of treating a "medical" illness, which is a more readily understood endeavor and more compatible with traditional Chinese medico-philosophical practices.

Concurrent use of Western and Chinese medicine. Out of a tradition of pragmatism, some Chinese American patients may simultaneously consult both Chinese and Western doctors, take both Chinese and Western medications, and even visit several health centers for the same complaints. In such a patient's mind, the simultaneous use of both Chinese and Western treatment modalities offers the advantages of making use of the best of both worlds. Chinese American patients often believe that Chinese medications have fewer side effects. Fortunately, many herbal medicines are harmless. But until their pharmacologic properties are ascertained, it is best to advise patients not to "mix" Western and Chinese medications to avoid unknown side effects.

Use of psychotropic medications.   The application of psychotropic medications in Asians has been amply discussed by Chien (see Chapter 14 on ethnopsychopharmacology). Because of differences in body weight and possible ethnic differences in drug metabolism and sensitivities, it should not be automatically assumed that drug dosages recommended for whites are equally valid for Chinese Americans. Until more data on comparative drug reactivity between various ethnic groups are in, it would appear prudent to start out with lower dosages when prescribing psychotropic medications for Chinese Americans.

Application of psychotherapy.   The authors of Chapter 4 on cross-cultural psychotherapy have addressed pertinent cross-cultural issues in psychotherapy. The application of a "talking cure" technique is alien to many Chinese Americans, and its application may require some education. However, this technique should not be hastily dismissed for Chinese Americans simply because of their initial reluctance to reveal intimate details, the presence of a language barrier, or an assumption of inapplicability based on differences in ethnic background between therapist and patient.

Conclusion

Chinese Americans compose a wide range of subcultural groups, with rich cultural heritage and divergent languages, values, behavioral norms, and idiosyncratic expression of distress. For English-speaking Chinese American patients acculturated to Western culture, their symptom patterns may generally be assumed not to differ significantly from those of the general white population. A Western-trained psychiatrist should have no difficulty correctly diagnosing the more common categories of psychiatric illnesses.

Tradition-bound, non-English-speaking, less acculturated Chinese Americans may adhere strongly to traditional Chinese values and beliefs that may influence the way they express their concerns and how they seek mental health care. Clinicians interested in delivering effective mental health services to Chinese Americans should be sensitive to possible variations of the illness experience within this group and learn to understand and treat their illnesses in the context of their unique cultural background.

References

Akutsu PD, Sue S, Zane NWS: Ethnic differences in alcohol consumption among Asians and Caucasians in the United States: an investigation of cultural and physiological factors. J Stud Alcohol 50:261–267, 1989

American Psychiatric Association: Diagnostic and Statistical Manual of Mental Disorders, 3rd Edition. Washington, DC, American Psychiatric Association, 1980

Bernstein RL, Gaw AC: Koro: proposed classification for DSM-IV. Am J Psychiatry 147:1670–1674, 1990

Bourne P: Suicide among Chinese in San Francisco. Am J Public Health 63(8):744–750, 1973

Carr JE, Tan EK: In search of the true Amok: Amok as viewed within the Malay culture. Am J Psychiatry 133:1295–1299, 1976

Chafetz ME: Consumption of alcohol in the Far and Middle East. N Engl J Med 271:291–301, 1964

Chen C: Current research on schizophrenia in Taiwan. Paper presented at the International Symposium on Psychiatric Research in Asia, San Francisco, CA, May 6, 1989

Cheng KK, Leung CM, Lo WH, et al: Risk factors of suicide among schizophrenics. Acta Psychiatr Scand 81:220– 224, 1990

Cheng TA: A community study of minor psychiatric morbidity in Taiwan. Psychol Med 18:953–968, 1988

Cheng TA: Sex difference in prevalence of minor psychiatric morbidity: a social epidemiologic study in Taiwan. Acta Psychiatr Scand 80:395–407, 1989

Cheng TA, Williams P: The design and development of a screening questionnaire (CHQ) for use in community studies of mental disorders in Taiwan. Psychol Med 16:415–422, 1986

Cheng TA, Williams P, Clare AW: Reliability study of the Clinical Interview Schedule (CIS) between British and Chinese psychiatrists. Bulletin of the Chinese Society of Neurology and Psychiatry 9:54–55, 1983

Chi I, Kitano HHL, Lubben JE: Male Chinese drinking behavior in Los Angeles. J Stud Alcohol 49:21–25, 1988

Chiu LPW: Attempted suicide in Hong Kong. Acta Psychiatr Scand 79:425–430, 1989

Compton WM III, Helzer JE, Hwu HG, et al: New methods in cross-cultural psychiatry: psychiatric illness in Taiwan and the United States. Am J Psychiatry 148:1697–

1704, 1991

Ewing JA, Rouse BA, Pellizzari ED: Alcohol sensitivity and ethnic background. Am J Psychiatry 131:206–210, 1974

Gaw A: John E. Fogarty International Center; an integrated approach in the delivery of health care to a Chinese community in America: the Boston Experience, in Medicine in Chinese Cultures (U.S. Dept HEW Publ No NIH-75-653). Edited by Kleinman A, Kunstadter A, Alexander ER, Gale JL. Washington, DC, U.S. Government Printing Office, 1975

Goedde HW, Harada S, Agarwal DP: Racial differences in alcohol sensitivity: a new hypothesis. Hum Genet 51:331–334, 1979

Hanna JM: Metabolic responses of Chinese, Japanese and Europeans to alcohol. Alcoholism: Clinical and Experimental Research 2:89–92, 1978

Hu C: China. New Haven, CT, Human Relations Area Files Press, 1960

Hwu HG, Yeh EK, Chang LY, et al: The Chinese Modification of NIMH Diagnostic Interview Schedule—reliability study and assessment of psychiatric symptoms (in Chinese). Psychological Testing 31:15–26, 1984a

Hwu HG, Lee CF, Lin HM, et al: The Family History Schedule: development and applicability. Bulletin of the Chinese Society of Neurology and Psychiatry 10:21–26, 1984b

Hwu HG, Lin HN, Yeh EK: A clinical, familial, and social study on Chinese psychiatric patients, part I: schizophrenia and mania. Taipei, Republic of China, Research Report of the National Science Council, 1987

Hwu HG, Yeh EK, Chang LY: Alcoholism by Chinese diagnostic interview schedule: a prevalence and validity study. Acta Psychiatr Scand 77:7–13, 1988

Hwu HG, Yeh EK, Chang LY: Prevalence of psychiatric disorders in Taiwan defined by the Chinese Diagnostic Interview Schedule. Acta Psychiatr Scand 79(2):136–147, 1989

Hwu HG, Yeh EK, Yeh YL: Risk factors of alcoholism in Taiwan Chinese: an epidemiological approach. Acta Psychiatr Scand 82:295–298, 1990

Jew CC, Brody SA: Mental illness among the Chinese: hospitalization rates over the past century. Compr Psychiatry 2:129–134, 1967

Kim BL: Asian Americans: no model minority. Social Work 18:44–53, 1973

Kitano H, Sue S: The model minority. Journal of Social Issues 29:1–9, 1973

Kleinman A: Depression, somatization and the "new cross-cultural psychiatry." Soc Sci Med 11:3–10, 1977

Lai HM: Chinese, in Harvard Encyclopedia of American Ethnic Groups. Edited by Thernstrom S. Cambridge, MA, Harvard University Press, 1980, pp 217–234

Lee MB, Rin H, Schmale AH: The cross-cultural comparisons of the nature and formation of psychosomatic symptoms between Taipei and Rochester. Paper presented at the World Psychiatric Association Regional Symposium, Copenhagen, August 19–22, 1986

Leighton AH: Relevant Generic Issues, in Cross-Cultural Psychiatry. Edited by Gaw AC. Littleton, MA, John Wright-PSG Pub Co, 1982, pp 199–236

Li F, Schlief Y, Chang CJ, Gaw AC: Health care for the Chinese community in Boston. Am J Public Health 62:536–539, 1972

Lin K, Kleinman A: Psychopathology and clinical course of schizophrenia: a cross-cultural perspective. Schizophr Bull 14:555–567, 1988

Lin KM, Kleinman A, Lin T: Overview of mental disorders in Chinese cultures: review of epidemiological and clinical studies, in Normal and Abnormal Behavior in Chinese Culture. Edited by Kleinman A, Lin T. Dordrecht, Netherlands, D Reidel, 1981, pp 237–271

Lin T: A study on incidence of mental disorders in Chinese and other cultures. Psychiatry 16:315–335, 1953

Lin T: Discussion: cultural aspects of mental health care for Asian Americans, in Cross-Cultural Psychiatry. Edited by Gaw A. Littleton, MA, John Wright-PSG Pub Co, 1982, p 69

Lin T, Lin M: Love, denial and rejection: responses of Chinese families to mental illness, in Normal and Abnormal Behavior in Chinese Culture. Edited by Kleinman A, Lin T. Dordrecht, Netherlands, D Reidel, 1981, pp 387–401

Lin T, Rin H, Yeh EK, et al: Mental disorders in Taiwan, fifteen years later, in Mental Health Research in Asia and the Pacific. Edited by Caudill W, Lin TY. Honolulu, HI, East-West Center Press, 1969, pp 66–91

Liu X: Psychiatry in traditional Chinese medicine. Br J Psychiatry 138:429–433, 1981

Lo WH, Lo T: A ten-year follow-up study of Chinese schizophrenics in Hong Kong. Br J Psychiatry 131:63–66, 1977

Marsella AJ, Kinzie D, Gordon P: Ethnic variations in the expression of depression. Journal of Cross-Cultural Psychology 4:435–459, 1973

Morgan HG, Burns-Cox CJ, Pocock H, et al: Deliberate self-harm: clinical and socio-economic characteristics of 368 patients. Br J Psychiatry 127:564–574, 1975

Nagoshi CT, Dixon LK, Johnson RC, et al: Familial transmission of alcohol consumption and the flushing response to alcohol in three oriental groups. J Stud Alcohol 49:261–267, 1988

Porkert M: The Theoretical Foundations of Chinese Medicine. Cambridge, MA, MIT Press, 1974

Rin H, Chu HM, Lin T: Psychophysiological reactions of a rural and suburban population in Taiwan. Acta Psychiatr Scand 42:410–473, 1966

Rin H, Schooler C, Caudill WA: Culture, social structure and psychopathology in Taiwan and Japan. J Nerv Ment Dis 157:296–312, 1973

Robins LN, Helzer JE, Croughan J, et al: National Institute of Mental Health Diagnostic Interview Schedule: its history, characteristics, and validity. Arch Gen Psychiatry 38:381–389, 1981

Sartorius N, Jablensky A, Shapiro R: Two-year follow-up of the patients included in the WHO International Pilot Study of Schizophrenia. Psychol Med 7:529–541, 1977

Sue S, McKinney H: Asian Americans in the community mental care system. Am J Orthopsychiatry 45:111–118, 1975

Sue S, Sue DW: MMPI comparisons between Asian-American and non-Asian students utilizing a student health psychiatric clinic. Journal of Counselling Psychology 21:423–427, 1974

Sung BL: Chinese American Manpower and Employment: Report to Manpower Administration, U.S. Department of Labor. Washington, DC, U.S. Government Printing Office, 1975

Tan E: Culture-bound syndromes among overseas Chinese, in Normal and Abnormal Behavior in Chinese Culture. Edited by Kleinman A, Lin T. Dordrecht, Netherlands, D Reidel, 1981, pp 371–386

Tsai M, Teng NL, Sue S: Mental health status of Chinese in the United States, in Normal and Abnormal Behavior in Chinese Culture. Edited by Kleinman A, Lin T. Dordrecht, Netherlands, D Reidel, 1981, pp 291–310

Tseng W: The nature of somatic complaints among psychiatric patients: the Chinese case. Compr Psychiatry 16:237–245, 1975

Tsoi WF: The prevalence of transsexualism in Singapore. Acta Psychiatr Scand 78:501–504, 1988

Tsuang MT: Psychiatric genetics in Taiwan. International Journal of Mental Health 1:221–230, 1972

U.S. Bureau of the Census: Census of Population, Vol 1, chapter C (PC80-1-C) and Vol 2, chapter 1E (PC80-2-1E). Washington, DC, U.S. Government Printing Office, 1980

Winfield G: China: The Land and the People. New York, William Sloane, 1948

Wolff PH: Ethnic differences in alcohol sensitivity. Science 175:449–450, 1972

Wolff PH: Vasomotor sensitivity to alcohol in diverse Mongoloid populations. Am J Hum Genet 25:193–199, 1973

World Health Organization: International Classification of Diseases, 9th Revision. Geneva, World Health Organization, 1978

Yang CK: Religion in Chinese Society. Berkeley, CA, University of California Press, 1961

Yang YY: Prophylactic efficacy of lithium and its effective plasma levels in Chinese bipolar patients. Acta Psychiatr Scand 71:171–175, 1985

Yap PM: The culture-bound reactive syndromes, in Mental Health Research in Asia and the Pacific. Edited by Caudill W, Lin T. Honolulu, HI, East-West Center Press, 1969, pp 33–53

10 Psychiatric Care of Indochinese Americans

J. David Kinzie, M.D.
Paul K. Leung, M.D.

The Indochinese are a diverse group of Southeast Asians from the old French colonial area that was called Indochina. They include Vietnamese, ethnic Chinese, Cambodians (Khmer), Laotians, Hmong, and Mien. They are identifiable as a group only because they came to the United States as refugees after the Indochina and Vietnam Wars. Differing from many other minority groups, they are of diverse ethnic origins and are among the most recent immigrants to the United States.

About 1 million Indochinese have come to the United States since 1975. Some of these refugees were highly educated, Western-trained Vietnamese professionals who adapted fairly well to life here and whose academic success in the American education system is well known. Other Indochinese refugees were rural people with little formal education in their own countries who made a long cultural, social, and educational leap resettling in the United States.

Frieze (1986) provides a good summary of the complicated history of the countries of origin of the Indochinese. Vietnam, for much of its history, has been influenced by China but became independent from it in the middle of the tenth century. Then Vietnam had its own territorial expansion, which included annexation of parts of Laos and Cambodia (the Khmer Empire), which was controlled by the Thais at that time. The language and religion of the Cambodians and Laotians have been influenced by India. The written language is in the Sanskrit script in Cambodia and the Pali script in Laos. The religion of both countries was strongly influenced by the Brahmanism of the Hindus as well as by Buddhism. Thus, this part of Southeast Asia came to be called Indochina. French rule over Indochina began in the middle of the nineteenth century and organized the region into separate political entities. The French concentrated on making Vietnam productive and economically viable but had only minimal influence on Cambodia and Laos. The

Vietnamese acted as public servants in areas of Cambodia and Laos, which added to the traditional fear and hatred the local populations felt toward the Vietnamese.

The Japanese occupied Indochina in 1941, but the French reestablished some control in 1945, which was challenged when nationalist Viet Minh troops engaged French troops in a struggle to reclaim the country in what became known as the Indochina War. By 1954, the United States was paying about 80% of the French war costs in Vietnam. In that year, the Geneva Agreement, signed by representatives of the Viet Minh and the French Union, essentially created two Vietnams, North and South, as a temporary expedient. The terms favored the Viet Minh. North Vietnam went to the Communist-backed government of Ho Chi Minh, and South Vietnam went to the French-backed government of Bao Dai. Reunification of Vietnam under one government was to have occurred through general elections scheduled for 1956. South Vietnam refused to participate in these elections, which the Communists were expected to win (The New Columbia Encyclopedia 1975).

Cambodia gained independence from France in 1953. Laos had been declared an independent neutral country in the Geneva Conference of 1954, but the deep divisions in the country made it impossible for it to function as a neutral state between pro-West Thailand and pro-Communist Vietnam. The escalation of the Vietnam War and the massive American involvement brought great changes in Vietnam, changes that spilled over into Cambodia and Laos. With the fall of Saigon and Phnom Penh in April 1975, the Communists effectively gained control over South Vietnam, Cambodia, and Laos. The Vietnam War had an enormous effect on all the countries in Indochina. All had undergone great devastation; not only had the land been scarred, but millions had died. Family and social life were disrupted, and there were marked economic losses. Members of the former regime were sent to "special reeducation camps" in South Vietnam, and many were never seen again. The most severe damage related to the Vietnam War was done in Cambodia. The Pol Pot regime initiated a radical reign of terror in which perhaps one-fourth of Cambodia's 7 million people died before the Vietnamese intervened in January 1979.

All of these upheavals resulted in waves of refugees leaving Indochina. The first wave occurred right after the fall of Saigon in 1975 and consisted mainly of well-placed administrators in the South Vietnamese government and military and of those who had the most to lose—Chinese and Catholics. The later waves included urban middle-class Vietnamese who complained of social and economic persecution and who feared internment and reeducation camps.

Although refugees from Cambodia did not really start coming to the United States until Pol Pot's control over the country was broken by the Vietnamese in 1979, their horror stories became known as they straggled into Thailand. Refugees from Laos, including both lowland Laos, Hmong, and Mien, also began escaping in several waves to Thailand after 1975, and many of these people stayed in refugee camps for a very long time.

From 1975 to 1988, a total of 839,865 Indochinese refugees had arrived in the United States—510,443 from Vietnam, 186,382 from Laos, and 143,040 from Cambodia. Because of the marked increase in birth rate in these groups, there are now more than 1 million Indochinese in the United States.

Indochinese refugees are one of the newest groups in the United States and have one of the briefest histories of interacting with Americans and the federal government. Indeed, the relationship between the refugees and the government is constantly evolving. Indochinese refugees all have one thing in common: they have been forced to leave their native countries because of political persecutions or military conflict. To Americans, these refugees are reminders of a controversial era in American history. As might be expected, such a large group of recent immigrants has had a varied reception in American society. In some areas, refugees have acculturated, found employment, excelled academically, and embraced American values. Others have not done so well and have remained marginal in terms of employment and integration. A third group has formed large communities where they live together, somewhat isolated from the mainstream culture. Examples of very large communities—Little Saigons—can be found in several American cities. In some areas, Indochinese have competed with other minority groups for jobs and social benefits and are subject to much discrimination. Their apparent success in some economic endeavors has resulted in their being attacked by other seemingly less fortunate minority groups.

Mental Health Services for Indochinese Refugees

A review of mental health services for Indochinese refugees indicates a lack of federal planning and foresight that has resulted in state services that are markedly uneven and poorly coordinated (Boehnlein 1987a). The federal government's initial approach after 1975 was to provide temporary solutions to refugee problems as well as some aid, but in 1980 the government's approach changed. With the Refugee Act of that year, individual states were given key responsibilities for planning, administrating, and coordinating the programs. These services have continued to provide uneven benefits for refugees, but the most glaring problem has been limited access to mental health services. Mental health services received a low priority in the Office of Refugee Resettlement and often have low priorities in individual states with inadequate resources for meeting the needs of their constituencies.

The economic climate where refugees have settled has greatly affected their health care, because many have only limited access to employment-related health insurance. Not only have barriers to access contributed to the worsening of existing mental disorders, but unemployment itself has created problems related to self-worth and role obligations within families. Because American policies have had direct and indirect effects on international events, including the number of Indochinese refugees entering the United States, a very good case can be made that a strong federal role in providing mental health services for Indochinese refugees is a moral imperative.

As we have been describing, a series of catastrophic events over the last 50 years have formed the background of the arrival of Indochinese in the United States: the Japanese occupation of Indochina, the wars of liberation from the French, the devastation caused by American involvement in Southeast Asia, the fall of governments in the region, the establishment of reeducation camps, and the horrors of Pol Pot. Finally, there were the difficult experiences many faced while escaping Indochina, living in refugee camps in a second country, and enduring refugee status in the United States. The Indochinese have suffered a history of trauma, social and cultural breakdowns, and the loss of family members, country, language, and culture. This history would impressionistically indicate that 1) the psychiatric disturbances and the mental-health needs of the Indochinese are greater than those of other minority groups and 2) because of their linguistic, cultural, and economic differences from the majority of Americans, these refugees would have less access to health care. Our current information indicates that both of these observations are true.

After their arrival in the United States, there has been widespread secondary migration by the Indochinese. The majority of the Indochinese immigrants now live in California, and more than half of these live in Southern California counties. The rest are unevenly distributed throughout the country. Information on age and education is lacking.

A large study of the mental health needs of Southeast Asians in California provided good demographic data for this population in the state (Gong-Guy 1987). Based on a large survey ($N = 2,773$), the data reveal a great diversity among Indochinese. Rural-urban differences are quite pronounced: for instance, 80% of the Hmong live in rural areas, whereas 63% of the Vietnamese live in urban areas. The Vietnamese averaged 10.5 years of formal education, the Hmong averaged 3.1, and the Laotians and Cambodians averaged in between. About 70% of the Vietnamese and 28% of the Cambodians are literate in English. Only 17% of the Cambodians and 14% of the Hmong were active in the labor force, compared with 52% of the Vietnamese. Overall, 65% of all Southeast Asian refugees were dependent on welfare.

In our clinic in Portland, Oregon, the patients' average age is about 40, and 60% are women. The level of education varies greatly among the Vietnamese, averaging about 8 years. The Cambodians average 2 years of formal education, and the Mien have an average of no formal education at all. Currently, most adults are fluent only in their native language, but young people who have been in the United States for a number of years are becoming increasingly conversant in English.

Epidemiology and Study Data

There is a marked paucity of epidemiologic studies on Southeast Asians in the United States, and none of them approach the sophistication of the Epidemiological Catchment Area studies. Nevertheless, some studies do give information about the problems present in Southeast Asian communities. Using the Cornell Medical Index (Brodman et al. 1949) with Vietnamese refugees, Lin and colleagues (1979) found that subjects had widespread symptoms of depression, anxiety, and somatic preoccupation. Furthermore, these symptoms continued to increase even 3 years after resettlement (Masuda et al. 1980).

The adjustment of the Hmong refugees in the United States was followed in a sophisticated longitudinal study, using self-rating scales (Westermeyer et al. 1989). Of the 100 Hmong studied, there was considerable evidence of acculturation and greatly reduced symptom levels for several symptom complexes. A large number, however, remained illiterate and uninvolved with the majority society. The study also showed that the subjects' depressive symptoms, somatization, and phobias improved over time, but anxiety, hostility, and paranoia changed little.

Beiser (1988) reported on a study of depressive symptoms among Southeast Asian refugees in Vancouver. In general, the longer the refugees had been in Canada, the fewer depressive symptoms they had. However, unattached Laotians and Vietnamese (there were no Cambodians in the study) experienced the highest levels of depression 10 to 12 months after arrival. For this group, depression still remained high even after 12 months. The ethnic

Chinese, who had access to a large like-ethnic community providing emotional support and reinforcing a sense of identity, had lower rates of depression that continued to fall over time.

Beiser (1987) has further suggested that refugees alter their time perception as an adaptive strategy. During times of acute stress, they focus on the present to the relative exclusion of the past and the future. As conscious awareness of past and future emerges, a risk for depression occurs.

A study in California using a psychological well-being scale showed marked differences in depression among the various ethnic groups (Rambaut 1985). The Khmer (Cambodians) showed the highest levels of depression, and the Khmer and the Hmong had much higher depression scores than did the Vietnamese and the Chinese.

Gong-Guy (1987) did a thorough community study to determine the mental health needs of Indochinese Americans in California. She found that the need for psychiatric services was moderate to severe for 31% of the Vietnamese, 54% of the Hmong, 50% of the Laotians, and 48% of the Cambodians. In addition, an estimated 10% of the refugees met the criteria for having posttraumatic stress disorder (PTSD). The greatest percentage of these—16%—were Cambodian.

Experienced psychiatrists using diagnostic criteria have rarely performed community surveys of nonpatients. One done of Cambodian adolescents showed extremely high rates of disorders: of 40 subjects, 50% had PTSD and 53% had a form of depressive disorder; 27 had at least one major DSM-III (American Psychiatric Association 1980) diagnosis (Kinzie et al. 1986).

Some data exist on the rates of various disorders among Indochinese who are actually in treatment. One of us (Kinzie and Manson 1983) studied 263 patients in the Indochinese Psychiatric Program and found that 19% had schizophrenia, 48% had a major depressive disorder, and 14% had anxiety or other disorders. A similar study, which also included the diagnosis of PTSD, was performed by Mollica and colleagues (1987). Of 52 patients, 71% had affective disorders, 50% had PTSD, and 10% had schizophrenia. Our most recent data are similar except that, of 322 patients, 72% have PTSD (Kinzie et al. 1990). Presumably, many more Indochinese have psychiatric disorders than those who seek treatment. It is likely that less symptomatic individuals may remain untreated. Other factors, including cultural biases against Western forms of treatment, may also deter some patients from seeking professional help.

Because the data come from different sources and because researchers use different methodologies, an accurate picture of mental illness in the various groups of Indochinese Americans is difficult to obtain. It is, nevertheless, clear that affective disorders and PTSD are highly prevalent in both community and clinical populations. Almost all studies indicate that Cambodians and/or Hmong have the highest level of distress and the greatest needs. It is possible that as many as 50% of the population have severe needs and/or are impaired by their psychiatric symptoms. The Vietnamese tend to be the least impaired in all the Indochinese groups studied; even so, their needs are quite significant when compared with those of mainstream Americans.

The Concept of Mental Illness

Mental illness, as characterized by psychosis, is heavily stigmatized in all Southeast Asian communities. Traditionally, having a mentally ill person in the family can bring shame on the entire family and can have social repercussions, such as social ostracism or difficulty in finding suitable marital partners for family members (see Chapter 12). Generally, mental illness is considered a family affair, which may explain, given the stigma, the difficulties families have in bringing relatives in for psychiatric help. Families tend to wait to seek help for mental illness until the relative's behavior becomes impossible to ignore or manage. At this point, the families are often extremely distressed or afraid. Often patients are admitted to the hospital in a severely agitated state when their families can no longer control their behavior.

In various Southeast Asian cultures, milder forms of mental illness, such as depression and anxiety, are not easily identifiable through objective behaviors, although the subjective states are frequently identified by individual patients. The tendency for many refugees to somaticize their psychological distress probably has many determinants but is partially related to the fact that these cultures do not make distinctions between mind and body. The symptoms of psychological distress, such as headache, backache, poor sleep, and poor appetite, are legitimate signs of disease and are not, as such, stigmatized. Indeed, reporting somatic symptoms may be one of the few ways some individuals can express their problems.

The traditional view of mental illness varies among different Southeast Asian cultures. The Vietnamese, strongly influenced by Chinese philosophy, have traditionally accepted a *yin-yang* concept of disease, according to which illness is attributed to an imbalance of forces, such as "hot" or "cold" (Lin 1980). (For a fuller description of traditional Chinese concepts of medical disorders, see Chapter 9.) Many Vietnamese speak of hot or cold influences causing their illnesses. These influences have more to do with abstract concepts about food properties than actual temperatures. Some Vietnamese hold more supernatural beliefs about illness and speak of various spirits that can invade the body. Spirits or forces can be let into or out of the body through coin-rubbing or cupping, which causes abrasions on the skin.

Many Vietnamese, particularly those who were in the first wave that came to the United States, were quite Westernized. Some were even physicians and accepted Western concepts of physical illness. But their apparent Westernization does not mean acceptance of Western psychological concepts. Ideas such as intrapsychic conflict, unconscious mechanisms, influence of life experience, or effects of stress and defenses against them are not readily understood in Indochinese American communities.

For Cambodians, two religious systems—Buddhism and the traditional religions—are relevant for understanding and curing illness. Almost all Cambodians are Buddhist, and their beliefs also contain elements of Brahmanism, which places emphasis on the life cycle and rebirth (Boehnlein 1987b). For Buddhists, life is painful, and problems individuals have in this life may reflect misdeeds they committed in their previous lives. This explanation has even been used for the terrible tragedies of the Pol Pot era: these were presumed to be related to something bad Cambodians had done in the past. However, many find little comfort in the notion that pain and suffering in the present can be relieved by a better life in the future. Therefore, Cambodians almost always hold traditional religious beliefs as well, because these relieve them of personal responsibility for illness. Within this framework, mental disorders are thought to be caused by supernatural spirits, ancestor spirits, or ghosts. Many Cambodians will still contact both Buddhist monks and traditional healers before seeing a Western physician.

Several studies have identified the beliefs Laotians hold about mental illness (Westermeyer 1988; Westermeyer and Wintrob 1978). Although Laotians are Buddhist, they have a wide variety of such beliefs. There were 54 explanations of insanity provided by Laotians. Fifteen identified supernatural causes, 15 physical causes, 14 social problems, and 10 psychological causes. Many self-evident factors such as familial problems were not mentioned, and illness was usually attributed to factors outside the individual's control. The Hmong, who are usually illiterate and animistic, had beliefs similar to those of the Laotians regarding illness and traditional methods of healing, although the Laotians had more complex theories and practices. The Mien are entirely animistic and believe strongly in supernatural causes. Their herbal medicines tend to be mild, and they have a strong aversion to most types of Western medicine. In one study (Kinzie et al. 1987), of all Southeast Asians, the Mien were the most noncompliant with Western medical treatment, and they remained noncompliant about taking Western medicines despite much education on this subject.

Traditional methods of healing are very common among Southeast Asians in the United States, even though its practice is limited by two factors: a lack of healers, particularly among the Cambodians, and the presence of a dominant society that disrespects their techniques. Our own experiences with traditional methods of healing are mixed. We have seen some Buddhist ceremonies give purpose to a patient's life and provide an understanding of suffering. But we have also seen other healers who have been naive or even brutal in their approaches—and they can be very expensive.

There is no Southeast Asian cultural paradigm for long-term healing or maintenance treatment such as there is in Western medicine. Nor is there a cultural analogy to psychological treatment involving relieving one's subjective state or exploring one's feelings. These experiences are new for Southeast Asians but can nonetheless be very useful.

The Expression of Mental Illness

The expression of mental illness in Indochinese people is curtailed by fear of stigmatization by their community, fear of being sent back to their country of origin, and lack of understanding of Western medical treatment. Not only is the expression of mental distress culturally inhibited, but even if these patients do reach Western physicians, their limited skills in English, interviewing techniques, and cultural understanding mean that many patients with psychiatric disorders are not referred to psychiatrists.

The fundamental cultural concept necessary for understanding Southeast Asian patients with mental disorders is that most present only with multiple somatic complaints. Symptoms often include pain, poor sleep, gastrointestinal complaints, and weakness without evidence of physical disease. Often, these patients receive a thorough and sometimes frightening evaluation involving multiple lab tests and procedures. A study of Vietnamese patients who presented with physical complaints at a family medicine clinic showed that most were also suffering from depression (Lin 1983). In our own clinical experience with more than 400 Southeast Asian patients, depressed patients usually present with somatic complaints. However, with acknowledgment of their distress and careful interviewing with trained mental health workers, patients can usually describe their subjective depressive feelings. Loss of country, language, and social position of the family all contribute to their depressive disorders.

Schizophrenia is also a common disorder in our psychiatric clinics. This is because most Southeast Asian patients with schizophrenia eventually come to medical attention and, because of the chronic course of the disorder, their numbers continue to grow. Currently 70 of our 400 active patients have schizophrenia. This is about 1% of the adult Indochinese population in our state. These patients are rarely violent and are generally hospitalized voluntarily. However, our experience with schizophrenic patients, especially single males, tends to show a chronic course of severe social and vocational impairment, even when their symptoms are well controlled with medicine.

The other "traditional" psychiatric disorders are seen infrequently among Southeast Asians. Organic brain syndrome and mental retardation, often from trauma or childhood diseases, are sometimes present. Generalized anxiety usually does not come to a psychiatrist's attention unless it is part of another disorder such as PTSD. Originally, little drug or alcohol abuse was apparent in Southeast Asians, but as American values, norms, and behaviors have become part of the refugees' life, alcohol dependence has become more frequent. Marital and family distress with occasional violence is in evidence as well, often resulting from alcoholism or the so-called generation gap. The rise of Asian gangs, with their intimidation and illegal activities, are also signs of increasing social disruption.

The most significant psychiatric disorders among Indochinese are caused by the traumatic experiences to which they were subjected. The appropriate treatment of refugees in the great majority of cases is closely related to the treatment of PTSD. As we mentioned previously, about 70% of our patients and perhaps 50% of the refugees in the general population have PTSD. This is not usually obvious at the time of the initial evaluation (we missed many cases), and patients rarely mention their severe traumas. Patients do not usually consider the primary symptoms of PTSD—startle reaction, nightmares, reexperiencing phenomena, and irritability—worth mentioning to a physician. Also, they consciously do not want to think about the traumas they experienced and avoid doing so. Moreover, psychiatrists have difficulty with these cases because of the time and emotional energy needed to listen to the terrible stories and the agony endured by the refugees.

Our studies (Boehnlein et al. 1985; Kinzie 1988) indicate that PTSD is a chronic disorder that has an episodic course, with some intrusive symptoms waxing and waning over time. Patients can be highly impaired by symptoms of recurrent nightmares, intrusive thoughts, irritability, poor sleep, and startle reactions. Avoidance behavior and numbing can lead to patients to withdraw from families and children, and some individuals seem incapable of sustaining ongoing relationships.

In our first 100 cases of Cambodians with PTSD, we found 7 with psychosis (Kinzie and Boehnlein 1989). This was a very impaired and disturbed group, and they were difficult to treat. It is now apparent that severe trauma can lead to psychosis in some refugees.

In the next section, we use three case studies to illustrate some typical patterns of presentation of severe psychiatric disorders in Indochinese patients. The second case study also demonstrates the effects of severe trauma. In our experience, most of the clinical pictures of our patients fit Western diagnostic categories. There are not any specific culture-bound syndromes in Indochinese refugees. However, some culturally determined behaviors and symptom interpretations can mask a patient's original presentation.

Case Study 1

History of present illness: K. L. was a 20-year-old married Laotian woman who was first referred to our emergency room. She was evaluated by a resident and found to be intoxicated. At the same time, she spoke abut her deceased grandfather being inside her. Her behavior caused the family to be very distraught, but there was little more that could be learned about her at the time of admission.

K. L. was hospitalized. Further evaluation revealed that several days prior to her admission, she had begun to act differently and to speak of her grandfather being inside her. Her grandfather had died many years before, and her family became convinced that, indeed, the grandfather's spirit had returned to the patient. The family was quite delighted at this occurrence and, knowing that the grandfather liked to drink, gave the young patient a moderate amount of whiskey to help the grandfather's spirit.

After she was detoxified in the hospital, it became apparent that K. L. had had a change in behavior for several weeks. She had become more withdrawn and agitated and was having auditory hallucinations and the delusion of being possessed by her grandfather's spirit. Her family gradually recognized that she had a mental illness that had existed over a period of time rather an acute culturally identified spirit possession.

Diagnosis and treatment course: K. L. was diagnosed as having schizophrenia. She was treated with antipsychotic medicine and socialization group therapy, and her family was given educational and supportive counseling. Her subsequent course has been chronic over a period of 10 years, with social withdrawal and affective incongruity but a decrease in active psychotic symptoms.

Case Study 2

History of present illness: When originally seen, S. A. was 38 years old. She was a Cambodian refugee brought because of "spirit possession" by her mother. During the original evaluation, the patient was so distressed and agitated that no real history could be obtained. A subsequent evaluation showed that she had recently been angry and depressed much of the time and actually felt that her mother had entered her body. This intrusion caused her to become very irritable and angry, and during these episodes, she would lose control.

Personal history: S. A.'s past history was very disturbing. She was born in a rural area in Cambodia, the third of five children. She worked as a secretary for 1½ years and married at the age of 17. During the Pol Pot regime, she was subjected to 4 years of forced labor. Her father died, and her husband was executed at the time she was in labor with her second child. S. A.'s child died of starvation, and her mother died of disease and starvation. She felt most distressed about the death of her mother, who was the person closest to her and who had helped her with the delivery of her child. In 1979, she left Cambodia and lived in refugee camps for 1½ years before coming to the United States.

Diagnosis and treatment course: At her original presentation, S. A. was extremely agitated and appeared to be in a dissociated state. But in the second interview, after a week of benzodiazepine treatment, she demonstrated a good fund of knowledge and a good memory for past events. She appeared to be numb and saddened about what she had suffered. Her symptoms included frequent nightmares, intrusive thoughts bout the past, startle reaction, irritability, and marked attempts to avoid all memories of the past or any events that would remind her of Cambodia.

S. A. was diagnosed as having depression and PTSD and was begun on treatment with imipramine and clonidine. She was frequently seen in individual therapy with support to reduce the outside stresses on her life and to give information about the origin of her symptoms. Later, socialization group therapy was added. She has had no more dissociative episodes, but she has had a chronic course with much exacerbation of her symptoms at times of stress despite being on medication.

Case Study 3

History of present illness: N. T., a 29-year-old Vietnamese single male, was originally hospitalized 10 years ago after he had immigrated to the United States. At that time he had anxiety and severe paranoia, thinking that he was going to be deported. He also reported feelings of impending death. He felt that Amy Carter was in love with him, but that other people were out to kill him. He had lost weight and had a sleep disorder.

At the time of his original hospitalization, an examination of N. T.'s mental status was not very fruitful because of his unfamiliarity with the English language. He appeared fearful and seemed to attend to voices during the interview. Throughout the hospitalization, N. T. appeared suspicious and withdrawn and continued to have delusions that he was going to die the following day. Later, it became clear that he had been having auditory hallucinations.

Personal history: N. T. grew up in Vietnam. He failed to complete his high school education and was inducted into the Vietnamese Army. After the fall of Saigon, he immediately came to the United States and worked at odd jobs. He tried to enroll in a junior college, but because of his poor English he withdrew from school. During this time he became more homesick and withdrawn and developed psychotic symptoms.

Diagnosis and treatment course: Over the next 10 years, N. T. was treated in the Indochinese Psychiatric Program and was maintained on antipsychotic medicine and supportive psychotherapy, but he remained socially isolated. He continued to show a flat affect and appeared tired in all of the interviews. Because of compliance problems, he was started on Prolixin Decanoate (fluphenazine decanoate) and continued on it for several years, up to the present. N. T. now participates in regular socialization group therapy to which he has responded well with better socialization. However, he still has some auditory hallucinations. During his treatment period, he has been socially isolated, and his only contacts are with the treatment team.

Treatment

Psychotropic Medications

Although there is no controversy surrounding the efficacy of psychotropic medications for Southeast Asians, much has been written about Asians needing less psychotropic medication. Early reports showed that Asians responded at much lower doses than non-Asians, and some pharmacokinetic studies showed dose-response differences among Asians compared to whites (Lin and Finder 1983). Such differences have not been found universally, and clinical studies are lacking. Our experience in treating Southeast Asian patients with antidepressant medications, as well as the experience of others, showed that noncompliance was such a big problem with all Asian groups that there is no way to detect whether differences in dosage are needed (Kinzie et al. 1987; Kroll et al. 1990). Once patients were taking medication, it seemed that they needed the same dosage of the antidepressant imipramine (at least 150 mg) to obtain the same therapeutic blood level as non-Asian patients. We also found that Mien patients were almost totally noncompliant despite many efforts to educate them about medication. We now strongly suggest that all Southeast Asian patients on antidepressants have a tricyclic antidepressant (TCA) blood level done early in treatment to determine compliance and to address directly any problems these patients may have with taking their medicine.

Likewise, regarding patients on antipsychotic medications (at least those patients with severe schizophrenia), we have found that they tend to need average American doses to gain clinical remission. Typically, our patients are on 24–40 mg of Trilafon (perphenazine) for control of symptoms. Perphenazine is well tolerated in this group, although noncompliance is still a problem; Prolixin Decanoate (fluphenazine decanoate) or Haldol Decanoate (haloperidol decanoate) has been very useful in this regard. Antidepressants and antipsychotic medicines cause patients to complain early in treatment, particularly about dry mouth, constipation, and postural hypotension. Much patient support is needed to work through these symptoms so that patients will stay on their medications. Desipramine, as a substitute for imipramine, is sometimes useful.

PTSD is difficult to treat because of its chronic and episodic nature. However, we have found imipramine to be very useful, because it helps with sleep disturbances as well as the accompanying depression. Recently we have found clonidine to be a very good adjunct; now, most of our patients are on imipramine and clonidine. This combination is well tolerated by patients and greatly relieves nightmares, irritability, and startle reaction (Kinzie and Leung 1989). There has not been much experience with prescribing of other medications to Southeast Asians, but at least theoretically, the antidepressants with fewer side effects, such as fluoxetine or bupropion, may have some advantages.

Psychotherapy

Psychotherapy with Southeast Asians is a difficult process. Most Western psychiatrists must conduct such therapy using an interpreter, because refugees typically have only a minimal ability to communicate in English. An interpreter adds an additional variable and may make the whole interaction more problematic. In our experience, the best approach is to have a well-trained mental health worker of the same ethnic background as the patient who works consistently with a psychiatrist and has a thorough knowledge of Western psychiatric concepts.

One of the most important aspects of psychotherapy is taking the patient's history. The therapist must be culturally sensitive and highly empathetic. The history must include a thorough background of the patient's life in his or her homeland, including the escape process, hardships endured in refugee camps, and the adjustment experience in the United States (Kinzie 1981). This information is necessary not only to be able to understand the patient but also to establish credibility with him or her. This may be the first time the patient has had the opportunity to tell his or her story, which makes taking a sensitive history of the traumas endured and of their effects on the patient even more imperative. A physical examination as well as a mental status examination put patients more at ease and provide a medical model that they can more easily understand.

In the first session, it is important for the therapist to try to understand the patient's view of his or her illness and to see whether a mutually acceptable model can be determined. In our therapy, we emphasize a stress model. We recall the stresses the patient has mentioned in the history and describe the way his or her body has reacted to the stresses to produce symptoms. This model is often understood easily by patients and incorporates life stresses and physical and psychological reactions.

For most of our patients, we have recommended open-ended, long-term supportive therapy. This format emphasizes regular, predictable contact through scheduled appointments and an ongoing personal relationship with common themes that carry over from session to session. These themes often include major symptoms, side effects, stressors, children, financial concerns, or adjustment problems to living in the United States. The therapist should provide a model of positive social behavior that includes clear communication, genuine calm, a constructive use of humor, and a realistic approach to solving many of the problems faced by refugees. Education of the family is needed to avoid their stigmatizing the patient.

In dealing with traumatized patients, it is important for the therapist to make the treatment situation as nonthreatening as possible and to avoid any suggestion of the interrogation the patient may have experienced previously (Kinzie and Fleck 1987). The therapist must be sensitive to the patients' needs to protect themselves by avoiding and by denying painful thoughts. This "numbness" to agonizing experience may be part of the behavior of these patients for a long time. It is necessary also to try to reduce the stresses in the lives of traumatized patients by ensuring that they have support from welfare agencies and other support groups to stabilize their incomes and living situations (Kinzie 1989).

It is very difficult for Indochinese patients to discuss stresses within their families. These are often taboo topics for discussion with outsiders, and the prohibitions are greater for these subjects than for talking about sex. Not only are patients dealing with social and economic stresses and those arising from their refugee experience, they are also trying to understand the way Americans handle problems such as raising children and dealing with changing standards of behavior and apparent cultural and generation gaps. These value differences between parents and children can be serious problems and are often difficult areas of family therapy.

Group Therapy

Group therapy of a very special nature can be useful as part of a total psychiatric program. Because the group process is influenced by cultural factors involving communication styles, respect for authority, and traditional social relationships, the most acceptable group activities are socialization experiences that encourage traditional practices and practical information. We have also found in our 4 years of experience in treating Indochinese patients through group therapy that being flexible, meeting concrete needs, and keeping a bicultural focus while maintaining individual sessions have contributed to acceptance by patients (Kinzie et al. 1988).

Herbal Medications and Traditional Healing

Several authors have described the prevalence and popularity of the use of herbal medicine in Asia (Ladinsky et al. 1987; Van Esterik 1988; Westermeyer 1988). In Indochinese refugee camps, traditional medical practices were accepted and encouraged, along with Western medical care (Hiegel 1981). Further, it has been noted that, in North America, Indochinese patients have continued their traditional healing practices, including the use of herbal medications (Golden and Duster 1977; Muecke 1983; Yeatman and Dang 1980).

In obtaining patients' histories, clinicians should try to obtain detailed accounts of the types and amounts of herbal or traditional medicines patients are taking in addition to any Western medications. Patients should be encouraged to offer their perceptions of the effects of such substances on the disease process. Further, clinicians should discuss very carefully with patients how using traditional or herbal healing methods may affect compliance with prescribed medications and treatment.

To avoid a direct confrontation between the two systems of healing, clinicians may wish to suggest to patients that, as a prudent practice, they should abstain from herbal medicines while taking Western medications, because the purity of herbal medications may be questionable. There are too few scientific studies of the side effects and action of herbal medicines. Clinicians should also know that, even though they may be advised against such practices, some patients will continue to use such culturally well-established methods of health care.

Issues With Family Therapies

Conflicts exist in any family or cultural structure. With the breakdown of a person's native culture and family and social networks, the conflicts are compounded. In Indochina, there are few publicly recognized and accepted professional avenues for managing conflicts that arise within a family. Therefore, the help of social workers, psychologists, and psychiatrists is not sought even by those who could afford it, and such conflicts are usually handled within the existing family and social networks. "Face-saving" and maintaining superficial harmony supersede the effort to resolve conflicts (Tran 1987).

In the process of adapting to a new way of life, Indochinese refugees who settled in this country began to experience many family problems. The necessity (and the ability) of the wife to contribute to the family economy resulted in contradictory pressures. As the wife's burden increased, so did her authority. In contrast, her husband's authority declined, and she no longer accepted his dominant position without challenge.

The traditional parenting method of the Indochinese endorses an authoritative role for the parental figure, who demands obedience from the children. This parenting style is, unfortunately, in conflict with the seemingly "democratic" parenting method of the dominant culture in the host society, under which children are, at least under "ideal" conditions, more often allowed to question authority and more often encouraged to strive for independence of mind. Another source of family conflict can be around providing care for elderly family members. The lack of culturally appropriate family, social, and community resources places the burden of care solely on the family and further strains their already overstressed lives.

In conducting family therapy, clinicians need to be aware that they will be placed in an authoritarian position (much like a village elder or respected teacher). The parents, when maintaining traditional values, may expect clinicians to promote that customary authority over all aspects of the children's lives. The children usually want the "freedom" and independence that they see in American children (especially adolescents). Clinicians must find a balance between these two desires. A good first approach is to show verbal and nonverbal respect to the parents and the culture from which they come. Then it is necessary to let all members of the family speak, modelling a form of democracy within the family. It is useful to provide information about "typical" American parenting. For example, American parents can love and guide their children without controlling all aspects of their lives, and American children usually understand the need for good study and work habits. This means, of course, that what is viewed as "freedom" often is a negotiated balance of study and social activities. Cross-cultural family therapy for refugees is a difficult procedure in which a series of changing forces are being balanced, clarified, and (one hopes) mutually negotiated (Kinzie et al. 1972).

Diagnostic Tests

Generally speaking, Indochinese patients are receptive to noninvasive radiologic and other diagnostic procedures. They often request or even demand that certain procedures be performed, sometimes inappropriately, to determine the etiology of their symptoms. For example, with the complaint of chronic headache, they may ask to have a head X ray. In the course of psychiatric treatment, it is not unusual for Indochinese patients to relate complaints that in general practice would be referred to primary care providers. Many Indochinese patients do not understand the American medical system, which tends to divide care according to specialties. For these patients, psychiatrists may wish to begin with an initial workup and to include, for example, an electrocardiogram, a chest X ray, gastrointestinal film, or basic blood tests. Before any diagnostic tests are performed, it is necessary for the clinician to explain the procedures carefully in order to secure patient compliance. This is especially true for invasive procedures or those that might involve risk to the patient.

The family should be involved in decision making, particularly the head of the family—be that the traditional figure of authority (i.e., the husband or father) or the family spokesperson. The spokesperson might be a son, daughter, relative, or friend who can speak English and thus act as a bridge from the family to the outside world. To secure cooperation from the patient and the family, it is necessary for the psychiatrist to be firm but sensitive in stating the need for, and the purpose of, any procedures.

Indochinese patients view blood as the essence of life. The loss of blood, regardless of the amount, is looked upon as a serious matter. Venipuncture for the purpose of testing is considered acceptable, although it may be reluctantly agreed upon (Hiegel 1981). Having blood drawn may cause an Indochinese patient to complain of fainting spells, fatigue, and other somatic discomforts. Generally, reassuring words from the doctor, bed rest, and a few nutritious sips of juice or broth will resolve these complaints. Test results should be discussed with patients in order to assure their cooperation in the future.

Use of Translators

Most clinicians would agree that translators provide a vital role in linking clinicians to patients in our health care system. They have been depicted as an indispensable element to the success of a specialty psychiatric clinic (Kinzie and Manson 1983), and their role has also been described as an ever-important leg of a therapeutic triad (Kinzie 1981). Given the reality of our current system, there will never be enough bilingual/bicultural clinicians to serve the needs of the increasing Indochinese population. To be effective with Asian patients, who may not be fluent in or even familiar with the English language, the Western-trained clinician must rely on a translator.

In general, the clinician should never rely on a patient's family members, friends, or other nonprofessionals to act as translators, except in emergency situations. The ideal translator is fluent in both the clinician's and the patient's languages and has the ability to identify with both host and native cultures. A translator must also have adequate training in the basic vocabularies of the health care and mental health fields and must be capable of interpreting the behavior, beliefs, and verbal and nonverbal languages of the patient in the context of culture.

Even an experienced translator should be oriented to the purpose of the interview or examination ahead of time. The translator should be cautioned against inclusion of unrelated information or screening out of materials as a result of the patient's irrational thought process. In some situations, the clinician should request a verbatim translation, especially while performing a mental status examination. During appropriate intervals, in order for the clinician to understand symptoms, complaints, behaviors, and nonverbal language, the translator should be asked to interpret the patient's statements in the context of Indochinese culture. Fundamental techniques for working with a translator have been well described by Kinzie (1981).

Based on what we have seen in our work with Indochinese patients, a conscious national effort should be undertaken to recruit and train health care and mental health care translators to ensure an ongoing supply of highly qualified professionals who can work with these and other ethnic immigrant groups.

Use of Psychiatric Consultants and Other Consultants

When clinicians deal with Indochinese patients, they need to bear in mind that the American system of rapid referral, or direct access to a medical specialist, is unfamiliar to them. In Asia, a person who lives in an urban area can usually expect to receive care from a generalist. The more severe cases are referred to a specialist, which in Indochinese cultures usually indicates a serious or even terminal condition. So far removed from specialists are people in rural areas in Indochina that they usually must rely on the mercy of the health care system and the political environment to obtain care from health workers with *any* formal medical training. Therefore, before an Indochinese patient is referred to a medical specialist, the patient and his or her family must receive a detailed explanation of the reason for referral so as to reduce their anxiety.

When a referral is made to a psychiatrist, it is best to tell the Indochinese patient that the referral is to a medical doctor who specializes in medical treatment of both emotional and mental difficulties. Appropriate explanations should be made before the referral, and it is extremely important to involve family members in this educational process. We have found that the "medical model" we have utilized in dealing with our Indochinese psychiatric patients has been well received (Kinzie and Manson 1983).

Hospitalization

As we have discussed, Indochinese Americans include different peoples. Each has its own culture, and each differs in the degree of its exposure to the Western medical system. The groups range from the Mien or Hmong, who lived in the hilly region of central Laos and who had limited access to Western medical facilities, to the Vietnamese who resided in big cities such as Saigon and who are familiar with modern health care systems.

Despite these differences, some generalizations can be made concerning hospitalization for Indochinese patients. First, before hospitalizing a patient, the physician should use every outpatient measure available to deal with the patient's disorder. Second, the decision to hospitalize should not be made without consensus among family members. Third, during the admission process, the physician should explain carefully the likely length of stay, the workup and what it involves, the array of tests involved, the preliminary treatment plan, and the expectations the facility has for the patient and the family. Staff on the ward should secure assistance from a professional translator/interpreter during the admission process and on a regular basis to ensure ongoing accurate communication with and for the patient.

A number of guidelines are relevant once the patient has been hospitalized. The family should be encouraged to visit during visiting hours and should be sensitively discouraged from having a member stay in the hospital with the patient except in an extreme emergency. Within the permissible limits, staff may choose to allow the family to bring in ethnic foods to supplement or replace Western-style meals offered to the other hospital patients.

During hospitalization, an effort should be made to review any treatment the patient may have received before admission, the different types and dosages of medication he or she may have been receiving, and the various health care providers the patient has seen. This assessment would enable the physician to understand the full spectrum of the patient's problems and to inform the patient as to the appropriateness of the prescribed treatment and medications. Further, such an assessment would make it possible to identify those who may be involved in the patient's health care after discharge and to coordinate plans for care with them.

Before discharge, the staff should hold a conference involving family members and other individuals who will have a part in caring for the patient. At this time, information gathered from the hospital stay should be discussed with the patient and family or other caregivers so plans can be made for a smooth transition to outpatient care.

Follow-Up Care

Our experience in Oregon strongly indicates that a well-staffed psychiatric clinic that is medically and psychosocially oriented and also specializes in caring for Indochinese patients is an excellent (if not the best) way to provide follow-up care for these patients. The development and progress of our clinic's program has been reported elsewhere (Kinzie and Manson 1983).

It is important to stress a point we made earlier concerning Indochinese patients seeking primary health care and psychiatric care from one provider. Some patients in the Indochinese Psychiatric Program in Oregon have used the clinic for primary care to monitor their general medical condition as well as a source of psychiatric treatment. It is not unusual for patients to seek care from their psychiatrists for hypertension, for adjusting their insulin or hypoglycemic agents for controlling diabetes mellitus, or for care for musculoskeletal ailments or viral respiratory infections. Although it is preferable to refer patients to other medical specialists, at times outpatient programs for Indochinese patients need to be flexible in order to accommodate the needs and perceptions of the patients.

References

American Psychiatric Association: Diagnostic and Statistical Manual of Mental Disorders, 3rd Edition. Washington, DC, American Psychiatric Association, 1980

Beiser M: Changing time perspective and mental health among Southeast Asian refugees. Cult Med Psychiatry 11:437–464, 1987

Beiser M: Influence of time, ethnicity, and attachment on depression in Southeast Asian refugees. Am J Psychiatry 145:46–51, 1988

Boehnlein JK: A review of mental health services for refugees between 1975 and 1985 and a proposal for future service. Hosp Community Psychiatry 38:764–768, 1987a

Boehnlein JK: Clinical relevance of grief and mourning among Cambodian refugees. Soc Sci Med 25:765–772, 1987b

Boehnlein JK, Kinzie JD, Rath B, et al: Post-traumatic stress disorder among survivors of Cambodian concentration camp: one year later. Am J Psychiatry 142:956–960, 1985

Brodman K, Erdmann AJ, Lorge I, et al: The Cornell Medical Index. JAMA 140:530, 1949

Frieze R: The Indochinese refugee crisis, in The Price of Freedom. Edited by Krupinsk J, Burrows G. New York, Pergamon, 1986

Golden JM, Duster MC: Hazards of misdiagnosis due to Vietnamese folk medicine. Clin Pediatr (Phila) 16:949–950, 1977

Gong-Guy E.: The California Southeast Asian's mental health needs assessment, California State Department Mental Health Contract #85-7628-2A-2, 1987

Hiegel JP: The ICRC and traditional Khmer medicine. International Review of the Red Cross 21:251–262, 1981

Kinzie JD: The evaluation and psychotherapy of Indochinese refugee patients. Am J Psychother 35:251-261, 1981

Kinzie JD: The psychiatric effects of massive trauma on Cambodian refugees, in Human Adaptation to Extreme Stress. Edited by Wilson JP, Hasel Z, Kahana B. New York, Plenum, 1988

Kinzie JD: Therapeutic approaches to traumatized Cambodian refugees. Journal of Traumatic Stress 2:75–91, 1989

Kinzie JD, Boehnlein JK: Posttraumatic psychosis among Cambodian refugees. Journal of Traumatic Stress 2:185–198, 1989

Kinzie JD, Fleck J: Psychotherapy with severely traumatized refugees. Am J Psychother 41:82–94, 1987

Kinzie JD, Leung P: Clonidine in Cambodian patients with posttraumatic stress disorder. J Nerv Ment Dis 177:546–550, 1989

Kinzie JD, Manson S: Five years experience with Indochinese refugee psychiatric patients. Journal of Operational Psychiatry 14:105–111, 1983

Kinzie JD, Sushama PC, Lee M: Cross-cultural family therapy—a Malaysian experience. Fam Process 11:59–67, 1972

Kinzie JD, Sack W, Angell R, et al: The psychiatric effects of massive trauma on

Cambodian children, I: the children. Journal of the American Academy of Child Psychiatry 25:370–376, 1986

Kinzie JD, Leung P, Boehnlein JK, et al: Antidepressant blood levels in South Asians. J Nerv Ment Dis 175:480–485, 1987

Kinzie JD, Leung P, Bui A, et al: Group therapy with Southeast Asian refugees. Community Ment Health J 24:157–166, 1988

Kinzie JD, Boehnlein JK, Leung PK, et al: The prevalence of posttraumatic stress disorder and its clinical significance among Southeast Asian refugees. Am J Psychiatry 147:913–917, 1990

Kroll J, Linde P, Habenight M, et al: Medication compliance, antidepressant blood levels and side effects in Southeast Asian patients. J Clin Psychopharmacol 10:279–283, 1990

Ladinsky JL, Volk ND, Robinson M: The influence of traditional medicine in shaping medical care practices in Vietnam today. Soc Sci Med 25:1105–1110, 1987

Lin EHB: Intraethnic characteristics and patient-physician interaction: "Cultural Blind Spot Syndrome." J Fam Pract 16:91–98, 1983

Lin KM: Traditional Chinese medical beliefs and their relevance for mental illness and psychiatry, in Normal and Abnormal Behavior in Chinese Culture. Edited by Kleinman A, Lin TY. Boston, MA, Reidel, 1980

Lin KM, Finder E: Neuroleptic dosage for Asians. Am J Psychiatry 140:490–491, 1983

Lin KM, Tazuma L, Masuda M: Adaptational problems of the Vietnamese refugees: health and mental health status. Arch Gen Psychiatry 36:955–961, 1979

Masuda M, Lin KM, Tazuma L: Adaptation problems of Vietnamese refugees, II: life changes and perception of life events. Arch Gen Psychiatry 37:447–450, 1980

Mollica RF, Wyshak G, Lavelle J: The psychosocial impact on war trauma and torture on Southeast Asian refugees. Am J Psychiatry 144:1507–1572, 1987

Muecke MA: In search of healers—Southeast Asian refugees in the American health care system. J Med 139(6):835–840, 1983

The New Columbia Encyclopedia. New York, Columbia University Press, 1975, pp 2890–2891

Rambaut RG: Mental health and the refugee experience: a comparative study of Southeast Asian refugees, in Southeast Asian Mental Health: Treatment, Prevention, Service, Training, and Research. Bethesda, MD, National Institute of Mental Health, 1985

Tran MT: Health and Diseases: The Indochinese Perspective. Paper presented at the HEW Mental Health Projects Grantee Conferences, Atlanta, GA, Chicago, IL, San Francisco, CA, and Seattle, WA, 1987

Van Esterik P: To strengthen and refresh: herbal therapy in Southeast Asia. Soc Sci Med 27:751–759, 1988

Westermeyer J: Folk medicine in Laos: a comparison between the two ethnic groups. Soc Sci Med 27:769–778, 1988

Westermeyer J, Wintrob R: "Folk" explanation of mental illness in rural Laos. Am J Psychiatry 136:901–905, 1978

Westermeyer J, Neider J, Callies A: Psychosocial adjustment of Hmong refugees during their first decade in the United States. J Nerv Ment Dis 177:132–139, 1989

Yeatman GW, Dang VV: Cao Gio (coin rubbing)—Vietnamese attitudes towards health care. JAMA 244:2748–2749, 1980

11 Psychiatric Care of Japanese Americans

June S. Fujii, M.D.
Susan N. Fukushima, M.D.
Joe Yamamoto, M.D.

I n this chapter, we describe the relationships between the factors that can affect the belief systems of Japanese Americans concerning mental health and illness and their attitudes toward and behaviors in treatment. The chapter also includes demographic data, information on epidemiology, psychopharmacology, and psychotherapy among Japanese American patients. In addition, several case studies are provided.

Japanese have been immigrating to the United States since the late nineteenth century. Over the years the term "Japanese American" has come to be used by historians and by the Japanese themselves, and it refers to permanent immigrants as well as American-born Japanese. This is the usage of the term that we employ in this chapter.

Japanese Americans include several generations. The *issei*, the first generation away from Japan, immigrated to the United States between 1885 and 1924 (Ichioka 1988). Their children are the *nisei*, the second generation away from Japan. The *kibei nisei* are second-generation individuals who were born in the United States to *issei* parents, sent back to Japan as children to live with relatives and go to school, and who eventually returned to the United States as young adults. Generations following the *nisei* are the third generation (*sansei*), fourth generation (*yonsei*), and fifth generation away from Japan (*gosei*).

For some groups of Japanese who have come to the United States, there are no specific terms. One of these groups is the wave of immigrants who came to the United States after 1965. Those members of the post-1965 immigration who did not become naturalized citizens will be referred to here

This work was supported in part by National Institute of Mental Health Grant 1 R01 MH44331-01, National Research Center on Asian American Mental Health. Our thanks to Zev Nathan, M.D., Ph.D., for his many helpful suggestions.

as "Japanese nationals." Another group consists of Japanese who reside temporarily in the United States. In the last two decades, Japan-born businesspeople have been sent by their companies to purchase prime real estate and to manage profitable institutions in the United States. These Japanese often raise their families in the United States. Their children retain Japanese citizenship but frequently become acculturated to American thoughts and mores.

The different generations away from Japan (*issei, nisei, sansei, yonsei, gosei*), the *kibei nisei,* and the Japanese nationals all have different degrees of assimilation and acculturation to the United States. "Assimilation" refers to adapting to the predominant culture of the mainstream without changing cultural attitudes or value identification. "Acculturation" involves changing value orientations (i.e., substituting and adhering to the values and attitudes of the mainstream rather than to ethnic cultural norms [Wilkerson 1982]).

In Los Angeles, there is an area called "Little Tokyo." Japanese nationals who reside there would be able to interact almost exclusively with other Japanese, speak only Japanese, and have all the comforts of being in Japan. These people would be able to adhere to the traditions and culture of their homeland while in the United States. Although they may interact with mainstream Americans on the job, these individuals are not changing their cultural identity—they are assimilating, not acculturating. However, the offspring of Japanese nationals, especially if they were born and reared entirely in the United States, would be immersed in American culture from an early age—at school, among non-Japanese friends, from the media—and may take on the cultural values and attitudes of the mainstream American culture. These children would be engaged in the process of acculturating. For such children, the process would not be absolute, because of the traditional cultural influence they may encounter at home.

The experiences of Japanese Americans differ depending upon where they live. Japanese Americans from Hawaii, the West Coast, and the East Coast have had unique upbringings, including variations in the ways their numbers relative to other racial groups have affected their lives. For example, Japanese are not considered a minority in Hawaii. The West Coast has an abundance of generations of various Asian groups born in the United States, whereas East Coast Asians are mostly Asian nationals who have come to the United States, generally for business reasons.

As can be seen, there are many different aspects of the Japanese American experience that must be considered by mental health professionals who wish to work more effectively with this heterogeneous group.

Traditional Belief Systems

Many Japanese Americans, especially the *issei,* have been affected by at least some of the following belief systems of traditional Japan: mythological legends concerning the divine origin of the emperor and people of Japan, Confucianism, Buddhism, Shintoism, and *bushido.*

Different accounts of the origin of the island nation of Japan have been handed down over the centuries through myths, traditions, and poetry. One version states that after heaven and earth were created, generations of gods were produced, including the god Izanagi and his consort goddess Izanami (Sansom 1962). As this pair stood on the rainbow bridge in Heaven, Izanagi dipped his spear into the ocean below, and the drops of water that fell from his spear tip congealed to form the sacred islands of Japan (Morton 1970).

In another version, the god and goddess married, and Izanami gave birth to the islands of Japan, as well as to the sea, rivers, mountains, and trees. The union also produced the gods and goddesses who ruled the land—the Sun Goddess, the Moon God, the Storm God, and the Fire God, among others.

These legends set the cornerstone for Japanese mythology. All things in nature were deified, as either gods or the offspring of gods. The sun, moon, mountains, rivers, trees, and even storms were considered divine (Sansom 1962). The emperor was also a divine descendant, as the imperial line stemmed in an unbroken succession from the gods. When Commodore Matthew C. Perry of the U.S. Navy visited Japan in 1853, the Japanese people considered themselves descendants of the gods (albeit this belief was not as strongly held as that of the divine origin of the emperor) and superior to other peoples. They also believed their land to be the realm of the gods (Latourette 1968).

Japanese thought and culture were also influenced by outside sources. The Chinese contributed to the written language of Japan and provided a basis for philosophy, ethics, and religion through the introduction of Confucianism and Buddhism (Latourette 1968). The values of Confucianism adopted in Japan included a belief in the importance of loyalty to one's lord or superior, obedience of children to their parents, and subordination of a wife to her husband.

Buddhism was the means by which the benefits of other civilizations (India, Central Asia, and China) were brought to the Japanese through philosophy, art, rituals, and architecture. The Zen sect of Buddhism, in particular, encouraged the repression of emotions (Latourette 1968), which may have had far-ranging effects in terms of expression of mental illness among the Japanese.

Shintoism, the indigenous religion of Japan, embraces the devotion to deities representing natural forces. Another Shinto tenet holds that the Emperor should be venerated as a descendant of the Sun Goddess. Shintoism is characterized by various ceremonies, including those to honor ancestors, to request blessings for the Japanese nation, and to request protection from evil.

Bushido (the ethical code of the military class) has also influenced Japanese culture. Loyalty was the paramount virtue of bushido. Bushido also promoted devotion to family, economy, simple living, and indifference to wealth. Self-control in the presence of pain was prized, as was personal honor. Any disgrace could be atoned for by suicide, which was regarded as the only honorable course of action in some situations. Every samurai (a member of the military class), was trained in seppuku (commonly referred to as hara-kiri), or ritual disembowelment. The highest test of character was the ability to perform this act calmly without flinching (Latourette 1968). Although bushido was intended for the military classes, the civilian population emulated the code as much as possible. Just as bushido influenced the citizenry, so were the ideals of Confucianism, Buddhism, and Shintoism adopted and modified by the Japanese through the ages.

Historical Background of Japanese in America

Most of the Japanese who immigrated to the United States came during the industrial and agricultural expansion that occurred after the American Civil War and before 1924, when the Oriental Exclusion Act was passed (Kitano and Kikumura 1976; Yamamoto 1982). The majority were young male laborers with limited education from the agricultural provinces of Fukuoka, Hiroshima, Kumamoto, Wakayama, and Yamaguchi (Kitano and Kikumura 1976). They settled in Hawaii and the West Coast states of California, Oregon, and Washington (Yamamoto 1982).

The history of the early Japanese immigrants can be divided into two broad time periods—1885 to 1907 and 1908 to 1924. The first period was characterized by dekasegi immigration, which involved Japanese who came, poor and empty-handed, in the hopes of achieving great wealth with which to return home to Japan.

In contrast, during the second period, immigrants who were laborers opted for permanent residency in the United States. The second-wave immigrants made the transition from laborers to farmers and other types of businessmen. After having relinquished the sojourner mentality, many of these farmers and proprietors of small businesses sent for wives from Japan (Ichioka 1988). Most were married through the "picture bride" custom in which relatives in Japan chose possible brides whose photographs were sent to the immigrant so that he might select a wife. Many factors were considered for the matches, including social standing and hereditary illnesses in the backgrounds of the potential bride and groom (Yamamoto 1982).

As the Japanese set down roots in the United States, anti-Japanese sentiments began to rise. This was exemplified by the formation of the Asiatic Exclusion League in 1905, at the instigation of labor leaders in San Francisco. This group aspired to halt Japanese immigration (Ichioka 1988). The hostility toward Japanese immigrants and the desire for their expulsion continued, as evidenced by laws and acts enforced during the early 1900s. In 1906, the San Francisco School Board was pressured by Mayor Eugene E. Schmitz into segregating Japanese school children (as well as Chinese and Korean children) into an Oriental Public School (Herman 1974). President Theodore Roosevelt's government filed two suits against the San Francisco School Board to force a reversal of the segregation order. The board only relented after President Roosevelt promised to drop the suits and find ways to limit Japanese immigration (Wilson and Hosokawa 1980).

The tide of anti-Japanese rhetoric continued. In 1913, the California Alien Land Law was enacted, effectively preventing Asian aliens from owning land and limiting their ability to lease land from white American landowners. Leasing of land was later permitted after these landowners made it known that they wished to lease to Japanese tenants.

In 1920, the Alien Land Act was passed (Herman 1974). This act prevented Japanese *issei* from buying land in the name of their *nisei* children who were American citizens. The Cable Act was passed in 1922 (Herman 1974). This act stated that a woman citizen who married an alien ineligible for citizenship would lose her own citizenship. If a white American or *nisei* woman married an *issei*, she would lose her citizenship. However, if a woman was divorced or widowed and if she was a white American, she could reapply for citizenship. If she was a *nisei*, she could not, because she was "of a race ineligible for citizenship" (Herman 1974, p. 15).

On March 15, 1924, the Immigration Exclusion Act was passed. It stated that all immigrants "ineligible for citizenship" were denied admission to the United States (Herman 1974, p. 16). It is noteworthy that this act limited all immigration to the United States but denied all immigration from Japan and Asia (Herman 1974). Thus, further Japanese immigration was effectively barred in 1924 (Ichioka 1988; Wilson and Hosokawa 1980).

As *issei* parents dealt with these antialien sentiments and laws, their children, the *nisei*, led a dual existence. On one hand, they lived in Japanese ghettos, which upheld the traditions of the motherland. They were expected to speak the Japanese language and behave as children in Japan would. After school and on Saturdays, the *nisei* were sent to Japanese school (*nihon-gakko*) where they learned Japanese manners, attitudes, and values. On the other hand, they were also expected to master the English language, do well in American schools, and socialize well with their American peers (Yamamoto 1968). The Japanese and American identities of these children were often in conflict. Even their citizenship status could reflect the ambiguity of their cultural position. Many *nisei* had dual citizenship in Japan and the United States; if they were born before 1924, they automatically had dual citizenship. In 1924, a law was adopted allowing dual citizenship only if a parent registered a child at the Japanese Consulate within 14 days of its birth (Ichioka 1988; Wilson and Hosokawa 1980).

Although the *issei* attempted to maintain a traditional Japanese family system, their *nisei* offspring often held a status within their families different from that of children in Japan. This difference in status was due to the *nisei*'s growing command of the English language and their parents' increasing reliance upon them to deal with difficult situations involving mainstream society (Wilson and Hosokawa 1980).

The *nisei* identity was an amalgamation of traditional Japanese customs and American ideas and attitudes. Connor (1974) supported this observation with a study of three generations of Japanese Americans that demonstrated that the *nisei* retain a Japanese identity and many of the values of their parents, especially when compared with their offspring, the *sansei*. Their "Japaneseness" was further reinforced by the anti-Asian prejudices that prevented highly educated *nisei* from obtaining jobs commensurate with their degrees. Many college-educated *nisei* worked as gardeners, clerks in fruit and vegetable stands, or returned to the Japanese ghettos to work in ethnic businesses (Yamamoto 1982).

Perhaps the greatest struggle the *nisei* had to face occurred during World War II. After the bombing of Pearl Harbor by the Japanese, Executive Order No. 9066 directed the incarceration of 117,000 mainland Japanese into internment camps located in Arizona, Arkansas, California, Colorado, Idaho, Utah, and Wyoming (Herman 1974; Wilson and Hosokawa 1980). Prior to this, the *nisei* had tried to become assimilated into the larger American community, but now their allegiance was questioned. In turn, many Japanese Americans questioned themselves about their loyalty to a country that would incarcerate its own citizens.

Though the *nisei* longed to believe in their future as Americans, the recognition they sought for their citizenship in this country was not forthcoming from the majority of Americans during World War II. The denial of their status as Americans was made painfully obvious by the fact that, although Germans and Italians were also classified as "aliens" by the U.S. War Department, provisions were made only for the internment of Japanese aliens and those American citizens of Japanese lineage. Despite this treatment by the government, most of the interned *nisei* pledged their loyalty to the United States, and from these numbers arose the all-*nisei* 442nd Regimental Combat Team, which became the most highly decorated unit in the war effort (Herman 1974; Koh 1990; Wilson and Hosokawa 1980).

At the end of World War II, the internment camps were closed and the Japanese were free to rebuild their lives. It was a time of difficult readjustment, especially for the *issei*, most of whom were elderly (Wilson and Hosokawa 1980). Many *nisei* who had resided on the West Coast before the war chose not to return to their former hometowns, where anti-Japanese sentiments still ran high. Relocation to areas further inland or in the Midwest was common.

Soon after World War II, Japanese Americans realized the achievement of many of their human rights goals. In 1948, President Truman signed the Japanese-American Evacuation Claims Act, which allowed a small compensation to evacuees for the material losses they had incurred. In 1952, the McCarran-Walter Act became law (Herman 1974). This act eliminated race as a consideration in American immigration and naturalization laws. The most significant official recognition of the violation of Japanese Americans' civil liberties and constitutional rights occurred August 10, 1988, when President Reagan signed legislation apologizing for the government's relocation of Japanese Americans during World War II. This bill provided for the establishment of a $1.25 billion trust fund to pay reparations to the former internees and/or their families ("President signs law to redress wartime wrong" 1988).

Demographic Data

According to the 1980 census, 716,331 Japanese lived in the United States. The Japanese American population increased by 18% between 1970 and 1980. Immigration accounted for fewer than 5,000 people annually during that period. California contained the largest number of Japanese Americans (268,818), and Hawaii was second (239,734). In California, Japanese

Americans were the third-largest Asian American group, whereas in Hawaii, Japanese Americans were the second-largest ethnic group and the largest Asian American group (Statistical Abstract of the United States 1989).

The 1980 census also showed that 27% of Japanese Americans were between 45 and 64 years old, 18.9% were 25 to 34 years old, and 17.4% were 15 to 24 years old. The percentage of foreign-born Japanese Americans was 28.4%. Of these, 81.6% had 4 years of high school education or more, and 26.4% had 4 or more years of college. There were 395,000 Japanese Americans in the civilian labor force, only 3% of whom were unemployed. The average family size was 3.59, and the median family income in 1979 was $27,354, which was higher than that for any of the following groups: other Asian Americans, Pacific Islanders, American Indians, Eskimos, or Aleuts. Only 4.2% of Japanese in the census were below the poverty level (Statistical Abstract of the United States 1989).

Epidemiology

There are few estimates of the incidence and prevalence of mental illness within the Japanese American community. Attempts to determine rates of mental illness are based on Japanese American usage of psychiatric facilities (generally hospitals), including the rate of admission and length of stay. This kind of data on utilization may lead to an underrepresentation of the true incidence and prevalence of mental illness within the Japanese American community, as we discuss below.

In the information one of us (J. Y.) cited on the utilization of mental health services in Hawaii, there was great variability in utilization rates per year from one ethnic group to the next (Yamamoto 1982). This study used the *1977 Hawaii Statistical Supplement,* which showed that among white Americans, the utilization rate was 711 patients per 100,000 population per year. Among the Chinese, it was 131 per 100,000; among the Japanese, 185 per 100,000; and among Native Hawaiians, 585 per 100,000. Both Japanese and Chinese Hawaiians used mental health services less often than the other groups. Unfortunately, these statistics from 1977 do not reflect any changes that may have occurred since. Further, Japanese Americans in Hawaii are the second largest ethnic group and the largest Asian American ethnic group. Thus, the experiences of Japanese Americans who live in Hawaii may not accurately reflect those of their mainland counterparts, who are an ethnic minority.

Mochizuki (1975) also documented Japanese Americans' usage rate of mental health services in Los Angeles as being far lower than that of their white American counterparts. Moreover, Kitano (1969a) reported a lower rate of psychiatric admissions for Japanese Americans in California: in 1965, the rate of admissions of Japanese Americans to state hospitals per 100,000 people was 60, compared with 180 for white Americans. Another study (Yamamoto 1982) reviewed the records at the Asian/Pacific Counseling and Treatment Center (APCTC) in Los Angeles and reported underuse of mental health services, probably because of the stigma attached to using them. More recent studies (S. Sue and McKinney 1975; S. Sue and D. W. Sue 1971, 1974) based on the utilization of community health services seem to corroborate a difference between Japanese Americans and white Americans in the use of mental health services. Further investigation is needed to determine whether stigmatization of mental illness is indeed the cause of the underusage of mental health services by Japanese Americans.

Using the Hopkins Symptom Checklist—90, Revised (SCL-90-R; Derogatis 1983), researchers in one study found that a cohort of California Asians that included Japanese Americans scored higher in the number of psychiatric symptoms reported than other Americans serving as controls (Yamamoto et al. 1983). The mean number of days until psychiatric care was sought was more for Asians than for the American controls. Moreover, Kitano (1969b) noted that some Asian families tend to keep family members with mental illness at home. It is possible that the lower rates of service usage and the increased length of time for seeking services may lead to an aggravation of a patient's mental illness. This pattern might also account for the observation made by some researchers that Asian patients seem to be more disturbed and require longer lengths of hospital stay than their white American counterparts (Kitano 1969b; Rogers and Izutsu 1980).

Kuo (1984) performed a population-based study to assess depression among Asian American groups in Seattle. He used the Center for Epidemiological Studies—Depression (CES-D) Scale (Radloff 1977) and found the prevalence of depression among Asian Americans was at least as high as that of the white American population. He also found underuse of services was not due to a lack of need for these services. On the contrary, his data revealed that Asian Americans had a lower mental health status (i.e., higher CES-D scale scores) than white Americans, particularly compared with other Asian immigrant groups. Kuo concluded that community support groups among Asian Americans may have reduced their need for dependence on public services and may have been a factor in their lower utilization rates of these services.

Besides the stigma associated with mental illness, investigations suggest that the differences in rates of utilization for Asians may be related to the following: inappropriate therapeutic methods, clinicians' inability to speak Asian languages, a cultural gap between patients and clinicians, Asians' presentation of symptoms in a physical rather than a psychological manner, patients' limited experience with concepts of mental health and illness, and patients' lack of awareness of mental health facilities or their accessibility (S. Sue and McKinney 1975; S. Sue and D. W. Sue 1971). Examples of symptom presentation are given in the "Case Studies" section of this chapter; therapeutic considerations and guidelines are given in the "Psychotherapy" subsection.

Kitano (1982) cited the work of Okano (1977), who conducted a mental health survey among Japanese Americans in Los Angeles. Okano found a general low awareness of ethnic community social service resources. He also discovered that ministers were listed as the primary resource for counseling of emotional problems. Relatives, friends, and the family doctor were mentioned more frequently than mental health professionals, and more than half of the sample stated they would work out emotional problems on their own.

S. Sue and McKinney (1975) studied Asian American patients who received care in community mental health facilities. They found that Asian Americans underused the mental health resources that were available to them. They postulated several factors to account for this. These included the stigmatization of mental illness and the possibility that the available forms of mental health services may not have met the needs and values of the Asian patients. The latter proposition was further supported by the investigators' findings that Asian Americans prematurely terminated treatment and had a high dropout rate (52%).

Although from these studies we can surmise trends in the epidemiology of mental illness in Japanese Americans, there continues to be a need for research specifically targeted at this group to determine what the true incidence and prevalence of mental illness are.

Mental Health: Myths and Realities

Japanese Americans are typically viewed as quiet, studious, hardworking, and polite. The mainstream mental health professionals' view of Japanese Americans is that they have a low incidence of mental and emotional difficulties (Caudill and Weinstein 1969; Henkin 1985). Henkin postulated that the low perceived incidence might be due to low *reported* figures rather than actually low numbers. Japanese who *do* have emotional problems are reluctant to seek help. In order to avoid the shame and humiliation an open acknowledgment of their illness would bring to themselves and their families, these individuals often prefer to hide their difficulties.

Stereotyping of Asian Americans has influenced past research. Maloney (1945) found that there was very little psychosis in Okinawa. Published in a major United States journal, his article concluded that this lack of psychosis was due to the fostering of an ideal mother-infant bond (Yamamoto 1982). This finding was later refuted by Wedge (1952), who compared Okinawans in Hawaii with other ethnic groups and found no significant difference in incidence of psychosis. Maloney's idealized mother-infant interaction was, therefore, not related to the incidence of psychosis among Okinawans. This example demonstrates how stereotyping might have played a role in generating false conclusions about a particular cultural group. Stereotyping of Asians may still affect the attitudes and research of professionals; therefore, further investigation is needed in this little-studied area.

Some in the mainstream may envision the typical Japanese American as the wealthy Japanese businessman who purchases American real estate or directs auto-manufacturing companies (as depicted in an American feature film *Gung Ho!*). Japanese wives are seen as obedient and Japanese children as compliant and excelling in their studies. But these simplistic images do not conform to a reality complicated not only by the individual variation in any population, but also by the strength of the relationships Japanese Americans and Japanese in America have with Japan and the United States. For example, Japanese Americans and Japan-born businesspeople are of two quite different populations. The Japanese who come to the United States for business reasons are not interested so much in acculturating as in assimilating. They intend to return to Japan and, therefore, maintain Japanese customs for themselves and their children. In addition, because educational opportunities are highly competitive in their homeland, many Japanese companies are establishing Japanese high schools in the United States with teachers recruited from Japan. These Japanese parents do not wish to find that their children have fallen behind in the Japanese school curriculum when they return to their homeland. In contrast, Japanese Americans are a group with various degrees of acculturation, often generationally determined.

It is important that clinicians and researchers understand the diversity of views that may be held by Japanese Americans. One example is that a sample of Japanese Americans may have differing views on the acceptability of seeking mental health treatment. On the whole, the younger generations appear more broad-minded about mental health issues. Representative sampling across generations might allow for a more accurate future assessment of the incidence of mental illness in this nonhomogeneous group of *sansei, yonsei,* and *gosei.*

The Stigma of Mental Illness

Rogers and Izutsu (1980) found that Japanese people in Hawaii only reluctantly sought mental health treatment, and families rarely sought hospitalization for a family member needing inpatient psychiatric care. Moreover, the psychotic patients brought to the attention of professionals were fewer than predicted on the basis of population, and they had severe and advanced symptoms that required longer hospitalizations than psychotic patients from other groups. Rogers and Izutsu concluded that the families probably attempted home care of these relatives as long as possible before seeking help, most likely because of the shame involved in having a mentally ill family member.

In Japanese culture, there has traditionally been much emphasis on the maintenance of family name and honor in order to avoid adverse social consequences. For example, it was not uncommon for marriages to be arranged between families of similar social class and economic background. A person whose family had hereditary medical illnesses, mental retardation, or psychiatric illness among any of its members would usually make a poor match or no romantic match at all.

Part of the stigmatization attached to any "defects"—be they physical, cognitive, or emotional—may stem from a common Japanese belief that their race was descended from gods and was, therefore, superior. The Japanese also believed that when the connection between heaven and earth was broken, of all the countries on earth, Japan was closest to heaven. Japan was, in fact, the country of the gods. This belief may account in part for the intense patriotism that characterizes the Japanese (Latourette 1968).

The Japanese have always had a strong identification with their country and their people, and they have been proud of being a homogeneous race. Lebra (1976, pp. 22ff) described the concept of identity being established through "belongingness" in the Japanese culture. In order to belong, the individual must conform to the group. Mental illness is seen as deviant in Japan, something that does not "belong" to the collective group and is, therefore, shameful. The family must hide a relative's illness because their association with a mentally ill member will identify *them* as different and not belonging. This viewpoint seems to have been transmitted to Japanese Americans, who apparently underutilize available mental health resources, probably because of the fear of stigmatization.

Because of the shame involved, most Japanese with emotional difficulties do not seek help from mental health professionals but instead present to their general practitioner with complaints of physical ailments. Most physical illnesses (except hereditary ones) have traditionally been socially and culturally acceptable to the Japanese, whereas psychiatric ones have not been (Ohnuki-Tierney 1984; Rogers and Izutsu 1980).

Folk Traditions and Traditional Psychiatric Care

Although there are folk traditions and indigenous therapies specific to Japan, they are not typically seen in the Japanese American community because of the acculturation that has occurred. For example, shamans (indigenous healers) appear to exert some influence on the treatment of mental disorders in Japan. Nishimura (1987) found that 80% of Japanese patients on a general mental hospital ward had visited shamans seeking divination before their admission to the hospital. These patients had differing diagnoses—close to 90% had schizophrenia or atypical psychosis, 75% had depression, nervous conditions or alcoholism, and 60% had epilepsy or organic mental disorders. Roland (1988) reported that one way a Japanese patient expressed resistance to psychoanalysis was by dropping out of treatment and seeking help from an indigenous healer.

Fox possession is a folk belief that frequently underlies the search for help from shamans in Japan. Although the *issei* have anecdotes about people who have been possessed by the spirit of a fox, this type of presentation is not currently seen in the Japanese American population. This is not surprising, because it is expected that, in the process of acculturating, some older folk beliefs will be lost and new meanings will be given to cultural folk concepts that are currently more relevant. A psychologist from Japan (O. Tabata, personal communication, October 1989) has observed that fox possession and use of shamans for this disorder is infrequent even in present-day Japan.

Folk healing is often used to treat physical ailments. Because Asians tend to express emotional illness or distress through physical symptoms, folk remedies have become prominent in treating psychosomatic ills. Kitano (1969a) described the undue concern of the Japanese regarding body functions, obsession with blood pressure, widespread usage of patent medicines, hot baths, masseurs, and acupuncture. In addition, the use of chiropractors and medical professionals to deal with psychosomatic symptoms is also quite common.

Concepts of Mental Health and Mental Illness

There are few data regarding Japanese Americans' concepts of mental health and mental illness. The stigma attached to psychologic difficulties probably inhibits discussion of such topics among people in this population, for fear that others will assume that either the discussant or someone in the discussant's family has a mental illness.

Asian Americans have a range of beliefs about the etiology of mental illness. S. Sue and colleagues (1976) found that Asian American college students felt that avoiding morbid thoughts could contribute to mental health. These students further believed that mental illnesses were caused by organic factors. Kitano (1970) reported that Japanese Americans considered mental illness inappropriate behavior or malingering and that these attitudes affected the use of mental health resources.

Degree of acculturation and the somatization of symptoms were investigated by Tanaka-Matsumi and Marsella (1976) in a study where associations to words the subjects considered equivalent to depression were compared among Japanese nationals, Japanese Americans, and white Americans. Japanese nationals associated the word "headache" with depression, whereas Japanese Americans and white Americans associated "loneliness" with depression.

Isomura and colleagues (1987) discussed the difficulties in treating second-generation and third-generation Japanese Canadians. Isomura and her colleagues found stigmatization of mental illness among their Japanese clients. The Japanese Canadians viewed mental illness as "inherited, contagious, or incurable" (p. 285) and saw psychiatrists as dealing only with severe mental illnesses. There was little interest in psychotherapy and psychodynamics among the Japanese, but they emphasized biological treatment methods.

Generational differences in attitudes toward psychotherapy were illustrated in an article by Isomura and colleagues (1987) with two cases involving Japanese Canadian children. One child had *issei* parents and the second had *nisei* parents. The *issei* parents were not psychologically minded, were referred to a psychiatrist by their child's school, complied reluctantly with this recommendation, and placed responsibility for their child's progress on the psychiatrist, from whom they expected concrete directives. The *nisei* parents, in contrast, were more willing to look at possible psychodynamic sources of difficulty with their child, requested a psychiatric referral for their child themselves, felt the responsibility for their child's progress lay with the family, and were willing to engage in family therapy with a psychiatrist. The authors commented on the need to recognize that the differences between these two Japanese Canadian families were based upon time of immigration and degree of acculturation.

Case Studies of the Expression of Mental Illness

The expression of mental illness among more-acculturated Japanese Americans is similar to that of the mainstream population in the United States (Yamamoto 1982). The *issei* and less-acculturated Japanese, however, may pose special clinical challenges. For the *nisei, sansei,* and *yonsei,* cultural factors may still play a part in the development or expressions of symptoms or in the acceptance of mental illness.

Case Study 1

One of us (J. S. F.) treated a Japanese woman, Ms. A., who had a delusional system involving a contraption in Japan that she believed shot laser beams into her body and made her ill. The woman fled Japan and came to the United States, hoping to get beyond the range of the machine's rays. She was hospitalized for inpatient psychiatric treatment and then was referred for outpatient care. At the time of the outpatient referral, she had been away from Japan for 1½ years.

Ms. A.'s auditory hallucinations and delusional system had been with her since she was in her early 20s. She presented to our hospital, through the walk-in medical clinic, with complaints of arm fatigue and abdominal pains. A medical exam and workup were negative, and the patient was referred for psychiatric evaluation. She was admitted to the psychiatric ward and treated with neuroleptics, with the resolution of her somatic complaints.

The auditory hallucinations and delusions remained. Ms. A. had never been treated for these symptoms in Japan. She had mentioned them once to her parents years ago and was told by them never to tell anyone else.

Ms. A. was an outpatient for nearly a year. She was always extremely deferential and polite but was marginally compliant with her medications. Exacerbations of her psychosis were always characterized by an increase in somatic symptomatology, which usually abated with medication adjustment and improved medication compliance by the patient.

Eventually Ms. A. wanted to return to Japan. Recommendations were made for her to continue psychiatric follow-up there. She declined, stating that her friends and relatives might think it "strange" and find her unacceptable. She did not want to ruin her chances of getting married and having a family. Instead, she stated she would rather return to the United States and be cared for here should she ever become "sick" again. The patient's concept of "sick" encompassed the somatic symptoms she complained about during an exacerbation of her psychoses. She felt that the machine in Japan was making her physically ill and was responsible for the voices that plagued her. She did not feel her problem was psychiatric in any way, even though her illness had been discussed with her many times and her somatic symptoms improved with psychotropic medications.

Ms. A. was diagnosed as having schizophrenia based on her auditory hallucinations and delusions. The difficulty in this case was not diagnostic; rather, it was in educating a patient whose cultural background did not easily allow acceptance of mental illness.

The importance of gathering history from family members was made very clear by the following case.

Case Study 2

An elderly Japanese *nisei* woman, Mrs. B., was being treated by one of us (J. S. F.) for depression on the geriatric psychiatry inpatient unit. Mrs. B. was always well groomed, well dressed, pleasant, polite, and quiet. She was a "model" patient on the ward, and she complied with all medications, ward routines, and activities.

Mrs. B.'s treating physician stated that he had had difficulty identifying DSM-III-R criteria for depression when he first interviewed her. Only after he had spoken with her family did he obtain the history of her increasing social withdrawal, changes in activity level, difficulty with sleep and appetite, and thoughts about ending her life.

The children of Mrs. B. explained to him that their mother wanted to put on a good "face" in public and in front of him, an authority figure, and so was a "model" patient on the ward. This case illustrates the phenomenon of the "model" patient in the presence of authority, which has been described by one of us (Yamamoto 1982). At home, where she need not fear blemishing the family honor, her true symptoms and feelings emerged.

It is also important to note that Mrs. B. was a *nisei*, a member of the "transitional" generation between the *issei*, who have adhered to traditional Japanese culture, and the *sansei*, most of whom do not speak or understand Japanese and are acculturated to American ways. This patient had both Japanese and American cultural values. Her American viewpoints allowed her to seek mental health assistance, but her Japanese views influenced her behavior in social situations, making diagnosis of her problem difficult.

A Japanese American family will often contain a family member's mental illness until a major social or family disruption occurs, as illustrated in this case study.

Case Study 3

A *nisei* man in his 30s, Mr. C., presented for treatment with one of us (S. N. F.) with a long history of bipolar illness that had emerged during his adolescence. It became quite apparent, when he described his large family, that the illness could be traced back at least two generations on his father's side and was affecting his siblings and various cousins. Among the family members affected were a grandmother who had hung herself and a granduncle who had committed *seppuku*. The patient's father had been a gambler, spendthrift, and womanizer who was eventually institutionalized after he became psychotic in his 60s. During this hospitalization, the father's diagnosis of manic depression was made.

Mr. C. himself was diagnosed following the institutionalization of his father. He stated that the family had had difficulties that they attributed to "bad blood" and tended to socialize mainly with the mother's family to "keep the lid on things." Although they were active in community affairs, they did not allow much intimacy on a personal basis. He noted that the family was never considered *kichigai* (crazy) and was accepted because its members were highly accomplished and generous. However, he recalled numerous incidents of his father's outrageous and often psychotic behavior with family members.

The relatives of Mr. C. were able to conceal effectively the extent of the family's psychological problems. It was only when Mr. C.'s father's symptoms became disruptive and possibly dangerous that outside help was sought. Even after education by mental health professionals, Mr. C. was unwilling to acknowledge the existence of mental illness within himself or the rest of his family. Despite having read extensively on bipolar disease and having had a favorable response to lithium, Mr. C. is continuing to have difficulty accepting the diagnosis of his illness.

The third (*sansei*) and fourth (*yonsei*) generations are acculturated into the mainstream population. They have an "American" identity and often marry outside their ethnic group. Compared with the cultural difficulties of the *issei* and *nisei*, their problems are more like those faced by the majority of Americans in their age groups. These problems include drug abuse, delinquency, personality disorders, neuroses and psychoses (Yamamoto 1982). However, cultural factors can still have significance in some cases, such as the one described in the following case study.

Case Study 4

A Japanese American woman in her 20s, Ms. D., had been experiencing palpitations, difficulty breathing, lightheadedness, and tingling in her fingers. She consulted an internist who diagnosed her as having panic attacks and then referred her to one of us (S. N. F.) for psychiatric treatment.

Ms. D. was the oldest of three siblings. Her mother had been a picture bride and her father a *nisei* who had made his living as the proprietor of a small grocery store. Her father had been living with his ailing mother, and the patient's mother became her mother-in-law's primary caretaker. There had been a great deal of tension between the two women, and the patient had grown up witnessing the difficulties her mother had experienced with her grandmother.

The symptoms Ms. D. experienced had arisen after she had become romantically involved in a relationship with a young man who was an only son and who was extremely close to his mother. Although her boyfriend was in his late 20s, he continued to live at home and was treated indulgently by his mother. Ms. D. felt that her relationship with her boyfriend was very threatening to his mother. During the course of the courtship, the boyfriend's mother became ill. The patient then became preoccupied with the thought of having to care for her boyfriend's mother as her mother had had to care for her grandmother.

At this point, Ms. D. began experiencing panic attacks. In her view, it would be unthinkable not to care for her boyfriend's mother. However, from her own observations and conversations with her mother, she also appreciated the problems in caring for a difficult mother-in-law.

Because of her physical and emotional difficulties, Ms. D. broke off the relationship with her boyfriend. Following this, her symptoms slowly resolved, and she was able to enter into another relationship and got along well with her new boyfriend's mother. Her new boyfriend had older brothers and sisters and was not expected to be primarily responsible for his aging parents. She did not reexperience panic symptoms in this new relationship.

Ms. D. presented very much like an "American" patient. She was willing to accept psychological interpretations of her illness without needing to deal with her symptoms in a purely somatic way. Her internal conflicts were colored by cultural expectations that children be involved intimately in an aging parent's care. For this woman, the important Japanese tradition of caring for aging parents was emphasized by three factors: her own mother's experience with her grandmother, her father's belief that a good wife cares for relatives, and the implicit expectations on the part of the prospective *nisei* mother-in-law. This case illustrates that cultural factors may play an important role in the dynamic presentation, but that treatment may proceed in a Western manner for more-acculturated Japanese Americans.

Alcoholism

Alcohol abuse has not been found to be a major problem among Japanese Americans. The incidence of alcoholism is lower among the Japanese community in Hawaii than among the rest of the population (Yamamoto 1982). Moreover, the *1977 Hawaii Statistical Report* showed fewer Japanese hospitalized for alcoholism than other ethnic groups (Yamamoto 1982). Rogers and Izutsu (1980) found that alcohol problems are minimal among the Japanese in Hawaii. The Japanese, along with other Asians, tend to have reactions to alcohol that include facial flushing, dyspnea, tachycardia, nasal congestion, and subjective discomfort (Yamamoto 1982, 1988). One of us (J. Y.) is continuing to study the possibility that cultural factors and the flushing response may be responsible for the low prevalence of alcohol abuse among Asian Americans.

D. Sue (1987) examined the genetic/physiological and historical/cultural factors that might account for the high rates of abstinence and low rates of alcoholism among Chinese and Japanese Americans. He recommended future investigation of within-group and between-group differences in order to shed further light on the drinking patterns of Asian Americans.

Suicide

Although suicide is considered deviant behavior in Japan, it is also deemed an honorable form of death, as we pointed out earlier—most likely related to the military code *bushido,* which associated voluntary death by *seppuku* or *hara-kiri* with "the honor of the ruling class and the elitism of feudal Japan" (Lebra 1976, p. 191). Because of this tradition, Westerners have assumed that the Japanese in America commit suicide more frequently than other ethnic groups. This has not proved to be so.

The Japanese in Hawaii have not been found to have more frequent suicides compared with other ethnic groups in the island state (Rogers and Izutsu 1980). One of us (Yamamoto 1976) studied suicides among Japanese in Los Angeles and did not find a higher incidence compared with non-Japanese inhabitants but did discover a difference between methods used by the unacculturated and more-acculturated Japanese. The unacculturated Japanese more often used "Japanese" methods—hanging, wrist-cutting, drowning, suffocating, and jumping. The more-acculturated Japanese Americans used "American" methods for killing themselves—guns and drug overdoses.

Case Study 5—A *Nisei* Suicide

A *nisei* woman in her 60s found it difficult to bear her perceived shame in a family matter. She came from a large family of 10 children. Because of the family's financial circumstances, all of the children had had to work at a very early age. The patient left home at age 15 to work in a factory. Although this was due to financial need, she had felt abandoned by her family, especially after they moved and did not inform her of their whereabouts.

As a young adult, the patient married another *nisei* whom she met in an internment camp during World War II. The couple had six children. When her husband was in his 50s, he became ill with lung cancer and passed away. When the patient was still upset and tearful 2 weeks after his death, she apologized to her family for still mourning her husband. She was apologizing for her lack of stoicism, a highly regarded attribute in Japanese culture.

The patient subsequently remarried. The union was problematical, and her new husband left the relationship. She felt abandoned, although she commented to family members that she realized she did not love him as much as she had her first husband. Her family urged her to seek psychiatric care, but she refused. She was ashamed and humiliated but appeared to be recovering from her loss. Although family members noted some distress in the patient, they were unaware of the severity of her shame and emotional difficulties.

Six weeks after her husband left, she hanged herself.

This case illustrates the cultural factors that influenced this woman. She was ashamed of her behavior after the losses of her spouses and sought to restore honor to her family. She chose to do this by suicide, and she used a Japanese method—hanging (Yamamoto 1976).

Alternative Expressions of Distress

Health professionals should be aware of the avenues that Asians may select to express stress or emotional difficulties. As mentioned previously, the Japanese tend to reveal stress through physical symptoms and problems. Fukui (1987) conducted a study to assess the impact of migration on the incidence of illness and health care–seeking behavior among Japanese residents in Boston. Fukui had his participants maintain a health diary. Despite his encouragement to do so, not one of Fukui's subjects recorded any emotional or psychological problems arising from the stresses of migration. The inverse relationship between the occurrence of health problems in these participants and their length of stay in the United States suggested the stresses of adjusting to a new environment and culture were expressed physically, not emotionally.

Although Japanese Americans and white Americans had similar responses in Tanaka-Matsumi and Marsella's (1976) somatization study, a study of white American and Asian American students showed differences between the two groups regarding direct expression of emotional problems. Tracey and colleagues (1986) discovered that Asian American students appear to find it more acceptable to express emotional difficulties through academic and vocational concerns rather than through emotional and interpersonal worries. They found that when Asian American students sought counseling, they focused on academic difficulties, whereas white American students identified emotional or interpersonal problems. Other studies have corroborated the difficulty that Asian Americans have in seeking psychological services. S. Sue and Kitano (1973) found that most Asian Americans were reluctant to admit personal difficulties and seek help. D. W. Sue (1973) noted that Asian Americans were taught to control how they expressed their feelings much more than their non-Asian counterparts. Webster and Fretz (1978) found that Asian Americans looked first to their families when they have emotional problems in order to maintain family honor.

Family Response to the Mental Illness of Its Members

As discussed earlier in this chapter, the stigma of mental illness makes individuals and families delay seeking psychiatric help for mental illness (Rogers and Izutsu 1980). Japanese society views mental illness as being correctable by the individual or with help from the individual's family. Therefore, when mental illness occurs, the family attempts to care for the afflicted member instead of seeking psychiatric assistance for him or her (Munakata 1985) and does so because family members wish to protect their social position as well as the marriageability of family members. A similar situation may exist in the United States. Kitano (1969a) cited an example (S. Terashima, unpublished data, 1958) of a Japanese American family who had a relative who was hospitalized for schizophrenia:

The patient, the youngest of five siblings, was not only rejected and neglected by his father, who was domineering, irritable and seriously alcoholic, but he was also isolated from friends in his childhood. The entire family was shut off from social relationships. . . . (Kitano 1969a, p. 7)

Within a Japanese American family, there is ordinarily high tolerance for unusual behavior from mentally ill family members, with external resources being used only if deviant behavior causes a major disruption. Hospitalization is considered a last resort (Kitano 1969a). However, once hospitalized, patients' families are cohesive and willing to participate in treatment plans for mentally ill family members (Yamamoto 1982). This is most often seen with the less-acculturated older generations who have usually lived their lives, even in the United States, within the interdependency of the family structure.

It is interesting to speculate on why mentally ill family members are kept within the family as long as possible. Wanting to conceal internal shame and maintain family honor probably figures significantly into the decisions made by a Japanese American family with a mentally ill relative. A family's compliance with treatment plans once a family member has been brought to the attention of mental health professionals may also be related to "saving face" in the eyes of professionals (i.e., being obedient to authority figures) in addition to expressing concern for the affected relative. In Japan, some families are unable to tolerate the humiliation of mental illness and the blemish it places on their family honor, and as a result they will disown mentally ill relatives who require chronic hospitalization. Kitano (1969b) believed it was possible for a Japanese American family to be slow in reaccepting a hospitalized member because of the shame involved.

Treatment

Psychopharmacology

Several reports have suggested that Japanese Americans and Asians in general do well on lower doses of psychotropic medication than Westerners. In one study (Yamamoto 1982), it was observed empirically that Japanese Americans tend to do well on maintenance plasma levels of lithium of 0.5–0.6 mEq, in contrast to the higher plasma levels recommended for a white American population. It was also noted that, in general, Asian American patients generally need less medication than white American patients, whether for depression or mania (Yamamoto et al. 1979).

Rosenblat and Tang (1987), in a retrospective drug history review, compared drug dosages for four commonly used psychotropic medications (amitriptyline, chlorpromazine, haloperidol, and trifluoperazine) in groups of matched Asian and white North American populations. The researchers found that although the original dosages of amitriptyline were the same for both groups, the maintenance dosages were significantly lower in Asians. In addition, lower dosages of chlorpromazine and haloperidol were needed for clinical improvement in Asians, but these did not reach statistical levels of significance.

Rosenblat and Tang (1987) also found that maintenance dosages of trifluoperazine were significantly lower in Asians than in white North Americans. In the second half of their study, data from a survey of psychiatrists in Asia and North America indicated that significantly lower dosages of chlorpromazine, phenelzine, diazepam, and chlordiazepoxide were being prescribed for Asians compared with white North Americans. Variations between these two groups in drug metabolism, side effects, and body weight may have resulted in the dosage differences.

Potkin and colleagues (1984) supported this hypothesis with their finding that Chinese schizophrenic patients in the People's Republic of China had plasma haloperidol levels that were 52% higher than the plasma levels for American non-Asian schizophrenic patients. The Chinese and non-Asian American patients were matched for sex and body weight. Both sets of patients adhered to fixed dosage schedules of medication—0.4 mg of haloperidol per day per kilogram of body weight for 6 weeks. The investigators concluded that the difference in plasma drug concentrations might explain why Asians are reported to require smaller dosages of neuroleptics compared with non-Asians, and why Asians appear to be more sensitive to neuroleptic-induced side effects.

Lin and Finder (1983) compared chlorpromazine doses for 13 Asian American and 13 white American patients matched for age, sex, diagnosis, and date of discharge. Mean maximum and stabilized chlorpromazine equivalent dosages were lower for the Asian American subjects than for the white Americans. In addition, the mean chlorpromazine equivalent doses associated with the first appearance of extrapyramidal symptoms were lower for Asian Americans.

Tien (1984) used three case histories to illustrate differences in the way Asian patients respond to medication. She concluded that Asians can easily develop adverse reactions or side effects even on dosages of psychotropic drugs that are smaller than are normally prescribed and that psychotropic drugs do not seem to be effective for some Asian patients.

Kalow (1986) reviewed drug metabolism reactions among various ethnic groups and found differences in conjugation reactions between white American and Asian groups who were given the same drug. Lin and co-workers (1989) studied haloperidol doses and serum concentrations in Asian and white American schizophrenic patients. They used fixed- and variable-dose regimens and found that the Asian patients required lower doses of haloperidol for optimal treatment of their condition and that the Asian patients exhibited extrapyramidal symptoms at lower medication doses. The researchers postulated that the difference between the two groups in terms of range of therapeutic haloperidol doses was due to ethnic differences in pharmacodynamics.

These studies demonstrate that Asians appear to require smaller doses of psychotropic medications and are more sensitive to their side effects than are white Americans. Overmedication on standard dosages of medication may be common and may lead to excessive or long-term side effects and ultimate noncompliance with medication. The studies discussed in this section suggest a trend in terms of Asian sensitivity to medications; however, the final chapter has not been written on this topic. There is still a need for more extensive controlled trials of medications comparing the responses of Asians and white Americans, as well as studies in which Japanese Americans are specifically examined as a group.

Psychotherapy

A Brief Summary of Relevant Cultural Factors

When clinicians are doing psychotherapy with Japanese Americans, it is important for them to recognize the variability in the extent to which Japanese values and socialization are parts of the patient's background. As we have pointed out earlier in this chapter, cultural values are determined to a great extent by the patient's generation, social class, education, geographic location, and personal experiences. The following is a brief summary of the most important cultural factors that may impinge upon therapy.

Clinicians in the United States should be aware of the concepts of *amae* ("passive love") and *shinkeishitsu* ("nervousness"), especially when treating Japanese patients who are less acculturated.

Doi's concept of *amae*.   In 1973, Doi published *The Anatomy of Dependence* on the subject of *amae*. Since then, there has been considerable study of *amae*, a Japanese form of "passive love" that Doi believed was a key to understanding the psychological structure of Japanese individuals and Japanese society as a whole. This concept has had some impact on therapy, as we will discuss later.

Amae is the noun form of the verb *amaeru*, which Doi (1962) defined as "to depend and presume upon another's benevolence." The term *amaeru* is associated with the Japanese word for "sweet" (*amai*) and is used to describe a child's attitude or behavior toward his or her parents, especially the mother. The dependency-need relationship may also exist between two adults, as Doi found in his psychiatric practice where his Japanese patients showed their wish to *amaeru* (Lebra 1976).

Other writers have expanded upon Doi's concept of *amae.* The role of expressing *amae,* referred to by the verb *amaeru,* has a complementary role in which one accepts another's *amae,* expressed by the verb *amayakasu* (Kumagai and Kumagai 1986; Lebra 1976). Both *amaeru* and *amayakasu* have "active" and "passive" stances. Active *amaeru* is the solicitation of the indulgence of another; passive *amaeru* is the acceptance of the indulgence of another. Active *amayakasu* is to pursue one's wish for indulgence; passive *amayakasu* is to accept another's wish for indulgence (Lebra 1976).

Shinkeishitsu neurosis is relatively common in Japan and has a wide variety of manifestations. Morita therapy (which we describe later) is the treatment of choice for *shinkeishitsu.* Kora, Morita's successor, classified *shinkeishitsu* into three different types (Lebra 1976):

- Type 1 is "ordinary" *shinkeishitsu* and is characterized by psychosomatic symptoms.
- Type 2 is "obsessional" or "phobic" *shinkeishitsu* and is characterized by fears, including fear of heights, fear of meeting another person's eyes, fear of not being able to be perfect, and fear of fainting.
- Type 3 is "paroxysmal neurosis" or "anxiety neurosis" *shinkeishitsu* and is characterized by palpitation seizures, anxiety fits, dyspneic seizures, and the like.

Morita postulated that *shinkeishitsu* neurosis was due to an "excessive concentration of attention." Doi disagreed, stating that the etiology was related to a "frustrated desire to *amaeru*" (Doi 1973, p. 19). Whatever the etiology, *amae* and *shinkeishitsu* are common in Japan. Clinicians in the United States may need to consider these entities when treating patients who are less-acculturated Japanese Americans or recent immigrants from Japan.

It has been noted that the *issei* retain Japanese values such as interdependency, hierarchical relationships, and the importance of empathy (Yamamoto 1982). The *nisei* have been more acculturated but are still preoccupied by the stigma of mental illness. In addition, because they are a transitional generation straddling two worlds, there may be conflict between two different value and cultural systems. The *sansei* and *yonsei* are more acculturated and often have values more like the American mainstream.

Social class factors are also important in therapy with Japanese Americans, particularly because the original immigrants were farmers, unsophisticated about mental health, and unlikely to seek out mental health resources (Yamamoto 1982). Geographic location is also important. The history of internment and lack of role models have been an important part of the Japanese American experience in the mainland United States. However, for Japanese Americans in Hawaii, who are an ethnic majority, life in America has been different. They experienced less racial discrimination and became leaders in government and in their communities.

A diversity of experience is also found even within generations in the form of differences in acculturation and group identification. Ford (1987) notes three categories of "social-psychological development" in minority students: traditional counselees who conform to family obligations with a high degree of obedience to parents; a marginal ethnic minority who have sacrificed their original culture to become assimilated and find themselves on the margin of two cultures; and the "ethnic pride" students who have rejected cultural assimilation and have accepted at least some traditional values but have modified others. These students demand a pluralistic form of integration into the majority culture.

Although it is important that cultural factors be taken into account in doing therapy, it is equally important to distinguish intrapersonal from culturally related problems and hybrids of the two. Marshall and colleagues (1983) and Henkin (1985) have noted the importance of distinguishing a personal problem from what may be in part a cultural difference. Other researchers described the opposite diagnostic pitfall of overinterpreting or explaining away symptoms on a cultural basis (Yamamoto and Chang 1988). Henkin (1985) also reported that mental health professionals should be aware of how Asians may cope with racism. Some Asians who are discriminated against on the basis of ethnicity may internalize this prejudicial treatment as being deserved for their individual shortcomings, when it is actually an issue of racism.

In doing therapy with Asians, some researchers advocated the importance of family participation, dealing with stigma, an educational approach, discussion of the duration of therapy, and explanation of medications (Yamamoto and Chang 1988). They also supported the use of "active empathy" in which the therapist is more directive and active in his or her interactions with the patient.

For short-term therapy, Henkin (1985) recommended a clear-cut structure. The role of the therapist should be established clearly and the counseling process should be explained, because many Japanese Americans do not have experience with counseling. Confidentiality should be assured and protected. It was also recommended that therapists refrain from making assessments for as long as possible and that they restate their understanding of patients' experiences to minimize misinterpretation.

Roland (1988) studied psychoanalysis in Japan and reported that it is possible to do analysis there if it is performed in a culturally sensitive way. He cited the cases of five Japanese patients to demonstrate that clear therapeutic progress was made and could be understood in psychodynamic terms, even though there was a minimum of interpretation, investigation, or even empathic reflections on the therapist's part. The therapist mainly conveyed empathy nonverbally.

The following case study illustrates some of the considerations important to therapy that were provided in this brief summary.

Case Study 6

Mr. E. was an elderly *kibei nisei* who was brought into treatment by his family upon the recommendation of another psychiatrist. He had fractured his hip and had undergone hip replacement surgery. He became increasingly depressed and felt that he was "a mechanical person." As Mr. E. became more depressed, he stopped taking care of his personal needs and spent much of his time either in an unresponsive state or moaning that he was a burden to his family and wanted to die.

His family took care of Mr. E. and did not seek psychiatric consultation for his depression, although he was getting extensive medical treatment. During his last medical hospitalization, he psychologically decompensated to the point of beginning to medically deteriorate. He was then transferred as an emergency case to the mental health unit of the hospital where he underwent a course of involuntary electroconvulsive therapy (ECT). Mr. E. responded quite dramatically to the treatment, becoming less depressed and more responsive to his environment. However, his treating psychiatrist, who was a white American, could not get the patient to communicate with him or agree to comply with continuing treatment and ongoing antidepressant medication. It was at this point that the patient was referred for treatment to a Japanese American psychiatrist (S. N. F.), because it was believed that he might do better with a therapist who was more sensitive to his cultural issues.

When Mr. E. first came to the office, he was accompanied by his wife and son. He insisted that they come to the consultation with him. Because of his memory loss after his ECT, they provided information about what his life had been like during the past several years, how he had responded to treatment, and what his major concerns were. After being educated about the nature of depression and the use of ECT and antidepressant medications, the family was able to encourage Mr. E. to start a course of antidepressants. On this medication, his depression continued to improve as did his ability to resume his chores at home.

After five family sessions, Mr. E. felt comfortable enough to see the therapist by himself. During his individual sessions, he was quite open regarding his concerns. He worried about being a burden to others and about individual family members and their relationships with each other. He also explored his guilty feelings that he had done something to cause his illness. He revealed that from an early age he had frequently been a caretaker and had intended to become a medical professional until World War II interrupted his plans. It was when he could no longer be a caretaker that his depression emerged.

One of the major therapeutic issues that faced this patient as his depression lifted was dealing with shame. He felt ashamed of his illness and the burden he believed it had placed upon his family. Culturally, shame plays an integral role in the discipline and appropriate group socialization of Japanese children. If a Japanese child misbehaves in public, he or she will commonly be reprimanded by a parent stating, "People are watching!" Parents inform the children that they are not only humiliating themselves but also staining their families' honor. Japanese nationals and less-acculturated Japanese Americans will be particularly sensitive to the issue of shame in regard to family status and honor.

Mr. E.'s case also illustrates some characteristic aspects of doing psychotherapy with a Japanese American patient. The family tolerated very high degrees of depression in their relative. They did not recognize the extent of his illness and did not seek psychiatric help until a radical intervention was called for. The family had been perplexed when the referring psychiatrist recommended further treatment for Mr. E., even though he had become socially withdrawn, psychomotor retarded, and unable to perform simple activities of daily living such as bathing. The family members did not understand that these were symptoms of depression, because mental illness is rarely addressed in Asian culture. They had preferred to attribute Mr. E.'s symptoms to physical problems. However, with education and support, the family was very helpful in involving him in therapy and seeing that he was compliant with treatment recommendations.

Initial therapy sessions involved family members, which included Mr. E., his wife, and one of their three children. The family talked and Mr. E. listened. Gradually, the focus shifted from the family unit to the patient so that he was able to engage in individual therapy.

It should be noted that at least part of each session was spent in attending to Mr. E.'s symptoms, consistent with a medical model, adjusting his medication, and providing suggestions and education to help him deal with his illness. Once a therapeutic alliance was established, however, he was able to deal with underlying issues that were contributing to his depression. It was then possible to work with his emotional conflicts and deficits from the past, enabling him to function better within his family and to accept his illness. It appears that involvement of the family was extremely important in establishing the therapeutic alliance. Besides the sensitivity to cultural issues, it is also interesting to speculate on the nature of Mr. E.'s transference to a Japanese American psychiatrist and how this might have contributed to his therapeutic alliance and ability to work in sessions.

According to Campbell's *Psychiatric Dictionary,* "transference" involves a patient's "projection of feelings, thoughts, and wishes" onto another person (usually the therapist), "who has come to represent an object from the patient's past" (1989, p. 771). Therefore, by definition, transference is a phenomenon that is defined by each individual's past experiences and is not the same for any two people. Transference is also a dynamic entity; it is constantly changing over the course of therapy.

There are different factors to consider in terms of the possible transference of Mr. E. discussed previously. Perhaps the visual familiarity of a Japanese American psychiatrist as opposed to a white American psychiatrist facilitated the patient's ability to trust and to feel comfortable divulging personal information about himself, thus encouraging the development of transference. It is also important to consider the degree of acculturation of the patient being treated as well as his or her needs as an individual. For example, less-acculturated Japanese American patients may not "believe" in psychiatry or may reject a psychiatrist who is not Japanese American because he or she is not Japanese. These patients may even reject a Japanese American psychiatrist who they may feel has "sold out" to the mainstream and is therefore incapable of truly understanding their more traditional thoughts and feelings.

As can be seen from this brief discussion, the issue of transference is a complicated one and beyond the scope of our discussion here. Transference is a highly individual phenomenon and should be approached as such when a clinician is working with a Japanese American, as with any other patient.

Japan-Based Therapies

Naikan and Morita therapies are two indigenous psychotherapies used in Japan (Lebra 1976). Naikan was developed by Ishin Yoshimoto in 1954 during his work with inmates in penitentiaries. It was then extended to patients with mental and physical illnesses. Naikan therapy involves a period of isolated introspection in which the patient may "discover" his or her true self. By reflecting on crucial relationships with significant others at various times in his or her life, the patient reflects on the care he or she has received by these significant others and how he or she hopes to repay this debt. At the end of the period of reflection, the patient has reconceptualized his or her life as having entailed dependency on a number of caretakers. The patient then acknowledges his or her social insensitivity and develops a sense of debt and gratitude toward others. Thus, Naikan aims to build moral constraints into the individual based on a sense of obligation.

Morita therapy was developed at the turn of the century. Morita described the emergence of the *shinkeishitsu* neurosis, and his therapy was specifically designed to deal with it. Morita therapy does not examine psychological conflicts or use therapeutic techniques such as dream analysis or transference (Ohnuki-Tierney 1984). It has its basis in Zen Buddhism and aims at liberating the patient from excessive self-preoccupation and intellectualizations, enabling him or her to live naturally and to accept things "as they are." This involves the patient's submitting to symptoms in defeat and resignation, "uniting" with his or her illness, and even being encouraged to enact or produce symptoms. Questions are discouraged, and the patient's direct experience is emphasized. Morita therapy is based on the belief that the self is not autonomous but should be submerged in nature or society.

For Morita therapy to be effective, the patient is removed from his or her environment and placed in a hospital. There are two major periods of treatment. The first phase lasts 5 to 7 days, during which the patient is in a state of total bed rest and isolation. There are no specific tasks to occupy the patient during this period. If the patient is left alone, the symptoms experienced are likely to intensify, according to Morita therapists, because he or she is presented with the maximal conflict between what he or she wishes to be and what he or she actually is. The patient is told to learn to live with suffering. Through the experience of despair and hopelessness, he or she comes to some form of self-acceptance. Thus, bed rest and isolation forces the patient to confront his or her relation to others and to acknowledge his or her existence as a part of group life.

The next phase of Morita therapy involves three stages, each lasting from

5 to 10 days and consisting of progressively harder work. In the first stage, light work is done, such as scrubbing the floor or picking up dead leaves. In the moderate stage, tasks are assigned that require more effort and patience. In the last stage, the patient learns to do whatever work is required in everyday life. Work therapy involves the patient's participation in group life, the assumption of a social role, and awareness that others depend on him or her and that he or she is useful to others.

Naikan therapy was originally developed to rehabilitate antisocial inmates into morally upright people, whereas Morita therapy was developed to transform patients with mental illness into healthy individuals (Lebra 1976). It is estimated that in the 1980s, Naikan and Morita therapies were utilized by less than 1% of the people who sought mental health services in Japan. In the United States, Reynolds (1989) has practiced Morita therapy and Naikan therapy (together referred to as "Constructive Living") since the early 1970s. There are Constructive Living centers located in Los Angeles, Hawaii, Salt Lake City, New York, San Francisco, Seattle, and Washington, DC. Reynolds has had success using the Constructive Living techniques with Westerners. Thus, Constructive Living may benefit Japanese of different generations as well as non-Asian patients.

Tabata states that psychoanalytically oriented therapy and pharmacotherapy are currently the most common forms of treatment in Japan (O. Tabata, personal communication, October 1989). The stigmatization surrounding psychodynamic psychotherapy has lessened among the younger generations. A Japanese psychiatrist's clinical orientation is often determined by the institution where he or she trained. For example, graduates of Jikei University favor Morita therapy, whereas Nagoya University graduates prefer psychoanalytically oriented psychotherapy.

Use of an Interpreter

Limited language facility is a problem specific to less-acculturated Japanese. Because psychiatric and psychological assessment rely heavily on verbal communication, language limitations can be particularly difficult for the clinician (D. Sue and S. Sue 1987). For clinicians who are not proficient in the Japanese language, interpreters become very important.

Studies by Ishisaka and colleagues (1985) and Marcos (1979) noted some of the difficulties that arise with the use of interpreters. Interpreters are often asked to translate questions into a language that does not contain corresponding words. Asian languages generally have few words to describe psychological problems. An additional difficulty is that the interpreters' own cultural beliefs and values might cause them to censor material a patient is disclosing that might be viewed negatively by the community. Interpreters have reported reluctance in asking patients about sexual matters, financial background, material that might be disrespectful to the clinician, and information related to suicidal or homicidal thoughts.

Marcos (1979) studied the various kinds of distortions that can occur through the use of an interpreter and identified three major forms of distortions. The first involved omissions, substitutions, condensation, and change of focus. The second involved the tendency of interpreters with little psychiatric knowledge to "normalize" a patient's thought processes or descriptions. In these cases, the clinician is unable to get a clear picture of the patient's mental status. The third type of distortion occurred when an interpreter's attitudes influenced the information given to the clinician. For example, family members who functioned as interpreters would tend to minimize the patient's psychopathology and to answer questions themselves without first consulting the patient. In order to attenuate these possible interpreter distortions, Marcos (1979) suggested that the clinician and the interpreter discuss the goals of the patient's evaluation and identify the areas to be assessed, including sensitive subjects that would be broached.

Hospitalizations

Japanese Americans view psychiatric hospitalization of a family member as a last resort. Usually the family is willing to work together on a treatment plan with mental health professionals to keep the family member at home unless the patient is a danger to himself or others.

The literature is sparse regarding the effects of psychiatric hospitalization on Japanese American patients and their families. One of the primary concerns for clinicians is the degree of acculturation of the patients and their families. The more-acculturated patients will have issues and concerns much like members of the mainstream population who require psychiatric hospitalization. Nevertheless, some of these patients may prefer having mental health professionals who are themselves Asians or who are familiar with Asian cultures and issues.

The less-acculturated patient, usually one of the *issei* generation or a Japanese national residing in the United States, poses different considerations. Ohnuki-Tierney (1984) wrote about the customs and conventions that surround a medical hospitalization in Japan. Family members are heavily involved, and they care for the patient's personal needs (furnishing fresh nightgowns, articles for the patient's hygiene, and objects for the patient's personal comfort in the hospital, such as favorite books and trinkets). The family is also responsible for providing the patient with preferred foods, and for receiving visitors. The Japanese patient typically receives many visitors, including relatives, friends, and neighbors. Fresh fruit and fresh cut flowers are usually the gifts of choice. Fruit is considered healthful, and cut flowers indicate the visitor's hope that the patient will be well enough to leave the hospital before the flowers wilt. Potted plants are never given, because such gifts may be interpreted as implying that a patient may "take root" in the hospital and require a long stay.

Family members are told of the patient's diagnosis, but the patient is never informed of it by his or her physician. Ohnuki-Tierney (1984) reported that this is preferred by both the patients and medical staff. Even Japanese physicians, when they became patients, preferred not to know their diagnoses. This is based on the belief that if a Japanese patient knew the truth about the illness, he or she might lose hope and deteriorate more quickly. The family and the patient's physician share this knowledge and remain supportive of the patient throughout the illness.

A psychiatric hospitalization is a different entity. For the Japanese in Japan, and the *issei* and Japanese nationals in the United States, there is stigma and shame regarding hospitalization attached to both patient and family. This disrupts the social rituals around hospitalization that ordinarily provide structure and support during a difficult time. The patient and family generally wish to keep the hospitalization secret and prefer not to have many visitors. In working with less-acculturated patients, it may be beneficial to provide the following:

1. A Japanese interpreter;
2. A Japanese American psychiatrist, or a consultation from a psychiatrist familiar with Asian dynamics and issues;
3. Visits from family members and others who provide social support whom the patient and family feel are appropriate (e.g., the patient's minister); and
4. The allowance of familiar personal effects and foods for the patient while he or she is on the ward (as permitted by the institution).

These measures may provide an atmospheric structure that is similar to a medical hospitalization—a situation that may be more familiar to both patient and family. This may enhance both the patient's and family's emotional comfort and treatment compliance.

Follow-Up Care

Acculturation is also a factor in follow-up care. Acculturated Japanese Americans will have follow-up issues similar to the mainstream in terms of outpatient therapy, medication visits, and compliance.

With less-acculturated patients, the clinician should establish and maintain communication with family members, who can often be important in the patient's compliance with medications and visits. Deference to authority figures does not guarantee compliance. The less-acculturated patient may be saying "yes" in the physician's office but be noncompliant with the treatment plan at home. The family can thus offer updates on the patient's progress in a familiar environment while helping the patient with his or her compliance. Contact with a clinician can also be psychologically supportive to the family itself. The clinician should educate the family about premonitory signs and symptoms of exacerbated illness so that a prompt hospitalization can be arranged if the patient shows signs of decompensation. Working together in this way may reduce the feelings of isolation and helplessness the family may feel if the patient deteriorates.

Involvement of the family may offset the high dropout rate that has been found among Japanese American outpatients (S. Sue and McKinney 1975). It is important for these patients to remain in follow-up, because most less-acculturated Japanese American patients only present to mental health professionals when their illness has become extremely severe.

Conclusion

The data presented in this chapter were based on a limited number of studies. Because of the paucity of literature on Japanese Americans and mental health and illness, there are some caveats to be considered. Some of the research cited did not deal only with Japanese Americans but also with other Asian American groups. Some studies assumed that Japanese immigrants were comparable to Japanese in Japan, when in fact they may make up a self-selected group whose members were willing to leave their homeland. Because a small number of researchers generate most of the investigations in the area of Asian American mental health, possible researcher bias must be kept in mind when reviewing the literature. Another type of researcher and clinician bias to consider is stereotyping of Asian Americans and how this may affect a mental health professional's attitude about the patient, including diagnosis and treatment recommendations.

Japanese Americans are heterogeneous. There are generational, cultural, and geographic differences that can affect these individuals and their families in terms of their view of mental illness, manifestation of symptoms, and willingness to seek psychiatric evaluation and care, as well as the treatment plans for these individuals and delivery of inpatient and outpatient care. However, it appears that the predominant factor is degree of acculturation. The various generations within the United States can also be designated by degree of acculturation. Clinicians can use the following as a framework when approaching a Japanese patient.

Less-acculturated patients (*issei*, Japanese nationals). An interpreter is usually necessary unless the mental health professional is fluent in Japanese. Members of this group would most likely prefer an Asian clinician or one who had an understanding of Asian issues. These patients will attach a strong stigma to psychiatric illness. They will be passive and deferential to authority figures, supplying little useful information. They usually do not come to the attention of mental health professionals on their own but are brought in by their families. The families are extremely important in terms of supplying history and symptom details. It is important to inquire about any folk beliefs or remedies that may have been considered by such patients. These patients will feel most comfortable with a medical model of care. They will opt for medications rather than psychotherapy (if given a choice), because this population prefers a passive stance, where the clinician has all the responsibility for their progress and they have little to none. Close communication with and cooperation of the families is imperative for the patients' compliance with treatment.

Moderately acculturated patients (*nisei*). The *nisei* maintain both Japanese and American cultural values. As members of a "transitional" generation, the *nisei* must constantly struggle with the experience of being between two different worlds. It is important to ask these patients if they had an internment camp experience during World War II and, if so, to explore further the ordeal of being American citizens who were locked up for being of a particular race. Such patients may have feelings of shame, anger, and distrust, especially if the clinician is non-Asian.

Although the *nisei* are more acculturated, there are degrees of variation within this population also. Most *nisei* are concerned about the stigma of mental illness and would prefer to turn to a physician, a minister, their family, or themselves if they have an emotional problem. They are often unaware of the mental health services that are locally available to them. They will most likely present to such a facility, either on their own or brought in by family members, when their illnesses become severe enough to pose a danger to themselves or to others. The majority of *nisei* are fluent in English (some *kibei nisei* are not) and will have no language problems with a non-Asian clinician. However, some may benefit from being treated by, or having a consultation with, an Asian clinician or a clinician familiar with Asian culture and issues. The family is important for treatment planning and compliance but may not be as necessary for structural support as with the less-acculturated Japanese. This population is generally compliant with treatment, but there may be a problem with premature termination of treatment. When dealing with the *nisei*, the clinician must keep in mind that, although they may appear acculturated in many ways, there may be small pockets of cultural differences that may affect the course of the patient's illness and treatment progress.

More-acculturated patients (*sansei, yonsei, gosei*).   The same caveat holds for this group as for the *nisei* (i.e., that the clinician not be beguiled into considering these persons identical to the mainstream population). Depending upon the acculturation of the family and family composition (e.g., did *issei* grandparents reside in the household?), these patients may have loci of cultural idiosyncrasies. On the whole, however, with the succeeding generations of Japanese in America, the view of mental illness, symptom presentation, seeking and receiving of mental health services, treatment plans, compliance, and involvement of family more closely resemble those of non-Japanese patients in the United States.

Issues to consider regardless of acculturation or generation include the following:

1. The prevalence of mental illness in the various diagnostic categories is probably the same among Japanese Americans as among the rest of the United States population. It is hard to assess the true incidence and prevalence of illness, partially due to the underusage of mental health services by Japanese Americans. For the less acculturated, this underutilization may be due to both stigma and lack of knowledge about available resources.

2. Japanese Americans with emotional difficulties often present with somatic complaints to their internists and family practitioners. It may be important for mental health professionals to do liaison work with their medical colleagues in terms of how to work most successfully with these patients.

3. Asian patients require smaller doses of psychotropic medications for optimal benefit and are more sensitive to side effects compared with white Americans. This is most likely due to ethnic pharmacodynamic differences.
4. Although suicide has been considered an "honorable" form of death throughout Japanese history, an increased incidence of suicide among Japanese Americans has not been seen.
5. Although Japanese Americans, especially those who are less acculturated, may prefer to consider mental illness as being due to biologic factors, it has been our experience that they can often work effectively in a psychodynamic fashion once a therapeutic alliance has been established.
6. Shame plays an important role in Japanese culture. A clinician working psychotherapeutically with a Japanese American patient may need to be less confrontational and work more slowly. As the Japanese American patient reveals more, he or she will feel more vulnerable to shame. Although this is true of non-Japanese Americans, we have found in our clinical encounters with this population that Japanese Americans seem to be more sensitive about this issue. Early termination is the undesirable outcome and can occur if a patient feels he or she has "lost face" in his or her therapist's eyes.
7. The family is a key factor for treatment of a Japanese American regardless of the degree of acculturation or the generation of the patient.

The research frontiers with regard to Japanese Americans and mental illness are vast. Data are needed on the incidence and prevalence of the various mental illnesses among Japanese Americans—data broken out by generation, degree of acculturation, geographic location, and gender. Further investigation is also needed in terms of the underutilization of the available mental health services (i.e., is it a question of stigma and/or provision of services that do not meet the needs of this population)? Further studies are also needed to examine the concepts and expectations of this heterogeneous group in terms of mental illness, available care, and clinician-patient relationship. More data on the stereotypes and attitudes of clinicians and their effect on the formulation and delivery of care to this population would also be useful.

Japanese Americans are a diverse group of individuals, each with his or her own style of adaptation to the mainstream culture. To treat this population effectively, the mental health professional must maintain an awareness of the common experiences of its members while simultaneously being attentive to the differences that can be culturally, generationally, or individually determined.

References

Campbell RJ: Psychiatric Dictionary, 6th Edition. New York, Oxford University Press, 1989, p 771

Caudill W, Weinstein H: Maternal care and infant behavior in Japan and America. Psychiatry 32:12–43, 1969

Connor JW: Acculturation and family continuities in three generations of Japanese Americans. Journal of Marriage and the Family Feb:159–165, 1974

Derogatis L: SCL-90-R Manual II. Towson, MD, Clinical Psychometric Research, 1983

Doi T: Amae: a key concept for understanding Japanese personality structure, in Japanese Culture: Its Development and Characteristics. Edited by Smith R, Beardsley R. Chicago, IL, Aldine Publishing, 1962

Doi T: The Anatomy of Dependence. Tokyo, Kodansha International Ltd, 1973

Ford RC: Cultural awareness and cross-cultural counseling. International Journal for the Advancement of Counselling 10:71–78, 1987

Fukui T: Health diary study of Japanese residents in greater Boston: variables related to high incidence of health problems. Cult Med Psychiatry 11:509–520, 1987

Henkin WA: Toward counseling the Japanese in America: a cross-cultural primer. Journal of Counseling and Development 63:500–503, 1985

Herman M: The Japanese in America, 1843–1973. Dobbs Ferry, NY, Oceana Publications, 1974

Ichioka Y: The Issei: The World of the First Generation Japanese Immigrants, 1885–1924. New York, Free Press, 1988

Ishisaka HA, Nguyen QT, Okimoto JT: The role of culture in the mental health treatment of Indo-Chinese refugees, in Southeast Asian Mental Health Treatment, Prevention, Services, Training and Research. Edited by TC Owan. Washington, DC, U.S. Department of Health and Human Services, 1985

Isomura T, Fine S, Lin TY: Two Japanese families: a cultural perspective. Can J Psychiatry 32:282–286, 1987

Kalow W: Conjugation reactions, in Ethnic Differences in Reactions to Drugs and Xenobiotics. Edited by Kalow W, Goedde HW, Agarwal DP. New York, Alan R Liss, 1986

Kitano HH: Japanese-American mental illness, in Changing Perspectives in Mental Illness. Edited by Plot SC, Edgerton RB. New York, Holt, Rinehart, & Winston, 1969a

Kitano HHL: Japanese Americans, The Evolution of a Subculture. Englewood Cliffs, NJ, Prentice-Hall, 1969b

Kitano HHL: Mental Illness in Four Cultures. J Soc Psychol 80:121–134, 1970

Kitano HH: Mental health in the Japanese-American community, in Minority Mental Health. Edited by Jones EE, Korchin SJ. New York, Praeger, 1982

Kitano HL, Kikumura A: The Japanese American family, in Ethnic Families in America. Edited by Mindel C, Habenstein R. New York, Elsevier, 1976

Koh B: Breaking the silence: oldest Japanese internees never spoke of the camps—

until now. Los Angeles Times, November 25, 1990, pp J1, J9

Kumagai HA, Kumagai AK: The hidden "I" in amae: "passive love" and Japanese social perception. Ethos 14(3):305–320, 1986

Kuo W: Prevalence of depression among Asian-Americans. J Nerv Ment Dis 172:449–457, 1984

Latourette KS: The History of Japan. New York, Macmillan, 1968

Lebra TS: Japanese Patterns of Behavior. Honolulu, HI, University of Hawaii Press, 1976

Lin KM, Finder E: Neuroleptic dosage in Asians. Am J Psychiatry 140:490–491, 1983

Lin KM, Poland RE, Nuccio I, et al: A longitudinal assessment of haloperidol doses and serum concentrations in Asian and Caucasian schizophrenic patients. Am J Psychiatry 146(10):1307–1311, 1989

Maloney JC: Psychiatric observations in Okinawa Shima, the psychology of the Okinawan and a psychiatric hospital in military government. Psychiatry 8:391–399, 1945

Marcos LR: Effects of interpreters on the evaluation of psychopathology in non-English-speaking patients. Am J Psychiatry 136:171–174, 1979

Marshall C, Wilson J, Leung P: Value conflict: a cross-cultural assessment paradigm. Journal of Applied Rehabilitation Counseling 14:74–78, 1983

Mochizuki M: Discharges and units of service by ethnic origin: Fiscal Year 1973–1974. County of Los Angeles Mental Health Service, Research and Information Section, E and R Rows and Columns 3(11):1–15, 1975

Morton WS: Japan, Its History and Culture. New York, Thomas Y Crowell Company, 1970

Munakata T: Japanese attitudes toward mental illness and mental health care, in Japanese Culture and Behavior: Selected Readings. Edited by Lebra TS, Lebra WP. Honolulu, HI, University of Hawaii Press, 1986

Nishimura K: Shamanism and Medical Cures. Current Anthropology 28:59–64, 1987

Ohnuki-Tierney E: Illness and Culture in Contemporary Japan. New York, Cambridge University Press, 1984

Okano Y: Japanese Americans and Mental Health. Los Angeles, CA, Coalition for Asian Mental Health, 1977

Potkin SG, Shen Y, Pardes H, et al: Haloperidol concentrations elevated in Chinese patients. Psychiatry Res 12:167–172, 1984

President signs law to redress wartime wrong. The New York Times, August 11, 1988, p A16

Radloff LS: The CES-D Scale: a self-report depression scale for research in the general population. Applications of Psychological Measurement 1:385–401, 1977

Reynolds DK: Flowing Bridges, Quiet Waters. Albany, NY, State University of New York Press, 1989

Rogers T, Izutsu S: The Japanese, in People and Cultures of Hawaii: A Psychocultural Profile. Edited by McDermott JF Jr, Tseng WS, Maretzki TW. Honolulu, HI, John A. Burns School of Medicine and the University Press of Hawaii, 1980, pp 73–99

Roland A: In Search of Self in India and Japan: Toward Cross-Cultural Psychology. Princeton, NJ, Princeton University Press, 1988

Rosenblat R, Tang SW: Do Oriental psychiatric patients receive different dosages of psychotropic medication when compared with Occidentals? Can J Psychiatry 32:270–274, 1987

Sansom GB: Japan, A Short Cultural History. New York, Appleton-Century-Crofts, 1962

Statistical Abstract of the United States 1989: Social and Economic Characteristics of the Asian, Pacific Islander, American Indian, Eskimo and Aleut Populations: 1980, 109th Edition. Washington, DC, Bureau of the Census, U.S. Government Printing Office, January 1989, p 39

Sue D: Use and abuse of alcohol by Asian Americans. J Psychoactive Drugs 19(1):57–66, 1987

Sue D, Sue S: Cultural factors in the clinical assessment of Asian Americans. J Consult Clin Psychol 55(4):479–487, 1987

Sue DW: Ethnic identity: the impact of two cultures on the psychological development of Asians in America, in Asian Americans: Psychological Perspectives. Edited by S Sue, NN Wagner. Palo Alto, CA, Science and Behavior, 1973

Sue S, Kitano HH: Stereotypes as a measure of success. Journal of Social Issues 29:83–98, 1973

Sue S, McKinney H: Asian Americans in the community mental health care system. Am J Orthopsychiatry 45(1):111–118, 1975

Sue S, Sue DW: Chinese-American personality and mental health. Amerasia Journal 1:36–49, 1971

Sue S, Sue DW: MMPI comparisons between Asian-American and non-Asian students utilizing a student health psychiatric clinic. Journal of Counseling Psychology 21:423–427, 1974

Sue S, Wagner N, Ja D, et al: Conceptions of Mental Illness Among Asian and Caucasian-American Students. Psychol Rep 38:703–708, 1976

Tanaka-Matsumi M, Marsella AJ: Cross-cultural variations in phenomenological experience of depression, I: word association studies. Journal of Cross-Cultural Psychology 7:379–396, 1976

Tien JL: Do Asians need less medication? J Psychosoc Nurs Ment Health Serv 22:19–22, 1984

Tracey TJ, Leong FTL, Glidden C: Help seeking and problem perception among Asian Americans. Journal of Counseling Psychology 33:331–336, 1986

Webster DW, Fretz BR: Asian-American, Black, and White college student's preferences for helping services. Journal of Counseling Psychology 25:124–130, 1978

Wedge BM: Occurrence of psychosis among Okinawans in Hawaii. Am J Psychiatry 109:255–258, 1952

Wilkerson AG: Mexican Americans, in Cross-Cultural Psychiatry. Edited by Gaw A. Littleton, MA, John Wright-PSG Pub Co, 1982

Wilson RA, Hosokawa B: East to America, A History of the Japanese in the United

States. New York, William Morrow, 1980

Yamamoto J: Japanese American identity crisis, in Minority Group Adolescents in the United States. Edited by Brody E. Baltimore, MD, Williams & Wilkins, 1968

Yamamoto J: Japanese-American suicides in Los Angeles, in Anthropology and Mental Health. Edited by Westermeyer J. Chicago, IL, Mouton and Company, 1976

Yamamoto J: Japanese Americans, in Cross-Cultural Psychiatry. Edited by Gaw A. Littleton, MA, John Wright-PSG Pub Co, 1982

Yamamoto J: Genetic, cultural and family factors in alcohol use in Asians. Paper presented at the 16th Annual Scientific Meeting of the American Association for Social Psychiatry Meeting, "Family, Culture, and Psychobiology," Washington, DC, October 16–17, 1988

Yamamoto J, Chang CY: Empathy and Transference in the Therapy of Asian-Americans. Paper presented at the Fourth Scientific Meeting of Pacific Rim College of Psychiatrists, Hong Kong, December 4–8, 1988

Yamamoto J, Fung D, Lo S, et al: Psychopharmacology for Asian Americans and Pacific Islanders. Psychopharmacol Bull 15:29–31, 1979

Yamamoto J, Fairbanks L, Kang BJ, et al: Symptom Checklist 90-R of normal subjects from Asian/Pacific Islander population. Pacific/Asian American Mental Health Research Center Research Review 2:6–8, 1983

12   Psychiatric Care of Korean Americans

Luke I. C. Kim, M.D., Ph.D.

K orean Americans are one of the fastest growing ethnic populations in the United States. The great majority of Korean Americans are immigrants who have arrived since 1965. In 1970, there were about 70,000 Korean Americans living in the United States; by 1980, the census registered 357,393. According to the 1990 U.S. Census (U.S. Bureau of the Census 1991), the count is now about 800,000.

The Korean People

The Koreans are an ancient and homogeneous people with a unique history, culture, and language distinct from both the Chinese and the Japanese. The founding of the first Korean states dates back to 2333 B.C.

Korea is a peninsula spanning 86,000 square miles, roughly the size of Minnesota. It is strategically located in the heart of northeast Asia, surrounded by the People's Republic of China, Japan, and the Russian Republic of the Commonwealth of Independent States. All three nations have long been interested in dominating Korea and using the Korean peninsula as a bridge through which to invade neighboring countries. Korea's national history has been the story of its struggle to maintain independence from such external interference (Choy 1979).

In the twentieth century, Korea was occupied by the Japanese from 1910 to 1945. After the end of World War II, the United States and the then-Soviet Union divided Korea into North and South Korea. The Korean War (1950–1953) erupted in the context of a Cold War struggle between the superpower camps. Unfortunately, Korea still remains divided, despite recent efforts to begin a dialogue toward unification of North and South Korea. Many Korean families are still separated because of this division.

Korea's geography as a natural bridge between the Asian mainland and Japan not only invited military attack over the centuries but also provided a cultural link between China and Japan. Confucianism and Buddhism, along with other aspects of art and culture, were introduced to Japan through Korea. However, Koreans have been able to maintain their own unique cultural identity in terms of language, art, custom, and belief in a common historical destiny (Choy 1979).

The Contemporary Collective Experience of Koreans

Historically, Koreans have experienced great strife and hardship. In this century alone, Korea has been under colonial rule or divided by foreign hegemony for more than 80 years. After the division of Korea at the end of World War II, several million Koreans escaped from the Communist-dominated North to South Korea. During the Korean War alone, Korea had more than 3 million military and civilian casualties.

Koreans have dealt with such social turmoil through various means. Confucian teaching has been a fundamental and traditional force in Korean culture, although in recent decades Christianity has gained strong influence. Self-reliance, self-discipline, and a strong work ethic are emphasized, and education and academic achievement are considered important steps in achieving success and social distinction (Yu and Kim 1983). In Korean society, the family is the dominant social unit, and respect for parents, elders, and teachers is inculcated in Korean young people.

Studying the lives of recent Korean immigrants in New York City, I. S. Kim (1981) found that the characteristic values and culture of Koreans tend to give them a head start in American life. However, Korean immigrants in the United States, like other immigrants, have experienced personal and institutional racial discrimination. Moreover, Korean immigrants are often regarded as the minority of minorities among Asian Americans. Because of their comparatively brief immigration history, Korean American immigrants have much less political and community clout than, for example, Japanese Americans and Chinese Americans have in some locales. In spite of their hard and determined work to establish themselves as American citizens, Koreans have been the object of hate crimes and interethnic conflict. This kind of difficulty is reflected in the tension in some neighborhoods between Korean immigrants and African Americans. This was amply demonstrated in the May 1992 Los Angeles riot, when much of Koreatown was destroyed.

The Korean Ethos

In order to better understand Korean people, it would be helpful if clinicians knew something about the ethos influencing Korean social attitudes and behavior.

Jeong. An emotive term referring to a special interpersonal bond of trust and closeness, *jeong* is an important word in the Korean ethos. There is no English equivalent for *jeong*. It encompasses the meanings of a wide range of English terms—feeling, empathy, affinity, compassion, pathos, sentiment, and love.

Jeong strengthens the bonding of relationships between friends, teachers and students, or parents and children. *Jeong* is considered an essential element in human life, promoting the depth and richness of personal relations. With *jeong,* relationships are made deeper and longer lasting. In times of social upheaval, calamity, and unrest, *jeong* is the only binding and stabilizing force in human relationships (K. W. Lee, personal communication, October 1989).

Haan. *Haan* refers to feeling anger, resentment, or a grudge. It is a form of a victimization syndrome in which *haan*-ridden Koreans feel victimized or unjustly treated. Some Korean psychiatrists think that *haan* is deeply imprinted in the collected subconscious of Koreans, who have endured much in their history. They make the analogy of the Jewish psyche and its connection to the Holocaust. *Haan* is an important and dynamic contributing factor to the manifestation of clinical depression, as well as to the culture-bound syndrome *hwa-byung,* which I discuss later in this chapter (Min and Lee 1988; Prince 1989).

Che-myun. *Che-myun* means "face-saving." As in other Asian countries, face-saving behavior is very important to Koreans in their public and social relationships. Maintaining *che-myun* protects the dignity and self-respect of the individual as well as of his or her family. Honor is considered an important concept to live by for Koreans, and the honor is maintained by *che-myun.* *Che-myun* helps to promote harmonious relationships. For example, face-saving may help a person to behave more gracefully and moderate his or her temper, even if that person is angry with someone else. *Che-myun* also promotes the development of mutual responsibilities and obligations, because a person loses face if he or she does not respond in a reciprocal manner. *Che-myun* is conducive to the development of a reciprocal bond and relationship between and among people.

Noonchi. In Western culture, verbal communication, explicitly and clearly expressed, is the main mode of communication. However, in Asian culture, communication is often subtle, indirect, and nonverbal. In Korean, *noonchi* means "measuring with eyes." It is an intuitive, sixth-sense perception of another person—a capacity for sizing up and evaluating another person through heightened awareness of, and sensitivity to, the person's gestures, facial expressions, and other nonverbal cues.

Palja. *Palja* means fate and destiny and is derived from the terminology of fortune telling. In traditional Korean society, a person's role and life status have been essentially predetermined, and people have little control over their lives. How, then, do they cope with the woes of life and their misfortunes? They accept their *palja* with a stoic, fatalistic attitude. Perhaps that is why religions such as Buddhism, Taoism, and even Christianity are highly appealing to some Koreans, because they help them accept *palja* more completely.

Muht. *Muht* is a Korean word meaning exquisite, beautiful, splendid, and elegant. A person of *muht* is someone who knows how to enjoy life and can appreciate nature, art, music, and poetry. The ethos of *muht* probably promotes the development of exquisite musical, artistic, and other cultural tastes and appreciation among Koreans.

The History of Korean Immigration to the United States

In terms of relationship with the West, Korea had remained the "Hermit Kingdom" until 1882 when Korea and the United States signed a treaty. Following the treaty, a team of Korean diplomatic envoys visited the United States in 1883 and 1884, and soon afterward, the first Korean legation was established in Washington, DC (Choy 1979; Hurh and Kim 1984).

The First Wave

Before 1903, about 50 Korean students, political exiles, and merchants had arrived individually on American shores. The first great wave of Korean immigration to America occurred from 1903 to 1905. By 1905, a total of 7,226 Korean immigrants (6,048 men, 637 women, 541 children) had reached Hawaii in 65 different ships. Another 1,033 Koreans immigrated to Mexico. The majority of immigrants who came from Korean port cities were young bachelors between the ages of 20 and 30 and were largely uneducated. They were recruited as laborers in sugar plantations in Hawaii. Because of the unbalanced gender ratio (10 men to every woman), frequent exchanges of photographs between prospective grooms in Hawaii and brides in Korea took place so that marriages could be arranged. As a result, 1,100 picture brides arrived from 1910 to 1924. Even so, many early male Korean immigrants (about 3,000) spent the rest of their lives as bachelors (Yu 1977).

Plantation life for these early immigrants was very hard because of segregation, low wages, extremely strenuous work, as well as language and cultural barriers. They endured this harsh life with hopes of returning to Korea someday. However, when Korea was occupied by Japan in 1910, they had no country to return to. Nevertheless, they remained very patriotic toward Korea. They started Korean language schools for their children, organized patriotic societies and military training centers, and sacrificed their own scarce funds to support Korean independence movements and the end of Japanese rule. (The well-known leader in Hawaii at that time was Syngman Rhee, who later established the Korean government-in-exile in Shanghai; he was elected as the first president of the Republic of Korea in 1948.)

Subsequent to their initial migration to Hawaii, some early Korean immigrants moved to the mainland. The 1930 U.S. census showed fewer than 2,000 Koreans on the mainland, most of them based in California. As I have mentioned, they were subjected to severe racial discrimination, and they were described as the "minority of minorities." Their life was a courageous, lonesome struggle in a hostile environment. Because the early Korean immigrants placed a high value on education, their children and grandchildren were encouraged to attain high levels of education, and many of them became successful professionals in the mainstream society.

The Second Wave

The second wave of Korean immigrants arrived in the United States between 1951 and 1964. This was a heterogeneous group: Korean wives of U.S. servicemen, war orphans, and students. A survey indicates that 37,063 Korean wives of U.S. servicemen arrived in the United States from 1950 to

1977. There are few studies of this "invisible" group. These Korean wives of U.S. servicemen were doubly marginal, both in the American society and in the Korean immigrant community. They suffered from culture shock, lack of education, isolation, poor communication in the family, a high divorce rate, and general alienation. There were some happy marriages, but physical abuse and mental health problems characterized many relationships, which often ended in divorce. After divorce, many of these women had economic difficulties because they lacked occupational skills (B. L. Kim 1978, 1980, 1981; Kitano and Daniels 1988).

Much less is known about Korean war orphans. Hurh and Kim (1984) indicated that 24,945 children were placed in Korean orphanages in 1950. Of these, 6,293 were adopted in the United States between 1955 and 1966, mostly through the Holt Adoption Agency. About 46% of those adopted were of white and Korean parentage, 41% were of full Korean parentage, and the rest were of African American and Korean parentage. Between 1962 and 1983, Americans adopted 45,142 Korean children (I. S. Kim 1987).

D. S. Kim (1977) conducted one of the few studies of adopted war orphans, in which he surveyed the self-concept of adopted Korean adolescents nationwide. The study revealed that adopted children were generally placed in middle-class, white, Protestant families living in rural areas or small cities. Most of the adopted children were assimilated into the American mainstream culture and showed little evidence of identifying with Koreans or Korean culture. Their self-concept was remarkably similar to the norms of other Americans. The study indicated that the adopted parents were generally satisfied with their Korean children. Overall, the placement of Korean children in American homes was regarded as "very successful" by the researcher.

A later study showed that the adopted children encountered some racial problems as they became older because of their Asian physical appearance. The adoptees were seen as Asian, yet they were almost totally cut off from other Asian ethnics and from Korean culture. Having to live with a dual identity but, for the most part, without ethnic support, they may have psychological problems as they grow older (Kitano and Daniels 1988).

The last group in the second wave of immigrants consisted of students who came to the United States to study at universities. About 6,000 came between 1945 and 1965. Although the data available for later years overlap with this data set, another survey showed that between 1953 and 1980, a total of 15,147 Korean students left for the United States with student visas (I. S. Kim 1987). In addition, there were at least 2,000–3,000 Korean physicians who were in training as interns and residents in American medical centers during this period. Although no accurate data are available, the majority of these students and physicians remained in the United States and succeeded in professional careers. Those who returned to Korea became leaders in their fields.

The Third Wave

The third large wave of Korean immigration was spearheaded by the Immigration and Naturalization Act of 1965, which raised the ceiling for the immigration quota among Asian countries. As a result, Koreans have become one of the most rapidly growing immigrant populations in the United States. This group of Korean newcomers is very different in composition from the previous immigrants.

Most of the latest immigrants consisted of young families with a mean adult age of 27.3 and an average household size of 3.8. The immigrants come from urban, middle-class backgrounds, and half of them are college graduates. About 50% of them held professional, technical, or managerial jobs in Korea. However, fewer than one-third of these professionals have found comparable jobs after their arrival in the United States. This downward mobility has resulted in an increase in the number of Korean owners of small businesses, such as dry cleaning stores, small groceries, fast-food restaurants, and other blue-collar or nonprofessional occupations.

During the period from 1966 to 1979, some 13,000 Korean medical doctors, dentists, nurses, and pharmacists entered the United States, and according to a 1980 survey, some 4,300 Korean immigrant doctors had resident status (I. S. Kim 1987).

Korean immigrants are evenly dispersed throughout the country, although they are more heavily concentrated in large urban areas such as Los Angeles, New York, Chicago, Baltimore, and Washington, DC. About half of them own homes in suburban areas.

Although only 25% of the population in Korea is Christian, 60%–70% of the new U.S. immigrants from Korea attend Korean ethnic Christian churches. There are more than 2,000 Korean churches in the United States. The rapid increase in the number of these Korean ethnic churches is quite remarkable. This phenomenon of attending ethnic Christian churches in a high proportion has not been found among other ethnic groups. Many Korean immigrants who were non-Christian in Korea may have been attracted to these Korean ethnic churches because they feel isolated and the ethnic church provides social and psychological support in addition to religious functions (Hurh and Kim 1988). Korean Christian churches seem to play the role of extended family to the otherwise isolated nuclear families, and they contribute an important function to social networking and community-building among Korean immigrants.

Sociopsychological Studies of Korean Immigrants

Hurh and Kim (1984, 1988, 1990a) conducted a series of sociopsychological studies on the adjustment process and mental health of Korean immigrants in the Los Angeles and Chicago areas. In one study, they conducted structured interviews with a sample of 631 Korean immigrants in the Chicago area and also administered four self-rating scales of mental health well-being to the same subjects. The four self-rating scales used were the Center for Epidemiologic Studies—Depression Scale (CES-D; Radloff 1977), the Health Opinion Survey (HOS; Macmillan 1957), the Memorial University of Newfoundland Scale of Happiness (MUNSH; Kozma and Stones 1980), and the Cantril Self-Anchoring Striving Scale, commonly known as the Cantril Ladder Scale (Cantril 1965; Hurh and Kim 1987, pp 24–26). Based on their findings, Hurh and Kim developed a model of the stages of adjustment following migration:

1. *The exigency stage:* The first 1 to 2 years of resettling were the most stressful, and the immigrants were most vulnerable during this stage. The factors that contributed most to their difficulties were economic hardship, culture shock, language problems, lack of social support, and family conflict.
2. *The resolution and optimism stage:* The immigrants' mental health and life-satisfaction improved the longer they stayed in the United States and the more confidence and mastery they gained in their new environment.
3. *The stagnation stage:* Their life-satisfaction reached a plateau around the 15th year or thereabouts after immigration. The life-satisfaction index remained flat or slightly decreased thereafter.

Reportedly the stagnation phase occurs because of identity ambivalence, or "existential limbo." This is a syndrome characterized by nostalgia and a desire to return to Korea and a feeling of relative deprivation and marginality compared with their white peer group. For example, many immigrant professionals realized that although they had achieved a certain level in the corporate hierarchy (i.e., middle management), they had no chance for more upward mobility. They felt that institutional racism worked against them as Asian immigrants. Many believed it would be more worthwhile and meaningful to return to Korea and contribute to the advancement of their fields there—and some did return.

Thus, these studies showed that the level of life-satisfaction over time produced an inverted J-curve. The exigency stage and the stagnation stage appear to be those that carry the greatest risk for mental and emotional problems.

Based on their research findings, Hurh and Kim (1988) also developed a conceptual model of the adaptation process called the "adhesive or additive mode of adaptation" of the immigrants (p. 238). They found that the ethnic attachment of Korean immigrants remains strong regardless of the length of their stay in the United States, and the degree of their education and acculturation to the mainstream society. In other words, the progressive Americanization of Korean immigrants and their strong ethnic attachment are not mutually exclusive. Americanization is "added on" to their "Koreanness" and does not eliminate or modify the original identification. The "adhesive adaptation pattern" indicates that the immigrants do not resist acculturation but rather seek to adopt the new culture whenever possible without discarding or weakening the old. This is an important finding in understanding the psychosocial life of these immigrants. In all likelihood, this model will apply only to the first-generation immigrants, and not to the second and third generations.

Hurh and Kim (1988, 1990b) also found that there are sex differences in the mental health correlates among Korean immigrants. For example, work-related variables, such as job satisfaction, occupation, and income, are strongly correlated with the male respondents' positive mental health. On the other hand, female respondents' positive mental health is more related to family life satisfaction, ethnic attachment variables (e.g., Korean church affiliation, kinship contact, reading of a Korean newspaper, etc.), and some Americanization variables (e.g., having a driver's license, being proficient in English, and having American friends). Little difference existed between the mental health of those females who are employed and those who are not. Moreover, high individual earnings are negatively related to the mental well-being of the employed females. The researchers interpreted the findings as providing evidence for the persistence of the traditional sex-role ideology (e.g., female as homemaker) among the Korean immigrants, as well as providing support for the validity of the adhesive mode of adaptation.

Epidemiologic Studies of Psychiatric Disorders Among Koreans

No systematic epidemiologic studies have ever been conducted on the prevalence rates of psychiatric disorders among Korean Americans in the United States. However, recent psychiatric epidemiologic data are available at the community level in Korea. It is possible that these data may not have generalization validity for Korean immigrants. Adjustment stress in the United States may be great enough that the prevalence rate for psychiatric disorders among Korean immigrants may be higher than that for people in Korea. Such was the case in a study of Eastern Europeans who migrated to England and the United States after World War II (Murphy 1965).

With this caveat in mind, I have included data from an extensive epidemiologic study by C. K. Lee (1988) of 5,100 randomly selected Korean subjects between the ages of 18 and 65 (by a two-stage cluster sampling method). They were 1,490 men and 1,644 women in Seoul and 974 men and 992 women in rural areas of Korea. In this study, the same structured interview tools were used as in the National Institute of Mental Health (NIMH) Epidemiologic Catchment Area (ECA) Project (e.g., a field-tested Korean version of Diagnostic Interview Schedule-III; Robins et al. 1981). Interviews were conducted by 78 trained interviewers, including 46 residents and medical students. According to the findings, the overall lifetime prevalence rate of psychiatric disorders, excluding substance abuse disorders and psychosexual disorders, was about 13.5%. When alcohol abuse or dependence and tobacco dependence were added to the tabulation, almost 40% of the subjects were found to have at least 1 of 20 DSM-III diagnoses (American Psychiatric Association 1980). The prevalence rate for alcohol abuse or dependence was 22% and for tobacco dependence, 20%. For drug abuse or dependence, the rate was 0.7%. This indicates that, although the use of alcohol and tobacco is high, drug abuse is not as serious in Korea as in the United States.

The lifetime prevalence rates were as follows: schizophrenic disorders, 0.46% (0.34% in Seoul and 0.65% in rural areas); affective disorders, 5.4% (with major depression 3.37%, manic episode 0.42%, and dysthymia 2%); and anxiety disorders, 9.5% (in Seoul, 5.26% for men and 12.7% for women; in rural areas, 5% for men and 15% for women). The anxiety disorders included phobic disorders (5.9%), panic disorder (1.68%), and obsessive-compulsive disorder (2.14%).

Thus, the overall lifetime prevalence of major psychoses, such as schizophrenia, major depression, and bipolar affective disorder, is about 6%, and the prevalence of anxiety disorders about 10%. One significant finding is that there were no marked differences in the overall prevalence of mental disorders between Koreans in Seoul and those in rural areas despite the regional environmental differences. If the USA-NIMH ECA data are compared cross-culturally with C. K. Lee's (1989) data, the prevalence rates of anxiety disorders of Korean subjects were higher than those for subjects in the United States, except for the prevalence rate of phobia cited in the Baltimore ECA.

Historically and Culturally Related Symptom Patterns

Studies in the 1960s (Chang and Kim 1973; Kim and Rhi 1976) indicated a high frequency of classical symptoms of conversion hysteria in Korea. The high frequency of hysteria was attributed to the peoples' poor medical knowledge, the traditional repression of sexuality and the inhibition of emotional expression in the typically large families. However, recent studies indicate that classical symptoms are being seen much less frequently. This change stems from recent Western modernization, including alterations in the family system, popularization of medical knowledge, and sexual liberation.

Common symptoms of schizophrenia also seem to have changed. During the Japanese occupation prior to 1945, the most frequent symptoms were agitated excitement and delusions of poverty. After 1945, grandiose delusions with political themes predominated. Persecutory delusions encountered more frequently recently include being victimized by secret agents, spies, communists, and high officials.

In Korean women, manifestations of a thinly disguised sexual theme are increasing, reflecting conflict between the rigid traditional sexual morality and recent sexual liberation. Depression is still frequently expressed in terms of somatic symptoms including insomnia, headache, and dizziness. Guilt feelings are often provoked in interpersonal relationships. These feelings are relatively easily produced among family members because of the traditional, interdependent way of life and the filial piety traditionally present.

In the past, the rate of admission of senile psychotic patients was relatively low, because Korean families provided protective environments for their elderly out of a tradition of respect. However, recent experience suggests a slight increase in the rate of admission to psychiatric facilities of patients with senile psychosis as a result of the gradual collapse of the large family system.

A recent survey shows that the number of patients with obsessive-compulsive disorder has increased, especially among young people. This can be attributed to their extremely competitive social and occupational lives and their high-pressured educational environments. However, because there are no previous study data to compare, it is difficult to say whether the increase in the number of patients with obsessive-compulsive disorder is really an increase in prevalence or just the appearance at the clinic of patients seeking help for their problems.

Outbreaks of suicides occur frequently among students following what they perceive as their failure in school, especially after being refused admission by an elite college. Among rural people, a mixture of anxiety, depression, hysteria, and psychosomatic symptoms often exists in the same patient; thus, clear subtyping is very difficult.

The Practice of Psychotherapy in Korea

Western-Style Psychotherapy

There is a relatively common perception that employing Western forms of psychotherapy with Koreans would involve great difficulty because Korean patients would not express their thoughts and feelings freely. Moreover, it has often been said that "talking therapy" is not effective with Asians. However, since the introduction of Western psychotherapy into Korea in the 1950s, some Korean psychiatrists trained in the United States and Europe have persistently used the Western psychotherapy in Korea. These psychiatrists have expressed the conviction that psychodynamically oriented psychotherapy is as effective with Korean patients as with Western patients. According to B. Y. Rhi, a Jungian analyst who treated both Korean and Western patients, the rates of success and failure in insight-oriented psychotherapy were the same for both Korean and Western patients (Rhi 1976). Koreans, especially those who are urban and educated, are becoming more Westernized and sophisticated in psychological knowledge.

Rhee (1975) believes that, based on his clinical experience, Western psychotherapeutic modalities such as psychodynamically oriented individual therapy, group therapy, and family therapy are applicable to Koreans, especially middle-class, educated people. He thinks that Korean patients express their emotions very freely and openly once a therapeutic relationship is established, allowing the development of an intense transference. Rhee has commented, however, that psychotherapy was even more effective when the

Western procedures were "grafted onto the already existing framework of the traditional culture, such as the Tao" (p. 910). Psychotherapeutic practice in Korea is not as well developed as in the United States, but psychotherapy has been gaining acceptance and popularity in recent years.

Eastern-Oriented Psychotherapies

Morita therapy and Naikan therapy were developed in Japan within the framework of Buddhism (Zen) and Taoism. Morita and Naikan therapies are examples of more culturally congruent psychotherapies in the Eastern tradition (S. C. Kim 1985a). Although currently they are not being practiced in Korea, other therapeutic approaches are being explored. I have observed the use of psychodrama in the following way: a shamanistic ceremony was played out for a patient so she could ventilate her emotions and come to terms with her ancestors and dead family members for reconciliation (shamanism is discussed in the next section). Another example has been the active interest in the development of a system of insight-oriented psychotherapy within the tradition of Buddhism and Taoism in Korea (Rhee 1975).

Why have some Korean and Korean American psychiatrists considered it important to devise psychotherapeutic methods that are based on Asian cultural views and philosophical traditions rather than Western ones? The answer lies in part in the differing Eastern and Western concepts and ideal images of the "self." Moreover, Eastern and Western worldviews are very different. The basic relationship between self and others in the East is based on a "centripetal-interdependent-holistic" orientation, while for the Westerner, there is a "centrifugal-independent-individualistic" emphasis (Chang 1982, p. 80; also see Chang 1988). The Asian or Asian American patient would tend to focus on relationships with others, cooperativeness, and harmony, whereas an American would emphasize the values of American individualism: being autonomous, assertive, independent, and competitive. These differences in the concept and sense of self are inextricably bound to social relations and culture, requiring different therapeutic goals and approaches for Easterners and Westerners, and for Asian Americans who stand in the great cultural divide between the two. Finally, compared with Westerners, Asian patients tend to have different assumptions about the relationship of human beings to the natural order. Their assumptions about life, health, and illness also differ, and, correspondingly, they have different expectations from psychotherapy.

In an effort to bridge the gap between the two cultures, a group of Korean

American psychiatrists in the New York area, for example, has been meeting weekly for more than 10 years to study Buddhism and explore ways of integrating Eastern thought into psychodynamically oriented psychotherapy (W. G. Im and H. S. Lee, personal communication, March 1990).

Traditional Concepts of Mental Illness and Folk Healing Practices

Koreans have been influenced by three different traditional concepts of disease and mental illness. They are derived from shamanism, traditional Chinese medicine, and Buddhism or Taoism. The practice of traditional healing methods still prevails, especially among rural Koreans.

From the common traditional perspective, mental illness is regarded as a supernatural intervention: an affliction caused by evil or vengeful spirits. However, Koreans may also hold other beliefs, including seeing mental illness as a result of hereditary weakness, character weakness, physical and emotional strain, or imbalance within the body of yin and yang (positive and negative energy systems as conceived by traditional Chinese medicine). Many Koreans believe that those who have mental illnesses are incurable and may have to spend the rest of their lives in a mental hospital. Stigma and shame are attached to mental illness, and all members of a family share in its impact. As in Chinese and Japanese societies, family members may encounter difficulty in finding a spouse because of the perceived undesirability of a family link with mental illness and its possible effects on future generations (C. Umeda, unpublished data, Asian Pacific Community Counseling, October 1987).

Shamanism

Shamanists believe that inanimate and animate objects are endowed with spirits, and that human misfortune results from an improper relationship with these spirits. Shamanists believe that disease arises at the behest of spirits for many reasons, including the violation of taboos. To cure a patient's ailments, a *mudang,* or a shaman, who is a qualified mediator between the spirits and the patient, is called in to perform the ceremony of *goot.* In this process, relationships with the spirits are harmonized (Chang and Kim 1973).

K. I. Kim (1982), a research psychiatrist, observed shamanistic healing ceremonies and evaluated 17 psychiatric patients treated by these healing sessions. Eight of the patients were said to be possessed by ancestral spirits, whereas the other nine had violated ancestral taboos. The patients participated in various healing ceremonies, ranging from the simplest form to the most elaborate form, *goot*. The *goot* ceremony takes 16 to 24 hours and is often spread out over several days. It begins with dancing and jumping and is accompanied by the beating of drums. The tempo gradually accelerates until a trancelike state is reached, leading into the second part of the ceremony in which the shaman delivers an oracle in a dignified manner to the audience. This brings participants and observers into the ceremony, which subsequently reaches a climax of emotional dialogue and total involvement. The third part is a repetition of the first in reverse, winding down the process and slowly bringing the shaman and the participants from the trancelike state back to reality. The ceremony is intended to invoke shamanistic gods who would mediate, forgive, and empower the patient.

In assessing the outcome of this form of healing, the investigating psychiatrists viewed the shamanistic treatment as only marginally and temporarily effective at best. Of 17 patients, four with anxiety disorders and one with schizophrenia reported experiencing temporary symptom relief. Of the eight patients with schizophrenia, six became more disturbed following the ceremonies. However, K. I. Kim (1982) believed that overall the shamanistic treatment was humanistic, cathartic, and anxiety-relieving. The treatment also had an effect of reconciliation in the interpersonal relationships of the family.

Another investigator (Rhi 1970a, 1970b) reported that rural people who had been treated by shamanistic ceremonies responded favorably in 38% of the cases, unfavorably in 8.7%, and remained unchanged in 52%. He also observed symbolic meanings of, and therapeutic elements in, the shamanistic ceremonies in which repressed feelings toward family members were well-ventilated through an encounter with the spirit of a dead ancestor. A philosophical tenet of shamanism may also have therapeutic value: shamanism views suffering as necessary for human maturation. Rhi described a shaman as repeating a song that told how an abandoned princess had obtained shamanistic power through long experience of suffering.

Traditional Chinese Medicine

The influence of classical Chinese medicine has been highly pronounced in Korea for many centuries. The use of Chinese herbal medicines and acupuncture is still popular. Even folk healing methods have incorporated some traditional Chinese medicines.

In the framework of traditional Chinese and Oriental medicine, human-kind is conceived of as a microcosm of the macrocosmic universe in which the rhythm of the cosmos affects the working of the human body. Health depends on the balance of *yin* and *yang,* proper adjustment of the body to its physical environment and a harmonious relationship between bodily functions and emotion (Gaw 1982). Each organ has been designated as having a certain set of emotional functions. The heart is the reservoir of pleasure and spirit; the liver is the seat of anger, courage, and the soul; the gall bladder is the locus of decision making and power; the spleen is the center of idea and will; and the kidney gives rise to fear. Depression is interpreted as the result of a malfunction (imbalance) of the liver and kidney. Treatment consists of restoring the balance of excessive and/or deficient energies (*ch'i*) of *yin* and *yang,* utilizing methods of acupuncture, moxibustion, digital massage, roots and herbal medicines, as well as the principle of moderation in living.

Many patients who visit a psychiatrist have already attempted acupuncture or treatment with herbal medicines, and sometimes concurrently. In a survey of 100 psychiatric patients who visited the Seoul National University Hospital Psychiatric Clinic, Rhi found that 66% of them had previously tried Eastern healing methods, including shamanistic sessions, faith-healing endeavors, and Chinese medicine in various combinations (Rhi 1973). Rhi also found that the more chronic the disorder, the greater the variety of remedies sought by patients.

There are no data on the effectiveness of traditional Chinese medicine in the treatment of mental illness, such as schizophrenia or mood disorders. Some favorable treatment responses have been anecdotally reported in cases of drug addiction and heavy cigarette smoking.

Buddhism

Buddhism flourished in Korea for many centuries and has asserted considerable influence on the thinking and attitudes of the Korean people. The essence of Buddhism is contained in the "four noble truths":

1. Life is suffering;
2. Suffering originates from undue desires;
3. Desire originates from ignorance and illusion; and
4. The road of salvation is to seek insight and attain enlightenment (nirvana, satori) by following the "eight noble paths." These paths include the right knowledge and the right action, which lead to a third path, that

of developing the right mind. Of many roads to the development of the right mind, the best approach is through concentration, meditation, and yoga (Chang 1982).

It should be noted that the movements of transpersonal psychology and self-help in the United States have shown much interest in meditation and yoga methods as part of their treatment strategies.

Taoism

Taoism advocates that people should be primarily concerned with the essential principle underlying the cosmic process—the Tao, or the Way. People must conform to the Tao. The key to understanding the Way is the doctrine of "no-action." This is not to be interpreted literally as meaning inaction; rather, it means doing what is most natural and spontaneous. It requires an attitude of acceptance of nature and natural process, whether in health or sickness, rather than trying to control, overcome, or manipulate nature. All healing arts must be in accord with nature: "Nature heals, and we (medicine) assist" (Chang 1982, p. 76).

Folk-Healing Practices

Religious and shamanistic beliefs are rather strong in the Korean people. Even common folk-healing methods contain many religious elements. Thus, the folk therapies include rare organic foods (ritually prepared), ceremonial purification of ancestral spirits, Buddhist chants, and prayer healing. Faith healing, religious counseling, fasting, and special prayer groups are often used for mentally ill people. Many families prefer to place their mentally ill members in mountaintop prayer centers, temples, locked religious facilities, or "Christian asylums" for patients with mental illness, rather than in psychiatric hospitals. When asked what kinds of treatment are needed for people who are mentally ill, many Koreans responded that isolation, rest, prayer, and penitence are key ingredients of therapy (Ahn and Rhi 1986).

In Korea there has been some syncretism of Christianity and shamanism in Christian faith-healing practices that have incorporated much of the shamanistic ceremonial component in their prayer meetings. For example, in Christian faith-healing meetings, repetitive words and movements characterize group singing or chanting that progresses from a slow to a fast tempo, leading to frenzy. At the peak of the frenzy, the minister may go around the room touching individual people, reciting incantations, shouting at the devil to leave, engaging in a dialogue with the devil, or declaring that the devil has left (K. I. Kim 1982).

Culture-Bound Syndrome

Hwa-byung

Hwa-byung has been known for many years in Korea as a folk medical term. It is an interesting Korean somatization disorder that is predominant among married women who are beyond middle age and of low social standing. K. M. Lin (1983) of the University of California at Los Angeles gave the first report in the English language literature of clinical cases of hwa-byung in the United States. There is some debate as to whether hwa-byung represents a culture-bound syndrome or not. For example, Prince (1989) asked, "How different and how characteristic do the somatic complaints have to be to warrant a different label?" (p. 140). But the fact is that hwa-byung is a uniquely Korean "mixed neurotic state" with characteristic symptoms that are culture-related. The term literally means "fire disease" or "anger disease." Within the framework of classical Chinese medicine, an excess of the fire element, one of the five basic elements, manifests behaviorally in an expression of anger.

Min and Lee (1986, 1988) studied 100 psychiatric outpatients at the Yonsei University Hospital in Seoul. These patients met the criteria both of having believed themselves to have hwa-byung and of other individuals (i.e., friends or relatives) having believed the patients have the disorder. One hundred fifty-seven patients without hwa-byung designations served as the control group.

The most frequent symptoms found in the hwa-byung patients were an oppressive and heavy feeling in the chest; a feeling of a mass in the epigastrium or abdomen; a feeling of something hot pushing up in the chest; a sensation of heat or hotness in the body (described as feeling like boiling, burning, or fire); sighing; headache; aches in the body; dry mouth; insomnia; palpitation; and indigestion. Ordinarily the patients expressed such somatic complaints. However, when they mentioned affective symptoms, the most common complaints were sad mood, nihilistic ideas, loss of interest, feelings of regret, suicidal ideas, and guilt. Other symptoms were an anxious mood, an impulse to rush out of the house, startling easily, loss of temper, and absentmindedness.

Interestingly, most of the *hwa-byung* patients expressed a view that *hwa-byung* has psychological causes. This means that lay people in Korea have a concept of the psychogenic nature of their physical symptoms. The most frequent subjective psychological state that the patients associated with *hwa-byung* was a feeling of anger and indignation because they had been treated unfairly and unjustly. Other feelings they reported included dissatisfaction, frustration, mortification, resentment, hate, worry, concern, pessimism, feelings of resignation, regret, anxiety, irritability, and disgust.

When *hwa-byung* patients were asked what they knew about the nature of this disorder, most of them answered that it develops as a result of bearing and suppressing *hwa* (fire, anger, resentment) for a long time. Some patients explained the etiology as follows: a mass is formed in the chest, and fire (heat) is generated in the chest, heart, or liver as a result of suppressing the feelings of *hwa* for too long.

Hwa-byung patients reported various life experiences which, they thought, were related to the development of the syndrome. The most frequently cited problems were familial: 72% indicated troubles with their spouses (indifference, extramarital affairs, alcoholism, domestic violence); 68% reported troubles with in-laws; 35% mentioned problems with children (the children were troublemakers, academic failures, or leaving home); and 25% identified chronic illness in the family.

When 56 subjects were randomly selected from the original 100 *hwa-byung* patients and evaluated clinically according to DSM-III criteria, the following diagnoses were obtained: 32 had major depressions; 31 had somatization disorders; 11 had generalized anxiety; 9 had dysthymia; 6 had phobic disorder; 5 had panic disorder; 4 had obsessive compulsive disorder; and for 5 no diagnosis was given. Many patients were given two or more diagnoses.

Korean psychiatrists believe that *hwa-byung* is psychodynamically related to the feelings of *haan,* an individual and collective emotional state of Koreans. The state is related to their cultural and historical experience of despair and anger associated with repeated military invasions, political and social suppression, and personal loss. Historically, Korea has been victimized by neighboring countries for many centuries. Politically and domestically Korea has been a class-conscious (*Yangban-Sangnom:* the ruling class and commoners) and chauvinistic society where the underclass, especially women, have endured much difficulty and hardship. Women have suffered from oppression by husbands, in-laws, and by society in general. These powerless people have had to suppress their feelings of anger and resentment and accept pervasive frustration for a long time. Interestingly, Korean shamanism

represents one important response to *haan*. Shamans are almost always female, and most of their clients are female. The shaman healing ceremony
appears to help patients release their *haan*.

Korean psychiatrists think that *haan* is "something accumulated, precipitated and formed in mass in the depth of mind in Korean people" (Prince
1989, p. 144). It is essentially a victimization complex. The syndrome of
hwa-byung and the concept of *haan* appear to be uniquely Korean.

Korean Americans and Psychiatric Care

Although we do not have any epidemiological data on the psychiatric disorders of Korean Americans, we have interesting information on Korean
Americans seeking mental health care at Korean American Mental Health
Services. This center is bilingually staffed and affiliated with the county-
funded Richmond Maxi Center in San Francisco. The clinic compiled data
on 65 Korean American patients treated between December 1983 and April
1986 (S. C. Kim, S. U. Lee, and K. H. Chu, unpublished data, March 1988).

The breakdown of the patients' clinical diagnoses was as follows: schizophrenic disorders, 17%; manic-depressive disorders, 9%; major depression,
8%; dysthymia, 22%; adjustment disorders, 13%; anxiety disorders, 9%; psychosomatic disorders, 8%; conduct disorders, 8%,; alcohol abuse, 3%; and
parent-child problems, 18%. Of these 65 patients, 45% were male and 55%
were female. Sixteen percent were age 17 or younger, 17% were 18 to 30, 30%
were 30 to 40, 19% were 40 to 50, 13% were 50 to 60, and 5% were over 60.
Twenty-five percent were single, 42% were married, 7% were widowed, 11%
were separated, and 15% were divorced. Twenty percent had interracial marriages. Thirty-six percent had less than a 12th-grade education, 31% had a
12th-grade education, 13% had some college education, and 20% had 4 or
more years of college. Most (92%) had been born in Korea, with a mean of
8.7 years of residence in the United States (ranging from 1 to 21 years). A
significant proportion were recipients of some type of social and/or medical
welfare: Social Security income, 15%; General Assistance, 8%; Aid to Families with Dependent Children, 5%; and Medicare/MediCal, 13%.

Forty percent of the referrals to the clinic were from the health system
(inpatient psychiatric and general hospitals, emergency services, and mental
health clinics), 16% were from the legal system (probation officers, attorneys,
and family court), 18% were from the social service and school systems, 15%
were referred by family and friends, 2% by clergy, and 9% were self-referred.

The above data suggest, as is the pattern with other Asian groups, that

Korean immigrants underutilize mental health services. The San Francisco Bay area is home to at least 50,000 Koreans. The fact that only 65 Korean patients came to the Korean mental health clinic during a 2½-year period indicates that the number of patients seeking psychiatric help is very underrepresentative of those in the area's Korean population who need mental health care. There may have been some Korean patients who have gone to other mainstream psychiatric clinics or private mental health professionals, but the number would be small.

Of great significance is the fact that only 9% of clients came to Korean American Mental Health Services on a self-referral basis. The majority of them received professional help voluntarily or involuntarily because of the urging and/or pressure of the family or outside agencies. From our observations, Korean patients seek psychiatric help only as a last resort when they are severely disturbed or in an acute crisis. Most likely, many of them have also tried herbal medicine, acupuncture, or Christian religious counseling before seeking Western psychiatric help.

Mental Health Needs

As the above data indicate, a wide range of mental health problems exist among Korean Americans: schizophrenia, manic episodes, major depression, suicide attempts, posttraumatic stress disorders, psychosomatic symptoms, adjustment difficulty, marital problems, intergenerational conflict, difficulty with impulse control, school behavioral problems, juvenile delinquency, alcohol abuse, spouse and child abuse, and violent behavior (S. C. Kim, S. U. Lee, and K. H. Chu, unpublished data, March 1988).

In the Korean American population, teenage drug abuse and delinquency, including gang involvement, have increased recently in Los Angeles and New York (Yu and Kim 1983). A study (Kiefer et al. 1983) also revealed that the mental health problems of the elderly in the Korean immigrant community have been increasing. When they studied elderly Koreans in San Francisco, Kiefer and colleagues found that this group experiences much emotional suffering and many adjustment problems due to language and cultural barriers, social isolation, and intrafamilial conflicts. Other studies of the Korean elderly in Los Angeles and Chicago confirmed these findings (K. O. Kim 1987).

The Asian Pacific Counseling and Treatment Center in Los Angeles also serves many Korean patients. However, due to its budget limitations, only severely mentally ill patients are accepted for treatment. Therefore, the center's data are not representative of the Korean American community's general mental health problems.

Engaging Korean American Patients in Therapy

Literature on psychiatric treatment and psychotherapy with Korean American patients is extremely limited. The following material is based primarily on the clinical experiences of S. C. Kim (1988), S. P. Kim (1988), and myself. S. C. Kim's writings in particular are extensively quoted throughout this section.

When talking about Korean American patients, it is easy to stereotype them. It is imperative that we evaluate them individually and modify our treatment approaches according to their background, educational level, and degree of Western acculturation. Even if we understand many ways in which these life experiences may affect individuals, we are still confronted with the question: How do we engage a traditionally oriented Korean patient in therapy? The engagement process is very challenging, because Korean American patients come from a background in which there is a strong cultural injunction against seeking psychiatric help.

Accepting the patient's inner reality. The fundamental premise in starting treatment with Korean or Asian patients is to accept their inner reality, such as fear of mental illness and stigma, as valid. They must feel that the therapist understands them and accepts their concerns as reasonable and valid. It is important to remember in treating Korean patients that psychotherapy and psychiatric treatment are foreign to most of them. Moreover, for these patients the concept of psychiatry automatically translates into "mental illness," which in turn is synonymous with "being crazy." Shame of exposing one's own problems or those of one's family to outsiders as well as fear of the stigma of "being crazy" are major cultural obstacles that might discourage a Korean American from seeking psychiatric help. Therefore, the engagement phase is a particularly crucial part of the therapeutic process.

The therapeutic relationship is largely a function of trust and faith in the therapist and the therapeutic process. It requires time to develop. We need to find ways of encouraging Korean American patients to stay in therapy over time, so that they can learn to feel more comfortable in the therapeutic relationship and develop a better understanding of the potential benefits of therapy.

Countering shame. It is useful to begin the therapy by empathizing with patients regarding their sense of shame and helping them to verbalize these feelings. Because the sense of shame can be very strong, it is especially important to assure patients of confidentiality and anonymity. Moreover, for Koreans and Asians, it is particularly useful to reframe their help-seeking as consonant with maintaining their family's good name. For example, the therapist can point out the patient's courage in seeking help and willingness to go beyond the cultural bias and inhibition against seeking necessary care. This kind of support not only expresses empathy and respect for the patient's subjective reality but also provides a reframing of his or her psychiatric distress and care-seeking. Such support minimizes the patient's sense of shame (S. C. Kim 1988).

Understanding the so-called "resistance."   Initial difficulties in developing trust, hesitancy in opening up, and tendency to give limited information have often been labelled as resistance rather than being attributed to Korean cultural values. Immediate openness, for example, is difficult for Korean patients, who have learned that premature disclosure of emotion to a stranger is a sign of immaturity and lack of self-control. The therapist needs to take time to parcel out what is cultural and what is personal in a patient's behavior. It is important to let trust develop over time and not to conclude prematurely that these cultural-behavioral manifestations represent resistance.

Employing the notion of "evaluation."   One way to engage Korean American patients in therapy is to employ the notion of "evaluation" instead of "therapy." The patient can usually more readily accept the rationale that a proper evaluation needs to be conducted before an appropriate treatment or solution can be found and that such an evaluation requires a few therapy sessions. Other ways of securing enough time for the patient to become sufficiently involved in therapy is to include medical and psychological evaluations and interviews with parents and relatives for collateral information over sessions.

Psychoeducation.   Many patients do not understand the concept of psychotherapy: how it works, why "talking" helps, how it differs from other folk-healing methods, and how they can cooperate in the therapeutic process. "Role induction," a form of psychoeducation, is, therefore, a necessary element of psychotherapy with Korean patients.

Somatic expression of symptoms.   For Korean Americans, especially elderly Koreans and women, somatic complaints are culture-syntonic means of expressing emotional conflicts. Direct interpretation of the psychological meaning of their somatic complaints would not make much sense to most patients. However, talking about the uniquely Korean folk medical term *hwa-byung* may pave the way for greater understanding and acceptance of the mind-body interaction. Because the psychosomatic nature of *hwa-byung* is commonly recognized, using it as an example may help patients understand how anger and stress can result in physical symptoms (S. C. Kim 1988).

Establishing authority and being directive.   The need to assume a directive stance in therapy, at least initially, makes sense when we remember that Asian culture is based on a patriarchal, vertical, and hierarchical structure. Within this culture, a high value is placed on respecting authority figures. Roles and relationships are well defined, and interpersonal behaviors are governed by strict rules. The patient expects the doctor to know what is wrong with the patient and what is the right way to correct it. By "directive," I do not mean being authoritarian, but rather being willing to assume the entrusted authority and use it wisely and benignly. One way of establishing authority and expertise would be for the therapist to use authoritative language, such as, "in my professional judgment . . . ," or "in working with many similar patients. . . . "

Multiple roles of the therapist.   It is often necessary for the therapist to assume multiple roles, especially working with patients who present with severe problems stemming from several hardships. The work frequently necessitates coordination, advocacy, case management, and psychoeducation, and requires time and active involvement of the therapist. Working with such patients can be a very draining emotional experience.

Becoming a loyal patient.   Despite the difficulty involved in engaging Koreans into therapy, many of them are likely to become loyal patients once they become engaged and come to trust the therapist. Also, though initially they may be unreliable in keeping appointments, later they become more regular and punctual.

Rapid development of positive transference.   There are certain types of Korean patients who tend to develop positive transference with the therapist rather readily and rapidly. Even before the initiation of psychotherapy, this kind of patient is willing to comply with the therapist's guidelines and expects to receive good care and attention. For the patient, the hierarchical relationship between the therapist and the patient has already been defined culturally, and the patient's role includes an orientation of reverence for authority. Out of deference to the therapist, such patients may be submissive and compliant and may not show much affective and verbal expressiveness. The therapist needs to understand these behavioral manifestations within their appropriate cultural context and not to interpret them in terms of resistance or severity of psychopathology. Despite the seeming security of a set role, patients may initially struggle with ambivalent feelings. On one hand, they want to present only the positive side of self to the therapist, thus saving face. One the other hand, they want to do whatever they are supposed to do according to the therapist's instructions. Only after several therapy sessions, with their therapist's assurance and continuing support, will patients become more trusting and spontaneous in their verbal and affective behavior. With cultural sensitivity and psychoeducation, a therapist can help patients become more comfortable and informal and less hierarchical in relationship to the therapist (S. P. Kim 1988).

Working together with family. Quite often patients come to the clinic with family members. It is extremely important to work with family members in the treatment of Asian patients (Shon and Ja 1982). Often treatment is initiated by family members, who can be helpful therapeutic allies, for example, in supervising the patient's medication compliance. It is often advantageous to begin therapy by addressing family members in the order corresponding to the hierarchy of power and social status prescribed by Korean culture. Also for strategic reasons, such as for better information-gathering, it is advisable for the therapist to conduct separate (rather than conjoint) interviews initially for couples and family members (S. C. Kim 1985b, 1988).

Psychotropic medication. Korean and Asian patients have mixed feelings about psychotropic medication. Some patients expect the doctor to prescribe medication for them. On the other hand, some patients may not be compliant in taking the medication as directed when it is prescribed. Depending on how they feel, especially about the side effects, they may arbitrarily reduce or stop taking their medication without informing the doctor. Asians are sensitive to the side effects of psychotropic medication. The latest psychopharmacology research on Asian patients has not firmly established previous clinical observations that Asian patients may require lower doses of psychotropic medication than non-Asians for a comparable clinical response and profile of side effects (K. M. Lin et al. 1989; Yamamoto and Fung 1979). However, in my practice, I start Asian patients on a low dosage and gradually increase it if necessary. Starting with a low dosage, warning the patient about possible side effects, and explaining the importance and benefits of taking the medication seem to encourage medication compliance for Asian patients.

Concurrent herbal and/or acupuncture treatment.   Traditionally-oriented Korean patients frequently ask the psychiatrist if it is permissible for them to continue herbal treatment and/or acupuncture while they are taking psychotropic medication. There is no empirical data to help us decide in approving or disapproving concurrent use of herbal and acupuncture treatment for patients who are on neuroleptics. In my practice, I explore the patients' attitude and feelings about the traditional treatment methods they are receiving, and what kind of meanings they attach to them. I also ask them how they would know which treatment is effective when they are receiving two or three different kinds of treatment at the same time. I encourage them to stay with the psychotropic medication. But if they have strong wishes to continue herbal or acupuncture treatment simultaneously, I have no objection to their continuing it. My personal opinion is that such traditional treatment methods are probably not effective for psychiatric disorders but can be helpful psychologically; at least, they are not harmful.

There are cases, however, in which an acupuncturist or herbal doctor had advised their patients not to take psychotropic medications because the Western medications are regarded as "too strong" or as "messing up" their *yin-yang* balance. In such cases, I would advise the patient to choose between the Western medication and the traditional method.

Applicability of psychotherapy.   Sue and McKinney's study (1975) of 17 community mental health centers in Seattle revealed not only that Asian Americans grossly underutilized mental health services, but also that of those who did seek services, 52% dropped out after the first sessions. Of the 48% who returned, the average number of therapy sessions attended was only 2.35. These statistics, which are not different from other urban areas, seem to imply the absence of the development of an initial relationship and alliance between therapist and client.

However, the experience of Korean American Mental Health Services in San Francisco (S. C. Kim, S. U. Lee, and K. H. Chu, unpublished data, March 1988) demonstrates that, with bilingual and bicultural staff and with culturally congruent modifications, psychotherapy appears to be effective and beneficial to Korean Americans. In spite of the clinic's services being short-term and crisis-oriented, most of the clients stayed in therapy for a meaningful period of time. The mean number of therapy sessions was 15.5, with a median of 8 and a range from 1 to 131 sessions.

Conclusion

In summarizing treatment approaches best suited for Korean Americans and Asian Americans, it is essential for a therapist to have a broader framework of what constitutes psychotherapy and treatment, so that his or her methods may be culturally sensitive and embrace certain therapeutic elements that are congruent and appropriate to Korean and Asian cultural and psychological needs.

References

Ahn DH, Rhi BY: Community leaders' reactions to mental disorder. The Seoul Journal of Psychiatry (Korea) 11(4):281–293, 1986

American Psychiatric Association: Diagnostic and Statistical Manual of Mental Disorders, 3rd Edition. Washington, DC, American Psychiatric Association, 1980

Cantril H: The Patterns of Human Concerns. New Brunswick, NJ, Rutgers University Press, 1965

Chang SC: The self: a nodal issue in culture and psyche—an Eastern perspective. Am J Psychother 36(1):67–81, 1982

Chang SC: The nature of the self: a transcultural view, Part I: theoretical aspects. Transcultural Psychiatric Research Review 25(3):169–203, 1988

Chang SC, Kim KI: Psychiatry in South Korea. Am J Psychiatry 130(6):667–669, 1973

Choy BY: Koreans in America. Chicago, IL, Nelson-Hall Publications, 1979, pp 1–43

Gaw A (ed): Cross-Cultural Psychiatry. Littleton, MA, John Wright-PSG Pub Co, 1982, pp 1–29

Hurh WM, Kim KC: Korean Immigrants in America. Cranbury, NJ, Fairleigh Dickinson University Press, 1984, pp 73–86, 138–155

Hurh WM, Kim KC: Korean immigrants in the Chicago area: a sociological study of migration and mental health. Interim Report for National Institute of Mental Health. Bethesda, MD, National Institute of Mental Health, October 1987

Hurh WM, Kim KC: Uprooting and adjustment: a sociological study of Korean immigrants' mental health. Final Report to the National Institute of Mental Health (Grant No. 1R01 MH40312-01). Bethesda, MD, National Institute of Mental Health, June 1988

Hurh WM, Kim KC: Adaptation states and mental health of Korean male immigrants in the United States. International Migration Review 24(3):456–479, 1990a

Hurh WM, Kim KC: Correlates of Korean immigrants' mental health. J Nerv Ment Dis 178(11):703–711, 1990b

Kiefer C, Kim SC, Cho K, et al: Mental Health of Korean American Elderly (Research Grant Report). Washington, DC, U.S. Department of Health and Human Services, 1983

Kim BL: The Asian Americans: Changing Patterns, Changing Needs. Montclair, NJ, Association for Korean Christian Scholars in North America, 1978

Kim BL: The Korean American Child at School and at Home. Washington, DC, U.S. Government Printing Office, 1980

Kim BL: Women in Shadows. La Jolla, CA, National Committee Concerned with Asian Wives of U.S. Servicemen, 1981

Kim DS: How they fared in American homes: a followup study of adopted Korean children. Child Today 6:2–6, 31, 1977

Kim IS: New Urban Immigrants: the Korean Community in New York. Princeton, NJ, Princeton University Press, 1981, pp 181–186

Kim IS: Korea and East Asia: premigration factors and the US immigration policy, in Pacific Bridges. Edited by Fawcett JT, Carino BV. Staten Island, NY, Center for Migration Studies, 1987

Kim KI: Christian faith-healing in Korea. Psychiatry Bulletin of Seoul National University Hospital 6:39–42, 1982

Kim KI, Rhi BY: A review of Korean cultural psychiatry. Transcultural Psychiatric Research Review 10:101–114, 1976

Kim KO: Effects of perceived control on the well-being of the Korean American elderly (Irvine Presidential Fellowship Research Report). Irvine, CA, University of California, 1987

Kim SC: Ericksonian hypnotic properties of Japanese psychotherapies: Morita and Naikan, in Ericksonian Psychotherapy, Vol I: Structure. Edited by Zeig JK. New York, Brunner/Mazel, 1985a, pp 565–581

Kim SC: Family therapy for Asian Americans: a strategic structural framework. Psychotherapy 22(25):342–348, 1985b

Kim SC: Therapy with Korean American clients. Paper presented at the annual meeting of the American Psychiatric Association, San Francisco, CA, May 1988

Kim SP: Transference and countertransference in psychotherapy with Asian Americans: cultural issues and therapeutic consideration. Paper presented at the annual meeting of the American Psychiatric Association, San Francisco, CA, May 1988

Kitano HL, Daniels R: Asian Americans: Emerging Minorities. Englewood Cliffs, NJ, Prentice-Hall, 1988

Kozma A, Stones MJ: The measurement of happiness: development of Memorial University of Newfoundland Scale of Happiness (MUNSH). J Gerontol 35:906–912, 1980

Lee CK: Psychiatric disorders in the Republic of Korea. Paper presented at the annual meeting of the American Psychiatric Association, San Francisco, CA, May 1988

Lee CK: The epidemiological study of mental disorders in Korea (XI): anxiety disorders. Seoul Journal of Psychiatry 14(1):36–44, 1989

Lin KM: Hwa-Byung: a Korean culture-bound syndrome? Am J Psychiatry 140(1):105–107, 1983

Lin KM, Poland RE, Nuccio I, et al: A longitudinal assessment of Haloperidol doses and serum concentration in Asian and Caucasian schizophrenic patients. Am J

Psychiatry 146(10):1307–1311, 1989

Macmillan AM: The Health Opinion Survey: techniques for estimating prevalence of psychoneurotic and related types of disorder in communities. Psychol Rep 3:325–329, 1957

Min SK, Lee HY: A diagnostic study on Hwabyung. Journal of the Korean Medical Association 29:653–661, 1986

Min SK, Lee HY: A clinical study on Hwabyung. Paper presented at the scientific meeting of the Pacific Rim College of Psychiatrists, Hong Kong, December 1988

Murphy HBM: Migration and the major mental disease, in Mobility and Mental Health. Edited by Lantor MB. Springfield, IL, Charles C Thomas, 1965

Prince RH: Review on a clinical study of Hwabyung by Min SK, Lee HY. Transcultural Psychiatric Research Review 26:137–147, 1989

Radloff LS: The CES-D scale: a self-report depression scale for research in the general population. Applied Psychological Measurement 1:385–401, 1977

Rhee DS: Research on psychotherapy of Korean patients. The New Medical Journal (Seoul) 13:901–925, 1975

Rhi BY: Folk psychiatry in Korea: concepts of mental illness among shamanistic society in Korea. Neuropsychiatry (Seoul) 9:35–45, 1970a

Rhi BY: Studies of shamanistic treatment of the dead in Korea: shamanism from the view point of analytic psychology. The New Medical Journal (Seoul) 13:79–94, 1970b

Rhi BY: A preliminary study on the medical acculturation problems in Korea. Neuropsychiatry (Seoul, Korea) 12:2, 1973

Rhi BY: Analysis in Korea with special reference to the question of success and failure in analysis, in The Proceedings of the 5th International Congress for Analytic Psychology. Edited by Adler G. New York, Putnam, 1976

Robins LN, Helzer JE, Croughan J, et al: National Institute of Mental Health Diagnostic Interview Schedule: its history, characteristics, and validity. Arch Gen Psychiatry 38:381–389, 1981

Shon SP, Ja DY: Asian families, in Ethnicity and Family Therapy. Edited by McGoldrick M, Pearce J, Giordano J. New York, Guilford, 1982

Sue S, McKinney H: Asian American in the community mental health care system. Am J Orthopsychiatry 45:111–118, 1975

U.S. Bureau of the Census: 1990 census summary report (1990-CPH-1), #003-024-07305-6. Washington, DC, U.S. Government Printing Office, 1991

Yamamoto J, Fung D: Psychopharmacology for Asian Americans and Pacific Islanders. Psychopharmacol Bull 15:29–31, 1979

Yu EY: Koreans in America: an emerging ethnic minority. Amerasia Journal 4:1, 1977

Yu KH, Kim LIC: The growth and development of Korean American children, in Psychosocial Development of Minority Children. Edited by Johnson-Powell G, Yamamoto J, Romero A. New York, Brunner/Mazel, 1983, pp 147–158

13 Psychiatric Care of Pilipino Americans

Enrique G. Araneta, Jr., M.D.

Τhe term "Filipino" refers to any native-born or naturalized citizen of the Republic of the Philippines (Las Islas de Filipinas). Because there is no "ph" sound in the native Malay-derived language, "Pilipino" has become the preferred term (Lott 1976). A person of Pilipino ancestry who is a citizen of the United States, either by birth or by naturalization, as well as any Philippine national who has obtained an immigrant status in the United States, is called a Pilipino American.

Although Pilipino Americans now make up the second largest group of the more than 7 million Asian Americans in this country, there is comparatively little information available about them (Johnson 1988). They have become the "forgotten" Asian Americans (Cordova 1973; Johnson 1988).

Racial and Cultural Roots

The Philippines is a tropical archipelago of some 7,000 islands located at the crossroads of the trade routes of Asia. The islands have attracted a variety of settlers and colonizers, which is reflected in more than 80 identified dialects and in the diverse racial and ethnic characteristics of the population.

The aboriginal tribes (the Australoid-Sakai and the Proto-Malay) are believed to have come to the islands between 30,000 B.C. and 15,000 B.C. The subsequent settlers included diverse peoples:

1. The tall, slender Mongoloids with tall noses from China, who brought an early neolithic culture (Indonesia Type A) around 6000 B.C. to 5000 B.C.;

The terms "Indonesia Type A and B" refer to the early and late neolithic cultures. Indonesia Type A refers to *early* neolithic cultural development from 6000 B.C. to 5000 B.C. Indonesia Type B refers to *late* neolithic cultural development from 1500 B.C. to 1000 B.C. (See Byers 1952, p. 2.)

2. The late neolithic seafarers (Indonesia Type B) who came from Indochina and South China around 1500 B.C. to 1000 B.C.;
3. The Copper–Bronze Age people who came from Indochina and South China around 800 B.C. to 500 B.C.; and
4. The Iron Age Malays from Borneo and Malaysia who came between 300 B.C. to 200 B.C., from whom are descended about 38% of the current population.

Between 700 A.D. and 1400 A.D., colonizers came in separate waves from Indonesia, Malaysia, Indochina, India, Borneo, and Java. Colonizers from Spain occupied the islands between 1521 and 1898, bringing other Europeans (including the Portuguese, Dutch, and British) and admitting immigrants from Arab-Persia, India, and China. American colonizers from 1898 to 1946 further contributed to the racial diversity and genetic pooling referred to as the "Filipino blend" (Beyer 1952). These successions of colonizers and settlers of the Christian era are believed to be the forebears of about 20% of the population.

The Spanish used military recruits from one area to subdue resistance or insurgency in another area of the country. This strategy not only facilitated control but also promoted regionalism and mutual distrust among the inhabitants (Quirino 1988). The Christian missionaries instilled in the people fear of retribution, submission to authority, and resignation to divine will. The concordance between the native beliefs and mythology and the brand of Catholicism that the missionaries taught not only facilitated compliance and conversion to Christianity but also provided the system of cultural assumptions from which the Pilipino colonial culture and identity would evolve.

Spanish rule lasted more than 350 years. During this period, many Spanish practices, traditions, and values were incorporated into the evolving "Philippine Christian culture" (Joaquin 1983), which remains relevant today. Also during this period, a feudal structure and patronage system were institutionalized to ensure the privileges of the colonizers and their supporters. The social, political, and economic institutions established were similar to those of other Spanish colonies in the Caribbean, Central and South America, and Mexico. Spanish, spoken and understood only by a select few, became the official language, and Pilipinos were given Spanish names. However, discontent sown by the unjust practices of the ruling minority spawned a succession of insurgencies that blossomed into the popular revolution of the *Katipunan* in 1897. Just as the uprising was on the verge of ousting the Spanish, the Spanish-American War broke out, and the Spanish surrendered to the Americans. Through the Treaty of Paris, the Philippines was ceded to the United States in 1898. This fomented the eruption of the Filipino-American War. In 3 years, more than 600,000 Pilipino lives were lost; and the evolving unity and national identity of the population, ignited by the *Katipunan* revolt against Spain, was again shattered. American colonial rule was maintained with the help of Pilipino mercenaries (later to become the Philippine Scouts) and was supported by the privileged class (*illustrados*). These realities further confounded the issues of loyalty, national interest, and national identity.

Westernization and the reinforcement of the colonial mentality were assured by a variety of measures. America established a public school system for Pilipinos in which the medium of instruction was English and the textbooks were written by American educators. Participatory democracy was introduced, based on a constitution patterned after that of the United States, and eventual independence was promised. English and Spanish became the official languages. Meanwhile, Philippine economic development was shaped toward meeting America's need for a steady market and a source of cheap labor and raw materials. For the Pilipinos, the eventual results of these economic and cultural forces were the promotion of Americanized cultural aspirations through education and the pervasive influence of Hollywood movies. Meanwhile, economic dependence was coerced through unfair trade treaties as gradual political independence was dispensed.

There were profound psychological and cultural consequences of this form of colonialism. The Pilipino self-concept as powerless and inferior was further ingrained, and the perceived dependence on the benevolence of envied Western masters detracted from the development of a strong national identity and solidarity. Pilipinos accepted their subservient, dependent, and mendicant role, perpetuating a "damaged culture" of dependency and passive resistance (Fallows 1987). For the immigrant Pilipino community in the United States, this colonial mentality detracted from its ability to organize and assert itself, resulting in political and economic stagnation (Lott 1976).

History of Pilipino Immigration to the United States

Contrary to popular belief, Pilipinos participated in the "American experience" long before the Philippines became a colony of the United States. In the early 1700s, Pilipino crew members, who deserted the Spanish galleons in Mexico or New Orleans, found their way into the bayous of Louisiana, where they eventually established a community around 1765 (Espina 1979). They became known as the "Manilenoes" (Manilamen), and by

1906 they numbered 2,000 (Espina 1980). These enterprising Spanish-speaking fugitives from Spain's galleon trade adjusted well among the ethnically diverse population of New Orleans and established the dried shrimp industry. Some intermarried with other ethnic groups, such as Germans, Irish, French, and American Indians.

Since the American occupation of the Philippines in 1898, three waves of Pilipino immigration to the United States are recognized. Between 1906 and 1934, Pilipinos came to this country primarily as laborers in the cane fields and pineapple plantations in Hawaii, in the vegetable farms and fruit orchards of California, and in the fisheries and canneries of Washington, Oregon, and Alaska. Some made their way to the railroads, factories, warehouses, and food service industries in Chicago and New York. They were lured by the promise of democracy and equal opportunity and the hope of financial advancement.

This wave of immigration ended with the Tydings-McDuffie Act of 1934, which established the Philippines as a commonwealth and changed the status of Pilipinos in the United States from "nationals" to aliens. The Act also imposed an annual immigration quota of 50 on Pilipinos. The estimated Pilipino population in the United States by 1935 was 175,000.

In 1946, through an act of Congress, Pilipinos who joined the United States Armed Forces during World War II were granted citizenship. Between 1946 and 1965, a second wave of immigration ensued. This wave consisted of recruits for the Armed Forces during the Cold War of the 1950s, war brides of Pilipino American and other servicemen, students seeking higher education, and professionals attracted by the rapid post-World War II technological and economic expansion. This wave brought an additional 75,000 to 80,000 Pilipinos to the United States.

Although the Marcos government sought help from the United States government to stop this "brain drain," the deteriorating political and economic situation in the Philippines did not avert yet another wave of immigration after October 3, 1965, when the Immigration/Naturalization Act of 1934 was amended. This immigration reform act, inspired by the civil rights movement, relaxed immigration quotas among Asians, smoothed the way for Pilipino family reunification, and attracted professionals and people with special skills needed in the expanding technological and economic growth of the United States. This surge of immigration continues. The new immigrants embrace cultural values compatible with the American focus on competition, upward mobility, and accumulation of material goods. Between 1965 and 1985, about 68,000 Pilipino immigrants arrived in the United States (Johnson 1988).

Demographic characteristics.   The 1990 census places the Pilipino American population in the United States at 1,406,770 (U.S. Bureau of the Census 1991a, 1991b). States with the highest concentration of Pilipino Americans are California (52.0% of Pilipino Americans), Hawaii (12.0%), Illinois (4.6%), New York (4.4%), New Jersey (3.8%), and Washington State (3.1%). In addition, Virginia has 2.5%, Texas 2.4%, Florida 2.3%, Maryland 1.4%, and Michigan 1.0%.

Since 1980, Pilipino American females have outnumbered males 52% to 48%. The foreign born have outnumbered the U.S.-born by more than 2 to 1.

Family and household characteristics.   According to Alegado (1987), 98% of Pilipino Americans are members of households, and 33% of Pilipino American families have more than five members. Pilipino American households have a greater percentage of extended families than any other ethnic group.

Marital characteristics.   Pilipino Americans have the highest rate of interracial marriage among Asian Americans. The majority of such marriages are contracted with white Americans and Hispanic Americans. The significantly higher rate of interracial marriage among Pilipino Americans compared with other Asian Americans has implications not only in terms of acculturation and assimilation but also in terms of intensity of ethnic identification and self-perception (Sue and Morishima 1982).

Educational characteristics.   Alegado (1987) estimates the percentage of Pilipino American females with some college training at 53%; for males, the estimate is 47%. The percentage that have not completed high school is estimated at 28% among foreign-born Pilipino Americans and 32% among those who are American-born.

Employment and income characteristics.   According to the U.S. Bureau of the Census, in 1980, among Pilipino Americans over 16 years of age, 72.5% were in the labor force (U.S. Bureau of the Census 1983; U.S. Commission on Civil Rights 1988). More members of Pilipino American families tend to be in the work force compared with members of white or African American families. However, 14% of Pilipino American families earned less than $10,000 and 20% earned less than $12,500 annually. On the other hand, 46% of Pilipino American families earned over $25,000. The median income per Pilipino American family in 1980 was $23,687, with a mean of $27,194 annually, which is higher than the average white household income of $20,800 ("America's Asians" 1989). However, among Asians, Pilipinos have a higher representation in the lower income categories.

Epidemiologic and Statistical Data

Prevalence of Mental Illness

Data on the prevalence of mental illness among Pilipino Americans remains woefully inadequate. Most of the available data are derived from studies of incidence of mental illness among Asian-Pacific Americans as a group.

Current data on the incidence of mental illness among Pilipino Americans have been derived mainly from their rates of admission and length of hospital stay, as well as their rate of utilization of mental health center services. These studies, cited by Sue and Morishima (1982), consistently found lower rates of treatment of mental disturbance among Asian Americans. On the other hand, Asian Americans who utilize mental health facilities were found to be more severely disturbed than white Americans who used mental health facilities (Sue and McKinney 1975).

An alternative to using mental health facility utilization rates for assessing incidence of mental illness is to use community surveys to estimate rates of psychopathology (Meinhardt and Vega 1987). However, according to Kuo (1984), the number "of population-based studies on Asian Americans is extremely small" (p. 450) to date. Further, the sensitivity of these tests for detecting psychopathology in different cultural groups may vary, and groups may vary in their reactions to being tested.

Interpretation of Epidemiologic Data

The most that can be said about the data on the rates and severity of psychiatric morbidity among treated cases is that Asian Americans, including Pilipino Americans, do not seek professional mental health care unless their problems become severe. This reluctance to be identified as needing professional mental health services has long been recognized. According to Tsai and colleagues (1982, p. 27), the most significant reasons for these attitudes and behavior among Asians are as follows:

1. Stigma related to mental disturbance. The fear of stigmatization results in the patient's as well as the family's reluctance to acknowledge the existence of mental illness.
2. Availability of alternative resources. These include churches, family

physicians, and family elders. Both Kitano (1969) and Kuo (1984) have suggested that these resources have reduced Pilipino dependence on mental health facilities.

3. Cost of mental health services.

4. Location and knowledge of service facilities. Kim (1973) reports that about 15% of male and 20% of female Asians (Chinese, Japanese, Koreans, and Pilipinos) did not know where to go for mental health services.

5. Hours of operation. According to Sue and Sue (1974), Asian Americans tend to work long hours. Among Pilipinos, a high percentage of adult family members work, making it difficult for them to use mental health services during "regular" office hours.

6. Belief systems about mental illness. Many Pilipino Americans still view mental illness as reflecting weakness of will, divine retribution, and effects of personal or ancestral misdeeds for which spiritual healers are more appropriate.

7. The cultural limitations of the mental health service. Lack of sensitivity to cultural beliefs and behavioral patterns by health providers often cause patients to terminate their participation in treatment, according to Flaskerud and Soldevilla (1986) who emphasize a "cultural-compatible approach" (p. 35).

Mental Health Needs of Pilipino Americans

Data based on population surveys show that the level of life satisfaction and perception of well-being is lower among Pilipinos than among Japanese Americans, Chinese Americans, or white Americans (Cabezas 1982). Kuo's (1984) study also shows a higher rate of depression for Pilipinos compared with these three groups.

Extrapolating from animal studies, Cassel (1974) noted, "Changes in group membership and the quality of group membership have been shown to be accompanied by neuroendocrine changes, particularly, but not exclusively, by changes in the pituitary and adrenocortical systems" (pp. 401–402)—changes that, according to him, influence vulnerability to illness.

Most émigrés experience the sociocultural discontinuity associated with immigration. The 100,000-plus Pilipino "old-timers," who were contracted as indentured laborers during the first three decades of this century, came to escape the oppressive feudal system in the Philippines and to find better economic opportunities. Instead they found that the Constitutional guarantees they learned in American-established schools in the Philippines had no reality for them in the United States. These "old-timers" found themselves facing a social Darwinism paradigm of race relations in which they were the objects of racial discrimination, social segregation, economic exploitation, and even violence (Bulosan 1946). Not having the right to vote, own property, or marry as they chose, they were discouraged from assimilating into American society (Lott 1976). The disparity between their expectations and their reality reduced many to total confusion. (Opler [1956] notes that higher rates of affective disorders and catatonic confusional states were observed among Pilipinos in Hawaii.)

In a similar predicament are Pilipino immigrants with limited language skills, such as relatives who immigrated under the family reunification law. Many are having difficulty adjusting to the American way of life, a problem that often leads to social isolation and alienation. Many from the less-Westernized provinces of the Philippines frequently find themselves assigned to menial jobs far below their training and experience ("America's Asians" 1989). However, conditioned to conformity by a culture that emphasizes communalism, many Pilipinos find themselves trapped in situations they are culturally unequipped to confront.

The conflict among different generations of Pilipino Americans is characterized by the clashes between traditional and Westernized cultural beliefs, values, and behaviors and differences in communication styles. This clash of values and behavior styles also threatens many interracial marriages (Atkeson 1970). Some traditional Philippine values and psychodynamics arising from the ideals of precolonial communalism, overlaid by the authoritarianism of feudalism and the coerciveness of colonialism, conflict with the egalitarian ideals and individualism of American society. This "cultural baggage" includes the following:

1. The primacy of family and small-group affiliation over the individual (Agpalo 1976). This value, strongly held by Pilipinos, inhibits free expression of dissent and tends to detract from the creativity and autonomy that are highly prized by Americans (Hollensteiner 1964).
2. The primacy of smooth interpersonal relationships (SIR) conflicts with the American ideal of openness and frankness.
3. An attitude of "optimistic fatalism" (Marsella et al. 1971) or *bahala na* is opposed to the American beliefs in future orientation, careful planning, and the drive for excellence and economic advancement through determined effort.

4. The sensitivity to slights and criticism, which springs from an exaggerated need for self-importance, *amor propio,* often leads to withdrawal and/or vengeance, in direct opposition to the American style of directness and sportsmanship.

5. The dread of *hija* (devastating shame; Bulatao 1964). This concern over face-saving is fostered by the use of ridicule and ostracism in child training and often inhibits competitiveness.

6. Conceding to the wishes of the group (*pakiki sama*) to maintain smooth interpersonal relationships does not afford the intellectually stimulating and broadening benefits of dissent.

7. The practice of *delicadeza,* or nonconfrontational communication most evident among females, is ineffectual in a society such as America's where directness is appreciated and competitiveness is encouraged.

8. *Utang nang loob,* or reciprocity of favors, that derives from the sentiments of gratitude and belongingness is incongruous in a society that gives primacy to individualism and the "bottom line."

These culturally conditioned sentiments and behaviors are irrelevant in today's American society. This is especially true for traditional Pilipino women, who are expected to be *mahinhin* (gentle and self-effacing) and who must adjust by deferring, by depending, by enduring, and by nurturing. Considering the added stresses associated with the effects of sociocultural discontinuity, subordinate minority status, and the lack of *bayanihan* (community working together) for support, Pilipino Americans confront a greater mental health risk than is reflected by current data on prevalence of psychopathology for this group.

Myth and Realities About the Mental Health and Mental Illness of Pilipino Americans

The paucity of well-substantiated data on the incidence of mental disorders or the general state of mental well-being of the Pilipino American population has led to conflicting speculations based on observations of small segments of this population. Those who see Pilipinos mainly in well-paying positions or in the successful practice of their professions believe that they are well-adjusted and have few psychological problems. The low rates of mental health service use by Pilipino Americans other than those individuals with psychoses should not be regarded as an indication that the incidence of neurotic and adjustment disorders is lower among members of this group. Indeed, Lapuz (1978) has noted that the overall incidence of neurotic disorders among Pilipinos in metropolitan Manila is comparable to data on white Americans of similar socioeconomic background in the United States.

To assume that Pilipino immigrants are better equipped to adjust to American society because of their long association and familiarity with Western culture is to overlook what Lott (1976) has pointed out—namely, that this long association has been in the context of a colonizer/colonized relationship and has resulted in the development of a "colonial mentality." The pervasiveness and persistence of this mentality reinforced by the social Darwinism paradigm of race relations have nullified the advantages that a Pilipino's familiarity with the American culture and language may have afforded.

The notion that Pilipino immigrants, having come from Asia with a predominantly Asian racial derivation, must therefore perceive themselves as Asian, react like Asians, and think like Asians is deceiving. Kuo's (1984) study on depression among Asians, as well as a study by Yamamoto and colleagues (1987), suggest that the Spanish Christian traditions are more deeply ingrained in the Pilipinos' perception of identity than is their Asiatic racial and cultural derivation. Although other Asians have grown up in cultures that evolved out of indigenous needs and their environment, Pilipinos have for generations lived, compromised with, and adjusted to a culture shaped by the political and economic goals of the colonial powers controlling the Philippines. Pilipinos are still struggling to define their cultural, racial, and historical identity. Compared with other Asians Americans such as Korean Americans, Japanese Americans, and Chinese Americans, Pilipino Americans have not achieved an equivalent cohesiveness and competitive stature educationally, financially, and politically ("America's Asians" 1989). Indeed, Pilipino Americans have difficulty keeping up with the image assigned to them as members of the "model minority."

Because average household incomes among Pilipino Americans have exceeded the mean for those of white Americans, it has been suggested that Pilipino Americans are no longer subjected to racial and social prejudice. However, comparisons based on family incomes are misleading; Pilipino families are generally larger and have more members working. In reality, the average personal income of Pilipino American males is lower than that of their white counterparts. If personal income was considered in relation to educational background and experience, Pilipino Americans, both male and female, would be considered relatively underemployed compared with white Americans ("America's Asians" 1989).

Difficulties in the task of adjustment to American society for Pilipino immigrants vary considerably according to individual degrees of cultural preparedness, which includes a host of innumerable factors (Tan 1987, pp. 1–2). For this reason, assessment of mental well-being or vulnerability to mental illness for Pilipino Americans will yield varying results related to sampling criteria and errors. Until more extensive and broader studies are undertaken, it is difficult to make generalizations about the mental health of Pilipino Americans.

As the "salad bowl" paradigm of race relations is supplanting the untenable "melting pot" paradigm, minorities are seeking to define their own "ethno-American" consciousness. As Evangelista (1988), in discussing the evolution of Pilipino American consciousness, reminds us,

> Class separation still exists among Filipinos in the United States. With the new immigration laws giving priority to professionals, highly educated immigrants become mainstream right away. On the other hand, the old-timers are older still, dying out, in fact, and usually dying in poverty. Their children, and others admitted under the family reunification laws, work on farms or in canneries, and are still relatively poor in a land of material riches. And perhaps because it is hard to be happy with yourself when you are poor in a rich country, or brown in a white country, the level of self-esteem in this group was often low. Filipinos in America were, in fact, frequently known to deny their ethnic background. (p. 42)

Further insight into Pilipino self-perception, confusion over identity, rage over having been exploited, low self-esteem, and brittle ego is offered in a poem by Fred Cordova that is quoted by Evangelista (1988):

> We say we are Filipino; we say we are
> American, so, who are we; more so, what
> are we; brown or white; or are we still
> "other"? . . . We are then marginal man,
> marginal woman, better yet, margarine,
> because we are being burnt, toasted,
> singed, braised, scorched, always to
> our detriment for someone else's
> benefit; thus, we party, dance,
> banquet, and, happy in our delusions
> of grandeur, we do not hurt as much
> with the pain of exploitation. (p. 52)

Stigmatization of Mental Illness: Cultural Origins and Manifestations

Among Pilipino Americans, the intensity of stigma regarding mental illness is reflected by the vehemence and indignation with which the occurrence of such illness is denied, and by the lengths to which families go to hide the presence of any disorder among their members. Several researchers (Flaskerud and Soldevilla 1986; Sechrest 1967; Sue and Morishima 1982) have noted that Pilipinos tend to keep mentally ill family members at home unless the severity of their symptoms pose a danger to themselves or others.

The cultural roots of this stigma are deep and pervasive. First, Pilipinos believe that only people who are dangerously insane and socially disruptive require psychiatric care. Therefore, apprehension and disdain toward anyone believed to be mentally ill persists. Second, the notion that mental illness is indicative of "bad blood" (*na sa dugo*) or a familial disorder is very strong in the Philippines. Third, having debilitating symptoms without demonstrable physical origins is seen as reflecting weakness of will, lack of moral courage, or frailty of character. Fourth, the notion prevails that symptoms without demonstrable physical origins and beyond conscious control indicate the influence of evil environmental forces or spirits such as *anitos*. These anthropomorphic spirits are believed to be agents of God that influence all the forces of the universe and the destiny of people on this earth. Persons affected adversely by *anitos* are therefore believed to have incurred God's disfavor through their own or their ancestor's misdeeds (Silliman 1964).

Folk, Traditional, and Mainstream Psychiatric Care

The persistence of a strong supernatural orientation predisposes Pilipinos to turn to indigenous spiritual healers for help in what they regard as problems involving supernatural affairs—a notion not unlike that popularized by some television evangelists. Sechrest (1964) observed that 50% of provincial school teachers in the Philippines still believe in *anitos*, 33% believe that indigenous healers can cure disease before which physicians are helpless, and 20% believe in the power of witches to inflict disease. Indigenous healers are the first to be consulted. Shakman (1969) cites the popularity of putative (psychic) surgeons, magicians (*bulo-bulo*), herb doctors (*herbalarios* or *arbolarios*), shamans, and masseurs among indigenous healers. Physicians are summoned only when death is imminent, and death often results. Death undermines the confidence toward physicians.

The effectiveness of indigenous healers employing magnetic healing and psychic surgery in alleviating conversion and psychophysiologic disorders fosters persistence of belief in traditional concepts of illness causation and treatment (Licauco 1981; Shakman 1969). This is exemplified by this case reported by Shakman (1969):

> A twenty-five-year-old college graduate speech teacher presented herself at a *spiritista* for a third time. She was unmarried. She stated that two months earlier she had developed such a sore throat that she could not speak above a whisper. She consulted a physician who treated her with an antibiotic by injection. When she failed to improve, she consulted the *spiritista*. He performed an "operation" on her throat which produced immediate and complete return of her voice. She suffered an identical reoccurrence of her illness exactly thirty days later. This time a physician was not consulted; the spiritual surgery was repeated with complete success. After another interval of thirty days, she presented once more with inability to speak above a whisper. She was observed on this occasion. She was not overtly anxious about her condition and her pharynx was not inflamed. A procedure was performed which was, according to the healer, identical to the two previous procedures. The patient lay on her back with the anterior surface of her neck free of clothing. After a prayer, the healer placed both hands over the thyroid and seemed to exert considerable pressure until blood mixed with clots squirted from beneath his hands. The blood was wiped away with cotton: the skin was unbroken. On sitting up, the patient had full return of her voice. (p. 282)

As industrialization progresses and technological skills and knowledge become increasingly indispensable for economic and social survival and advancement, Western scientific concepts are becoming increasingly more relevant to the coping problems experienced among Pilipinos. Excessive reliance on supernatural influences on one's fate is slowly eroding as competitive self-determination is taking hold (Marsella et al. 1971). In Manila, emotional and adjustment disturbances are being seen more and more as problems of coping style and perception of environmental stresses, according to Lapuz (1977, 1978). In the United States, Flaskerud and Soldevilla (1986) report an increasing number of Pilipinos seeking help in community mental health facilities despite their "subscribing to natural and unnatural disease categories of illness causation" (p. 33).

The effectiveness of spiritual healers (those employing magnetic healing and psychic surgery) is interpreted by most American observers as the result of the power of suggestion (Licauco 1981; Shakman 1969).

Conceptualization of Mental Health and Mental Illness

In Philippine folk medicine, illnesses are not differentiated into mental and physical categories. Rather, illness is conceived of as the disruption of the harmonious functioning of the whole individual—physical, mental, and spiritual—in its interaction with its natural, social, and spiritual environment.

Factors believed to cause mental illness by various segments of the Pilipino population include witchcraft; evil spirits; situational stressors; malign magic; divine retribution for disregarding taboos; deficient vital force (bisa); loss of soul; inadequate or unfavorable food, water, or climate; malposition of internal organs; disordered flow of blood to the head; and diseases of the body (Shakman 1969; Tan 1987). Among the Westernized group, physical and emotional strain or exhaustion, sexual frustration, sexual excess, unrequited love, lack of self-discipline, weakness of character, and inherited constitutional defects are acknowledged causative factors.

Expression of Mental Illness

Opler (1956) substantiated Kraeplin's observation that mental disorders show a differential frequency of occurrence from one culture to another. Schlesinger (1981) notes that symptoms are profoundly influenced by the culture to which a patient belongs. However, he emphasizes,

> Psychiatrists and anthropologists alike state that major patterns of abnormal behavior seen by Western psychiatrists are found in societies throughout the world. However, there are significant differences in presentation, frequency of occurrence, distribution, and social ramifications of such deviant behaviors. (p. 26)

Sechrest (1964) identified the most common manifestations of mental illness among Pilipinos. He noted that among males, aggressive and/or destructive behavior, unpleasant delusions, impaired sleep and unkempt appearance, "sadness," and somatic complaints are the most common symptoms in order of enumeration. Among females, the order is somatic complaints, such as impaired appetite and sleep; quarrelsomeness; provocative behaviors; shouting, dancing, and singing; and incoherence and visual hallucinations. According to Lapuz (1978), Pilipinos with mental illnesses overwhelmingly present with psychosomatic and hysterical conversion symptoms and explosions of inappropriate behavior.

Among the functional psychoses, it has been reported by Flaskerud and Soldevilla (1986) in the United States and by Varias (1960) and Sechrest (1967) in the Philippines that the ratio of the incidence of schizophrenia in relation to affective disorders is greater among Pilipinos than the ratio reported for the general United States population.

Among Pilipino Americans with schizophrenic disorders, paranoid symptoms predominate. As with other ethnic groups with strong supernatural orientations, influence by malevolent spirits, witches, and demons dominate the Pilipino patient's unpleasant delusions. The propensity for destructive, provocative, or violent behaviors is well documented for this group (Flaskerud and Soldevilla 1986; Guthrie 1967; Sechrest 1967; Varias 1960). Among the poor Pilipinos who had recently immigrated and were admitted to the Hawaiian State Mental Hospital system, Opler (1956) noted a significant number of psychotic patients who exhibited apathy, withdrawal, negativism, and mutism, and who often had ideas of reference. However, whether this symptom complex represents catatonic schizophrenic disorder or "social breakdown syndrome" is not clear.

The prevalence of major depressive disorders among Pilipinos is very likely grossly underestimated. This is because only "difficult" or "peculiar" behaviors are considered to be in need of psychiatric intervention and because of a "particular cultural tendency among Pilipinos to deny the presence of depression" (Lapuz 1978, p. 47). Pilipino culture places a special premium on endurance and silent suffering (Bulatao 1963). According to Flaskerud and Soldevilla (1986), 46% of the Pilipino patients they reviewed somatized their emotional problems.

As noted by Lapuz (1978), it is only when the classic symptoms of psychotic depression become apparent that Pilipinos who are depressed come to the attention of health care providers. The frequency of manic patients being brought for mental health care in the Philippines as well as in California (Flaskerud and Soldevilla 1986) suggests that the incidence of manic-depressive disorder among Pilipinos is probably comparable with the incidence in the general American population.

Mania among Pilipinos is characterized more often by defiant and destructive behaviors and hypersexuality rather than by gregariousness, creativity, and enhanced productivity.

Organic mental disorders are the more readily recognized and accepted mental disorders among Pilipinos. Perhaps this is because virtually every Pilipino family has had an elderly, often senescent member living at home. Thus, symptoms of organic brain dysfunction are familiar to many who grew up in a Pilipino household. Medical care is, therefore, more likely to be sought relatively early in the evolution of an organically based disorder, without too much apprehension about stigma to the family. Organic mental disorders are reported as second in frequency to schizophrenia among the psychotic disorders seen in mental health facilities in the Philippines (Varias 1959, 1960). Because of the demographic effects of the ongoing immigration of young working-age Pilipinos into the United States, the proportion of organic mental disorders is likely to show a temporary decline among Pilipino Americans and would be significantly lower than the proportion of such disorders among people in the Philippines.

According to Lapuz (1978) and Reyes and Lapuz (1963), the overall incidence of neurotic disorders among patients seen in Manila appears comparable to incidences observed in most studies in the United States. But Lapuz has noted that anxiety disorders, conversion disorders, and obsessive-compulsive, dissociative, and psychophysiologic disorders were more common in the Pilipino sample than in the American sample. The propensity for somatization and psychophysiological symptoms reported by Duff and Arthur (1967) among naval recruits also has been attributed by Lapuz (1978) to the cultural acceptance of "poor health" as an adequate excuse for almost any self-indulgence, including medical attention.

According to Reyes and Lapuz (1963), the predominant personality structure observed among their patients was a hysterical character. Paranoid personality patterns were reported to be frequently encountered as well. This is to be expected in a culture that still believes in witchcraft and supernatural influences (Shakman 1969) and in the notion that destiny is largely shaped by external forces.

Differentiating dysthymic from panic disorders among Pilipino patients using the standard DSM-III-R criteria (American Psychiatric Association 1987) is often difficult. A patient's somatic symptoms of anergia and sleep difficulties are often overshadowed by complaints of panicky feelings, palpitations, and anger over perceived oppressions. The stigma associated with depression, as deserved punishment or as an indication of character weakness, may be the trigger mechanism for panic attacks that delay the recognition of the underlying characteristic symptoms of depression.

The incidence of suicide among Pilipinos is not known. The notion of suicide as a mortal sin is very deeply engraved in the Pilipino conscience through a Catholic upbringing. Threats of suicide may reflect manipulative maneuvers directed at controlling others. Although premeditated suicide is probably rare among Pilipino Americans, sudden, impulsive, self-destructive behaviors are being reported with increasing frequency, especially among the young.

Although the use of alcohol is popular at Pilipino gatherings, alcohol abuse and alcoholism is reported to be relatively low by Western standards. Among women, alcohol use is very rare and is still generally considered to be socially unacceptable. It is equated with promiscuity and low moral standards in most circles. Although alcohol and drug use (marijuana, heroin, and cocaine) among Pilipinos has not become a significant mental health issue, the incidence of casual use among the young is reported to be increasing (Quejas 1983). Tuason, a mental health worker, reports that among the Pilipino American and other Asian American populations in New Mexico, diagnoses of substance abuse, panic and anxiety disorders, and depression are common in both men and women (Scheck 1990).

Culture-Bound Syndromes in Expression of Mental Illness

Culture-bound syndromes are symptom complexes believed to be found exclusively in certain cultures. Two such syndromes attributed to Pilipinos and other Malay-Indonesian groups are *latah* and *amok*.

Latah is known in the Philippines as *mali-mali* or *silok* (Simmons 1980). Those people exhibiting the syndrome respond to minimal stimuli with an exaggerated startle response, often shouting expletives or sexually denotative words. Often such an episode is accompanied by echolalia, coprolalia, or compulsive obedience to commands or imitation of the actions of others.

> A case of *mali-mali* that I observed was that of a middle-aged homemaker whose husband was having an affair with her cousin. Instead of becoming indignant and angry over the situation, the aggrieved woman acted as if nothing were amiss and remained generally cheerful and affable. However, if she were approached when she was in a pensive mood or lost in thought, she would get startled easily and exclaim "*Ay bilat, bilat, bilat*" (Visayan for "Oh, cunt, cunt, cunt"). She would then compulsively repeat whatever she heard (echolalia). This behavior would only stop when everybody around would be quiet for a minute or two until the woman had calmed down and regained her composure.

Although the characteristic set of interactive behaviors described here as *mali-mali* is widely believed to be culture-specific, syndromes of "easy startle" followed by sets of repetitive behaviors have been observed among other unrelated ethnocultural groups. Syndromes essentially like *mali-mali* have been reported in Burma (*yuan*), Thailand (*bah tschi*), Siberia (*myriachit* or *ikota*), among the Ainu of Northern Japan (*imu*), and among the French Canadians of Maine (jumping mania). Simmons (1980) has demonstrated that the stereotyped behaviors among people with hyperstartle are the results of culture-specific exploitation of a neurophysiologically determined behavior potential.

Another culture-bound syndrome that Pilipinos share with their Malaysian cousins is the well-known *amok*. In this syndrome, a person who has been brooding over what he or she perceives as an irreparable wrong done to the individual, his or her family, or his or her religious beliefs would suddenly go on a rampage without any apparent provocation. Such an individual is often described as not being him- or herself and acting as though possessed. The person who is *amok* will indiscriminately attack anyone within reach, usually with a bolo. This relentless homicidal assault may last several hours. If the *amok* or *juramentado* is not maimed or killed, he or she will eventually collapse in exhaustion and lapse into a stupor and on awakening will be virtually amnesic of the episode.

Although it was once the general belief that this irrational outburst of homicidal behavior was peculiar to the Malays, reports from the world press indicate that instances of mass murders associated with a dissociative episode are widespread. The massacre at a McDonald's restaurant in California and the campus killings by a sniper in the carillon tower of a Texas university are but two well-publicized examples of *amok* in the United States. Many more instances of war veterans who in a "flashback" (dissociative state) act out their warrior roles with devastating results have been reported.

Gomez (1982) describes what he calls an "exclusively Puerto Rican syndrome known as *ataque*." This syndrome consists "of bizarre seizure patterns usually considered psychogenic in nature" and may include "a display of histrionics or aggression on the part of the patient, and sometimes culminating in stupor" (p. 124). In dynamic terms, this attack is explained as an "opportunity for a physical release of accumulated repressed anger" (p. 124). Perhaps because of similar role definition and social restrictions imposed on women by Spanish colonial culture, a syndrome known as *atake ng nerbyos* with the same symptoms as the Puerto Rican *ataques de nervios* is not uncommon among Pilipino women. However, this is but one variety of culturally conditioned hysterical conversion reaction used by Pilipino women to displace and ventilate frustration and anger. A more common form for displacing frustration that has evolved is compulsive shopping or compulsive gambling (Lapuz 1977). This seems to have proved more effective in discouraging financially successful husbands from maintaining a traditional mistress (*querida*).

Folk or Traditional
Categories of Mental Illness

According to Tan (1987), a distinction between physical and mental disorders is not made in the traditional or folk conceptualization of illness in the Philippines. Illnesses are viewed as caused by the disruption of the harmonious functioning of body, life-force (*liget* or *bisa*), and spirit within the individual, as well as in his or her relations with the group and the spirit world. Therefore, Philippine categories of illness are distinguished not so much on the basis of somatic or psychological signs and symptoms but rather on concepts related to their perceived causation. There are three major folk theories of illness causation: the mystical, the personalistic, and the naturalistic (Tan 1987).

Mystical Causation

Illnesses attributed to mystical causation include *usug*, which is believed to result from contact with a person with a stronger life-force. This is usually manifested by general weakness and increased suggestibility. Another disorder of mystical causation is "soul-loss." This may manifest in the form of withdrawal, irrationality, indifference, bad dreams (*hupa*), and nightmares (*bangungut*) that are believed to result in death if the victim is not able to awaken during the attack. The *bangungut* syndrome was first reported in the medical literature in 1917 and has been the subject of medical investigation by Santa Cruz (1951), Nolasco (1957), and Aponte (1960). Researchers from the U.S. Department of Health and Human Services' Centers for Disease Control have investigated sudden deaths among Southeast Asian refugees, mostly Loatians, whose deaths appear to have characteristics similar to the Pilipino *bangungut*. Those researchers have been unable to establish the exact cause of death other than physiologic cardiac failure (Centers for Disease Control 1981).

Mystical retribution (*gaba*) involves the notion of immanent justice (i.e., "As ye sow, so shall ye reap"). *Gaba* is usually manifested in a form similar to the misery one may believe oneself to have inflicted on another. Depression and psychophysiological disturbances such as insomnia, asthma, gastrointestinal disturbance, impotence, and chronic pains and headaches are often attributed to *gaba*.

Personalistic Causation

Personalistic causes of illness are divided into two groups: the supernatural (animistic) and the human (malign magic). Animistic beliefs attribute the existence of life-force or "life-stuff" to animate as well as inanimate objects. This "life-stuff" may manifest as ghosts (*multo, tomawo*) or "souls" of the dead. The potential malevolence of ghosts is proportionate to the sentiments aroused in a person at the instant of his or her death. Unbaptized or aborted children may "haunt" the living and cause depression, hallucinations, or even suicide.

Other supernatural entities representing life-force, other than those of the dead, are believed to participate in the maintenance of proper functioning of social and ecological systems. These entities are known as *dwendes, anitos, enkantos, kapres, haan tao,* and *santermos*. Activities that offend these spirits or entities are believed to result in illness, usually in the form of psychophysiological disorders (Tan 1987).

Personalistic illnesses are believed to be induced by specially gifted and trained human agents called variously *mankukulam* in Tagalog, *tomay* in Ilokano, and *hiwit* in Visayan. These shamanistic workers cause illness by implanting objects that cause discomfort and malfunction in the victims. The resulting illnesses are successfully treated by enlisting the help of another specially trained and gifted shaministic worker or spiritual (i.e., psychic) healer who possesses the skills to extract the offending object. This procedure often results in the dramatic disappearance of excruciating pain and dysfunctional behaviors.

Other syndromes associated with malign magic are possession and poltergeist. These phenomena are fairly common in the Philippines, even in urban Manila. Bulatao (1982, 1986), a clinical psychologist who has investigated a number of these cases with the use of hypnosis, found these phenomenon to fit the category of dissociative disorders, wherein the afflicted act out the impulses of their alter-egos and subconscious selves. Bulatao also reports good results with hypnotherapy.

Naturalistic Causation

Diseases caused naturalistically are thought to stem not from machinations of angry beings, but rather from such natural forces or conditions as cold, heat, winds, dampness, exposure to stress, and above all, from the ability of these factors to upset the balance of basic body elements (Foster and Anderson 1978). Wind (*hangin*) is believed to cause *pasma* (rheumatism or joint pains), *pilay loming* (muscular pains), or *tampal-tampal* (urticaria).

Diet is believed to cause illnesses by affecting the shifting and malposition of internal organs or upsetting the balance of their function. Respiratory and gastrointestinal disorders are linked to injudicious consumption of "cold" foods such as fruits, whereas *singaw* (eruptions in the mouth and/or skin) are linked with "hot" foods. The idea that infections cause illnesses is generally accepted, though concepts of the infective agents may vary from those of Western medicine. Stress and exposure to physical or psychological strain are generally accepted as illness-producing. *Kabuhi* and *lanti* are "fright illnesses" similar to the Mexican *susto*. People with these disorders present with social withdrawal and alienation, insomnia, pervasive anxiety, depression, and "flashbacks" suggestive of a posttraumatic stress disorder. Other stress-related disorders include *pasma sa kaon,* which results from prolonged hunger disturbing the organismic balance and which may manifest in physical or behavioral changes or both. Like *uget* (bad feelings in the heart; a "heartache" that discourages eating), resignation, passivity, and withdrawal are prominent symptoms.

Folk Healers and Mainstream
Mental Health Providers

According to Licauco (1982) and Shakman (1969), a great variety of indigenous healing is popular in the Philippines. The role of traditional healers in Pilipino communities in the United States is also significant. In most cases they are regarded not only as healers but also as spiritual leaders (Licauco 1982). The most popular forms of healing include the following:

1. Psychic surgery, which enjoys a great following in the Philippines and Brazil, is gaining popularity in this country (Licauco 1982).
2. The use of herbs by herb doctors who heal by application of medicinal plants topically or by ingestion as a brew. These concoctions are often

used to relieve agitation and to promote sleep (Concha 1982; Quisumbing 1951).

3. The use of manipulation of muscles, joints, and bones by *manghihilot* or bonesetters. These procedures are believed to relieve pain, reduce anxiety and tension, and improve state of mind.

4. Magnetic healing, which consists of passing the magnetic healer's hands over the affected area while the healer prays, meditates, and reportedly is possessed by a supernatural being. This technique is credited with restoring the normal flow and balance of life-force and is good for somatic symptoms and disturbed moods and disorganized thinking. This form of healing is common in this country but is known by many different names.

5. *Bulo-bulo,* a procedure where the practitioner extracts the causative agent of disease from a person by blowing into a glass of water which is passed over the patient, particularly over his or her affected body part. The appearance of color, stones, insects, and other objects in the water signifies removal of the causative agent of the disease and often produces immediate relief.

6. Reflexology or zone therapy, in which the healers use massage along acupuncture meridians. This is believed to restore the balanced flow of the life-force. Some of their maneuvers show close similarity with acupressure.

7. The repositioning of internal organs by massage has many proponents, especially in the treatment of hysterical women.

8. Mystical healing and "white" witchcraft use prescribed rituals to counteract the influence of malevolent spirits, malign magic, and the possession phenomenon.

The notion that the folk healer is sought only by people who hold similar traditional concepts of disease causation, such as poorly educated Pilipino immigrants, is not entirely valid. Even relatives of physicians seek the help of indigenous healers. Unfortunately, no scientifically controlled study has been conducted to measure the effectiveness of traditional healers in symptom relief and rates of cure of medically authenticated cases. The work of Licauco (1981) and Lava and Araneta (1983) would indicate that the effectiveness of some of these healers is not limited to psychophysiologic or conversion disorders. A report by Singer and Ankenbrandt (1980) is inconclusive.

Mainstream medicine and the psychiatric establishment publicly condemn so-called folk healers. In the United States, where many of these healers come under the sponsorship of religious groups to perform spiritual healings, they are often sued for "practicing without a license" and are jailed. Except for a few Pilipino physicians who have established working relationships with selected healers in the Philippines, mutual rejection and avoidance characterize the relationship between mainstream health workers and Philippine folk healers (Licauco 1982). This is unfortunate, because folk healers can, indeed, be efficacious in treating some disorders (Shakman 1969).

As the number of folk healers increases in the United States through the efforts of local religious groups, it seems unavoidable that mainstream medicine will have to form some sort of contact or even reach some type of accommodation with them. This will at least afford mainstream medical professionals the opportunity to reach those patients who choose faith healers as their primary source of help and to ensure that the patients' serious physical problems are not overlooked. More important, it behooves mental health workers to determine whether these healers can, indeed, provide a culturally appropriate resolution of patients' problems, whether through suggestion or other as yet unidentified mechanisms. After all, to effect a resolution of psychiatric disorders, traditional practices that reflect an understanding of the mystical beliefs of indigenous concepts about existence, development, identity, and self-image are essential for those who live by these beliefs. In my own experience in Guyana, working with a local Kali healer proved very helpful, especially in dealing with cases of adjustment disorders, neurotic family interactions, and psychophysiological disorders (Singer et al. 1979).

Family Response to Mental Illness of a Family Member

A response consistently noted among Pilipino families reacting to a relative's mental illness is an initial refusal to accept the possibility of the illness's existence. During this initial phase, a family attributes the uncharacteristic behaviors or moodiness to the effects of normal disruptions and vicissitudes in the human condition. Unfavorable circumstances and events, disturbed relations, exhaustion, and deprivation of gratification are often blamed. This attribution of the disturbance to external causes, according to Lapuz (1978), reflects a cultural propensity that can be traced back to childhood conditioning (blaming the *tomawo, kapre,* or *dwende*).

Following this initial denial phase, the next family response usually consists of concerted efforts to convince the patient and themselves of the susceptibility to change of naturalistic factors that may have led to the illness. "Prescriptions" include rest cure, avoidance of mental stress, building physical and moral strength by going to church, praying, making spiritual offerings, gratifying physiological needs, indulging the patient's wishes, and encouraging thoughts of contentment and peace (Lapuz 1978).

If still no improvement occurs, a period of tolerant accommodation follows. The paramount concern at this point is to prevent the patient from causing embarrassment to the family. Progressively stricter disciplinary measures, including isolation or seclusion in his or her room, are imposed on the patient in order to avert publicly embarrassing situations. At this point, the family begins to consider the need for external sources of help. Also, at this time, divergence in concepts of illness causation lead to diverging paths in the help-seeking behaviors among the more traditionally oriented families and the more Westernized ones.

The families that are more traditionally oriented are more likely to seek a priest, a spiritual counselor or healer, a psychic surgeon, and other folk healers for assistance. This is in keeping with their belief in possession, malign magic, or witchcraft as the likely agent of mental illness. The rationale given for the choice of spiritual healers over Western medical resources is that these healers are believed to be effective in mediating between physical and spiritual disruptive forces within the individual and the various forces of the spirit world. Also, folk healers are less expensive. If the treatment succeeds, then the patient never gets to see a medical doctor. However, if the ministrations of these healers do not achieve the desired results, then the patient is taken by a family elder to a medical doctor, usually a general practitioner. It is through this general practitioner that the patient and his or her family eventually become involved with mental health workers. Psychiatric referral is still strongly resisted by both patient and family alike.

According to Flaskerud and Soldevilla (1986) and Bucton (1984), by the time Pilipino patients reach Western mental health care providers, usually through referral by general practitioners, their mental disturbance has become chronic and severe, or explosive acting out behavior has occurred. This is especially true of people with affective or psychotic disorders.

However, because conversion hysteria and psychophysiological disorders make up the predominant psychiatric syndromes among Pilipinos (Flaskerud and Soldevilla 1986; Lapuz 1978; Shakman 1969; Varias 1963), then the delay in the psychiatric referral of these cases is probably of little significance. According to Wittkower and Warnes (1974) and Frank (1972), results with the use of Western psychiatric treatment modalities in treating these cases have not produced any better results than those of indigenous healers.

Treatment of Pilipino American Patients

Although the perception of psychological stress and adjustment demands are culturally influenced, the neuroendocrine, cardiovascular, and other somatic changes associated with mental illness are measurable and amenable to accepted psychiatric somatic remedies. These treatment modalities are applicable to all patients with mental illnesses, even those from differing ethnocultural origins, so long as the remedies are adjusted differentially and introduced judiciously.

Psychotropic Medications

According to Flaskerud and Soldevilla (1986), Pilipino psychiatric patients are quite accepting of medications because of their familiarity with American medicine. These researchers, in fact, advocate the use of medications to attract Pilipino patients to continue coming for treatments. Lin and Finder (1983) reported that effective weight-standardized neuroleptic dose ranges for Asian patients (including Pilipinos) were significantly lower than those for their white counterparts. Lin and Finder also noted the occurrence of extrapyramidal symptoms at lower doses for Asian patients. These findings were supported by various researchers (Binder and Levy 1981; Murphy 1969; Yamamoto et al. 1979), but other studies yielded contradictory results. However, caution is necessary in titrating the dosage of psychotropic medications (including lithium and antidepressants) for Pilipino patients because of the alienating consequences of unpleasant side effects. I recommend that clinicians start with a small dose and instruct patients to raise this gradually by a specific amount at predetermined safe intervals so that the recommended therapeutic dose is not reached until the next scheduled visit. The other alternative is to assess the patient's drug response at more frequent intervals. This assessment can then be used to establish rapport and initiate talk therapy.

Psychotherapy

Psychotherapy with Pilipino patients requires a fairly broad understanding of their ethnocultural diversity and their unique initial response pattern conditioned by long years of colonization, strong kinship ties, child-raising practices, and degree of Westernization.

According to Ponce (1974) the initial approach should be authoritarian. This conforms to the patient's conceptualization of the doctor as a *patrón*, a "superior," or an "expert." The patient will initially concentrate on physical complaints, which are seen as properly the concern of a physician. Somatic measures that can afford immediate relief should be discussed and initiated. Meanwhile, it is important to inquire about the patient's assumptions and beliefs about the cause of the illness. If he or she is reticent, it may be because of fear of ridicule and the belief that interpersonal conflicts and problems of the spirit world are properly dealt with by priests, spiritual advisors, and psychic healers. It is essential that the clinician not belittle these beliefs; rather, the patient should be treated with compassion and respect and encouraged to talk about them. The clinician must remember that workable accommodations between differing beliefs are always possible and that relieving a patient's symptoms rather than changing a patient's beliefs is the primary task of this therapy.

According to Lapuz (1978), a Pilipino patient will seek to establish familiarity and close personal ties with his or her psychiatrist. This is a normal cultural reaction (i.e., to gain a *patrón* or powerful ally). The inappropriateness of this sought-after alliance has to be clarified with the patient without alienating him or her. To fail to clarify the essence of the therapeutic relationship may limit the patient's disclosures to those the patient believes the *patrón* wishes to hear.

Although Lapuz (1978) believes that most Pilipino patients may be helped to "self-actualize," most still feel compelled to reconcile their individual fulfillment with family values. Rather than concentrate on internal conflicts experienced by the patient, I find it useful to encourage the patient to be involved with activities that will make him or her feel better. The patient wants direction and needs help in evaluating and formulating personal interactions with his or her milieu. The expert giving instruction therapy is culturally syntonic. Occasionally, patients outgrow the need to link their identity with the family and become ready to emancipate themselves from the family and their traditional cultural milieu. This often is effected by finding employment in some distant place to avoid the issue of individual aspirations versus family loyalty. The issue of loyalty is of great concern to Pilipino patients because of cultural emphasis on interdependence and communality. This issue may be more productively dealt with in a group therapy setting.

Hypnotherapy and Cognitive Therapy

Bulatao (1982) has found that the Pilipino proclivity to deference and the need to conform makes Pilipino patients highly susceptible to hypnosis. Bulatao has used this therapy effectively in patients with "spirit possession" or "poltergeist."

Cognitive therapy is quite effective but is generally difficult to implement with Pilipino patients, except within the context of their group affiliation and religious convictions. Pilipinos tend to be very religious, and religious precepts constitute the major premise in their rationale system.

Direct suggestions, where the secondary gains of the symptoms have been discussed and/or relinquished, is often dramatically helpful in Pilipino patients with conversion disorders.

Herbal Medications

Herb doctors (*herbalarios* or *arbolarios*) are among the most common of the Pilipino folk healers. However, in the absence of tropical medicinal plants that abound in the Philippines, I have yet to hear of a practicing *arbolario* in the United States. There are many Pilipino psychiatric patients who consult Chinese herbal medicine practitioners and health food stores for treatment of their "nervous" disorders. Although I have not heard of or read about any serious adverse drug interaction, I do not encourage the simultaneous use of herbal medicine with psychotropic drugs. Fortunately, the quantity of active ingredients in most herbal potions is often relatively mild and innocuous. The dosages of "supplements" recommended in health food stores are more alarming, and I advise patients to consult the approved minimum daily requirements.

Collaboration With Folk Healers

I have personally always found working with folk healers to be challenging, instructive, productive, and essential. Otherwise, how can clinicians possibly improve our insight into and management of patients who share the folk healer's beliefs? It is necessary to remember that Western medical interventions deal mainly with the proximal causes and manifestations of a problem that patients may regard as a complex physical-social-spiritual problem involving not only themselves but also their family, social network, and their relations with the spirit world. Belief in the distal or ultimate causes of patients' distress may require removal or neutralization of a spell, appeasement of the spirit world, and restoration of familial and social unity. These tasks are best dealt with in association with spiritual leaders and/or indigenous folk healers. Meanwhile, clinicians can offer suggestions based on the most up-to-date understanding of illness causation. Often, folk healers are also eager to learn.

Issues in Family Therapy

Close family ties are highly valued by Pilipinos. They tend to resent intrusion by outsiders (i.e., therapists) and especially object to family conflict being exposed to outsiders. Pilipinos tend to regard members who expose family problems to outsiders as acting disloyally. Consequently, family therapy for Pilipinos constitute a delicate operation that can easily become unproductive if the tradition of deference to elders (to prevent loss of face) and notions of *delicadeza* and *amor propio* are not taken into account during family therapy (Sue and Morishima 1982). Progress in family therapy with Pilipinos is possible if emphasis is placed on the appropriateness of role definition and task assignment rather than on exploring attitudes and feelings among family members toward one another. By focusing on the restructuring of roles and tasks, the sense of close ties can be preserved while affording opportunities for role expansion and individual growth, without getting enmeshed in the issue of loyalty among people sensitized to it.

Another difficult issue for Pilipino families is the question of emancipation and individual rights versus family welfare. Is family solidarity more important than individual fulfillment? Here, the tradition of consensus born of communalism is very important. Pilipinos believe in conforming to group expectations. By appealing to the recognized leader of the family to allow members' input in the formulation of goals for the greater glory and security of the family, breaking down the authoritarian pattern of interaction may be achieved and increased opportunity for individual fulfillment secured.

Other Aids to Treatment

Diet as therapy.   The notion that diets influence both the physical and emotional well-being of individuals is still popularly held by Pilipinos, as it is by most people in our society. Certain effects are attributed by Pilipinos to "cold" foods that are the inverse of those resulting from "hot" foods. Securing a list of these food categories may be helpful in order for a clinician to be able to recommend a culturally acceptable, nutritious, balanced diet.

Diagnostic tests. The use of diagnostic tests is generally not considered objectionable by Pilipino patients, because they are fairly well acquainted with Western medical diagnostic and treatment procedures. For most, the major concern is cost.

Ethnic caseworkers. The use of ethnic caseworkers has been found to be absolutely essential on the West Coast in securing accurate information and in promoting patient confidence and cooperation. These caseworkers also ensure that patients properly understand explanations and instructions that are highly valued by authority-oriented Pilipino patients.

Consultants. Use of medical and psychiatric consultants by caseworkers is generally welcomed, because Pilipinos generally have a high regard for authority. Issuance of prescriptions (magic potions) would further enhance patients' confidence and positive anticipation.

Hospitalization. Generally, Pilipinos see psychiatric hospitalizations as ominous and very likely permanent. If hospitalization is contemplated, the patient and his or her family need to be seen together, and the purpose and benefits of this step clearly explained and exhaustively discussed. The notion of permanence derives from the fact that psychiatric hospitalization in the Philippines has always been reserved for very severe and often irreversible chronic cases or for violent patients. To a Pilipino family, a patient's hospitalization will most likely denote isolation from society rather than restoration to a more healthy level of functioning.

Follow-up care. Follow-up care is very important but is sometimes difficult for Pilipino patients because of the cost of health care and the need for transportation. Because most Pilipino household members are employed outside the home, taking the patient for clinic visits is often difficult. Also, the notion of prolonged care is new to Pilipinos, who are used to seeing doctors only for immediate symptomatic relief of acute problems. Furthermore, the notion of rehabilitation, self-actualization, and enhancement of function beyond pretreatment levels is quite new to most Pilipino Americans. It requires a great deal of skill and patience to keep Pilipino patients in extended follow-up care for these purposes.

Conclusion

Pilipinos make up a racially, ethnically, and culturally diverse group of people. Although some live according to tribal traditions and beliefs, others are more at ease in American society than in Philippine society.

The circumstances of their existence in this country have subjected Pilipino Americans to emotional stresses that some believed would increase their susceptibility to mental illness. The overprotective and restrictive Pilipino child-rearing practices and traditional cultural values added obstacles to Pilipino Americans' optimum adjustment to American society. Intergenerational conflict in Pilipino American families is escalating as acculturation and assimilation increase.

The incidence of paranoid schizophrenia has been noticeably higher among Pilipinos as compared with other Asian groups. Psychophysiologic and other somatization disorders are also high in comparison with white Americans and African Americans. Depression is believed to be underestimated because of the value that Pilipinos place on the virtue of endurance. Anxiety and related disorders are believed to approximate, if not exceed, the incidence rate for the general population in the United States. Suicide and alcohol and drug abuse are believed to be well below the national average, although there are indications that this may be changing, especially among third-, fourth-, and fifth-generation Pilipino Americans.

There are special issues that need to be taken into account in the treatment of mental illness among Pilipinos. Among these are proportionately lower dose ranges for psychotropic medications, interference between traditional family values and Western psychotherapeutic process and goals, negative attitudes toward psychiatric hospitalization, lingering belief in mystical and personalistic theories of disease causation, and responsiveness to a variety of folk healers. An ongoing problem is that current systems of mental health service delivery are not well adapted to meet the needs of Pilipino Americans and the special problems that they face.

My discussion in this chapter has emphasized that any therapeutic approach to mental illness among Pilipino Americans must take into account their cultural conditioning. In psychotherapy, the patient's belief system and conceptual style are dealt with. These are culturally conditioned and, therefore, responsive to culturally defined behavior modifiers rather than diagnosis-specific remedies. The probability of stunting cultural development by reinforcing ethnocultural adaptive style has been feared as a possible drawback of culturally oriented psychotherapy. However, experience in collaborative efforts has shown such work to be more often progressive than regressive and productive of an integrated cultural and community development (Singer et al. 1979).

Throughout their history in the United States, there was never a lack of desire among Pilipinos to assimilate into American society. Barriers to their assimilation erected by the host country have been responsible for Pilipino Americans forming unions and social organizations for their collective security. What is interesting is that this process is strengthening rather than weakening as the "melting pot" paradigm of race relations is giving away to the paradigm of "ethnic pluralism" or the "salad bowl" concept of constructive coexistence. This would suggest that major obstacles to the mental health of Pilipino Americans stem from their sense of vulnerability over their perceived and actual subordinate status in this society, reminiscent of their colonial history.

References

Agpalo R: The politics of Philippine modernization, in Psychopathology. Edited by Lapuz L. Quezon City, Philippines, New Day Publishers, 1976

Alegado D: Profile: U.S. Filipinos in the 1980s. Katipunan, September/October 1987, p 11

American Psychiatric Association: Diagnostic and Statistical Manual of Mental Disorders, 3rd Edition, Revised. Washington, DC, American Psychiatric Association, 1987

America's Asians. The Economist, June 3, 1989, pp 23–25

Aponte G: The enigma of "Bangungot." Arch Intern Med 52:1258–1263, 1960

Atkeson P: Building communication in interracial marriage. Psychiatry 33:396–408, 1970

Beyer O: The Philippine Saga, 3rd Edition. Manila, Capital Publishing House, 1952

Binder R, Levy R: Extrapyramidal reactions in Asians. Am J Psychiatry 138:1243–1244, 1981

Bucton L: Filipinos and mental health: seeking help. Philippine News, April 4–10, 1984, pp 11–14

Bulatao J: Personal preferences of Filipino students. Proceedings of the Symposium on the Filipino Personality. Manila, Psychological Association of the Philippines, 1963, pp 8–18

Bulatao J: Hiya. Philippine Studies 12:424–438, 1964

Bulatao J: Local cases of Possession and their cures. Philippine Studies 30:415–426, 1982

Bulatao J: A note on Philippine possession and poltergeist. Philippine Studies 34:86–

101, 1986

Bulosan C: America Is In The Heart. New York, Harcourt Brace & Co., 1946

Byers HO: The Philippine Saga, 3rd Edition. Manila, Capitol Publishing House Inc., 1952

Cabezas A: In Pursuit of Wellness. San Francisco, CA, Department of Mental Health, 1982

Cassel J: Psychiatric epidemiology, in American Handbook of Psychiatry. Edited by Arieta S. New York, Basic Books, 1974, pp 401–410

Centers for Disease Control (U.S. Department of Health and Human Services): Sudden, unexpected, nocturnal deaths among Southeast Asian refugees. MMWR 30(4):581–584, 589, 1981

Concha J (ed): Philippine National Formulary, 2nd Edition. Manila, National Science and Technology Authority, 1982

Cordova F: The Filipino-American: there's always an identity crisis, in Asian-Americans: Psychological Perspectives. Edited by Sue S, Wagner N. Palo Alto, CA, Science and Behavior Books, 1973, pp 136–139

Duff D, Arthur R: Between two worlds: Filipinos in the U.S. Navy. Am J Psychiatry 123:836–843, 1967

Espina M: Seven generations of a New Orleans Pilipino family, in Perspectives on Ethnicity in New Orleans. Edited by Cooke J. New Orleans, LA, Committee on Ethnicity in New Orleans, 1979, pp 33–36

Espina M: Asians in New Orleans, in Perspectives on Ethnicity in New Orleans. Edited by Cooke J. New Orleans, LA, Committee on Ethnicity in New Orleans, 1980, pp 63–66

Evangelista S: Filipinos in America: literature as history. Philippine Studies 36:36–53, 1988

Fallows J: A damaged culture. Atlantic Monthly, November 1987, pp 49–58

Flaskerud J, Soldevilla E: Pilipino and Vietnamese clients: utilizing an Asian mental health center. J Psychosoc Nurs Ment Health Serv 24(8):32–36, 1986

Foster G, Anderson B: Medical Anthropology. New York, Wiley, 1978

Frank J: Common features of psychotherapy. Aust N Z J Psychiatry 6(1):30, 1972

Gomez A: Puerto Rican Americans, in Cross-Cultural Psychiatry. Edited by Gaw A. Littleton, MA, John Wright-PSG Pub Co, 1982, pp 109–136

Guthrie G: Philippine temperament, in Six Perspectives on the Philippines. Edited by Guthrie G. Manila, Benchmark, 1967

Hollensteiner M: Social control and Filipino personality. Proceedings of the Symposium on the Filipino Personality, Psychological Association of the Philippines, Manila, 1964, pp 23–27

Joaquin N: Quijano de Manila: Discoveries of the Devil's Advocate. Manila, Cacho Hermanos, 1983

Johnson L: The migration waves of Filipinos. Rice 1(11):37–39, 1988

Kim B-L: Asian-Americans: no model minority. Social Work 18(3):44–53, 1973

Kitano H: Japanese-American mental illness, in Changing Perspectives in Mental Illness. Edited by Plog S, Edgerton R. New York, Holt, Reinhart, & Winston, 1969, pp 256–284

Kuo W: Prevalence of depression among Asian-Americans. J Nerv Ment Dis 172(8):449–456, 1984

Lapuz L: Filipino Marriages in Crisis. Quezon City, Philippines, New Day Publishers, 1977

Lapuz L: A Study of Psychopathology. Quezon City, Philippines, New Day Publishers, 1978

Lava J, Araneta A: Faith Healing and Psychic Surgery in the Philippines. Manila, Philippine Society for Psychical Research Foundation, 1983

Licauco J: The Magicians of God. Manila, National Book Store, 1981

Licauco J: The truth behind faith healing in the Philippines. Manila, National Book Store, 1982

Lin K, Finder E: Neuroleptic dosage for Asians. Am J Psychiatry 140(4):490–491, 1983

Lott J: Migration of a mentality: the Filipino community. Social Case Work 57:165–173, 1976

Marsella A, Escudero M, Gordon P: Stress, resources, and symptom patterns in urban Filipino men, in Transcultural Research in Mental Health. Edited by Lehre W. Honolulu, HI, University of Hawaii Press, 1971, pp 148–171

Meinhardt K, Vega K: A method for estimating underutilization of mental health services by ethnic groups. Hosp Community Psychiatry 38:1186–1190, 1987

Murphy HBM: Ethnic variations in drug response: results of an international survey. Transcultural Psychiatric Research 6:5–23, 1969

Nolasco J: An inquiry into "Bangungot." Arch Intern Med 99:905–912, 1957

Opler M: Culture, Psychiatry, and Human Values: The Methods and Values of a Social Psychiatry. Springfield, IL, Charles C Thomas, 1956

Ponce D: The Filipinos of Hawaii, in Peoples and Cultures of Hawaii. Edited by Teng W, McDermott J, Maretzki T. Honolulu, HI, University Press of Hawaii, 1974, pp 34–43

Quejas S: The role of non-governmental organizations in the prevention and reduction of drug abuse. Republic of the Philippines Dangerous Drugs Board, Bulletin on Narcotics 35(3):53–62, 1983

Quirino C: The Spanish Colonial Army: 1878–98. Philippine Studies 36:381–386, 1988

Quisumbing E: Medicinal plants of the Philippines. Manila, Department of Agriculture and Natural Resources, 1951

Reyes B, Lapuz L: The practice of psychiatry in the Philippines. Journal of the Philippines College of Physicians 1(3):161–165, 1963

Santa Cruz F: The pathology of "Bangungot." Journal of the Philippine Islands Medical Association 27(7):476–481, 1951

Scheck A: Treating mental illness in Asian patients said to require cultural knowledge and insight. Clinical Psychiatric News 18(8):1, 24, 1990

Schlesinger R: Cross-cultural psychiatry: the application of Western-Anglo psychiatry to Asian-Americans of Chinese and Japanese ethnicity. J Psychosoc Nurs Ment Health Serv 19(9):26–30, 1981

Sechrest L: Symptoms of mental disorder in the Philippines. Proceedings of the Symposium on the Filipino Personality. Manila, Psychological Association of the Philippines, 1964, pp 28–45

Sechrest L: Philippine culture, stress, and psychopathology. Transcultural Psychiatric Research Review 4:18–22, 1967

Shakman R: Indigenous healing of mental illness in the Philippines. Int J Soc Psychiatry 15:279–287, 1969

Silliman R: Religious beliefs and life at the beginning of the Spanish regime in the Philippines. Dumaguete City, Philippines, College of Theology, Silliman University, 1964

Simmons R: The resolution of the Latah paradox. J Nerv Ment Dis 168(4):195–206, 1980

Singer P, Ankenbrandt K: The ethnography of the paranormal. New Directions in the Study of Man 4:19–34, 1980

Singer P, Araneta E, Naidoo J: Learning of psychodynamics, history, and diagnosis management therapy by a Kali cult indigenous healer in Guyana, in Spirits, Shamans, and Stars: Perspectives From South America. Edited by Browman D, Schwarz R. The Hague, Mouton Publishers, 1979, pp 157–178

Sue S, McKinney H: Asian-Americans in the community mental health care system. Am J Orthopsychiatry 45(1):111–118, 1975

Sue S, Morishima J: Mental Health of Asian-Americans. San Francisco, CA, Jossey-Bass, 1982

Sue S, Sue D: MMPI comparisons between Asian-Americans and non-Asian students utilizing a student health psychiatric clinic. Journal of Counseling Psychology 21:423–427, 1974

Tan M: Usug, Kulam, pasma: traditional concepts of health and illness in the Philippines. Quezon City, Philippines, Alay Kapwa Kilusang Pangkalusuan, 1987

Tsai M, Teng L, Sue S: Mental status of Chinese in the United States, in Mental Health of Asian-Americans. Edited by Sue S, Morishima J. San Francisco, CA, Jossey-Bass, 1982

U.S. Bureau of the Census: General Population Characteristics: 1980 (No PC 80-1-B1). Washington, DC, U.S. Government Printing Office, 1983

U.S. Bureau of the Census: Subject Report: Asian ord Pacific Islander Persons by Groups for the United States: 1990. Washington, DC, U.S. Government Printing Office, 1991a

U.S. Bureau of the Census: Subject Report: Race and Hispanic Origin for the United States: 1990 and 1980. Washington, DC, U.S. Government Printing Office, 1991b

U.S. Commission on Civil Rights: The Economic Status of Americans of Asian Descent: 1980. Washington, DC, U.S. Government Printing Office, 1988

Varias R: Cases of mental illness known to a group of public mental health workers.

Philippine Journal of Public Health 4(3):114–122, 1959

Varias R: Cases seen at Cubao Mental Hygiene Clinic. Philippine Journal of Public Health 5(3):130–134, 1960

Varias R: Psychiatry and the Filipino personality. Proceedings of the Symposium on the Filipino Personality, Psychological Association of the Philippines, Manila, 1963, pp 17–22

Wittkower E, Warnes H: Cultural aspects of psychotherapy. Am J Psychother 28:566–573, 1974

Yamamoto J, Fung D, Lo S, et al: Psychopharmacology for Asian-Americans and Pacific Islanders. Psychopharmacol Bull 15:29–31, 1979

Yamamoto K, Soliman A, Parsons J, et al: Voices in unison: stressful events in the lives of children in six countries. J Child Psychol Psychiatry 28(6):855–864, 1987

14   Ethnopsychopharmacology

Ching-Piao Chien, M.D.

Since the introduction of modern psychopharmacology in the mid-1950s, impressive amounts of data have been accumulated on the psychological, sociological, and pharmacological aspects of drug treatment. Although some cultural and ethnic data for patients undergoing drug treatment were reported in the early literature on psychopharmacologic drug use, only in the last decade has modern technology been available for measuring the plasma level and pharmacokinetics of various psychotropic drugs in different ethnic groups.

Since the immigration laws were changed in 1965, there has been an influx into the United States of refugees from all over the world, of whom a particularly large proportion are Indochinese. During this period, American society has become more multicultural and multiethnic. Such a trend is not limited to the United States but can also be observed in many other industrialized countries. The need to provide adequate and effective health care for these new immigrants cannot be met without appropriate knowledge of and familiarity with their ethnic and cultural characteristics.

Transcultural psychiatry has thus become a popular topic at national and international psychiatric conventions. More and more major residency training programs have incorporated transcultural psychiatry into their educational curricula, and psychopharmacology has been the major focus of the biological aspect of this field. Transcultural psychopharmacology is a discipline that seeks to determine the relative importance of and relationships between sociocultural, environmental, genetic, biological, and physiological variables in psychopharmacologic treatment and research (Itil 1976).

My primary focus in this chapter is on the differences, if any, between Asian and whites in the dosages, pharmacokinetics, and pharmacodynamics of psychotropic drugs. I also provide some background information on Asian immigrants and their cultural traits. First, the trend of the immigration pattern in the United States over the last half century is reviewed. Second, cultural characteristics in relation to drug therapy are discussed, and then well-established ethnic variations in metabolic processes are presented. Next, the literature on dosages, pharmacokinetics, and pharmacodynamics

413

are reviewed for four major psychotropic drug categories: neuroleptics, antidepressants, antianxiety agents, and lithium. Finally, based on this literature review, the myth that Asians require a lower dosage of psychotropic drugs is discussed.

Patterns of Immigration Into the United States

Although the United States is said to be a nation of immigrants, the immigration laws of earlier times did not provide equal opportunity for certain ethnic groups to settle in the United States. The Chinese Exclusion Act in 1882 and the National Origins Act in 1924 virtually halted Asian immigration into the United States from the late 19th century through the first half of the 20th century. The McCarran-Walter Act of 1952 allowed some easing of the restrictions against Asian immigration. Changes in the immigration laws in 1965, which took effect in 1968, abolished the national origins quota system in favor of one giving preference to family members of people already in the United States and to workers with needed skills. This was the turning point for Asian immigrants, to whom the gateway to the United States had been so tightly closed for more than half a century (Gardner et al. 1985).

Analysis of legal immigrants admitted to the United States by region of birth reveals that, from 1931 to 1960, only 5% of the legal immigrants were Asians, whereas more than half were Europeans (Gardner et al. 1985). From 1960 to 1969, the percentage of immigrants from Latin America increased to 38%, and the highest percentage of immigrants was still of European background. During this period, Asians made up more than 12% of immigrants. However, from 1970 to 1979, the Asian share increased to 34% of all legal immigrants, whereas the percentage of European immigrants decreased to only 19%. In this period, Latin Americans immigrants were the most numerous, amounting to 41% of the total.

From 1980 to 1984, the immigration pattern changed drastically. Asians accounted for 40% of the immigrants, Latin Americans 35%, and Europeans 12% (Gardner et al. 1985). This remarkable increase in Asian immigrants was partly the result of changes in American immigration laws in 1965 and to the influx of Indochinese refugees after the Vietnam War ended in 1975. The sudden increase in Asian Americans in the United States has created culture shock for some new immigrants. A remarkable number of studies have been made of the psychosocial and cultural features of Asian Americans, particularly of Indochinese refugees over the last decade (Owan et al. 1985).

The need to understand the psychobiological and sociocultural character-istics of Asian Americans has never been so great. Along with closer collab-oration in international psychiatric research, more data are needed on ethnicity and psychopharmacology. Transcultural psychopharmacology, which was first studied in the late 1950s, has been limited mostly to interna-tional comparisons. Now with the availability of so many different ethnic populations in the same region, or even in the same hospital, comparisons can be readily made within the same ward milieu, with the same staff, and with standardized rating instruments and laboratory procedures.

Culture, Pharmacology, and Mental Disorders

According to Webster's *Third New International Dictionary* (1986), culture is defined as

> a complex of typical behavior or standardized social characteristics peculiar to a specific group, occupation or profession, sex, age, grade, or social class. It is the body of customary beliefs, social forms, and material traits constituting the distinct tradition of a racial, religious, or social group.

Explaining the relationship between culture and psychopharmacology is a complex scientific task. Not only must psychosocial, educational, eco-nomic, and political factors be considered, but the effects of biological vari-ables, including genetic factors, customary dietary patterns, and the nutritional states of specific groups, must also be accounted for. Because the topic of culture and psychopharmacology is, in and of itself, a complex and formidable one, space limitations in this chapter makes it necessary to en-courage the reader to review publications devoted exclusively to the discipl-ine of culture and psychopharmacology (Itil 1976; Lin et al. 1986).

Differences in socioeconomic class have been found to be related to dif-ferences in patients' receiving appropriate psychiatric treatment as well as differences in attitudes of patients toward mental illness and their preference for pharmacotherapy instead of psychotherapy. If a patient's orientation to-ward mental illness is based on a genetic and neurochemical model, then pharmacotherapy will be viewed as an essential element in the treatment of mental illness. Without medication, such patients may feel they are not get-ting appropriate treatment for their mental illness. Therefore, it is important in the therapeutic contract to discuss and clarify what patients' expectations for therapy are. They must also be prepared for any side effects. If they are not, the side effects may be interpreted as indicating that the drugs are harming the body, and patients may discontinue medications unilaterally (Chien and Yamamoto 1982).

In a study of Southeast Asian refugees, Kinzie and colleagues (1987) found that, although there was no detectable tricyclic antidepressant in patients' blood, they nonetheless complained of drug side effects. This "reverse placebo effect" of patients' experiencing drug side effects without pharmacologic cause can be observed in a high proportion of Southeast Asian refugees.

There are a number of drug-related beliefs Asians often hold. For example, some Indochinese expect that medication is only for the acute phase of illness and to be used for a short time. When chronic maintenance medication is prescribed, patients may not continue the drug for fear either that they may become addicted to the medication or that long-term use of "chemicals" might harm the body (Kroll et al. 1990).

Herbal Medicines

Asians commonly hold the belief that Eastern herbal drugs, which are products of natural plants, are not as harmful or toxic as Western medicines are. Therefore, with the belief in the *yin-yang* balance of the universe and the body, some Asian patients may combine herbs with Western psychotropic drugs without telling their psychiatrists. The interactions of herbal and psychotropic drugs have not been well studied. But herbal drugs are likely to cause or to intensify side effects if they contain an atropine-like substance that is known to produce anticholinergic effects. Patients may also decrease the dosage of psychotropic drugs by themselves without obtaining the permission of or even talking with their treating physician. They may reduce the dosage, either combining the drugs with herbal medicines or not.

The traditional belief in Eastern herbal medicines, which consist of several herbs, have accustomed Asians to polypharmacy. Physicians in Japan, China, Korea, and Taiwan often practice polypharmacy and usually do not disclose the content of medicines to patients. The philosophy behind this practice is that, because they are mysterious, unknown drugs have more appeal to patients and therefore will be more therapeutic. In some Asian countries, drugs can be prepared and sold to patients by a physician right at the physician's clinic. Drugs in different kinds of tablets and colors are usually put together in a single package without any indication of the name of the drug or its strength, as is required in the United States. There is a traditional belief in

China and Japan that a good doctor is skillful in combining different kinds of drugs. Therefore, polypharmacy, which is discouraged in the United States, is widely practiced and accepted in Asia.

Western Drugs in Developing Nations

The availability of psychotropic drugs in developing nations has to do with economics. Choice of psychotropic drugs is limited, and those available may be in generic categories. Even in the United States, where many drugs (either generic or marketed under commercial names) are readily available and their quality is ostensibly tightly controlled by the Food and Drug Administration, the bioequivalence of generic drug and innovator's drugs is still a controversial matter (Ansbacher 1988; Carey 1989; Ingersoll 1989). The generic products manufactured in different countries or by different companies in the same country may not have the same bioequivalence because of a lack of a standardized quality control system. Therefore, the same dosage of generic drugs manufactured by different companies may result in different plasma levels and produce different levels of side effects.

Culture, Emotional Expressiveness, and Relapse Rate

The relapse rates of symptoms of schizophrenia and affective disorders have been reported to be significantly correlated with the degree of emotional expressiveness of the family members or significant others of the patients (Karno et al. 1987). High levels of expressed emotion (EE) were correlated with a higher relapse rate, whereas low EE levels were correlated with a lower relapse rate, even when the patients were not on medication. Karno and colleagues further reported that white American families tend to have the highest EE levels, followed by British families. The EE levels of Mexican American families are lower than either white American or British families. When a comparison of relapse rates was made among many cultures all over the world, it was found that the EE level of the patient's family may be an important factor (Lin and Kleinman 1988).

Ethnicity and Metabolic Variation

There are differences related to race in biological response to food and drugs. The inability to digest milk sugar (lactose) is one of the better-known conditions correlated with race. Groups that lack the enzyme lactase, which is needed to digest milk sugar, will experience bloating, flatulence, cramps, and diarrhea after drinking milk. Lactose intolerance has been reported in 94% of Asians, 90% of African blacks, 79% of American Indians, 75% of African Americans, 50% of Mexican Americans, and 15% of white Americans (Bose and Welsh 1973; Dill et al. 1972; Duncan and Scott 1972; Leichter and Lee 1971; McCracken 1971; Sowers and Winterfeldt 1975).

Tolerance of alcoholic beverages is also known to vary among ethnic groups. Alcohol is first oxidized to acetaldehyde by the alcohol dehydrogenase (ADH) enzyme, then acetaldehyde is oxidized to acetic acid by acetaldehyde dehydrogenase (ALDH; Stamatoyannopoulos et al. 1975). There are two variants of ADH enzyme. A high-activity variant converts alcohol to acetaldehyde quickly, whereas a low-activity variant converts it slowly (Kalow 1982). Those who have the high-activity ADH variant and who are also deficient in ALDH enzyme oxidize alcohol to acetaldehyde quickly. They then experience a long period of high blood acetaldehyde levels, because the breakdown of acetaldehyde is delayed because of their deficiency in the ALDH enzyme. A high plasma level of acetaldehyde induces many of the symptoms of alcohol intoxication, including facial flushing and certain psychomotor symptoms (Mizoi et al. 1979). Because of a deficiency in the ALDH enzyme, sizable numbers of Asians and American Indians experience a rapid onset but a slow decrease of blood acetaldehyde levels (Goedde et al. 1983), and they have a low tolerance to alcoholic intake.

A well-known beta-receptor blocker, propranolol, has been studied in Chinese and white populations (Zhou et al. 1989). It was found that although the Chinese subjects excreted propranolol faster than the white subjects, the effect on heart rate and blood pressure of low plasma levels of propranolol was significantly different in the two ethnic groups. Chinese subjects had lower blood pressure and a slower heartbeat than white subjects. Although these data provide some evidence that there are indeed variations in metabolic processes among different ethnic groups, whether this variation occurs with psychopharmacologic agents remains to be explored. The following section reviews the literature on ethnic differences in response to psychotropic drugs.

Neuroleptics

In earlier literature, Yamamoto and colleagues (1979) reported that the dosage of neuroleptics was generally lower for Asians than for whites. Lin and Finder (1983) also reported that the dosage for Asian patients was significantly lower than that given to white patients when the maximum dose and stabilized dose (discharge dose) were compared. Subjects for this study came from the acute psychiatric inpatient population at the Harbor-UCLA Medical Center, which serves metropolitan Los Angeles. The incidence of extrapyramidal side effects (EPS) did not differ significantly between the Asian and white populations, because the lower dosage was given to Asian patients in this study.

However, findings that conflicted with those of Lin and Finder (1983) have been reported by several investigators. Binder and Levy (1981) compared the neuroleptic dosages of a sample of Asian and white inpatients at the Langly Porter Neuropsychiatric Institute in San Francisco. They found no differences in neuroleptic dosage, yet a higher rate of EPS was observed among the Asians. At the Metropolitan State Hospital, Sramek and colleagues (1986) used the same method as Lin and Finder (1983) did. The researchers found no differences between Asians and whites in the maximum and stabilized dosages or in the EPS of the two groups.

In 1986, we conducted a study in Taiwan with the aim of comparing the dosages of neuroleptics being given to Taiwanese patients with those of white American and Asian American patients as reported by Lin and Finder (1983) and Sramek and colleagues (1986). We studied the maximum and stabilized dosage of three major psychiatric hospitals in Taiwan and found that the maximum and stabilized dosages for Chinese patients at those hospitals were about as high as the dosage for white patients in the United States (Chien and Lu 1987). Lu and I and our team (Lu et al. 1987) then compared the maximum and stabilized dosages of Asian, white, African American, and Hispanic inpatients at the San Francisco General Hospital. The overall comparison again showed no statistically significant difference among the four ethnic groups. However, when the study group was subdivided into the new immigrants—those who had been in the United States less than 5 years—and immigrants who had been in the United States longer than 5 years, both Asians and Hispanics showed significant differences when compared with whites and African Americans. A lower dosage was given to the new immigrants compared with the less recent immigrants.

The data from Metropolitan State Hospital, which Sramek and colleagues (1986) originally reported as showing no difference in the dosages of neuroleptics given to white patients and Asian patients, was reevaluated with length of stay (less than 5 years versus more than 5 years) as a new variable. Indeed, with this new variable, a statistically significant difference in dosage was found. As in the San Francisco General Hospital study by Lu and colleagues (1987), lower dosages were given to new immigrants. These findings are of special interest to clinicians, because no ethnic difference could be found when each ethnic group was studied as a whole, yet significant differences surfaced when length of stay in the United States was used as a discrete variable for statistical analysis. Obviously, the length of stay of immigrants deserves to be explored as a variable in future work.

Pi and colleagues (1986; Pi and Gray 1988) surveyed the neuroleptic dosages used in several Asian countries and found that dosages given to patients in Japan and Korea are equal to or even higher than dosages given to white patients in other countries. His findings are consistent with the findings of our 1986 survey in Taiwan (Chien and Lu 1987). These results point to the fact that the neuroleptic dosages given to patients in Asia now are much higher than those observed many years ago.

Questions Related to High Neuroleptic Dosage in Asia

The high neuroleptic dosages used in Asia poses interesting questions. Are Asians more tolerant of a higher dosage because their diet has become much more Westernized in recent years? Or is there no difference in the receptor sensitivity of Asians and whites? Are the EPS suppressed because the dosage is raised to a level that precludes the manifestation of EPS? Or has the practice of pharmacotherapy by Asian psychiatrists become Westernized? Are the neuroleptics used in Asia less potent than those used in the United States? These questions remain to be answered.

Although dosage surveys have resulted in conflicting and inconclusive findings, more objective evaluation has been possible with pharmacokinetic studies. Potkin and colleagues (1984) reported that schizophrenic Chinese patients had a 51% higher plasma level of haloperidol than non-Asian American schizophrenic patients (mostly whites) when both groups were given oral haloperidol in a dose of 0.15 mg per kilogram of body weight. In a study using nonschizophrenic control subjects, Lin and colleagues (1988a) also demonstrated that Asian American subjects had higher plasma levels of haloperidol and prolactin than white subjects when given the same oral dosage as used in the Potkin study. It is intriguing to note that recent Asian American immigrants in the study had a higher plasma level of haloperidol and prolactin than the American-born Asians.

However, when Lin and colleagues (1989) repeated the same study using a schizophrenic population instead of nonschizophrenic control subjects, they failed to show a significant difference in the plasma level of haloperidol between Asian and white subjects. In this study, the researchers concluded that although there was no difference in pharmacokinetics, a pharmacodynamic difference was demonstrated by Asians. This group had higher EPS scores than whites in the fixed-dose phase, in which both groups received 0.15 mg per kilogram of body weight per day. The dosage was then adjusted clinically at the neuroleptic threshold level at which each patient did not require anticholinergic medication and manifested minimal extrapyramidal symptoms. The optimal dose was also determined, which was the dose at the point of lowest total Brief Psychiatric Rating Scale (BPRS) score (Overall and Gorham 1962). With this clinically determined dosage manipulation, Lin and colleagues found Asians in their sample required only one-third to one-half of the dosage of white subjects, with a resultant serum concentration of haloperidol one-half that of the whites. There was no difference in EPS between the two groups when the Asian subjects received this low dosage.

Chang and colleagues (1987) studied the conversion rate of haloperidol to reduced haloperidol. They reported that the Chinese subjects in their study had a slower rate of conversion compared with the reported conversion rate for whites. The researchers attributed the slower conversion of haloperidol to the higher serum level of haloperidol observed in the Chinese subjects. This report is intriguing and should be replicated for two reasons. First, the conversion rates used in the study were not all evaluated by the same laboratory. To eliminate the possibility of introducing a confound into the data, conversion rates should all be evaluated by the same laboratory. Second, the positive correlation between clinical improvement and the ratio of reduced haloperidol to haloperidol reported in this study (Chang et al. 1987) would suggest that either the greater the level of reduced haloperidol, the more the patient improved, or the lower the level of serum haloperidol, the more the patient improved. Because reduced haloperidol has been considered to be of less therapeutic potency than haloperidol, the findings of Chang and colleagues are difficult to explain.

In conclusion, the findings of dosage comparisons of Asian and white patients by American or international studies are inconsistent. In recent surveys, Asians in the United States or abroad were found to have received the same dosage as whites. This finding suggests that there may be an increase in the neuroleptic dosage given to Asian patients, whereas the contrary might be the case for the dosage for white patients.

The pharmacokinetic comparisons of Asians with whites have been limited primarily to studies of haloperidol, because it produces a simple metabolite (i.e., reduced haloperidol). Moreover, there are only a few such studies. The research of Potkin and colleagues (1984) and Lin's research (Lin et al. 1988a) is the most representative in this field. Lin's data, when normal subjects were used, were consistent with those reported in the Potkin study. However, Lin's subsequent study (Lin et al. 1989) using schizophrenic patients as study subjects revealed findings inconsistent with those of the Potkin team. More studies are needed that use larger samples representative of the population of patients using haloperidol.

Antidepressants

Yamashita and Asano (1979) surveyed the tricyclic antidepressant dosages used for patients in 10 Asian countries and reported that daily dosages ranged from 75 mg to 150 mg, which is about one-half of what white American patients received. Although the low dosage used for Asians suggests low tolerance by this ethnic group, more data on the plasma level of tricyclic antidepressants such as clomipramine, desipramine, and nortriptyline have been reported successively for interethnic comparison. Allen and colleagues (1977) reported higher clomipramine plasma levels in East Asian (Pakistani and Indian) male volunteers than in male British volunteers after both groups had been given single doses of either 25 mg or 50 mg of clomipramine on two separate occasions.

Rudorfer and colleagues (1984) reported that plasma clearance of desipramine among Chinese control subjects was significantly slower than in their white counterparts when both groups had been given a single 100-mg oral dose of desipramine. The researchers found a trimodal distribution of desipramine clearance among the study subjects (i.e., there were low-, intermediate-, and high-clearance groups). The white subjects were all in the intermediate- to high-clearance groups and the Chinese were all in the low- to intermediate-clearance groups. This finding should be taken as a caveat that sample bias may influence the outcome depending on whether the study subjects are drawn from the low- or high-clearance groups.

Kishimoto and Hollister (1984) compared the pharmacokinetics of nortriptyline in Japanese Americans and white Americans. The Japanese American subjects showed significantly higher area under the curve (AUC; 1,150 ng × hr/ml) compared with the white Americans (730 mg × hr/ml), even though the Japanese subjects received only 50 mg of desipramine while the white subjects received 75 mg. There was essentially no significant difference between the two groups in elimination half-life, clearance, or volume of distribution, although Kishimoto and Hollister found that Asians reached peak serum concentration significantly faster than whites. Pi and colleagues (1989) repeated the study with only minor modification of the methodology.

The researchers again found no difference between the two groups except that the *white* subjects reached peak serum concentration *faster* than the Chinese subjects. They also found some trend toward trimodal distribution in serum concentration as had been reported by Rudorfer and colleagues (1984).

Gaviria and colleagues (1986) studied the pharmacokinetics of nortriptyline in Hispanic and white American control subjects. These volunteers were given a single oral dose of 75 mg of nortriptyline. The researchers did not find significant differences between the two ethnic groups, although they did find large interindividual differences. They postulated that pharmacodynamic differences rather than pharmacokinetic differences could be attributed to the previous reports of hypersensitivity in Hispanics.

In conclusion, despite the objectivity of pharmacokinetic measurement, reports from investigators in this field are not consistent. All the studies used tricyclic antidepressants; monoamine oxidase inhibitors (MAOIs) were not used in any systematic controlled studies. Despite earlier reports conducted on the basis of dosage comparison, there has been a shift toward plasma level and pharmacokinetic comparison that did not consistently support the hypothesis that Asians require less tricyclic antidepressants, although some studies suggested such a trend. Perhaps larger sample sizes are needed so that representative numbers of slow, intermediate, and fast drug excreters are included to eliminate sample bias.

The data from control subject samples should not be readily compared with data from depressive patients because of the difference in tolerance to psychopharmacological drugs between control subjects and psychotic patients as observed in clinical practice. The same doses of a psychotropic drug given to a person who does not have a mental illness and to a severely psychotic patient usually result in different tolerances; greater sedation and more side effects are experienced by control subjects. Clinically, a higher dosage is often administered to sicker patients, and the dosage is usually decreased as the patients improve. It is therefore desirable that, in the future, patient samples be used if such findings are to be applied to clinical practice.

Antianxiety Agents

Studies in this field are scarce and mostly focus on benzodiazepines. The clinical dosage surveys and comparisons between Asian and white subjects are weak and inconclusive. But the pharmacokinetic studies by Ghoneim and colleagues (1981) and Lin and colleagues (1988b) provide examples of very useful ethnic comparisons of antianxiety agents. Ghoneim and colleagues (1981) used diazepam for 12 white and 13 Asian volunteer control subjects and measured the kinetic variables. The researchers found significant differences between the two ethnic groups, with Asians showing slower total body clearance, a smaller volume of distribution, and higher serum levels of diazepam and its metabolite, desmethyldiazepam. Although the Asians seemed to be slow excreters of the drug, there was no difference in the level of sedation noted.

Lin and colleagues (1988b) compared the pharmacokinetics of alprazolam in 28 Asian control subjects (14 foreign-born and 14 American-born) and 14 white control subjects. Alprazolam was administered both orally and intravenously to all subjects. The researchers found a higher peak concentration of plasma alprazolam (C max) and a greater AUC in both groups of Asian subjects compared with the white subjects. Even adjustment to the body surface area was made by covarying the AUC, but the statistical significance still remained for po-C max and iv-AUC. However, the pharmacokinetic parameters for the two Asian subject groups stayed essentially the same. The latter finding is of special interest because of the difference found between these two Asian groups when neuroleptic (i.e., haloperidol) pharmacokinetics were studied by Lin and colleagues using the same laboratory. This finding may suggest, for clinical purposes, that new Asian immigrants might be more intolerant of neuroleptics than American-born Asians. However, the tolerance of these two groups was the same when they were both given benzodiazepines. This example indicates that ethnic findings for one drug category cannot be generalized to another drug category, and thus justifies a review of the ethnic variations for all psychotropic drug categories, as I have attempted in this chapter.

In conclusion, studies of antianxiety agents were limited only to benzodiazepines. Diazepam and alprazolam were used in interethnic comparisons of subjects, revealing slower elimination by Asian control subjects than by their white counterparts. Although the limited number of studies suggest lower doses of benzodiazepines are required by Asians, more studies are needed using clinical samples before a definite conclusion can be drawn.

Lithium

The need for special attention to ethnic differences during lithium treatment was aroused by the report of Takahashi and colleagues (Takahashi

1979; Takahashi et al. 1975). The researchers claimed that nearly 70% of manic patients in a study conducted in Japan responded to lithium when the plasma level was below 0.86 mEq/l, whereas no patients responded at such a level in a Veterans Administration collaborative study conducted in the United States primarily with white patients. As for treatment of depression, Japanese patients responded to lithium at 0.41 mEq/l, whereas U.S. patients required a plasma level higher than 0.7 mEq/l. Takahashi (1979) concluded, "Japanese patients require a lesser amount of lithium carbonate for the same degree of efficacy and respond to a lower serum lithium level than their U.S. counterparts" (p. 35).

However, this issue was debated in a symposium entitled "Transcultural Psychopharmacology in Depression: East and West." Prien (1979) questioned whether the patient selection criteria, the major clinical efficacy, and the adverse reactions were comparable in Japanese and American studies. Basing his remarks on Honda's report, Prien expressed doubt that there was a pharmacokinetic difference between the two ethnic groups (Honda and Suzuki 1979). He further commented that the absence of standardized evaluation scales measuring side effects and clinical efficacy across cultures, coupled with a lack of basic dose-response studies in the United States, made it difficult to interpret the Takahashi team's findings.

Six years later, Chang and colleagues (1985) reported on the pharmacokinetics of lithium response in 22 Taiwanese and 30 white patients diagnosed with bipolar disorder. After each subject was given a single oral dose of 900 mg of lithium carbonate, the researchers found essentially no difference in any of the kinetic parameters calculated for the two ethnic groups.

Healthy Afro-Caribbean and white male volunteers were compared by Shelley (1987) using a study design similar to that of Chang and colleagues (1985). Shelley found no significant differences between these two ethnic groups in terms of either pharmacokinetics or side effects. It is regrettable that he did not examine the red blood count (RBC)/serum lithium ratio between African Americans and whites (Chang et al. 1984; Okpaku et al. 1980; Ostrow et al. 1986; Trevisan et al. 1984).

Yang and colleagues (1989) also reported on the pharmacokinetics of a single oral dose of 900 mg of lithium carbonate given to each of 22 manic Taiwanese Chinese patients. The researchers compared their data with that of Danish researchers and concluded that there was no statistically significant difference in lithium pharmacokinetics between Danish and Taiwanese subject groups (Nielsen-Kudsk and Amidsen 1979). Because lithium carbonate is excreted through the kidneys and not through the liver, where various enzymes can affect the metabolism of neuroleptics, antidepressants, and antianxiety agents, the findings so far indicate that the mechanism for eliminating salts such as lithium and sodium might be the same among different ethnic groups. As to why different clinical dosages have been used in different cultures, more studies are needed to clarify whether psychosocial parameters such as tolerance and acceptability of manic-depressive behavior and drug side effects differ among cultures, and/or whether biological parameters such as pharmacodynamics—receptor sensitivity differ among various ethnic groups. As Prien (1979) pointed out, more data are needed for basic dose-response studies in different ethnic populations.

In summary, lithium carbonate is the only psychotropic agent for which there is clearly no pharmacokinetic distinction between Asians and whites. This is probably because its elimination is via the kidneys and not the liver, as liver metabolism involves many enzymes. Dosage differences, if any, might be due to psychosocial factors rather than pharmacokinetic factors. As to the pharmacodynamic difference (receptor sensitivity), more data based on systematic controlled studies are needed before a conclusion can be made.

Conclusion

This review of the literature revealed inconsistent and conflicting reports in dosage surveys and pharmacokinetic studies of neuroleptics used to treat Asian and white patients. Some conflicting results have been found in the pharmacokinetic studies of tricyclic antidepressants. There have been relatively few studies of antianxiety agents, and these have been primarily of benzodiazepines. However, the latter reports are consistent in demonstrating pharmacokinetic differences between Asians and whites. The pharmacokinetics of lithium carbonate, which is excreted through the kidneys and not subject to liver metabolism, seem to be similar for Asians and whites.

The notion that Asians require a lower dosage of psychotropic drugs than whites cannot at this point be supported unequivocally for all four major categories of psychotropic drugs except benzodiazepines, which still need more confirming clinical studies. In future ethnopsychopharmacology studies, larger samples of subjects, preferably from patient populations, must be used to allow adequate representation of subjects who are slow, intermediate, or fast excreters.

The discipline of ethnopsychopharmacology is still in its pioneer phase. With the availability of standardized pharmacokinetic measurement, more objective information should soon be available in this exciting field. Meanwhile, clinicians are advised to take a prudent approach and to provide individually tailored dosages for their patients, irrespective of those patients' racial or ethnic backgrounds.

References

Allen JJ, Rack PH, Vaddadi KS: Differences in the effects of clomipramine on English and Asian volunteers; preliminary report on a pilot study. Postgrad Med J 53(suppl 4):79–86, 1977

Ansbacher R: Generic drugs: bioequivalence and bioavailability. JAMA 259(2):220, 1988

Binder RL, Levy R: Extrapyramidal reactions in Asians. Am J Psychiatry 26:1320–1322, 1981

Bose D, Welsh J: Lactose malabsorption in Oklahoma Indian. Am J Clin Nutr 26:1320–1322, 1973

Carey J: How far has the cancer spread at the FDA? Business Week, Sept. 18, 1989, pp 30–31

Chang SS, Pandey GN, Zhang M, et al: Racial difference in plasma and RBC lithium levels. Paper resented at the 137th annual meeting of the American Psychiatric Association, Los Angeles, CA, May 7–11, 1984

Chang SS, Pandy GN, Yang YY, et al: Lithium pharmacokinetics: interracial comparison. Paper resented at the 138th annual meeting of the American Psychiatric Association, Dallas, TX, May 19–24, 1985

Chang WH, Chen TY, Lee CF, et al: Low plasma reduced haloperidol/haloperidol ratios in Chinese patients. Biol Psychiatry 22:1406–1408, 1987

Chien CP, Lu FG: Ethnopsychopharmacology. Proceedings of the 3rd biennial meeting of the Pacific Rim College of Psychiatrists, Tokyo, April 1987

Chien CP, Yamamoto J: Asian American and Pacific Islander patients, in Effective Psychotherapy for Low-Income and Minority Patients. Edited by Acosta FX, Yamamoto J, Evans LA. New York, Plenum, 1982, pp 117–146

Dill J, Levy M, Wells RF: Lactase deficiency in Mexican-American males. Am J Clin Nutr 25:869–870, 1972

Duncan I, Scott E: Lactose intolerance in Alaskan Indians and Eskimos. Am J Clin Nutr 25:867–868, 1972

Gardner RW, Robey B, Smith PC: Asian Americans: growth, change, and diversity. Population Bulletin 40(4):5, 1985

Gaviria M, Gil AA, Javaid JI: Nortriptyline kinetics in Hispanic and Anglo subjects. J Clin Psychopharmacol 6:227–231, 1986

Ghoneim MM, Korttila K, Chiang CK, et al: Diazepam effects and kinetics in Caucasians and Orientals. Clin Pharmacol Ther 29:749–756, 1981

Goedde H, Agarwal DP, Harada S: Population genetic studies on aldehyde dehydrogenase isozyme deficiency and alcohol sensitivity. Am J Hum Genet 35:769–772, 1983

Honda Y, Suzuki T: Transcultural pharmacokinetic study on Li concentration in plasma and saliva. Psychopharmacol Bull 15(4):37–39, 1979

Ingersoll B: FDA finds problems at 10 of 12 firms being probed in generic-drug scandal. Wall Street Journal, September 12, 1989

Itil TM (ed): Transcultural Neuropsychopharmacology. Istanbul, HZI Neuropsychiatric Foundation, 1976

Kalow W: The metabolism of xenobiotics in different populations. Can J Physiol Pharmacol 60:1–9, 1982

Karno M, Jenkins JH, de la Selva A, et al: Expressed emotion and schizophrenic outcome among Mexican-American families. J Nerv Ment Dis 175(3):143–151, 1987

Kinzie JD, Leung P, Boehnlein JK, et al: Antidepressant blood levels in Southeast Asians: clinical and cultural implications. J Nerv Ment Dis 175:480–485, 1987

Kishimoto A, Hollister LE: Nortriptyline kinetics in Japanese and Americans (letter). J Clin Psychopharmacol 4:171–172, 1984

Kroll J, Linde P, Habenicht M: Medication compliance, antidepressant blood levels and side effects in Southeast Asian patients. J Clin Psychopharmacol 10:279–282, 1990

Leichter J, Lee M: Lactose intolerance in Canadian west coast Indians. American Journal of Digestive Diseases 16(6):809–813, 1971

Lin KM, Finder E: Neuroleptic dosage in Asians. Am J Psychiatry 140:490–491, 1983

Lin KM, Kleinman AM: Psychopathology and clinical course of schizophrenia: a cross-cultural perspective. Schizophr Bull 14:555–567, 1988

Lin KM, Poland R, Lesser I: Ethnicity and psychopharmacology. Cult Med Psychiatry 10:151–165, 1986

Lin KM, Poland RE, Lau JK, et al: Haloperidol and prolactin concentrations in Asians and Caucasians. J Clin Psychopharmacol 8:195–201, 1988a

Lin KM, Lau JK, Smith R, et al: Comparison of alprazolam plasma levels and behavioral effects in normal Asian and Caucasian male volunteers. Psychopharmacology (Berlin) 96:365–369, 1988b

Lin KM, Poland RE, Nuccio I, et al: A longitudinal assessment of haloperidol doses and serum concentrations in Asian and Caucasian schizophrenic patients. Am J Psychiatry 146(10):1307–1311, 1989

Lu FG, Chien CP, Heming G, et al: Ethnicity and neuroleptic drug dosage. Poster presented at the annual meeting of the American Psychiatric Association, Chicago, IL, May 12, 1987

McCracken R: Lactase deficiency: an example of dietary evolution. Current Anthropology 12(4–5):479–517, 1971

Mizoi Y, Ijiri I, Patsuno Y: Relationship between facial flushing and blood acetaldehyde levels after alcohol intake. Pharmacol Biochem Behav 10:303–311, 1979

Nielsen-Kudsk F, Amidsen A: Analysis of the pharmacokinetics of lithium in man. Eur J Clin Pharmacol 16:271–277, 1979

Okpaku S, Frazer A, Mendels J: A pilot study of racial differences in erythrocyte lithium transport. Am J Psychiatry 137:120–121, 1980

Ostrow DG, Dorus W, Okonek A, et al: The effect of alcoholism on membrane lithium transport. J Clin Psychiatry 47:350–353, 1986

Overall JE, Gorham DR: The Brief Psychiatric Rating Scale. Psychol Rep 10:799–812, 1962

Owan TC, Bliatout B, Lin KM, et al: Southeast Asian Mental Health: Treatment, Prevention, Services, Training and Research. Rockville, MD, National Institute of Mental Health, 1985

Pi EH, Gray GE: Psychopharmacology: A cross-cultural perspective on Asian-Caucasian differences. Paper presented at the 4th scientific meeting of the Pacific Rim College of Psychiatrists, Hong Kong, December 4–8, 1988

Pi EH, Jain A, Simpson GM: Review and survey of different prescribing practices in Asia, in Biological Psychiatry, 1985. Edited by Shagaas C. New York, Elsevier, 1986, pp 1536–1538

Pi EH, Tran-Johnson TK, Walker NR, et al: Pharmacokinetics of desipramine in Asian and Caucasian volunteers. Psychopharmacol Bull 25(3):483–487, 1989

Potkin SG, Shen Y, Pardes H, et al: Haloperidol concentration elevated in Chinese patients. Psychiatry Res 12:167–172, 1984

Prien RF: Discussion, in Transcultural psychopharmacology in depression: East and West. Psychopharmacol Bull 15(4):35, 1979

Rudorfer MV, Lan EA, Chang WH, et al: Desipramine pharmacokinetics in Chinese and Caucasian volunteers. Br J Clin Pharmacol 17:433–440, 1984

Shelley RK: Are there ethnic differences in lithium pharmacokinetics and side-effects? Int Clin Psychopharmacol 2:237–342, 1987

Sowers M, Winterfeldt E: Lactose intolerance among Mexican Americans. Am J Clin Nutr 28:704–705, 1975

Sramek JJ, Sayles MA, Simpson GM: Neuroleptic dosage for Asians: a failure to replicate. Am J Psychiatry 143:535–536, 1986

Stamatoyannopoulos G, Chen S, Fukui M: Liver alcohol dehydrogenase in Japanese: high population frequency of atypical form and its possible role in alcohol sensitivity. Am J Hum Genet 27:789–796, 1975

Takahashi R: Lithium treatment in affective disorders: therapeutic plasma level. Psychopharmacol Bull 15:32–35, 1979

Takahashi R, Sakuma A, Ito K, et al: Comparison of the efficacy of lithium carbonate and chlorpromazine in mania: report of The Collaborative Study Group on Treatment of Mania in Japan. Arch Gen Psychiatry 32:1310–1318, 1975

Trevisan M, Ostrow D, Cooper RS, et al: Sex and race differences in sodium-lithium counter-transport and red cell sodium concentration. Am J Epidemiol 120:537–541, 1984

Webster's Third New International Dictionary. Chicago, IL, Merriam-Webster Inc., 1986, p 552

Yamamoto J, Fung D, Lo S, et al: Psychopharmacology for Asian American and Pacific

Islanders. Psychopharmacol Bull 15:29–31, 1979

Yamashita I, Asano Y: Tricyclic antidepressants: therapeutic plasma level. Psychopharmacol Bull 15(4):40–41, 1979

Yang YY, Yeh EK, Chang SS, et al: Maintenance lithium levels could be lowered: based on Taiwanese and Danish studies. Journal of the Formosan Medical Association 90(5):509–513, 1991

Zhou HH, Koshakji RP, Silberstein DJ: Racial difference in drug response. N Engl J Med 320(9):565–570, 1989

15 Psychiatric Care of Mexican Americans

Cervando Martinez, Jr., M.D.

Mexican Americans are this country's second largest ethnic minority, numbering about 13.3 million people (1990 U.S. census projection), but for various reasons, their achievements are usually unrecognized and they are sometimes misunderstood. Most live in the Southwestern United States away from the centers of communication, money, and power. They tend to be poor, not very well educated, and generally disenfranchised. The history of Mexican Americans distinguishes them in several ways from other Hispanics—Puerto Ricans, Cubans, and other Latin Americans.

First, there is a history of war between Mexico and the United States. This war, considered unjust by many, was motivated by American avarice and resulted in the acquisition of most of the Southwest, a territory occupied at the time by Spaniards and by Mexican and American Indian peoples of the Southwest. There followed years of fighting, stealing, chicanery, and strife between those called "Anglos"* and the people of Mexican and Spanish descent in the Southwest. The strife has continued into the present and still raises its ugly head occasionally.

The modern conflict has taken many forms: struggles between unions and business owners, job discrimination, immigration restrictions and crackdowns, school segregation, and electoral disenfranchisement (Montejano 1987). (An outline of the history of Mexican American immigration is presented in Table 18–11.) For example, unionizing efforts in Southwestern states have been directed primarily at Mexican Americans in low-paying jobs. In California, the effort to unionize the farm workers led by Cesar Chavez was long and arduous. During the 1950s, the copper mine workers in southern Arizona went through this process. In the 1940s, the pecan shellers of San Antonio, led by Emma Tenayuca, received national attention. Workplace discrimination in the Southwest has largely involved Mexican Americans.

---

*In many parts of the Southwest, the term "Anglo" is used to describe all white people, with the full realization that not all whites are Anglo Americans.

American Indians and African Americans have also experienced this injustice, among others; but because Mexican Americans are the largest minority in the Southwest, they have faced the brunt of the problem there.

The countless dilemmas of immigration in the United States seem to take on the form of a Gordian knot. These dilemmas have primarily involved Mexicans in this century and will probably do so into the next. There have been many waves of immigration from Mexico during times of revolution or economic crisis in Mexico and during periods of economic boom or war in the United States. These have usually been followed by efforts to stem the flow of immigrants—in the past, through deportations and other repressive measures, and more recently, by the complex mechanisms of the Simpson-Rodino Immigration Law. There are conflicting opinions about whether the present law has slowed immigration. But no one expects immigration, in either direction, to become much less than what it is now: the most central experience in the lives of many Mexican Americans.

Segregation in the Southwest included the establishment of separate schools for Mexican American children. This official practice continued through the 1960s and 1970s and has left a heritage of barely literate generations, underfunded school districts, and high dropout rates. For Mexican Americans, voting strength, the essence of democracy, has been watered down, circumvented, or frankly attacked by means of poll taxes, gerrymandering, and at-large elections. In this context, it is important to recall that the majority of Mexican Americans, although descendants of immigrants in many cases, are not themselves foreign born.

Although Mexican Americans and Anglos have lived side by side in the Southwest for generations, there remains a residue of distrust from the years of frank conflict. Because there are few African Americans in the Southwest, racism has often manifested itself as antagonism toward Mexican Americans. Thus, some Mexican Americans feel a complex ambivalence toward Anglos because of this history of war, conflict, discrimination, and racism. Other Mexican Americans (perhaps more accurately called Mexicans living in the United States) who have arrived more recently may not have this historically derived attitude. But having been raised in Mexico, they may have been similarly influenced by that country's national attitude toward the United States: admiring the *gringo* and resenting him as well. Unlike Puerto Ricans, thousands of Mexicans in the United States never become American citizens. They travel frequently to Mexico and retain their Mexicanness in the United States. Unlike Cuban Americans, Mexican Americans can return to their native or ancestral land almost at will. The border between the United States and Mexico is 2,000 porous miles long, with an incalculable number of crossings, legal and illegal, being made every day.

Mexican Americans are a heterogeneous group found throughout the country and concentrated in the Southwest and Chicago. The largest number live in Los Angeles and Chicago. The diversity of Mexican Americans may obscure their similarities, but the characteristics they hold in common are powerful ones and have particular relevance to psychiatric care.

The vast majority of Hispanics in the Southwest consider themselves to be, and are, of Mexican origin. However, in New Mexico and elsewhere, many Hispanics trace their lineage to the Spanish colonists and eschew the term "Mexican." These two different concepts of identity have political, sociocultural, and economic roots in Mexico's history. At the time of the conquest by Cortés and the Spaniards in the 16th century, Mexico had an enormous indigenous population that had developed a complex and refined culture and had built wondrous cities. Bernal Díaz del Castillo, one of Cortés' men, described Mexico (Tenochtitlán) the capital of the Aztec empire, thus:

> During the morning we arrived at a broad Causeway and continued our march towards Iztapalapa, and when we saw so many cities and villages built in the water and other great towns on dry land and that straight and level Causeway going towards Mexico, we were amazed and said that it was like the enchantments they tell of in the legend of Amadis, on account of the great towers and cues and buildings rising from the water, and all built of masonry. And some of our soldiers even asked whether the things we saw were not a dream. (Díaz del Castillo 1956, pp. 190–191)

Although at the time of the conquest the Aztec empire was dominant, many other Mexican civilizations had existed, risen in influence, and eventually declined. Some, like the Mayas, extended to what is now Central America. The Olmecs, Mayas, Toltecs, and others built monumental city-states, elaborated complex religious systems, encoded their ideas in glyphs, measured time, and in many other ways contributed to the rich and elaborate indigenous culture that the Spaniards encountered. The Spaniards, of course, brought with them their own powerful traditions. Strongly Catholic and imbued with a conquering spirit fresh from the successful struggle to expel the Moors from Spain, they came to subjugate and to convert. The Spaniards triumphed, at least on the surface; but unlike what occurred in the United States, the Indian presence in Mexico was not removed. Instead, it was absorbed and incorporated.

> The Christianity brought to Mexico by the Spaniards was the syncretic Catholicism of Rome, which had assimilated the pagan gods, turning them into saints

and devils. The phenomenon was repeated in Mexico: the idols were baptized, and in popular Mexican Catholicism the old beliefs and divinities are still present, barely hidden under the veneer of Christianity. Not only the popular religion of Mexico but the Mexican's entire life is steeped in Indian culture—the family, love, friendship, attitudes toward one's father and mother, popular legends, the forms of civility and life in common. The image of authority and political power, the vision of death and sex, work and festivity. Mexico is the most Spanish country in Latin America; at the same time it is the most Indian. Meso-American civilization died a violent death, but Mexico is Mexico thanks to the Indian presence. (Paz 1979, p. 140)

During the colonial period, settlement, exploration and exploitation, intermarriage, and expansion continued. Missions and forts were established in the more sparsely populated, harsher Northern provinces and in these regions there resulted an isolation from the essentially Indian Mexico, both culturally and politically. But the Spanish colonists in Northern Mexico encountered another native population: the North American Indian tribes. In some areas this confluence resulted in amalgams of peoples and cultures. Later, the Spanish Mexicans encountered a third group: the westward-moving Anglos. During the Texas war for independence from Mexico, many Spanish Mexican Texans fought on the side of Texas and later served with distinction in government and commercial life. In other parts of the Southwest, many of the descendants of the Spanish Mexican settlers stayed after the Southwest territory was taken by the United States. Because of this history, their descendants do not feel particularly connected to Mexico.

In the late 18th century, generations of *criollos* (people born in Mexico but of Spanish parents) began to seek a Mexican identity and independence from Spain. The father of Mexican independence, Miguel Hidalgo, was a *criollo* priest. In the early 19th century, the struggle for Mexican independence from Spain continued. In the next 50 years, this struggle included the campaign against the Texans, the war with the United States, occupation of a weakened Mexico by foreign troops (the French), and finally, an externally imposed emperor, Maximilian.

After the French were driven out, Benito Juárez, a Oaxacan Indian lawyer and supreme court justice, became president and instituted far-reaching political changes intended principally to separate church and state and ensure stability and self-government. During the second half of the 19th century, Mexico was governed by Porfirio Díaz, a former Juárez general who maintained power and permitted foreign exploitation and development of his country's resources. Great fortunes were amassed (unfortunately, most of them in the United States) while in rural Mexico the landless (*peóns*) were tied to enormous self-sufficient ranches (*haciendas*). Migration to the United States was stimulated by the *hacienda* system and other economic factors.

The Mexican revolution of 1910 was driven by various forces. Zapata and his followers in the South had an almost messianic desire for land. Others also fought against the cruelty and injustice of the old system, or for a new form of government, for glory, or for their own self-interest. The present quasi-democratic, single-dominant-party system evolved in the 1930s.

At the beginning of the 20th century, Mexico had a largely rural population dominated by a peonage system. The country was sprinkled with colonial, European-style cities of some wealth and governed by an authoritarian government supported in the background by a still powerful Catholic hierarchy. The revolution upset this order, and it had repercussions in the United States, mainly in the form of an almost continuous migration of the poor, displaced, or frightened seeking to escape the economic turbulence and war of the next decade. The system that eventually evolved in Mexico has not been successful in effective land distribution or fair economic development; great inequality of wealth and opportunity has persisted, further stimulating migration.

Thus, at least in this century, the story of Mexican Americans in the United States has been closely tied to occurrences in Mexico and to the resulting migrations back and forth. Furthermore, to understand the social and cultural conditions of Mexican Americans, one must have an understanding of parallel conditions in Mexico.

In Mexico, high levels of illiteracy and minimal education have persisted, especially among the rural poor. Although immigrants to the United States have been from all social classes, the majority have been from poorer, often rural areas. Life in such communities today can be a tense mixture of the traditional and modern existing side by side: Someone from a small Mexican town that still has no running water and relies on agriculture can see the world through television and listen to its music with a Sony Walkman. The poorer Mexican states and the Northern ones provide many of the immigrants to the United States. They come across the border to seek a better life or for adventure; they are imbued with the work ethic, are law-abiding, and generally do not depend on governmental programs. Many return to Mexico with a nest egg or simply to be with their families. The movement back and forth across the border is enormous, creating problems of hardship and separation, but also serving as the mechanism for the infusion of Mexican and Latin culture into the United States and for the reverse diffusion of American culture into Mexico. In fact, the border region has been viewed by some as a unique bilingual, bicultural zone of increasing economic and political importance to both nations (Fernandez 1977).

Early Studies, Modern Implications

There has been a considerable amount of research on people of Mexican origin in the United States, particularly if the fields of sociology, anthropology, education, and psychology are included in addition to psychiatry. Critical reviews of much of this work exist (Vaca 1969). Some of these studies and reports date back to the 1930s and are not reviewed here in depth; however, some of the issues they dealt with are still highly relevant.

The first of these issues has to do with the educational and academic achievement of Mexican American children. Several of these early studies focused on the lower scores of Mexican American children on IQ tests given in English and attempted to explain these scores on the basis of theories of genetic inferiority, social factors (poorer schools, less English fluency), or cultural values that were not conducive to higher achievement. This issue of lower educational accomplishment remains important and controversial to this day.

Although the mean level of education of Mexican Americans has increased since the 1930s, it remains considerably below that of Anglos (8 versus 12 years). Also, the dropout rate among Mexican American school children is unacceptably high. Some estimates peg it as high as 40% between the first and twelfth grades, although admittedly this is a difficult phenomenon to measure accurately. The problem remains an issue for obvious reasons of equity and fairness. But it is also relevant because it is apparent that as the population of Mexican origin in the Southwest grows (and it is the fastest growing of the ethnic groups), it behooves these states to ensure that this group not have large pockets of poor, undereducated, undertrained members who would constitute a potential underclass that could put an economic drag on their communities.

Bilingual education remains a contentious issue and has been one of the factors motivating the "English-only" movement. However, bilingual education, a product of the 1960s and 1970s, arose as a reaction to discriminatory practices such as separate schools for Mexicans and Anglos, punishment for the use of Spanish in school, and the shunting en masse of Mexican children into technical or vocational rather than academic programs. Furthermore, Spanish-language use, especially in the Southwest, has been and probably will be tenacious. Literally thousands of children of Mexican origin, even those whose parents and grandparents were born in the United States, continue learning Spanish first in the home.

Thus, the challenge of providing a school environment where children who are poor and not fluent in English can thrive educationally will remain. Besides inadequate educational programs, there are two other proposed explanations for the academic underachievement of Mexican Americans: genetic inferiority and cultural orientation. The former no longer receives much support, at least openly, although from time to time the issue still arises. The latter remains a controversial and commonly used explanation for poor achievement. Indeed, the study of the culture of Mexican Americans has been ongoing and relates directly to issues in psychiatric care, as I discuss later.

The study of the culture of Mexican Americans has also led to controversy because many scholars, particularly Mexican Americans, have thought that much of this work presents stereotypes and is reductionistic (Montiel 1973). The work on the cultural characteristics of individuals and families has been based, to some extent, on Mexican writers describing aspects of the Mexican national character (Paz 1961; Ramos 1962). Their analysis, using an historical-psychoanalytic frame of reference, has attempted to explain certain commonly observed Mexican traits in terms of the country's history. These and other writers emphasized several aspects of Mexican history that they believed contributed to characterological developments: the conquest and subjugation of the Indian population of Mexico by the Spaniards, and later, the large-scale intermarriage of the two peoples resulting in a *mestizo* people (mixture); the persistence of national female deities—Tonantzin for the Indians and Guadalupe since colonial times; and the history of conquest by war and economic dependence on the United States. These and many other historical and cultural developments are thought (by Ramos, for example) to contribute to a Mexican sense of inferiority and its compensatory mechanisms. Paz sees the Mexican male (*macho*) as a closed, defensive figure whose sense of masculinity can be easily threatened.

> The Mexican whether young or old, *criollo* or *mestizo,* general or laborer or lawyer, seems to me to be a person who shuts himself away to protect himself: his face is a mask and so is his smile. In his harsh solitude, which is both barbed and courteous, everything serves him as a defense: silence and words, politeness and disdain, irony and resignation. . . . (Paz 1961, p. 29)

Paz goes on to explain the historic origins for the Mexican life views exalting resignation, stoicism, and indifference toward suffering. Two of

Mexico's greatest heroes, Juárez and Cuauhtemoc, are legendary partly because of this. Paz's rich analysis of Mexico leads him to conclude that the Mexican female ideal also has certain distinct characteristics.

> Despite her modesty and the vigilance of society, woman is always vulnerable. Her social situation—as the repository of honor, in the Spanish sense—and the misfortune of her "open" anatomy expose her to all kinds of dangers, against which neither personal morality nor masculine protection is sufficient. She is submissive and open by nature. But, through a compensation mechanism that is easily explained, her natural frailty is made a virtue and the myth of the long-suffering Mexican woman is created. (Paz 1961, p. 38)

The following Mexican family pattern has been described as the dominant one: the unquestioned supremacy of the father and the self-sacrifice of the mother (Diaz-Guerrero 1955). Diaz-Guerrero also points out the sharply delineated sex-role expectations and their everyday manifestations. For example, young boys are raised to be aggressive, girls submissive; adolescent boys court an idealized woman who is not necessarily considered a sexual object and simultaneously seek out other women for sexual gratification; the woman is traditionally raised to be self-sacrificing. Diaz-Guerrero presents epidemiologic results (albeit crude ones by today's standards but yet strikingly prescient ones) that conclude that the Mexican woman, as a result of these role pressures, has a greater tendency to report more nervousness, depression, and other symptoms of distress.

These and other astute observations about Mexican individual and family characteristics should not be too readily dismissed. They are certainly generalizations, and one can always point to many exceptions: not all Latin men are strutting *machos*, and not all women are martyrs. The individual and family observations of Mexican Americans grew out of these Mexican reports and can be similarly criticized: they describe a rural individual or family, whereas most modern Mexican Americans are urban; many exceptions exist; Mexican Americans are not homogeneous. However, despite these criticisms, it is important to take these generalizations into account because, although it is true that both Mexico and the Southwestern United States are rapidly modernizing and its people (especially the younger generations) are becoming acculturated, very strong residues of these values and traits remain, especially in older or recently arrived individuals and families. (An outline of cohort experiences of Mexican American elders is presented in Table 18–12.) If nothing else, this can result in intergenerational value conflict, as has been described for Cuban Americans (Szapocznik et al. 1978).

Conflict between persistent traditional values and more modern values in individuals and families may be responsible for individual and family psychopathology. For example, a Mexican American woman in her 30s who was raised as a child in rural Mexico and is married to a childhood sweetheart may now find herself living in Los Angeles and aspiring to work outside the home. She may be raising "modern" teenagers and facing other life choices and problems whose resolution conflicts with her traditional values. Depressed mood, even depressive disorder, tension and somatization, and other problems, may ensue.

Modern Studies, Early Implications

The recent and more strictly psychiatric studies of Mexican Americans build upon earlier themes and issues. The former interest in exploring whether differences in academic achievement are explainable by genetic factors, by problems in the system, or by culturally mediated processes led to a similar, decades-long series of works on the underutilization of mental health services by Mexican Americans and its attendant explanations. The rich studies on Mexican character and Mexican American cultural values directly and indirectly led to a search for differences in the expression and prevalence of psychopathology—differences that could be explained by culturally determined patterns in male/female expected role behavior and family dynamics.

Underutilization of Mental Health Services

More than 30 years ago, Jaco (1960) observed that Mexican Americans were underrepresented in psychiatric treatment facilities in Texas. His findings were confirmed by others in different areas (Bachrach 1975), and this has remained a consistent finding into the present (Hough et al. 1987). However, it has been observed that this underusage phenomenon disappears in smaller communities where the proportion of Mexican Americans is much greater, such as the border city of Laredo, where close to 90% of the population is Mexican American (Trevino et al. 1979). Nevertheless, because the majority of Mexican Americans live in large cities (with Los Angeles having the largest concentration of people of Mexican descent outside of Mexico City), the problem of utilization remains of concern.

To explain this underusage of mental health facilities, the following hypotheses have been explored (Karno 1966).

1. Mexican Americans experience the same or almost the same rates of mental disorders as Anglos do. But there are institutional and other barriers to their access to services, such as discriminatory practices, lack of money, and seemingly more pressing life problems.
2. Mexican Americans seek help for mental disorders, as well as other problems, from alternative providers, such as general medical practitioners, priests, folk healers, or health care providers in Mexico.
3. Mexican Americans have a lower incidence and prevalence of the disorders that come under treatment in the psychiatric facilities. This hypothesis has three corollaries:
   a. Mexican Americans perceive mental disorders differently and thus present themselves to treatment less often.
   b. There is something about the family and social structure of Mexican Americans that may buffer or protect an individual against stress and mental illness, and people with mental illnesses are also better accommodated or supported in their social milieu.
   c. Mental disorders express themselves differently and are responded to differently among Mexican Americans.

Prevalence of Psychiatric Disorders

The epidemiologic question about whether Mexican Americans have different rates of mental disorders is a complex one (Roberts 1987). Logic may dictate that a group undergoing marked social stresses (migration and separation, language accommodation, and socioeconomic disadvantage relative to the dominant culture) would consequently experience higher rates of certain stress-related disorders. However, it also appears as though the Mexican American family and social structure provide a relatively supportive, buffering environment (Griffith 1984; Keefe 1979), thus neutralizing some of the stress effects. The relationship between the acculturation process and the development of psychopathology has also been difficult to disentangle.

Several hypotheses have been put forth:

1. That the less acculturated experience more stress and hence more disorder because they are not equipped to deal with the new culture (Fabrega et al. 1968);
2. That the more acculturated and more Anglicized experience more stress and dysfunction because of alienation from, and loss of, the supportive "mother" culture (Graves 1967); and

3. That there is a curvilinear relation between acculturation and mental health (i.e., that those bicultural individuals who have integrated both sets of values are at least risk for mental disorder).

The most definitive work bearing on the question of prevalence of mental disorders among Mexican Americans is the Los Angeles part of the Epidemiologic Catchment Area (ECA) study (Karno et al. 1987). The group conducting this study examined the relationship of acculturation, mental disorder, and immigrant status and found that *higher* acculturation was associated with higher lifetime rates of phobia, alcohol abuse/dependence, and drug abuse/dependence (Burnam et al. 1987). There were also striking differences in rates of disorders among native-born compared with immigrant Mexican Americans. The immigrants had lower rates of the above disorders as well as of two affective disorders and anxiety disorder. When the immigrants alone were examined for acculturation and mental disorder, it was found that those who were more acculturated differed from the less acculturated only in having more drug abuse or dependence—presumably an effect of the dominant Los Angeles culture where the highest national rates of drug abuse or dependence were found.

Thus, we find little support for a stress-related model of mental disorders, at least when immigration is considered the stressor. Instead, the findings seem to support the notion that those who immigrate may be the more adaptable or robust, and with time (and acculturation), changes occur that may result in higher rates of certain disorders. As the immigrant is first exposed to the new culture, the use of drugs rises, especially in men. This may be because of the more extensive exposure to drugs that occurs in the United States; reports about drug use in Mexico indicate very low prevalence, except in certain border cities.

With a longer stay in the United States and with greater acculturation, Mexican American men in particular may be prone to heavy drinking, whereas Mexican American women may become symptomatic with anxiety and depression. Fabrega and colleagues (1967) demonstrated in clinical studies that Mexican men and women express internal distress differently: the men by excessive drinking and perhaps aggressive behavior, the women more directly through depression and anxiety. The almost prescient description by Madsen (1964) of the "alcoholic *agringado*" is likewise supported by the contemporary ECA study. He described *agringados* in south Texas: men who had become like *gringos,* deserting their culture and its traditions and values and as a result finding meaninglessness and alienation.

It must also be pointed out that the Mexican immigrant in the United

States is usually relatively better off financially than his or her peer left behind in Mexico. Most Mexican immigrants to the United States come to work, because they believe they can make a better living in the United States. Many also do not come with the idea of staying forever but merely of saving money and returning home. Thus, the stress model of mental illness may apply better to Mexican Americans who have been in this country longer and who, because of more long-term goal frustration, develop problems.

In addition to the higher rate of alcohol abuse/dependence in Mexican American men, the ECA study (Karno et al. 1987) found a very high rate of current phobia in Mexican American women over age 40 and a higher rate of cognitive impairment in general among Mexican Americans than in non-Hispanic whites. The latter finding is probably explained by the fact that cognitive impairment was measured with the Mini-Mental State Exam (Folstein et al. 1975), a procedure vulnerable to bias from language, education, and cultural factors. The differential rate of phobic disorders in older Mexican American women has not been completely explained, but it may be a different manifestation of an underlying problem that affects both Mexican American men and women: they have traditional values but must live in a modern society.

Also in accord with previous work (Katon et al. 1982), the ECA group reported a relationship between somatization symptoms (not necessarily somatoform disorder) and dysthymic and depressive disorders, especially in older Mexican American women (Escobar 1987).

Barriers

Explanations for underusage of mental health facilities by Mexican Americans other than that of lower prevalence of disorders have not been extensively explored. Several hypotheses to explain the lower admission rates for patients with psychotic illness have been advanced. One of these focuses on cultural factors. The Mexican American family provides a more supportive, tolerant environment, thus either protecting its members from stress and illness or, if the illness prevalence is indeed the same, tolerating the disordered behavior longer. In either case, the result is less—or delayed—hospitalization. Such complex cultural influences are difficult to disentangle by focused research, although some attempts to do so have been made. Several investigators have examined whether Mexican American patients who are mentally ill are more seriously ill at the time of admission into the treatment system than their non-Hispanic white counterparts (Cuellar and Roberts 1984). Other investigators report that, compared with mainstream

American patients, Mexican American patients have a significantly more negative view of psychiatric hospitalization and treatment (Lawson 1982).

The question of how Mexican Americans perceive and respond to mental illness is likewise a complex one and is related to the question of perception of health and illness in general. Karno and associates concluded that there are significant differences between Mexican Americans and Anglos in how mental illness is defined, explained, and dealt with (Edgerton and Karno 1971; Karno and Edgerton 1969). In the researchers' studies using clinical vignettes and involving surveys of community residents, Mexican Americans tended to define mental illness in more traditional "illness" terms and to see it consequently as a medical problem subject to psychiatric intervention. Karno and Edgerton also divided their Mexican American respondents according to the language of the interview, assuming that Spanish preference signified a more traditional, less-acculturated orientation. Sharp differences were found between the two groups: the more traditional Mexican Americans, as predicted, held more conservative views about mental illness. They were more likely to believe in the inheritance of mental illness, in the benefit of prayer in treatment, and in the protective role of the family in the care of the mentally ill. The Mexican Americans who responded to the survey in Spanish were more likely to favor family care, in addition to psychiatric treatment, for seriously mentally ill people, as opposed to care outside the home.

It has also been fairly well demonstrated that Mexican Americans, particularly the less acculturated, are able to maintain both folk and "modern" concepts of disease causation and treatment and that their health-seeking behavior (use of medical practitioners versus use of folk healers) for what is considered a physical disorder is guided by this understanding. Thus, if the symptom pattern suggests to them a folk disease (e.g., *susto* or magical fright), the first recourse may be a healer; if the clinical condition suggests modern treatment, this is sought. There are, of course, ambiguous conditions, some of which may be attributed by lay people to "modern" illness (e.g., psychosis), some to a folk explanation (e.g., *susto*), and some to willful misconduct (e.g., substance abuse). Other conditions may not necessarily be seen as abnormal, such as personality disorders or adjustment disorder.

Clinical Considerations

Conducting clinical work with Mexican Americans, particularly those who speak limited English and are not acculturated, can be difficult and challenging. The patient's limited English (and often the therapist's limited

Spanish) may cause both to decide not to enter into treatment; or they may do so, but halfheartedly and with negative expectations. As I discuss in the next section, language need not present an insurmountable barrier. However, even assuming adequate language compatibility, there are additional social and cultural considerations that should be kept in mind. Many of these issues have not been documented by rigorous research and probably never will be; these observations are based on the anecdotal evidence of clinicians and others. Not all Mexican Americans will present with similar cultural dynamics, but I contend that even the most acculturated will be dealing with some of these issues and concerns, although at different levels. The more traditional, less acculturated patient will still be embedded in his or her family, religion, and language of origin. At the other extreme, the acculturated Mexican American may not be so culturally grounded and may have left these roots behind; but he or she may therefore have to deal with this lack and its resulting effects, particularly on self-identity and relationships with parents and children.

There are many aspects of Mexican and Mexican American culture such as cuisine, social customs, and the arts that impinge only indirectly, if at all, on the clinical situation. Most of these characteristics contribute in a global, cumulative fashion to the person's sense of cultural and ethnic identity. In the past, things Mexican were usually not held in high esteem by much of the dominant Anglo society. As a result, many Mexican Americans experienced ambivalence toward and conscious rejection of parts of their culture. To avoid this disapproval some parents, with great effort, stopped teaching their children Spanish (Rodriguez 1980).

Some customs may have subtle clinical relevance. The formality built into the Spanish language, which has formal and informal pronouns and verbs, carries over into social relations. For example, the *usted* form of address is formal and is used with older persons or with peers whom one does not know well. This form of address may be changed to an informal form (*tú*) by mutual tacit agreement. Generally, however, it is considered improper to address a person in a professional relationship by the informal form unless the person is a child or an adolescent. Thus, in a clinical situation, it is advisable to address older Mexican American patients as Mr., Miss, or Mrs. (*señor, señorita,* or *señora*).

Also, culturally relative beliefs concerning respect and honor may be strongly held by many Mexican Americans, particularly ones with more traditional values. Showing respect, particularly for elders and persons of authority, is something that is considered very important; any lack of it, actual or perceived, may be cause for apology. Honor, which can be violated by social indiscretions, involves the self and family and if compromised may be the source of considerable torment and guilt, as the following case illustrates.

Case Study 1

H. L. is a 28-year-old mother of three who is from a small rural community in northern Mexico and is being treated for a recurrent depressive disorder. She improved after coming to treatment and after she had become more comfortable, she brought up a new complaint: a persistent lack of sexual pleasure. She associated this difficulty to having been raped as a teenager by an older man and to the resulting response of her parents. As she recalls, they had felt that the honor of the family was harmed by this occurrence. Mrs. L. felt blamed for this and eventually felt forced to leave the community to compensate for this dishonor.

Other problem areas affected by culture include family relations. Particularly in couples where traditional, more restrictive role definitions are maintained, considerable conflict may occur. The most common clinical situation involves the traditional man married to a woman who feels overrestricted and is struggling for greater equality. There may be considerable emotional conflict caused by such situations affecting both the woman and the man. This and other clinical problems were examined in an interesting study of clinicians who were surveyed regarding the kind of cultural situations encountered in their practice (Lopez and Hernandez 1987). When working with Hispanic patients (presumably mainly Mexican Americans, because the study was done in California), these therapists reported marital conflicts, gang related behavior, psychosis, and alcohol use as having significant cultural components. These results conform to the areas that have been reported in the literature and in personal communication from other clinicians.

Language

Most Mexican Americans speak two languages with varying degrees of fluency. Depending upon where they live in the United States, their fluency in either language will vary greatly. In some areas there will be Mexican Americans who speak no Spanish and in other areas those who speak no English, but the majority will speak both. The group who speak no Spanish will be larger the greater the distance from the border, because of intermarriage and assimilation, especially of the young. But there are many young

Mexican Americans—multigenerational citizens of the United States—who still learn Spanish first and grow up bilingual. Likewise, monolingual Spanish speakers are either recent arrivals from Mexico or older people who, although American born, have lived insular lives in a *barrio*.

The quality of the Spanish bilingual Mexican Americans speak is often good. There is the mistaken idea that people who are bilingual do not speak either language well. Especially along the border, the Spanish spoken is very much like Mexican Spanish, but there is a great deal of mixing of the two languages at many levels. English words have been converted to Spanish (car to *carro*, watch to *watchar*) and are used both formally and as slang. The same process, of course, has been going on for hundreds of years in the Southwest, where Spanish and Indian words have been incorporated into English. In daily discourse, the two languages are often used in a mixture of words, sentence fragments, and phrases that linguists call code switching.

This movement back and forth from language to language takes many forms and is multidetermined. In daily conversation, these fluctuations are determined subconsciously, often for convenience and speed: "*dame el chart*" (give me the chart) is said instead of "*dame el expediente*," because chart is a better-known term and easier to say than *expediente*. At other times, particularly in clinical situations, the choice of language will be determined by dynamic factors (Rozensky and Gomez 1983). A predominantly Spanish-speaking patient, when being interviewed by an English-speaking psychiatrist, may resist speaking in English. This resistance may be just that—an attempt to avoid dealing with painful issues—or it may reflect repeated frustrations and/or fatigue. However, during the course of an interview, especially a family session, a patient's switching to one language or the other may be an attempt to conceal feelings or deceive the therapist or a family member. Moreover, the second language may be used as a device for avoiding feelings. In the analytic literature, there are case reports of patients who during analysis are able to access certain memories and affects only in the native language.

The question of whether there is more or less psychopathology expressed in the native language or the second language in bilingual Hispanics has been of considerable theoretical and practical interest. The original reports (Del Castillo 1970) indicated that bilingual patients expressed less psychopathology in the second language (English), perhaps because the effort involved in speaking it suppressed the expression of symptoms. However, subsequent studies (Marcos et al. 1973) demonstrated the opposite with bilingual Hispanic schizophrenic patients. They demonstrated more psychopathology when attempting to communicate in English, the language in which they were less fluent. These authors point out that the process of speaking in a language of less fluency results in seeming disturbances of organization and integration of thought that can be interpreted as manifestations of a thought disorder. Finally, in a study specifically with bilingual Mexican American schizophrenic patients, it was found that significantly more psychopathology was expressed during the Spanish-language interview (Price and Cuellar 1981). It was further concluded that the wider the discrepancy in a patient's verbal fluency in English and Spanish and the more he or she fluctuates from a balance bicultural status, the more likely it is that language will have an effect on the expression of psychopathology and diagnosis.

In situations where a Spanish monolingual patient has to be evaluated by an English-speaking psychiatrist, an interpreter may be the only recourse. However, interpreters interject another level of complexity into the diagnostic process, which may result in distortion, omission, and errors. These can be minimized by proper training and debriefing (Marcos 1979).

As has already been pointed out, there is a small but significant minority of Mexican Americans who are monolingual in Spanish or strongly Spanish-language dominant. The majority are bilingual with varying degrees of fluency. Although most of the clinical language issues are similar to those described previously for Spanish-dominant Hispanic patients, other questions are relevant for bilingual patients. For example, in a true bilingual person, is psychopathology expressed equally in both languages? What are the significance and meaning of language switching? Are certain memories and feelings more accessible in one language or the other? Answers to these questions are not available or perhaps even possible, but they do arise frequently when working with the spectrum of bilingual Mexican American patients.

Religion

Religion affects the lives of Mexican Americans in profound and paradoxical ways. The Mexican religious historical experience has been a complex and tumultuous one. The indigenous population had highly systematized and pervasive religious systems before the arrival of the *conquistadores*. The Spaniards conquered for gold and religious conversion, though which of the two took precedence is a matter of great debate. The resulting clash and then amalgamation of the two cultures (particularly their religious elements during the next 200 years) occurred in a political context that included the equally complex history of the Mexican Catholic church, which had great wealth and power. The prolonged struggle for independence by the Mexican republic included the necessity of stripping the church of its power. This in turn led to further armed struggle (the Cristeros war) in this century.

A strongly Catholic people, an officially outlawed but still influential church, and a secular government have been at a standoff until the present. From this background we have Mexican Americans in the United States, still predominantly Catholic in affiliation, imbued with Mexican Catholic images, symbols, and beliefs during their development, and living in communities where the church has a strong presence in arenas outside the purely religious (i.e., education, politics, and human services). Furthermore, in both the United States and Mexico, the influence of nondenominational evangelical groups is rising and has particular clinical significance.

Consideration of a Mexican American patient's religious life is an important part of complete care and management (Bach-y-Rita 1982). There are many ways in which religious life can assume significant clinical relevance. One of the most common is the situation where a patient, raised in the church and believing in the importance of its practices, has fallen away from religion. In psychiatric patients, this dislocation from the church has usually occurred during the course of the illness for one or more of several reasons. The patient may have been involved in substance abuse or had troublesome interpersonal relations, including divorce. The patient may have thought, said, or done self-defined blasphemous acts or just not had time to remain concerned and dedicated to the demands of the church. Often a patient feels that because of these or other indiscretions, the church no longer wants or will accept him or her.

If the patient is still religious, as rehabilitation occurs, attention should be given to assisting him or her in becoming involved in church life once more. After assessment of the patient's previous religious life (including baptism, education, communion, and attendance at confession) and present orientation (alienated, but interested is the usual stance encountered), specific recommendations can be made. These may be coupled with interventions to reduce resistance, usually due to guilt about past transgressions. The use of a pastoral counselor may be particularly useful at this point, because this person can speak as a representative of the church and can appreciate the patient's clinical condition as well. The relieving of guilt for past behavior by confession, the rejoining of the familylike environment of a parish, and the resumption of the self-enhancing influence of prayer can result in improvement in the quality of life of the psychiatric patient.

Mexican Catholic religious references are often characteristic of the thought content of many patients, particularly references to the Virgen de

Guadalupe, the patron saint of Mexico and a ubiquitous presence in Mexican and Mexican American life. There is one well-known element of the legend of her appearance to an Indian in the 16th century that psychiatric patients have sometimes strongly identified with. The Virgen de Guadalupe is believed to have appeared to Juan Diego who then informed the Bishop of Mexico City, but the latter did not believe the Indian man's story. So, the dark-skinned saint then had to send her mantle with its imprinted image of her as proof. The saint's message not being believed by the Spanish authority may resonate with the life experiences and personal dynamics of some patients who may feel they have not been listened to, understood, or believed.

Psychotic and obsessional patients may incorporate elements of cultural myths, legends, and beliefs into their thought content. For example, the Guadalupe legend and occasionally another Mexican legend, *La Llorona* (the crying woman), are laden with dynamic possibilities that some women may identify with. The latter is the legend of a woman who kills her children and then wanders the streets at night crying (*llorando*).

The non-Catholic evangelical churches are growing rapidly in many parts of the Southwest and present an interesting dilemma. They establish themselves among the poorest of the poor and are successful in attracting many recently immigrated families, to whom they provide an accepting, supportive, familylike environment. However, because of their fundamentalist views, these congregations are extremely intolerant of deviant behavior, reject and ostracize nonconforming members, and can espouse beliefs that are against Western medicine. There are some like the successful system of churches in Texas founded by a former heroin addict, Jimmy Garcia, whose sole mission is to the addict and his or her family.

In closing this section on religion, I would like to mention the repeatedly observed epidemiologic phenomenon of a significantly lower risk of suicide among Mexican Americans. Although it is important to note that there are major problems in drawing conclusions from suicide data, Hoppe and Martin (1986) and Sorenson and Golding (1988) report lower rates of completed and attempted suicide and lower rates of suicidal ideation among Mexican Americans. Hoppe and Martin (1986), in their study of rates of completed suicides, noted a rise from the 1970s to the 1980s among Mexican American women equal to a rise for non-Hispanic white woman, but with lower overall rates for Mexican Americans. Sorenson and Golding (1988) examined community rates of suicidal ideation and suicide attempts using Los Angeles ECA data (Karno et al. 1987). Although documenting significantly lower rates of both in this community sample, the researchers could not identify strong correlations with immigrant status and acculturation.

One hypothesis to explain the lower rates is that Mexican Americans have a relatively intact and functional social structure. There is a great deal of data to support this hypothesis, including the facts that there are proportionally fewer single women with children and more families living with parents. However, another relevant cultural factor may be one often observed clinically. When a depressed Mexican American patient who has contemplated suicide is asked what kept him or her from proceeding with the contemplated action, a very common response is "I know it is a sin and God would punish me."

Folk Medical Beliefs and *Curanderismo*

The roles of the folk system of health beliefs and folk healers (*curanderos*) in Mexican American health care have been controversial. There have been repeated observations by clinicians (Gomez and Gomez 1985; Ripley 1986; Stenger-Castro 1978) of the roles played by this system in the health-seeking behavior of their patients. They report that a large number of their patients attribute some symptom patterns to folk illnesses and consequently seek the services of a folk healer, the *curandero* or *curandera*. The two most common folk illnesses with direct psychiatric implications are *susto* (magical fright or soul loss) and *mal puesto* (hex).

Soul loss has been described throughout the Americas in different manifestations and presents as a state of agitation, anxiety, increased startle, insomnia, anorexia, excessive worry, and fear (Rubel 1978). Both the family and the afflicted person can usually identify a specific fear-inspiring occurrence (e.g., being surprised and frightened by a snake) that triggered the reaction. Once the folk diagnosis is made, the ill person is taken to a *curandero*. This healer provides a ritual intended to summon the soul back to the body, because soul loss, occurring at the time of the frightening experience, is considered the underlying causative mechanism. It is not known how commonly the condition is believed to occur among Mexican Americans in the United States. It is reported in almost all anecdotal accounts of current folk-medical behavior, but its exact clinical implications are not known. Presumably many of the occurrences represent transient episodes; but it is not known, for example, whether there is a subpopulation of Mexican Americans (the ECA-reported phobic group) who are chronically anxious but who have been categorized by the folk system as having *susto* and are treated largely in that system or are untreated.

Mal puesto means a hex placed on someone, usually because of jealousy. The hex can result in any kind of misfortune to the victim, and most "cases" probably do not come to any medical attention. However, it has been the experience of some psychiatric clinicians (Stenger-Castro 1978) that, if explored carefully, a Mexican American patient's history may often reflect significant experience with this folk illness. The most common way that *mal puesto* may present is illustrated by the following case.

Case Study 2

A. R. is a 24-year-old Mexican American single man who was seen in the outpatient clinic after hospitalization for persistent psychotic symptoms. He reported that all his life he had felt "threatened" by others and consequently had been an aloof, guarded, and suspicious person. Yet he had progressed in school, graduated from high school, and worked in various blue-collar jobs until 4 years previously, when he gradually developed auditory and visual hallucinations. He described hearing a lion telling him that he was going to die and also thought that God was speaking through him. He also began to see shadows and objects out of the corner of his eyes. He eventually became more and more agitated, believed that the messages he was receiving from the radio were real. One day Mr. R. left his parent's home abruptly and went to the river downtown with the intention of drowning himself. However, his parents followed him, brought him home, calmed him, and shortly thereafter took him to the first of his visits with a *curandero*.

His parents thought that he had a hex placed upon him by a girl whom he had briefly dated several years before and who had called him afterward but toward whom Mr. R. had not responded with interest. It was their belief that she had asked a witch (*bruja*) to place the hex on Mr. R. through a picture he had given her because she was jealous of his new girlfriend.

Mr. R. saw the *curandero,* a middle-aged man, five or six times, and his condition improved. He said, "As I got to trust him, I felt better and went back to work." During their visits, the *curandero* asked Mr. R. questions, applied some oils, and recited prayers. He contrasted the *curandero's* questions with those in the psychiatric interview and remarked that many more were asked in the latter even though it was itself brief. After returning to work, however, Mr. R.'s visits to the *curandero* ceased and, after several weeks, his symptoms worsened. He returned to the *curandero* once more, but his symptoms persisted and he was brought instead to the hospital.

In this case the emerging psychotic illness is attributed by the family at first to a folk illness, and the services of a folk healer were sought. The *curandero's* suggestive, supportive, and religiously based treatment produced some temporary relief in a young man who felt a sense of trust, support, and understanding. Because his delusional and hallucinatory symptoms had religious elements, it is not surprising that he felt comfortable with the *curandero*'s religious healing techniques (prayers, use of holy palm, incantations). Eventually, as A. R.'s psychosis continued, assistance was sought in the scientific mental health care system.

It should be repeated that Mexican Americans may use both folk and scientific medical explanatory systems to explain illness. In the case of a clearly physical disorder (fever and vomiting) that has an unclear etiology, a folk explanation and treatment may supersede the scientific. In the case of a clearly organic illness such as a fracture, where the etiology is obvious, the reverse will occur. However, in cases where the cause is not at all clear as in a psychosis, the first resort may be to the folk healer and may be continuous, with a search for a supernatural etiology (hex) and cure. Often both systems are used concurrently for psychiatric disorders; but a clinician may not be aware of this, unless he or she explores the question carefully with patient and family.

There have been seemingly conflicting reports about how much folk healers are used by Mexican Americans. Clinicians, including nurses, pediatricians, and psychiatrists, note that the folk belief system and *curanderos* figure prominently in their patients' health-related behavior (Gonzalez-Swafford and Gutierrez 1983; Martinez 1977). On the other hand, epidemiologists examining a healthy community sample are not impressed by the percentage of their subjects who report the use of *curanderos*—usually under 10% (Edgerton et al. 1978; Sugarek 1984). It should be noted that the epidemiologists do not benefit from the greater trust and openness that are usually characteristic of doctor-patient relationships. However, there is agreement that the folk system exists and that it represents an aspect of Mexican American life with psychiatric implications. The same system has been described extensively in Mexico and throughout Latin America.

Treatment Considerations

The psychiatric treatment of Mexican Americans presents several challenges and opportunities. Because they are the largest ethnic minority in some Western cities (Los Angeles, Denver) and are a majority in others (Albuquerque, San Antonio), private and public health care professionals should be interested in accessible and appropriate services. Some psychiatric institutions in the Southwest have attempted to address this problem by developing special programs for Mexican American patients.

Program Adaptations

There are several adaptations that can be made so that psychiatric programs are more accessible to Mexican Americans. Which adaptation is implemented depends on the degree of interest of the institution, the resources available, and, to some extent, the size of the Mexican American population served. The first of these is simply the hiring of Spanish-speaking mental health professionals so that, at a minimum, an accurate initial assessment can be made and appropriate treatment provided. In some facilities, there may only be one clinician who is proficient in Spanish and this person may treat most of the Hispanic patients, particularly those not fluent in English. However, other programs may want to assemble a more substantial number of Spanish-speaking professionals and organize them and others into a special program for their Mexican American or Spanish-speaking patients (Heiman et al. 1975). In some communities there may not be a sufficiently large pool of Mexican American mental health professionals for this purpose; as a result, people from other Latin countries or Spain will be hired. Furthermore, except for a few cities in the Southwest (e.g., San Antonio), most cities with large numbers of Mexican Americans also have large numbers of people from the rest of Latin America, particularly Central America. Thus, the common factors between staff and patients will be language and Latin culture.

Under such conditions, some difficulties may ensue. Even though the staff are from Latin America, they may not be familiar with the nuances and details of Mexican and Mexican American culture and how it affects behavior. The Mexican American patients may initially respond hesitantly, even to fellow Latinos, because of educational and social-class differences. However, these and other problems are relatively minor compared with the issue of language. Moreover, even the availability of Mexican American professionals may not guarantee ideal cross-cultural communication between patients and staff. For example, staff members' language fluency may be less than ideal, and they may be fairly acculturated and thus not very responsive to the needs of a much less acculturated patient. A case in point would be a young acculturated Hispanic professional woman who may not fully appreciate the intensity of the dilemma and conflict experienced by a similarly young but less-acculturated Mexican woman in the United States who is torn between working outside the home, caring for her children, and attending to her husband's and family's traditional expectations. Similarly, a Mexican American male professional may not appreciate parallel issues in his women patients but also may not understand the traditional Mexican American man's emphasis on respect and masculine role functions and activities.

The configuration or assignment of Hispanic staff within an institution is also important. In some circumstances, enough Spanish-speaking staff are available at all levels of care. However, many facilities may not have this luxury and may want to develop a Hispanic, Latino, Mexican American, or Spanish-speaking component. In hospitals, these components have taken the form of special Latino or Hispanic units (Dolgin et al. 1987). Not only are most if not all of the staff and patients on such a unit Hispanic, but the milieu is *Hispanicized*. The physical environment is decorated and arranged with a Latin touch. The importance of the Hispanic family as a source of support is appreciated, and special efforts are made to involve the relevant members in decision making. Staff training for treatment team members on such a unit would include a special emphasis on other cultural elements that affect patient care.

These units for Hispanics have been developed in several different types of institutions. Some have been organized in state hospitals as 24-hour units (San Antonio, Pueblo) or as day programs (St. Elizabeth's). Other programs are 24-hour units in general hospitals, such as the Latino Unit at the San Francisco General Hospital (A. G. Lopez, E. Carrillo, E. Pierantoni, et al., unpublished data, November 1990). In some outpatient clinics, a Spanish-speaking clinic, component, or team has been developed. The method of referral of patients to these units may vary. Some units treat all Hispanic patients in the institution regardless of clinical condition, language use, or level of acculturation; others, such as the Bilingual-Bicultural Unit at the San Antonio State Hospital, accept patients only after acute treatment and stabilization and select only the more Spanish-dominant and unacculturated. In this institution, more than half of the patients are Mexican American.

Some institutions may be unable or unwilling to hire Latino professionals and may instead choose to use interpreters. The use of interpreters for psychiatric treatment and evaluation may seem intuitively inappropriate. However, Acosta and Cristo (1981) demonstrated the usefulness of interpreters in a program they developed in a large outpatient clinic, where a cadre of community residents was trained to serve as interpreters for the professional staff. Growth occurred in the number of Spanish-speaking patients attending the clinic, and follow-up evaluation revealed that the patients, contrary to the therapist's expectations, felt adequately helped and understood.

There are other issues and problems involved in delivering services adequately to Mexican Americans. Geographic accessibility is important for obvious reasons. Many Mexican Americans are poor and use public transportation. In some communities there is a great reluctance to travel, even by car, outside the perimeters of familiar, usually Mexican, neighborhoods. Printed materials used in clinics should be in Spanish and English. A session orienting a patient to the clinic and to the types of problems treated may be especially useful (Acosta et al. 1980). Similarly, clinical staff can receive specific orientation to their patients' sociocultural needs in order to enhance their effectiveness. Such an orientation program has been shown to be effective in improving staff knowledge, sensitivity, and effectiveness in their work with patients (Acosta et al. 1982).

Psychotherapy

In individual therapy with Mexican Americans, several specific issues and problems recur. To begin with, there are specific issues involving language that are of interest in conducting dynamic psychotherapy. As I mentioned earlier, the work of Marcos and colleagues (e.g., Marcos et al. 1973) has been important in understanding the role of language in evaluating psychopathology in Spanish-dominant bilingual patients. The implications of these findings to psychotherapy have also been elucidated (Marcos 1976). The language barrier is described as having a detachment effect so that emotionally charged material is verbalized without display of the expected or accompanying emotion. Therefore, the abreactive or cathartic process is more difficult and problematic. A second outcome of the detachment effect, especially in obsessional patients, may be a reinforcement of obsessive defense mechanisms resulting clinically in preoccupation with diction, the use of cliches, and other avoidances. Third, Marcos repeats what others have observed: in the bilingual's intrapsychic world, there can be certain threatening or emotionally charged areas originally encoded in the first language that can only be revealed in the safer second language.

Although the work of Marcos and colleagues was with non-Mexican–Hispanic bilingual patients, its results appear to have usefulness for other bilingual patients, particularly those that learned Spanish first and then English. It should be kept in mind, however, that Mexican American bilinguals can be roughly divided into two groups: those born in Mexico who migrate to the United States in childhood or later, and those born in the United States who learned Spanish relatively simultaneously with English. The implications drawn from the Marcos study may apply only to the former, more Spanish-dominant group of bilingual Mexican Americans, because these are probably more similar to the Spanish-dominant Hispanic patients he described.

Because Mexican Americans tend to be overrepresented among the poor and published reports about psychotherapy with Mexican Americans are more likely to be based on observations made in public clinics, descriptions of psychotherapy with Mexican Americans emphasize issues relevant to all low-income patients. These observations include the fact that somatization is common: specific help for social problems is sought; symptomatic relief is expected; and directive therapies are considered particularly useful (Boulette 1976). However, other studies of Mexican Americans in psychotherapy have reported that they have preconceived notions about psychotherapy very similar to those of Anglos (Acosta 1979).

Acosta and his colleagues have also developed some additional therapy guidelines for work with Mexican Americans (Acosta et al. 1982). They recommend that therapists provide "substantial expressions of friendliness and encouragement" (p. 68) so that their Mexican American patients will find it easier to discuss their feelings and problems. The reason for this is to attempt to overcome the normal reticence that a Mexican American, especially one who is not very fluent in English, may have upon initiating therapy with a non-Latino therapist. The concept of *personalismo* has been used to describe the Latin tendency to seek the personal touch, the small informality. This Latin quality coexists paradoxically with the need for formality described previously. It is also suggested that therapists make special efforts to have Mexican American patients express disagreement with them. This suggestion is based on the observation that many Mexican Americans still adhere to traditional values that call for unquestioned acceptance of authority, or at least outward acquiescence. This may result in a tendency to want to take a passive role in therapy rather than a more collaborative one. This attitude may be welcome at first, because it may result in better compliance; however, in the long term, it is probably better that the therapist attempt to develop a more balanced therapist-patient relationship.

Any techniques used in therapy should be tailored specifically to the individual patient. A given Mexican American patient can fall anywhere on the continua of acculturation, language preference, and psychopathology; therefore, general guidelines such as those given here need to be used judiciously and selectively. For example, it would not make sense to treat an overly shy, English-dominant, acculturated Mexican American with too much *personalismo*. Sue and Zane (1987) in a very thoughtful review of this problem have described the conundrum thus:

> Perhaps the most difficult issue confronting the mental health field is the role of culture and cultural techniques in psychotherapy. We believe that cultural knowledge and techniques generated by this knowledge are frequently applied

in inappropriate ways. The problem is especially apparent when therapists and others act on insufficient knowledge or overgeneralize what they have learned about culturally dissimilar groups. (p. 38)

Similar observations can be made about group psychotherapy with Mexican Americans. It has been recognized that group therapy can be an effective modality for Spanish-speaking patients, especially those from working-class backgrounds, particularly if certain modifications in therapy are made (Normand et al. 1974; Olarte and Masnik 1985). These include flexibility in scheduling and attendance, a more directive educational approach, provision of assistance with social problems and medication needs, and judicious use of therapist self-disclosure. Biweekly meetings may be better attended than weekly ones, because they would fit better into patients' busy schedules.

The effective use of group therapy with low-income Mexican Americans has also been reported (Herrera and Sanchez 1976). These authors reported the successful use of assertiveness training, modeling, and behavior rehearsal. Additionally, they noted the common problems of marital discord because of role strain resulting from the tension engendered in a marriage as the woman seeks greater freedom but is confronted by a husband with traditional expectations.

Family Therapy

One of the distinctive aspects of Latinos in the United States is their persistent familism. That is, even in the face of acculturation, they continue to maintain certain familial patterns related to their cultural heritage (Rueschenberg and Buriel 1989). For Mexican Americans these involve aspects of respect for authority, traditional family roles, and the protectiveness of the family. These elements are rooted in and reinforced by Mexican Catholicism. Specific techniques of family therapy with Mexican Americans have not been fully developed. However, the exploration of Hispanic family therapy has been most extensively done by Szapocznik and associates (1981, 1983, 1988) in Miami in their work primarily with Cuban American families and individuals. Using a systems approach that incorporates Cuban values, they have developed specific techniques to treat depressed elders, adolescent drug users and their families, Cuban families in crisis, and human immunodeficiency virus (HIV)-infected gay Hispanic men. They have described several models of intervention with these groups derived from structural family therapy (Minuchin and Fishman 1981) and modified for use with Cubans.

The work of Szapocnik and colleagues (1981, 1983, 1988) is particularly valuable because it has a strong theoretical base, is derived from astute and extensive clinical observations, and takes into account the complexities of real-life family interactions. Instead of simply viewing the Hispanic family as basically supportive, which it is, these clinicians have also described how pathological family processes such as enmeshment can develop and be treated. The researchers place particular emphasis on understanding family power balances based on traditional role expectations and then working within their context. For example, they caution therapists to respect the authoritative role of the father. Even when this role seems unreasonable, it is important to form an alliance before attempting to change patterns of interaction. The use of such techniques with Mexican Americans has not been reported on, but there are such strong similarities in the family patterns of Cuban Americans and Mexican Americans that the techniques could be used with this latter group as well.

The use of pastoral counselors or ancillary therapists in therapeutic work with Mexican Americans may be particularly helpful because of the strong role of religion in many patients' lives. The pastoral counselor carries a dual authority as therapist and as representative of the church. He or she can also address certain issues from a spiritual perspective, something not usually done by psychiatrists. Efforts to relieve guilt, inspire hope, or encourage the will to live may be more persuasive if conveyed by a representative of the Higher Being. In my work, I have found the pastoral counselor particularly helpful with patients experiencing conditions that include some aspect of complicated bereavement, as the following case illustrates.

Case Study 3

C. T. is a 54-year-old Mexican American woman whose husband died suddenly in her arms of a stroke. Following his death, she became withdrawn and intermittently mute. She talked to him and saw him in her mind. Weeks went by and these and other symptoms persisted. She reported frontal headaches, weakness, and numbness of her left side, apathy, and continued "trances." Finally, she was admitted to the inpatient unit for further evaluation. Neurological evaluation was entirely normal. She appeared withdrawn and would intermittently become partially mute and preoccupied, reporting that she "saw" her husband and that he was with her. Staff and family repeatedly emphasized to her that he was dead. Her children even showed her videotapes of the funeral. She was prescribed 100 mg of nortriptyline per day and was released after 3 weeks to the day-hospital program. Her condition, although not as extremely withdrawn, remained poor.

Several attempts were made to have Mrs. T. verbalize her inner experiences, but she could only say that she felt that her husband was still with her. Finally, the pastoral counselor (a Mexican American woman) began seeing her. During their second visit, Mrs. T. explained that she still felt her husband's presence and saw his image in her mind and that she did not want to let go of it. She had not said goodbye and was resistant to doing so. Working patiently yet persistently, the pastoral counselor told Mrs. T. to wave goodbye to her husband. A half-hearted yet definite wave of the hand occurred, followed by uncontrollable crying and then relief. A dam had been broken. It was emphasized that Mrs. T. needed to continue this process, and during the ensuing days she showed remarkable improvement.

The pastoral counselor not only has a great deal of experience working with grieving individuals in a general hospital but can also, with all sincerity and ease, make statements to patients like Mrs. T. that their loved one is in heaven and that he or she is watching. These reassurances may facilitate the working through of the grief.

Pharmacotherapy

In using psychotropic medications with Mexican American patients, there are several sociocultural and biological considerations. The first of these is that Mexican American patients who live close to the U.S./Mexican border often go to Mexico to obtain medications. In Mexico, psychotropic drugs are less tightly regulated and cheaper than in the United States. The lower costs make available medications that might not otherwise have been affordable. Also, certain psychotropics (e.g., clomipramine) were available in Mexico before they were in use in the United States. But this cross-border practice may result in problems and complications. Fewer restrictions on drugs in Mexico may enable American citizens to abuse prescription drugs, and these people may then have to be treated in the United States. Amphetamines, barbiturates, and anxiolytics, in particular, may be abused.

There does not appear to be a general rule about the receptiveness of Mexican Americans to the use of psychotropics or other therapeutic modalities. Receptiveness probably depends most on individual personality characteristics. Impressionistically, it may be concluded that, at least among less-acculturated, lower-income subgroups, there may be a tendency to expect medication for immediate symptom relief or because medications represent a more concrete and direct form of assistance. However, the few studies that have examined therapy expectations even in public clinics have found surprisingly high levels of expectation among Mexican Americans for the verbal therapies.

Possible greater sensitivity of Hispanics to psychotropic drugs has been reported in terms of clinical response and side effects (Marcos and Cancro 1982). One study of Colombians supported this impression (Escobar and Tuason 1980). However, a study comparing the pharmacokinetics of nortriptyline in Hispanic (Mexicans in the United States) and Anglo control subjects found no significant differences in the two groups (Gaviria et al. 1986). If the clinical observations of greater sensitivity are real, then at least for this drug, the difference may be because of receptor hypersensitivity.

As with patients from all ethnic groups, the prescribing of psychotropic medication to Mexican Americans requires skill and care. Several recurrent problems need to be appreciated. First of all, when many Mexican Americans hear the term drug or *droga* in Spanish, they associate it to drugs, drug abuse, and drug addiction. They then become concerned about whether the psychotropic medication being prescribed produces dependence or addiction. This response should be anticipated and appropriate explanation and assurance given. Calling the drugs medication, medicine, or another similar term may avoid this problem altogether.

A second common occurrence is concern about single daily dosing, ingesting more than one kind of medication at the same time, and use of high-milligram pills. The underlying worry in these cases has to do with taking too high a dose of medication and fear of overdosing, poisoning, or excessive sedation. Anticipation of these concerns and explanations usually allays a patient's fears. In general, Mexican Americans appear to be good compliers with medications, particularly for the more severe (especially psychotic) disorders. This may be related to the underlying perception of mental illness as an illness requiring medical intervention. This basic attitude appears to be more common among Mexican Americans than among Anglos (Karno et al. 1969).

Treatment Outcome

Mexican Americans present an intriguing situation in regard to the outcome of mental illnesses, particularly schizophrenia. As has been pointed out previously in this discussion, they share many sociocultural characteristics with the people of Mexico, a relatively underdeveloped country. The course of schizophrenia has been shown to be more benign in underdeveloped countries of the world (Sartorius 1978). Reasons for this are thought to include warmer, less judgmental family bonds, lower expectations for independence from the family, and greater likelihood that a chronically impaired individual might find a rewarding, somewhat functional social niche.

Expressed emotion (EE), the family variable thought to be related powerfully to relapse and outcome, has been extensively studied in Great Britain and to some extent in the United States. Interestingly, Karno and associates completed a study of EE in the families of Mexican American schizophrenic patients in southern California (Karno et al. 1987). They found a lower level of EE in the sample of Mexican American families compared with Anglo American families. As in other studies, the researchers found the relapse rate in the Mexican American high-EE families significantly higher than in the low-EE families, but the relapse rate among the Mexican American high-EE families was not as high as among families of Anglo American and British patients. The authors speculate that because Mexican American families tended to be larger, the harmful effects of strongly expressed emotions may be buffered by the presence of other family members.

These same investigators report some interesting qualitative differences in the responses of the families of Mexican American schizophrenic patients (Jenkins et al. 1986). They noted that, rather than expressing irritability and anger at the patient, these families often expressed feelings of sadness, sorrow, and pity, accompanied by caring behavior. These responses may be related to several culturally determined attitudes about schizophrenia: that it is a "real" illness and that it is out of the patient's control. These attitudes, along with the strong notions about family protectiveness, responsibility, and support, result in what has been described previously as the Mexican American tendency toward greater tolerance and compassion for people with mental illness.

Conclusion

Some general considerations about the history of Mexican Americans and implications for psychiatric diagnosis and treatment have been presented in this chapter. My hope is that, as a result, clinical skills for working with Mexican Americans will be improved and enriched. At the least, clinicians will have been helped to develop a more complex, multidimensional cultural perspective. Ideally, this perspective is one in which the individual Mexican American patient is, of course, seen not only as a human being with a developmental history and psychopathology, but also as a person who has what can best be called Latinness and Mexicanness, with both the latter qualities interacting with the former processes. This cross-cultural perspective or sense is difficult to define, measure, or teach. However, if this discussion has been able to help the reader get even one step closer to this goal, then it has achieved its aim.

References

Acosta FX: Pretherapy expectations and definitions of mental illness among minority and low-income patients. Hispanic Journal of Behavioral Sciences 1(4):403–410, 1979

Acosta FX, Cristo MH: Development of a bilingual interpreter program: an alternative model for Spanish-speaking services. Professional Psychology 12:474–482, 1981

Acosta FX, Evans LA, Yamamoto J, et al: Helping minority and low-income psychotherapy patients "tell it like it is." J Biocommun 7(3):13–19, 1980

Acosta FX, Yamamoto J, Evans LA: Effective psychotherapy for low-income and minority patients. New York, Plenum, 1982

Bach-y-Rita G: The Mexican-American: religious and cultural influences, in Mental Health and Hispanic Americans: Clinical Perspectives. Edited by Becerra B, Karno M, Escobar JI. New York, Grune & Stratton, 1982, pp 29–40

Bachrach LL: Utilization of state and county mental hospitals by Spanish Americans in 1972: Statistical Note No. 116 (DHEW Publ No ADM-75-158). Washington, DC, National Institute of Mental Health, Division of Biometry, 1975

Boulette TR: Assertive training with low income Mexican-American women (Psychotherapy with the Spanish-Speaking: Issues in Research and Service Delivery, Monograph #3). Los Angeles, CA, University of California—Los Angeles, Spanish Speaking Mental Health Research Center, 1976, pp 67–71

Burnam MA, Hough RL, Karno M, et al: Acculturation and lifetime prevalence of psychiatric disorders among Mexican-Americans in Los Angeles. J Health Soc Behav 28:89–102, 1987

Cuellar I, Roberts RE: Psychological disorders among Chicanos, in Chicano Psychology. Edited by Martinez JL, Mendoza RH. New York, Academic Press, 1984

Del Castillo JC: The influence of language upon symptomatology in foreign-born patients. Am J Psychiatry 127(2):160–162, 1970

Díaz del Castillo B: The Discovery and Conquest of Mexico. Edited by Garcia G. New York, Farrar Straus & Cudahy, 1956

Diaz-Guerrero R: Neurosis and the Mexican family structure. Am J Psychiatry 112(6):411–417, 1955

Dolgin DL, Salazar A, Cruz S: The Hispanic treatment program: principles of effective psychotherapy. Journal of Contemporary Psychotherapy 17(4):285–299, 1987

Edgerton RB, Karno M: Mexican-American bilingualism and the perception of mental illness. Arch Gen Psychiatry 24:286–290, 1971

Edgerton RB, Karno M, Fernandez I: Curanderismo in the metropolis, in Hispanic Culture and Health Care. Edited by Martinez RA. St. Louis, MO, CV Mosby, 1978, pp 172–182

Escobar JI: Cross-cultural aspects of the somatization trait. Hospital and Community Psychiatry 38(2):174–180, 1987

Escobar JI, Tuason VB: Antidepressant agents: a cross-cultural study. Psychopharmacol Bull 16:49–52, 1980

Fabrega H, Rubel AJ, Wallace CA: Working class Mexican psychiatric outpatients. Arch Gen Psychiatry 16:704–712, 1967

Fabrega H, Swartz JD, Wallace CA, et al: Ethnic differences in psychopathology, I. Clinical correlates under varying conditions. Arch Gen Psychiatry 19:218–225, 1968

Fernandez RA: The United States-Mexico Border. Notre Dame, IN, University of Notre Dame Press, 1977

Folstein MF, Folstein SE, McHugh PR: Mini-Mental State: a practical method for grading the cognitive state of patients for the clinician. J Psychiatr Res 12:189–198, 1975

Gaviria MA, Gil AA, Javaid I: Nortriptyline kinetics in Hispanic and anglo subjects. J Clin Psychopharmacol 6(4):227–231, 1986

Gomez GE, Gomez EA: Folk healing among Hispanic Americans. Public Health Nurs 2(4):245–249, 1985

Gonzalez-Swafford MJ, Gutierrez MG: Ethno-medical beliefs and practices of Mexican-Americans. Nurse Pract 8:29–34, 1983

Graves TD: Acculturation, access, and alcohol in a tri-ethnic community. American Anthropologist 69:306–21, 1967

Griffith J: Emotional support providers and psychological distress among Anglo- and Mexican Americans. Community Ment Health J 20(3):182–201, 1984.

Heiman EM, Burruel G, Chavez N: Factors determining effective psychiatric outpatient treatment for Mexican-Americans. Hosp Community Psychiatry 26(8):515–517, 1975

Herrera AE, Sanchez VC. Behaviorally oriented group therapy: a successful application in the treatment of low income Spanish-speaking clients (Psychotherapy with the Spanish-Speaking: Issues in Research and Service Delivery, Monograph #3). Los Angeles, CA, University of CaliforniaLos Angeles, Spanish Speaking Mental Health Research Center, 1976, pp 73–84

Hoppe SK, Martin HW: Patterns of suicide among Mexican-Americans and Anglos, 1960–1980. Social Psychiatry 21:83–88, 1986

Hough RL, Landsverk JA, Karno M, et al: Utilization of health and mental health services by Los Angeles Mexican-Americans and non-Hispanic whites. Arch Gen Psychiatry 44(8):702–709, 1987

Jaco EG: The social epidemiology of mental disorders: a psychiatric survey of Texas. New York, Russell Sage Foundation, 1960

Jenkins JH, Karno M, de la Selva A, et al: Expressed emotion in cross-cultural context:

familial responses to schizophrenic illness among Mexican-Americans, in Treatment of Schizophrenia. Edited by Goldstein MJ, Hand J, Hahlweg K. Berlin/Heidelberg, Springer-Verlag, 1986, pp 35–49

Karno M: The enigma of ethnicity in a psychiatric clinic. Arch Gen Psychiatry 14:516–520, 1966

Karno M, Edgerton RB: Perception of mental illness in a Mexican-American community. Arch Gen Psychiatry 20:233–238, 1969

Karno M, Jenkins J, de la Selva A, et al: Expressed emotion and schizophrenic outcome among Mexican-American families. J Nerv Ment Dis 175(3):143–151, 1969

Karno M, Hough RL, Burnam MA, et al: Lifetime prevalence of specific psychiatric disorders among Mexican-Americans and non-Hispanic whites in Los Angeles. Arch Gen Psychiatry 44(8):695–701, 1987

Katon W, Kleniman A, Rosen G: Depression and somatization: a review. Am J Med 72:127–135, 1982

Keefe SE, Padilla AM, Carlos MI: The Mexican-American extended family as an emotional support system. Human Organization 38(2):144–152, 1979

Lawson HH, Kahn MW, Heiman EM: Psychopathology, treatment outcome and attitude toward mental illness in Mexican-American and European patients. International Journal of Psychiatry 28:20–26, 1982

Lopez S, Hernandez P: When culture is considered in the evaluation and treatment of Hispanic patients. Psychotherapy 24(1), Spring 1987, pp 120–126

Madsen W: The alcoholic agringado. American Anthropologist 66(2):355–361, 1964

Marcos LR: Bilinguals in psychotherapy: language as an emotional barrier. Am J Psychother 30(4):552–559, 1976

Marcos LR: Effects of interpreters on the evaluation of psychopathology in non-English-speaking patients. Am J Psychiatry 136(2):171–174, 1979

Marcos L, Cancro R: Pharmacotherapy of Hispanic depressed patients: clinical observations. Journal of Psychotherapy 26:4, 1982

Marcos LR, Alpert M, Urcuyo L, et al: The effect of interview language on the evaluation of psychopathology in Spanish-American schizophrenic patients. Am J Psychiatry 130:549–553, 1973

Martinez C: Curanderos: clinical aspects. Journal of Operational Psychiatry 8(2):35–38, 1977

Minuchin S, Fishman HC: Family Therapy Techniques. Cambridge, MA, Harvard University Press, 1981

Montejano D: Anglos and Mexicans in the making of Texas, 1836–1986. Austin, TX, University of Texas Press, 1987

Montiel M: The Chicano family: a review of research. Social Work 22–31, 1973

Normand W, Iglesias J, Payn S: Brief group therapy to facilitate utilization of mental health services by Spanish-speaking patients. Am J Orthopsychiatry 44(1):37–42, 1974

Olarte SW, Masnik R: Benefits of long-term group therapy for disadvantaged Hispanic outpatients. Hosp Community Psychiatry 36(10):1093–1097, 1985

Paz O: The Labyrinth of Solitude, Life and Thought in Mexico. New York, Grove Press, 1961

Paz O: Reflections: Mexico and the United States. New Yorker, 17 September 1979, pp 136–150

Price CS, Cuellar I: Effects of language and related variables on the expression of psychopathology in Mexican-American psychiatric patients. Hispanic Journal of Behavioral Sciences 3(2):145–160, 1981

Ramos S: Profile of Man and Culture in Mexico. Austin, TX, University of Texas Press, 1962

Ripley GD: Mexican-American folk remedies: their place in health care. Tex Med 82:41–44, 1986

Roberts RE: An epidemiologic perspective on the mental health of people of Mexican origin, mental health issues of the Mexican origin population in Texas, in Proceedings of the Fifth Robert Lee Sutherland Seminar in Mental Health. Austin, TX, Hogg Foundation for Mental Health, 1987, pp 55–70

Rodriguez R: Aria: a memoir of a bilingual childhood. The American Scholar 50(1):25–42, 1980

Rozensky R, Gomez MY: Language switching in psychotherapy with bilinguals: two problems, two models, and case examples. Psychotherapy: Theory, Research and Practice 20(2):152–160, 1983

Rubel AJ: The epidemiology of a folk illness: susto in Hispanic America, in Hispanic Culture and Health Care. Edited by Martinez RA. St. Louis, MO, CV Mosby, 1978, pp 75–91

Rueschenberg E, Buriel R: Mexican-American family functioning and acculturation: a family system perspective. Hispanic Journal of Behavioral Sciences 11(3):232–244, 1989

Sartorius N, Jablensky A, Shapiro R: Cross-cultural differences in the short-term prognosis of schizophrenic psychosis. Schizophr Bull 4:102–113, 1978

Sorenson SB, Golding JM: Prevalence of suicide attempts in a Mexican-American population: prevention implications of immigration and cultural issues. Suicide Life Threat Behav 18(4):322–333, 1988

Stenger-Castro EM: The Mexican-American: how his culture affects his mental health, in Hispanic Culture and Health Care. Edited by Martinez RA. St. Louis, MO, CV Mosby, 1978, pp 19–32

Sue S, Zane N: The role of culture and cultural techniques in psychotherapy: a critique and reformulation. Am Psychol 4(1):37–45, 1987

Sugarek NJ: Curanderos in San Antonio (letter). Nurse Pract 9:61, 1984

Szapocznik J, Scopetta M, Kurtines W: A cross-cultural comparison of Cuban and American values. J Consult Clin Psychol 48:961–970, 1978

Szapocznik J, Santisteban D, Hervis O, et al: Treatment of depression among Cuban American elders: some validational evidence for a life enhancement counseling approach. J Consult Clin Psychology 49:752–755, 1981

Szapocznik J, Kurtines W, Foote F, et al: Conjoint versus one person family therapy:

some evidence for the effectiveness of conducting family therapy with one person. J Consult Clin Psychol 51:889–899, 1983

Szapocznik J, Perez-Vidal A, Brickman A, et al: Engaging adolescent drug abusers and their families into treatment: a strategic structural systems approach. J Consult Clin Psychol 56(4):552–557, 1988

Trevino EM, Bruhn JG, Bunce H: Utilization of community mental health services in a Texas-Mexico border city. Soc Sci Med 13A:331–334, 1979

Vaca NC: The Mexican-American in the social sciences. El Grito 3(1):17–50, 1969

16   Psychiatric Care of Puerto Ricans

Ian A. Canino, M.D.
Glorisa J. Canino, Ph.D.

T his chapter focuses on mental health considerations for two groups of Puerto Ricans: those living in the mainland United States, particularly in New York, and those living in Puerto Rico. We begin by presenting some background information and an updated review of relevant mental health information about these two populations.

Background History

Puerto Rico

Christopher Columbus arrived in Borinquen during his voyage to the New World in 1493 and found the island inhabited by the Taino Indians. He named it San Juan Bautista (St. John the Baptist) in honor of Prince Don Juan, son of the Catholic King and Queen of Spain.

The process of colonization started on the island in 1508. It was then that Juan Ponce de León, the first governor, reached the northern bay of the island, which he called Puerto Rico. Soon after, a colonial ordinance called a *repartimiento* was instituted; 5,500 Indians were enslaved—ostensibly in order to convert them to Christianity, but in reality to place them into forced labor. This ordinance, together with European disease epidemics, would have a devastating effect on the native Indian population. By 1550, there were 10 plantations on the island for processing sugar cane. West African Blacks, imported by Portuguese slavers, provided a solution to the gradually diminishing supply of Indian labor.

Spain's strict mercantile policies initially curtailed Puerto Rico's economic growth. Spain allowed the island to keep only one port open, and Puerto Rico was forbidden to trade with non-Spanish powers. This prohibition eventually precipitated a lucrative illicit trade and, as a consequence, an underground black market. By 1765, the islands' population had grown to 45,000; by the turn of the century, mainly because of immigration, the population had tripled.

Spain placed more importance on the naval development of San Juan, which had been fortified to resist pirate attacks, than to the island's economic development. As a result of Napoleon's invasion of Spain in 1808, Spain was forced to undergo a complete reorganization of its colonial government and to initiate a series of reforms. These reforms allowed Puerto Ricans to gain status as Spanish citizens. In addition, a university was founded, and tariffs on machinery and tools were dropped. By the 19th century, Puerto Rican trade had grown significantly, partly because in 1824 Puerto Rican harbors were conceded the right to admit non-Spanish merchant ships.

Slavery was finally abolished in Puerto Rico in 1873. However, for more than a century before this, there had been an odd inconsistency in slavery policy: since 1750, slaves running away from other countries had been admitted to Puerto Rico as free men and women and allowed to earn wages.

After a period of enduring colonial dictators and a severe cholera outbreak, the people on the island developed a growing separatist fervor. Although Spain allowed Puerto Rico to draft a colonial constitution, no new concessions were granted. In September 23, 1863, a group of Puerto Rican supporting autonomy for the island took the town of Lares and proclaimed the short-lived Republic of Puerto Rico. Spain quelled this attempt at independence and continued its colonial rule.

By 1897, the Spanish Prime Minister was overwhelmed by the severe financial burden of the colonies on an impoverished Spain. He declared Puerto Rico an autonomous state, allowing the Spanish-appointed governor only restricted powers. As this process was occurring, the Spanish-American War exploded, and in July 1898, 16,000 American soldiers landed on Puerto Rico. Puerto Rico became a protectorate of the United States, with a population reaching 1 million by the turn of the century.

The Foraker Act of 1900 allowed for a governor of Puerto Rico, appointed by the President of the United States, an Executive Council composed of North Americans and Puerto Ricans, a House of Delegates, and a Resident Commissioner. The latter was chosen by the Puerto Rican people to represent the colony in the House of Representatives in Washington, DC, but had no vote. The first American governors effected a change over to American currency on the island and promoted trade with the United States.

In 1917, the Jones-Shafroth Act granted American citizenship to all Puerto

Ricans. However, the island's politics had, over time, become divided into pro-American and anti-American factions. In the 1930s, the views of the anti-American faction were best expressed by Pedro Albizu Campos, who stated that the claims of the United States on Puerto Rico were illegal, because the island was already autonomous at the time of the occupation.

Luis Munoz Marin, initially a strong advocate for independence from the United States, later reversed his position and proposed a plan for the long-term economic development of the island contingent upon its continued union with the United States. In 1948, Munoz became the governor of the island. He advocated turning Puerto Rico into an associated free state, a position that represented a compromise between the factions mentioned above.

Munoz's proposal was endorsed in 1950 by President Truman as Public Law 600. During the Munoz governorship, Operation Bootstrap was implemented. It was aimed at developing an economy based on tourism and industry, with a program of tax incentives designed to attract industries. During Munoz's governorship, perspectives proliferated on what the status of the island should be. The Popular Party advocated a commonwealth status, the New Progressive Party was in favor of statehood, the Puerto Rican Independence Party was in favor of autonomy, and the Socialist Party was in favor of communism.

Puerto Ricans in the United States

Even before the Spanish-American War, there were Puerto Ricans in the United States. Notably, there was a Puerto Rican political group working from New York to gain independence of the island from Spain. By 1910, there were 1,513 Puerto Ricans living on the mainland, with one-third of them in New York City. More came during World War I and then during the 1920s seeking job opportunities. By 1930, there were 53,000 Puerto Ricans on the mainland. After declines in the size of the Puerto Rican population during the Great Depression and World War II, movement to the mainland began again in large numbers. It reached its peak in the 1950s. Among the factors thought to explain the large migration waves were the population increase on the island, Puerto Rico's surplus labor force, economic pressures to seek better opportunities, lack of legal or political restrictions on migration, and easy transportation (Rodriguez 1989). Puerto Rican migrants were different from European migrants in that they arrived in the United States as citizens, served in the United States armed forces, had a Caribbean cultural and ethnic background, and had easily accessible transportation back to their country of origin (Ramos and Morales 1985).

The initial groups of migrants settled for agricultural and industrial jobs and resided mainly in New York City. There, they lived in Brooklyn, East Harlem, the Lower East Side, and the South Bronx. During the 1950s and 1960s, a host of community organizations such as ASPIRA, the Puerto Rican Forum, the Puerto Rican Community Development Project, and the Puerto Rican Family Institute were created (Fitzpatrick 1971).

Until 1964, Puerto Ricans in New York State were required to take a literacy test for English before they were permitted to register to vote. The test was ruled out by the Civil Rights Act of 1965 that allowed Puerto Ricans not literate in English to register if they showed evidence of having completed 6 years of schooling in Puerto Rico. By 1965, Puerto Ricans in New York City had elected a Puerto Rican, Herman Badillo, as Bronx Borough President. He later became the first elected Puerto Rican Congressional representative. By 1966, Puerto Ricans constituted 12.5% or more of the public school population in New York City (Fitzpatrick 1971).

After 1965, a much greater dispersion of Puerto Ricans across the United States was evident. By 1980, the majority were living outside of New York State, and more than 40% lived outside of Puerto Rico (Uriarte-Gaston 1987). Today large Puerto Rican communities are concentrated in New Jersey, Connecticut, Chicago, and Miami.

In the last 15 years or so, New York has undergone a transition from a major manufacturing center to a postindustrial economy based on service industries. Puerto Ricans had been employed in the most vulnerable segments of the manufacturing sectors: the durable goods and the garment industries. As a result of their employment vulnerability, the New York City fiscal crisis, credentialism, and the federal government's withdrawal of funds from alternative action programs and other forms of social spending, Puerto Ricans in New York have been severely affected (Rodriguez 1989).

In the last decade, there has been an acceleration in the shift of traditional lifestyles in Puerto Rico. There is more frequent travelling and exposure, better education, and the daily impact of the mass media at all social levels. For those Puerto Ricans who by birth or settlement have lived in the United States for a long time, returning to Puerto Rico means having to confront themselves with their own acculturation process. They often do not speak Spanish, and their socialization processes differ from those of Puerto Ricans. For many other Puerto Ricans, their ethnic identity is "neither here nor there": they do not feel fully comfortable in either country. Some are able to become truly bicultural and bilingual, whereas others deny their cultural roots, changing their names and refusing to speak their native tongue.

Demographic Characteristics

Puerto Ricans in Puerto Rico

The estimated total population of Puerto Rico in 1987 was 3.3 million people, an increase of 0.5% over the population in 1986 (Departamento de Salud 1989). The gross per capita income as of July 1988 was $4,600 (Oficina del Gobernador 1988), and the official unemployment rate for 1989 was 14.4% (Departamento de Trabajo 1989). Sixty-seven percent of the population in 1988 was receiving public assistance income (Departamento Servicios Sociales 1988). The median age of the population in 1986 was 28. The percentage of the population younger than 15 years of age was 27.8%, and 9.9% were 65 or older (Departamento de Salud 1988).

During 1987–1988, 38.4% of males and 39.8% of females graduated from high school, and 7.7% of males and 7.5% of females finished college (Departamento de Educación 1987–1988). The urban and rural dropout rate for eleventh graders was 23% and for twelfth graders, 37% (Departamento de Educación 1988–1989).

Puerto Ricans in the United States

Of all Puerto Ricans on the mainland, those in New York have been among the most extensively studied. The following data therefore refer to those Puerto Ricans living in New York City.

In 1985, there were 2.56 million Puerto Ricans residing in the United States (Current Population Report: Population Characteristics 1985). Puerto Ricans constitute 12.67% of the total population of New York City. More Puerto Ricans were born in the United States (49.4%) than were born in Puerto Rico (48.1%). Recently reported data from the 1980 census in New York City indicate that 60.6% of New York City's Hispanics were Puerto Ricans; Cubans, Mexicans, and other Hispanics constituted the other groups (Canino et al. 1988).

In a comparison of Puerto Ricans and non-Puerto Rican Hispanics in New York City (Mann and Salvo 1988), important differences have been reported. One of these was in the percentage of single women who were heads of households. More than 26% of the city's families were classified as headed by "female householders, with no spouse present"; of these, 43.5% were Puerto Rican women and 32.1% were other Hispanic women.

Another difference between Puerto Rican and non-Puerto Rican Hispanics was in median age. Puerto Ricans had a median age of 23.4 years, and other Hispanics, 26.7 years. Both groups were considerably younger than the total New York City population, which had an overall median age of 32.6 years.

The lowest average educational achievement for Hispanic groups in the city was recorded for Puerto Rican females, with 9.7 years of school completed. Of other Hispanic males, 47.6% graduated high school, but only 36.8% of Puerto Rican males did so. Of Puerto Ricans, 13.3% went to college compared with 23% of other Hispanic males. The percentages graduating in each group were 13.3% and 4.3% for other Hispanics and Puerto Ricans, respectively. Neither Puerto Rican nor other Hispanic females reached the level of education of their male counterparts. Puerto Ricans and other Hispanics aged 25 and over of both sexes had significantly fewer median years of school completed than did the general population.

The average number of children ever born to Puerto Rican women was 3.03 and for other Hispanics, 2.35 (completed fertility rates). In addition to lower fertility levels and higher educational attainment, a higher percentage of other Hispanic women were in the labor force. Labor force participation is reflected in the fact that less than 20% of other Hispanic households received public assistance in 1979 compared with 39% of Puerto Rican households.

The annual income for Puerto Rican households was $8,200; it was $12,000 for other Hispanics (the city median was $13,859). More than 47% of Puerto Rican households earned less than $7,500 per year, compared with 32% of other Hispanic households. Rodriguez (1989) suggests that Puerto Ricans in New York City have had to relocate more often than other groups, thus causing displacement and negative effects on education, jobs, income, support networks, and community organizations. Puerto Ricans have to cope with other stressful experiences as well: needing to learn a new language, dealing with prejudice and discrimination, and having to adapt to ways associated with living in large urban centers.

A large proportion of Puerto Ricans still speak Spanish at home. At the same time, a larger proportion of Puerto Ricans (70%) indicate that they speak English well to very well compared with other groups of Spanish origin (60% of Cubans and 42% of Mexicans; English Proficiency of Latinos 1980).

Of the specific factors that characterize Puerto Rican history, several have created particular difficulties for Puerto Ricans. The continuous impact of a variety of cultures and races, consistent economic difficulties and transitions, and the powerful influence of colonizing countries have created sociocultural, economic, and political stresses.

Historically, the Spanish colonizers discriminated and abused the native Indians and later the African slaves. As the races mixed, there was discrimination based on shades of skin color and on white Spanish versus Indian or African features. In spite of the growing number of Puerto Ricans born of mixed parentage and the consequent creation of the *criollo* (indigenous Puerto Rican), those Puerto Ricans who could claim purer Spanish blood considered themselves better and superior. As the island was ready to become fully autonomous from Spain and ready to forge its own national identity and pride as a country, it became part of the United States during the Spanish-American War. Many of the North American governors continued to discriminate against native Puerto Ricans. A process of equal impact eventually occurred in which all that was American was better, reaching its worst consequences by the intermarriage of Puerto Ricans with white North Americans in the belief that this was to "better their race and opportunities."

After World War II and the concomitant overpopulation on the island, Puerto Ricans arriving to the United States and already born as full citizens had to once more confront open discrimination through frequent comments about their "secondary citizenship" and their allegedly being "loud, lazy and unreliable." In order to survive, many Puerto Ricans changed their names, intermarried, and tried to deny their language and heritage. Others decided to fight. These stressors were often compounded by the consequences of the necessary but extremely rapid process of industrialization and urbanization occurring in Puerto Rico during the 1940s and 1950s. People left their small towns and extended networks and frequently had to learn new skills. Many did well; others became dwellers of the sprawling city slums. Still others, dreaming of new opportunities, came to the shores of this country. Many adjusted and found jobs; others became dwellers of inner city ghettos. Family members were divided in this process. Some were left in small towns, others in big cities; some were left in Puerto Rico, and others came to the "mainland." Further differences evolved as some were born and raised in Puerto Rico, while others were raised in the United States with little knowledge of their language and their culture. Back-and-forth migration was to cause further stressors on the families.

It is difficult to ascertain the effects of colonization, discrimination, industrialization, migration, and acculturation, both within the island and within the United States, on the mental health/illness diathesis of this population. It is even more difficult to assume it had no impact in the development of Puerto Rican strengths as well as vulnerabilities as an ethnic group. The relevance of these factors is thus crucial when preventive and educational programs are implemented or socioculturally sensitive treatment interventions instituted. For that sector of the population at high risk for mental illness or those who already have a mental disorder, these added stressors may have had an impact on symptom expression, disease exacerbation or remissions, and long-term prognosis. Political and economic shifts will have direct consequences on allocation of funds for mental health programs. These, in turn, if not socioculturally specific, will not allow for adequate and effective treatment interventions.

The purpose of the two subsequent sections, one on epidemiology and the other on the sociocultural values in the Puerto Rican population, is to describe a state-of-the-art profile of those Puerto Ricans at risk for or who already have mental disorders. These sections will add to the aforementioned social factors epidemiologically relevant factors and sociocultural nuances that have to be considered in any prevention or treatment intervention program. However, the economic and political implementation of these findings is beyond the scope of this chapter.

Epidemiologic Data

Epidemiologic studies are crucial for the accurate understanding and care of the mental health needs of Puerto Ricans and other Hispanics. Despite this, there is still a paucity of epidemiologic studies of Puerto Ricans in the United States as well as in Puerto Rico, and the evidence provided by these studies is not yet conclusive.

One of the difficulties encountered in reviewing epidemiologic research among Puerto Ricans (as well as other populations) is that the findings from these studies are seldom comparable because of differences in illness definition, techniques of ascertainment, or methods of examination. Even subtle differences in diagnostic definitions can have a major impact on illness rate estimations. Conversely, the same definitions applied to data gathered with different diagnostic interviews in the same population can also influence rates. For example, most epidemiologic studies have reported higher rates of mental illness among mainland Puerto Ricans compared with other ethnic groups in the United States (Srole and Fisher 1962).

Impairing Symptoms and Psychiatric Diagnosis

Dohrenwend's (1966) study of a sample of New York City Jewish, black, Irish, and Puerto Rican populations found that Puerto Ricans had significantly higher rates of impairing mental health symptoms than any of the other groups. Attempting to explain these findings, he postulated that

Puerto Ricans were willing to express more distress than the other groups (Dohrenwend and Dohrenwend 1969).

Haberman (1970), reanalyzing these data, found other important variables as well. Women and respondents with lower incomes and less education were more likely to report more symptoms than men and those with higher socioeconomic status. In explaining the differences found for Puerto Ricans, Haberman postulated that these subjects may not have seen the questions in the instruments as indices of deviant or socially undesirable behavior, while other groups did. He concludes suggesting different cutoff scores for defining caseness in multiethnic populations. In a follow-up study, Haberman (1976) found that Puerto Ricans in Puerto Rico indicated more symptoms than Puerto Ricans in New York. However, the number of symptoms declined with the length of time the subjects had lived in New York City, suggesting a variety of explanations, including the effect of acculturation on the reporting of symptoms.

Finally, Krause and Carr (1978) found that Puerto Ricans in the Midwest were more likely to admit psychiatric symptoms than members of other ethnic groups. Within the Puerto Rican subsample, higher reports of symptoms were also related to subjects' having less education, being older, being female, having migrated more recently, and having high anomie scores.

This group of early studies on the epidemiology of mental disorders among Puerto Ricans and other ethnic groups used symptom scales to determine psychiatric morbidity. Those who scored above a certain cutoff point in the scales (determined by comparing psychiatric patients' ratings with those of nonpatients) were considered as having a mental illness. These symptom scales were composed mostly of somatic, psychotic, depressive, and anxiety measures and excluded items relating to substance abuse and personality disorders. It is not surprising that women invariably scored higher in these scales and for many years were believed to be at higher risk of mental illness. Evidence from population-based studies of specific psychiatric disorders in five communities in the United States (Epidemiologic Catchment Area [ECA] Studies) has revealed a significantly higher prevalence of anxiety, somatic, and depressive disorders among women (Robins and Regier 1991). However, the ECA showed that substance abuse disorders and antisocial personality are considerably more frequent among men (Robins et al. 1984). In the ECA studies, the Diagnostic Interview Schedule (DIS) developed by Robins and colleagues (1981) was used.

More recent evidence from a population-based study on the island of Puerto Rico suggests other explanations for the apparently higher rates of psychiatric symptoms reported earlier. This investigation used a methodology similar to that used in the ECA studies; however, a translated, adapted, and validated version of the DIS was used. The DIS is a structured psychiatric interview that can be administered by lay interviewers. Diagnoses from the instrument are made by computer algorithms that implement various diagnostic criteria, including criteria for 25 DSM-III (American Psychiatric Association 1980) diagnoses. The results of this study showed no true difference in either the lifetime or 6-month prevalence rates of most psychiatric disorders for island Puerto Ricans as compared with members of five other United States communities (G. Canino et al. 1987b). An exception to this was the fact that island Puerto Ricans showed higher rates of somatization. When island Puerto Ricans were compared with Mexican Americans and non-Hispanic whites from Los Angeles, Puerto Ricans showed significant higher rates of somatic symptoms (I. A. Canino et al., in press; Escobar et al. 1989). Although further research is needed to confirm these findings, they are suggestive of a possible ethnic influence in the manifestation of somatization among Puerto Ricans.

Although the prevalence rates for most psychiatric disorders did not significantly differ between island Puerto Ricans and residents of the United States, some risk factors differed. For example, alcohol abuse and/or dependence was found to be 12 times more frequent in males than in females in Puerto Rico as compared with the United States, which was four times more frequent in males (G. Canino et al. 1992). A strong sex differential was also obtained for the diagnosis of dysthymia. In Puerto Rico, dysthymia is four times more prevalent in women than in men, but in the United States, it is twice as prevalent (G. Canino et al. 1987a; Weissman et al. 1991).

Important differences between this study and the earlier ones are the use of DSM-III criteria for estimating psychiatric morbidity, and the fact that the results could be extrapolated with a considerable degree of confidence to the entire adult population of Puerto Rico aged 17 to 64. The use of complex, stratified sampling procedures and a response rate of 91% permitted this kind of extrapolation (See G. Canino et al. 1987b for more details). Thus, differences in methodological and nosological criteria may, in part, explain some of the differences in results in prior studies.

Others (Rogler et al. 1989) have attempted to explain these differences by claiming that the DIS only measures a limited number of disorders and, as a result, prevalence rates ought to be lower. Although this is a valid argument, it probably does not explain the difference in results between the earlier and more recent findings, because, as previously stated, the symptom scales used in the earlier studies were also limited in scope. In fact, the early symptom scales did not include items on alcohol abuse and dependence, one of the more prevalent disorders in both the ECA and Puerto Rico studies (G. Canino et al. 1987b; Robins et al. 1984).

Another plausible explanation has been given by Rogler and colleagues (1989). He has stated that it is possible that Puerto Ricans in Puerto Rico report more symptoms than other ethnic groups and, therefore, score high on dimensional measures of psychopathology, but they actually have rates of mental disorders similar to those of other communities and ethnic groups. However, this last hypothesis has been discarded by recent evidence provided by Shrout and colleagues (in press). Psychiatric disorders and symptoms of Mexican Americans and non-Hispanic whites from Los Angeles were compared with those of island Puerto Ricans, controlling for education level, number of household residents, age, and gender. The results indicated no significant differences between island Puerto Ricans and the other two groups regarding mean number of symptoms. The only exception to this was somatic symptoms, which were more prevalent among Puerto Ricans, as had been previously reported (I. A. Canino et al., in press; Escobar et al. 1989).

Cultural Syndromes of Puerto Ricans

Ataques de nervios (nerve attacks) have been described in the literature for more than 30 years as a culturally defined syndrome typical of Puerto Ricans and other Hispanic groups (Abad and Boyce 1979; De La Cancela et al. 1986; Fernandez-Marina 1961; Garrison 1977b). They are dramatic episodes in which the person trembles, begins to shout, sometimes becomes aggressive, and then falls to the floor. The most common symptoms described are trembling, heart palpitations, loss of consciousness, memory loss, paresthesia, dizziness, and fainting spells. Thus, the characteristic episode is a combination of somatic and panic symptomatology.

A qualitative and quantitative analysis of the Puerto Rican psychiatric epidemiology data set was done (G. Canino et al. 1987b) to determine the extent to which symptoms related to *ataques de nervios* may have influenced the responses to the somatic items and the DIS. Preliminary analyses suggest the possibility that the excess of somatic symptoms observed among island Puerto Ricans may be related to this syndrome (Guarnaccia et al., in press).

In another psychiatric epidemiology study, *ataque de nervios* was directly studied in the adult population of the island (ages 17–67). The results of this study showed that 16% of the population admitted having experienced at least one *ataque de nervios* in their lives (Guarnaccia et al., in press). Furthermore, 12% of the population reported that the *ataques* were so impairing that either they had to consult a doctor about them or they had considerably affected their daily functioning. As expected from results of previous research in this area, *ataques de nervios* were more prevalent among women over the age of 40, of low socioeconomic background and low levels of education, and who are widowed, separated, or divorced. Contrary to expectations, more than 63% of those who reported an *ataque de nervios* met diagnostic criteria for either an anxiety or depressive disorder. The findings raise questions about the contention that *ataques* are "normal" expressions of distress and suggest the possibility that the syndrome might be a cultural idiom used by Puerto Ricans to describe episodes of depression and anxiety. The fact that the correlates of *ataques* are the same correlates as those of anxiety and depression further supports this possibility.

Mental Health Care Utilization of Puerto Ricans

The mental health care utilization patterns of island Puerto Ricans have also been reported as part of the epidemiological study one of us conducted (G. Canino et al. 1987b). Among those who met criteria for a DIS/DSM-III disorder within the previous year, only 17% utilized the mental health sector or a specialist in mental health, whereas 47% visited a nonpsychiatrist physician. Twenty-one percent visited both a mental health specialist and a physician for mental health problems, and another 21% used both the health sector and spiritualists for their mental health problems (Martinez et al. 1991).

Those individuals who reported to have sought the help of spiritualists at some time in their lives were more likely to report symptoms of depression or somatization than those who did not seek help from a folk healer. Those with more psychiatric symptoms were also more likely to work outside the home; they were more likely to be in the lowest income quartile and were more likely to visit mental health specialists (Hohmann et al. 1990).

In a study of island Puerto Rican poor, Alegria and colleagues (1991) reported on mental health utilization patterns. The results of the study indicated that of the 30% of the island poor population in need of mental health services, only 32% received any mental health care in the previous year. Of the 30% in need, 22% used the physical health sector to deal with their mental health problems, compared with 18% who sought care in the mental health sector. The results suggested that nonpsychiatrist physicians are the main gatekeepers to mental health treatment on the island.

In a study analyzing health-seeking behavior of Hispanics in New York (of which the largest group were Puerto Ricans), the results indicated that acculturated Hispanics were more likely than unacculturated ones to use mental health services (Rodriguez 1987). There was a correlation between subjects' use of services and subjects' perceptions of problems with agencies; therefore, instead of indicating barriers to patients' use, critical perspectives predicted service utilization. This finding was explained by the fact that those who had used services would be more likely to criticize them. Contrary to the alternative resource theory that extended family and community networks would substitute for the need to seek outside resources, for the Hispanic and African American subjects in the study, integration into the social network provided advice and referral information that made it more likely that they would seek services. In terms of mental health services, private therapists and prevention programs were reported as the most underutilized, whereas outpatient services and nonpsychiatric physicians were the most widely used.

Psychiatric Epidemiology in Children and Adolescents

A major psychiatric epidemiologic survey of children in Puerto Rico was completed in 1986 and the main findings have been reported (Bird et al. 1988). The study used the same household probability sample used a year earlier in an epidemiologic survey of the adult population (G. Canino et al. 1987b). The survey used the Child Behavior Checklist (Achenbach and Edelbrock 1983) as a screening instrument, and prevalence rates were estimated on the basis of clinical diagnoses and other measures provided by child psychiatrists during the second stage of the study.

Results of the survey showed that the prevalence of DSM-III child diagnoses in the island (for children ages 4 through 16) was around 49%, which is higher than that observed in other community studies in Canada and Australia (Offord et al. 1987; Verhulst et al. 1985). However, when impairment was taken into account in the definition of maladjustment, similar levels were observed across studies (from 16% to 18% in Puerto Rico, depending on severity of impairment). The factors that were most strongly associated with psychopathology in Puerto Rican children were the following:

1. Having a low socioeconomic status;
2. Being male;
3. Being in the age range of 6 to 11;

4. Having failed in school;
5. Having a poor medical history; and
6. Living in a stressful household environment (Bird et al. 1989).

Of the 16% of children who met DSM-III criteria and were highly impaired functionally, 26.3% received some type of mental health service, the majority of which was provided by either a school social worker or a psychologist. This means that 73.7% of the children who had severe or moderate psychiatric impairment were not receiving any type of intervention for their condition, in spite of the fact that 92% of the psychiatrists, 46% of the teachers, and 79% of the parents considered them to be in need of psychiatric services. Only 4.6% of the total population of children and adolescents had used some type of mental health service in the past 6 months.

A study of Puerto Rican children in New York City found that they had a higher frequency of symptoms in the categories of sleep and articulation problems, physical problems, inadequate intellectual development, anxiety and fears, and anger and belligerence (Canino et al. 1988). Slightly larger populations of Puerto Rican than white children were diagnosed during the initial interview for this study as learning disabled or having transient situational (reactive) and behavioral disorders. The data for this study had been collected by city mental health facilities during fiscal year 1976–1977. The study offered a limited psychiatric profile of the children, because it was based purely on secondary data analysis and did not attempt to find a true prevalence of psychiatric disorders.

Ethnocultural Values of Puerto Ricans

Values that have often been described in Puerto Rican culture are *personalismo,* or the need to relate to people and not to institutions, *respeto,* or respect, *verguenza* and *orgullo,* or shame and pride, and *confianza,* or trust (Rogler and Cooney 1984). Another frequently mentioned value is the importance of family. This value consists of family interdependence and loyalty among members, reinforcing cooperation over competition. The needs of the individual are subordinate to the needs of the family (Ramos-McKay et al. 1988). Many studies have underlined the family's crucial role in Puerto Rican society. It has been described as facilitating rural to urban migration and as the primary setting for the care of people with mental illness (Rogler and Hollingshead 1975).

The Puerto Rican family has also been described as having clearly demarcated sex roles. Traditional sex roles have been framed in two codes: *machismo* and *marianismo*. Culturally, *machismo* means that the male is responsible for the welfare and honor of the family; he is the provider. *Marianismo* means that females are considered spiritually superior to men and, therefore, are capable of enduring suffering better than men are (Gomez 1982). On the mainland and in certain sectors of Puerto Rico, increased alternative means of support for women and high rates of male unemployment may function to undermine this traditional role structure. In many families, the myth of the strong male authority figure contrasts sharply with the reality of a subculture where the female may be the source of income through government help or the only consistent and present force in single-parent families. The literature on Puerto Rican woman has been scant. Most of the research, however, tends to confirm the hypothesis that Puerto Rican women, who are rigidly entrenched in adhering to traditional values as the norm, experience more conflict and maladjustment than those who are either less traditional or live in a family context with fewer intergenerational differences.

Torres-Matrullo (1976) investigated the relationship between acculturation and psychopathology in mainland Puerto Rican women. Her study demonstrated that poorly acculturated women as compared with highly acculturated women were more likely to exhibit symptoms such as aggression, hostility, isolation, loss of self-esteem, and personal inadequacy. The implication of this study is that Hispanic women on the mainland, who adhere more strictly to traditional values (as do nonacculturated women), tend to be less well-adjusted than less traditional or nontraditional Puerto Rican women.

This hypothesis was confirmed by Gonzalez's (1978) study of the relationship between sex role and mental health among island Puerto Rican women. She found that the university-educated females who were nontraditional in their sex role attitudes were more adjusted than both homemakers and female mental patients. Conversely, Puerto Rican women who had been diagnosed as neurotic or depressive and were receiving treatment had significantly more traditional sex-role expectations than the homemakers and students who were not neurotic or depressed. The homemakers scored (in a scale of self-actualization) as significantly more actualized than the female patients but lower than the less traditional university students. Gonzalez interpreted these results as due to the rapid industrialization and modernization experienced in Puerto Rican society in recent decades. The more traditional women were of lower socioeconomic class and were significantly older than the university students, having lived their youth in an agricultural Puerto Rico, where the traditional female role was valuable and adaptive to the societal structure. Puerto Rico's reality is now very different. The strict female traditional role is not as valued, and the life-styles of daughters are incongruent with the traditional roles held by their mothers. If this interpretation is correct, then it is not the adherence to traditional values per se that may precipitate psychological disorders, but the conflict experienced by traditional women who live in a society and family context where less traditional values are reinforced (Canino 1982b).

Canino (1982a) found that, when sex-role values were measured, both husband and wife reported traditional patriarchal attitudes. When these same families were both extensively interviewed, however, and observed making decisions, the more prevalent marital transaction was shared decision making. Inflexible dominance of one spouse over another was only observed in dysfunctional family systems. Additionally, Munoz (1979) interviewed a sample of married and divorced Puerto Rican women about marital decision making. The women reported that men dominated all decisions (sex frequency, personal growth, social activities, budget expenses) except for household tasks and child-raising. Because only women were interviewed, the more complex interpersonal reality that appears when the couple is interviewed was not portrayed.

Puerto Rican families have been described as maintaining a high degree of control over their offspring. Their child-raising techniques have also been depicted as conventional and imperative (i.e., they emphasize respect for authority, obedience conformity, and the use of power-assertive techniques). Their migration to the mainland United States, however, is said to have challenged such authority patterns. Some (I. A. Canino et al. 1987) argue that the weakening in parental control that occurs when the family migrates is due to the rapid adoption by Puerto Rican children of the more symmetrical organization of the American family. In American families, there is more equality for the mother and more independence for the children. Others (Robles et al. 1980) argue that, in addition, parental controls and authority are also threatened by the role reversal that is likely to occur when Spanish-speaking parents have to depend on their English-speaking children in many activities of daily living. This role reversal is said to lead to a questioning and weakening of parental authority. This phenomenon is also likely to affect the parent-adolescent relationship when both the child and parents were born in Puerto Rico.

Case Study 1

M. P., age 14, was referred to a mental health clinic by her school for occasional truancy and defiant behavior in the classroom. The school had previously requested a parents' conference to discuss this problem, and M. had served as the translator between the English-speaking officials and her Spanish-speaking parents. M.'s parents felt, as do many Puerto Rican parents, that the school, as an extension of the family, should discipline her. The school felt otherwise. Mr. and Mrs. P. perceived the school as hostile and intrusive. They fluctuated between severely punishing their daughter and siding with her against the school. The problems were compounded when Mr. P. was told that M.'s truancy was due to her "escapades" to meet a boyfriend. Mr. P. reacted by demanding that M. be home earlier than before, by withdrawing permission for his daughter to leave the household unless accompanied by a family member, and by accusing his wife of not raising her correctly.

M. openly rebelled, citing the behavior of her peer group and accusing her father of ridiculous and old-fashioned attitudes. The once-normally enmeshed, culturally acceptable pattern, whereby young girls are overly protected and discouraged from independent behavior, had broken down. In addition, M. was bilingual and had become the translator for the parents in their relations with outside institutions. As a "parentified" child with many responsibilities, it was difficult for her to assume a more submissive, dependent, and "respectful" role.

In response to her increasing protestations and lack of respect, Mr. P. forced his daughter to stay at home and eventually did not even trust her to go to school. Mr. P. became increasingly overprotective toward his daughter and developed difficulties with his wife concerning child-rearing practices. M.'s need to differentiate and express autonomous behavior had been curtailed. From the family's perspective, M. had brought *verguenza* to her family and had broken the prescribed mores of *respeto* and *dignidad* (self-worth of the family [Canino and Canino 1980, pp. 539]).

The Puerto Rican family has been described as providing an extended network that often includes neighbors and other relatives. As part of the extended family system, *compadrazgo* is a network that establishes two sets of relationships: one between the *padrinos* and *ahijados* (godparents and their godchildren), and the other between the godparents and the parents who become *compadres* (coparents). Godparents are supposed to assist their *ahijados* in case of emergencies, especially at their *compadres'* deaths.

Contrary to these popularly held beliefs, more recent studies of Puerto Ricans on the island and in New York City have been unable to verify the importance of the *compadrazgo* network as a help-supplying system (Rogler and Cooney 1984). Recent studies suggest that social changes in Puerto Rico are diminishing the traditional bonds of help between neighbors and friends. Divorce, working parents, lack of leisure time, living in large apartment buildings, urbanization, and acquisition and acculturation of American values have affected these traditions. In San Juan, these bonds are weakest among families at the bottom of the stratification heap (Caplow et al. 1964). Rogler and colleagues (1983) have suggested that these traditional bonds are attenuated in New York as well.

In an intergenerational study of residentially and maritally stable Puerto Rican families in New York, the authors found that the greatest intergenerational changes have occurred in the following order of frequency: socioeconomic status, language used at home, values and self-concept, and bicultural preferences (Rogler and Cooney 1984). The study suggested that the married-child generation still retained symbolic bonds with Puerto Rico, although these individuals were raised in the mainland. In the study, level of education and age of arrival were considered to be very important variables. The married children's socioeconomic status as defined by educational and occupational attainments were higher than those of their parents. Nevertheless, this did not cause any loss of intergenerational family solidarity. As education level increased, knowledge of English and Spanish increased but daily use of Spanish decreased. The subjects with more education were less fatalistic, less family oriented, and more modern. Age of arrival had no effect on these variables but had an important influence on ethnic self-identification and was related to language ability and usage. The subjects who had arrived at a younger age reported a greater ability with and more frequent usage of English.

There is thus considerable variation in values in Puerto Rico and in New York (Leavitt 1974). A number of factors, including migration status, rate of male unemployment, and increased alternative means of support for women, have modified these traditional concepts (Canino et al. 1988).

Indigenous Healing

This section describes the most frequently studied indigenous-healing practice in the Puerto Rican population: *espiritismo* (spiritism).

The origins of *espiritismo* can be traced to Hypolyte Rivail, a French physician and educator, who, in 1869, published *The Book of Spirits* under the pseudonym Alain Kardec (1869/1951). This book and his other works were widely read and translated into several languages. The belief in spirits was then referred as telepathy and occultism. Scientific attempts were made to research these psychic phenomena, and international congresses were established. Spiritism influenced some of the beliefs held by Christian Scientists and Theosophists. Some postulate that parapsychology as we know it today had its roots in the spiritism of that time.

Kardec (1869/1951) taught that in every human being there is a soul undergoing an evolutionary process during the person's lifetime. People must do their utmost to perfect their spirits and to develop their *facultades,* or faculties, so their spirits can lead them through life. Different levels are achieved through *pruebas* (trials), which may consist of hardships or difficulties. The level of spiritual development that people can reach in the spiritual evolutionary process depends on how they deal with these trials throughout their lives. Among Puerto Ricans, Christian beliefs in the soul and purification, combined by the animistic beliefs of Indian and African ancestors, allowed for the easy introduction of these principles into their culture.

Present-day Puerto Rican *espiritismo* can be seen as functioning on several levels. There is a continuum of adherence from intellectual to folk spiritualist beliefs, with the vast majority of *espiritistas* at some point between the two extremes (Salgado 1974). Those in the educated classes insist that their adherence to *espiritista* beliefs is scientific, experimental, and philosophical. They are well-versed in Kardec's writings, theosophy, Rosicrucian doctrines, and the psychoanalytic literature, and attempt to distinguish between their beliefs and those of the lower socioeconomic classes. Their Kardecian mediums are known as *espiritistas,* whereas others of lesser sophistication are referred by them as *espiriteros.*

In a second category is a group of *espiritistas* whose activities are reminiscent of Protestant revivalist meetings in North America. The *Fraternidad Surcos* is typical of this category. It carries out weekly "healing" services with prayers and laying on of hands. Other groups have organized prayers and rituals drawn from the Catholic denomination and ceremonies reminiscent of the Catholic Mass.

A third category incorporates more long-standing indigenous beliefs involving witchcraft, magic, and the ritualistic use of herbs and potions, all of which purportedly affect the influence of spirits. This group utilizes old Indian practices, *curanderismo* and, particularly in New York City, practices from *santerismo,* a well-established Afro-Caribbean religion mainly practiced among Cubans.

Previous studies have indicated that Puerto Ricans use spiritism as indigenous therapy, network therapy, a community support system for people with chronic schizophrenia, and as an outlet for the anxiety caused by economic and interpersonal stressors (Garrison 1977a; Harwood 1977; Rogler and Hollingshead 1961, 1965). Attempting to explain why Puerto Ricans still occasionally practice *espiritismo,* many authors have stated that *espiritistas* are accessible, charge reasonable fees, offer concrete solutions to problems, communicate in the same language as their clients, and use the extended family system in their healing processes (Lubchanski et al. 1970; Ruiz and Langrod 1976).

Garrison (1971) conducted a study of 14 *centros* (centers for the practice of *espiritismo*) in which she found an active caseload of 570 clients versus an active caseload of 350 patients in mental health clinics of the same area. The same patterns of attendance were reported for the *centros* as for the mental health clinics: 43%–50% did not return after the first visit; 45% attended only 2 to 5 sessions; and only 5%–13% attended more than 5 sessions.

Various observations were made of the spiritists' approach to clients with emotional complaints. Garrison (1971) noted that the mediums interpreted the symbolic significance of visions, frequently based their comments on postural cues or visible evidence of tension, and gave direct attention to and support for mood and feeling states. She found that the mediums asked multiple questions regarding interpersonal relationships and that their revelations covered physical as well as physiological and emotional symptomatology. They generally inquired if the client had already visited a doctor.

Case Study 2

A. J., age 10, was referred to a Hispanic mental health center with a presumptive diagnosis of childhood-onset schizophrenia. The diagnosis was of visual and auditory hallucinations and social withdrawal. Careful inquiry revealed that, 2 years prior to consultation at the center, A. J. had been taken to a spiritualist because of a sleep disturbance. In the child's presence, the spiritist informed the family that an evil spirit was disturbing the child at night and recommended that two pans of clear water be kept under the child's bed to cleanse the room of spirits. Nine months prior to the psychiatric consultation, the child's grandmother, with whom she had been very close, died. The so-called hallucinations consisted of hypnagogic phenomena in which the child saw and heard the grandmother's spirit, who visited her at night. Clinical assessment revealed no evidence of psychotic illness but, rather, a prolonged grief reaction. (Bird and Canino 1981, p. 732)

Assessment and Treatment

In view of the many variables, both social and cultural, that may affect the mental health status of the Puerto Rican population and the paucity of research in treatment specificity and efficacy, this section offers general guidelines to the clinician treating Puerto Rican patients. The benefits of therapist-patient ethnocultural similarities in comparison to other therapist-patient variables still need to be validated. The importance, though, of the therapist's effectiveness based on his or her credibility (Sue 1981) and his or her sensitivity to the patients' ethnocultural background cannot be underestimated (Griffith 1977).

One of us has suggested that the clinician should first ask about dietary habits, major holidays, musical and religious interests, and community activities, and then should inquire about child-rearing practices, cultural attitudes toward teaching, disciplining, and health-seeking behavior (Canino 1985). In addition, and when relevant, the clinician must evaluate the impact of migration, the degree of acculturation, and the patient's particular language, community, and family structure with the concomitant ability of these factors to offer support or to cause stress.

Sociocultural Context for Therapy

All clinicians must have a genuine interest in the personal meaning sickness has for the patient as well as a working knowledge of the patient's cultural environment. Suggestions have been made that therapists, indigenous healers, priests, and ministers work together and teach each other whenever feasible (Abad et al. 1974; Bluestone and Purdy 1977). For such an exchange to be most helpful, more knowledge is needed of the specific reasons for help-seeking behavior, client characteristics, and utilization rates for those patients going to ministers or healers and for those availing themselves of mental health professionals.

Assessment and treatment of those Puerto Ricans arriving in the United States and perhaps of those born and raised in the United States and returning to Puerto Rico must address issues of their ethnic self-identity, changing sexual role behavior, and binguality.

In terms of the impact of migration on self-identity, three therapeutic goals have been described in the literature. These are directed at helping patients who are undergoing cultural transitions to reconsolidate their ethnic sense of self:

1. Reflecting or mirroring to the patient the ethnocultural aspects of self;
2. Educating the patient through a reformation of his or her ethnocultural identity; and
3. Helping the patient integrate and resolve the conflicts between the two cultures (Comas-Diaz and Jacobsen 1987).

Arrival in another culture confronts Puerto Ricans with different sex-role expectations. Conflicts develop surrounding dating, sexual expression, and issues related to authority and submission. These conflicts are often determined by whoever produces more income in the new culture. Some authors (Sluzki 1979) believe that traditionally Hispanic males take an instrumental role, whereas Hispanic women take an affective one. They believe that because of the economic forces and the availability of marketable skills, there is often a reversal of roles for many Puerto Ricans arriving in the United States. This often causes multiple stressors. A family therapy model for these families has been suggested (Canino and Canino 1982), as in the following case.

Case Study 3

N. R., a 16-year-old Puerto Rican girl, was referred to a community mental health clinic for treatment after a suicide attempt. N. is one of six children in an intact migrant family who had moved 7 years earlier from Puerto Rico to an American industrial city. The family complained of N.'s temper tantrums, during which she destroyed dishes and glasses and damaged some furniture. Mrs. R. charged that her daughter was disrespectful, did not obey her, and did not help her with household chores. N. criticized her parents (who were both in their early 40s) for being too restrictive and old-fashioned and for not allowing her to go out.

Mrs. R. had been hospitalized the previous year for depression and a suicide attempt. She devoted her days to cooking and cleaning and complained that her husband would not take her out, but instead spent all of his time at the bar playing dominoes with his friends. Mrs. R. did not speak or understand English, although she had lived in the United States for many years. Her isolation and dependency were exacerbated by the fact that her extended family had remained in Puerto Rico and she had not cultivated friendships that could replace this essential support system. She relied for support only on the family; she was guarded and suspicious about using any outside resources, such as friends or community organizations. Mr. R., on the other hand, had worked in a restaurant for many years (although he had been unemployed for 2 years when N. was brought in for treatment). He understood and spoke English, had a network of Hispanic and American friends, and had adjusted to his community. (p. 301)

The issue of language is particularly important for Puerto Ricans who migrate to the United States and speak Spanish as a primary language. Language-related issues may be relevant for therapy with those who return to

Puerto Rico after having been raised in the mainland and who speak English as a primary language. Nevertheless, most of the literature reviewed here refers to the Puerto Ricans in New York. The general principles, however, are probably applicable to both groups. A study of bilingual patients found that for those whom Spanish was the primary language, there was less contact with the interviewer and more withdrawal (Marcos 1976). Compared with the ratings these patients received when they were interviewed in Spanish, they were rated as having more pathology when interviewed in English. In another study in which the clinicians' ethnicity was held constant, the opposite was found: patients were rated as having more psychopathology in the Spanish interviews compared with the English ones (Price and Cuellar 1981).

When people use a language other than the dominant one in a particular culture, they make more frequent pauses and use more clichés, and they pay greater attention to how things are said instead of what is said. When a patient is using the nondominant language, there may also be distortions in expressed affect (Marcos and Urcuyo 1979). Some bilingual patients have stated that their perception of themselves varies somewhat according to which language they use (Marcos et al. 1977). If they learned their second language later in life, they may have less access to early memories while using their second language (Rozensky and Gomez 1983). Pitta and colleagues (1978) recommend a technique called language-switching to help bilingual patients express overwhelming emotionally laden material. They are encouraged to switch to their second language when more self-observance and more tolerable levels of anxiety are necessary, but the bilingual therapist may switch to the primary language when the patient is using intellectualization and avoiding emotions and early memories.

If the therapist is monolingual and needs to use an interpreter, Marcos (1979) advises the therapist to be aware that there may be errors associated with the interpreters' attitude toward the patient, language competence, translations skills, or lack of psychiatric knowledge. Marcos (1979) strongly recommends that the therapist and interpreter meet before and after therapy in order to clarify any misconceptions.

Socioeconomic Status and Therapy

Cobb (1972) cited some of the inadequacies of the literature on lower socioeconomic groups: the absence of a common definition of socioeconomic status; difficulties in specifying and evaluating treatment programs for these populations; the absence of sufficient studies comparing the effectiveness of treatment approaches with specific subgroups of lower socioeconomic patients; and finally, the absence of multivariate research approaches. Despite the scientific limitations of the literature, it does contain insights that may be very important clinically.

In assessing and treating Puerto Ricans, particularly those subjected to the greatest socioeconomic stresses who seek help at public mental health clinics, the clinician must be aware of a series of factors in addition to those which have already been discussed.

Meers (1973) expressed some of the difficulties of distinguishing psychopathological behaviors from behaviors that are socially or ethnically normal or deviant. Working within a psychoanalytic model, he described how the sociocultural milieu of inner-city populations exposed them to early and chronic distress, contributing in some cases to the impairment of ego functions. Often symptoms and coping behaviors that are reactive to external distress are difficult to differentiate from those derived from internalized conflicts. Meers also cited the added complications of intrauterine damage as well as postnatal nutritional deficits in some members of these groups. His observations led him to conclude that many of the clients he saw discharged anxiety or tension through action and utilized the defenses of identification with the aggressor and isolation of affect. He acknowledged particular difficulties in the analysis of those clients where drive discharge was either supported or encouraged by their environment.

Murphy and Moriarty (1978), in discussing the strengths of inner-city children, stated that some of the children in their study developed self-protective tactics and measures to reduce stress. These include limiting or fending off excessive stimulation; controlling the impact of the environment through strategic withdrawal, delay, and caution; and selecting and restructuring their environment.

In an article describing psychotherapy for these children, Graffagnino and colleagues (1970) strongly support therapy concurrent with special school and environmental interventions. They caution therapists about their own countertransference in the form of feeling inadequate and being overwhelmed by the chaotic background of these children. They recommend an approach incorporating total medical care, increasing social levels, promoting minority-group acceptance, and educating the parents in appropriate behavioral responses to their children.

In terms of adult outpatient facilities in lower socioeconomic areas, Phillipus (1971) recommends that facilities have the following characteristics:

1. Geographical accessibility;
2. Crisis orientation with no waiting list;
3. Bilingual staff;
4. Community involvement;
5. Liaison with medical services; and
6. A drop-in room for immediate accessibility.

Bluestone and Vela (1982) outline some important factors to consider in the psychotherapy of inner-city Puerto Ricans. They mention the cultural concept of time as it relates to appointments, cultural reactions to authority figures, and difficulties with the modulation of anger. They mention the patient's need to form an affectionate and familiar relationship with the therapist and the frequent wish that the therapist will solve all his or her problems. Bluestone and Vela recommend the use of humor, proverbs, and metaphors and suggest that therapists help these patients become more verbally assertive. For economically stressed, inner-city Puerto Ricans, De La Cancela and colleagues (1986) offered a dialectical therapy model. In this work, they help patients recognize their socioeconomic reality and how it leads to either contradictory, interactive, adaptive, or maladaptive behaviors. The following case study attempts to integrate all these ideas.

Case Study 4

C. S., a 35-year-old Puerto Rican woman, had arrived in New York City 5 years ago. She came to the emergency room because of a recent episode of profuse sweating, fast heart beating, motor twitching, agitation and screaming. Mrs. S.'s family stated it looked like a seizure. Her husband, a 40-year-old Puerto Rican man born and raised in New York, seemed genuinely concerned. The English-speaking neurologist had already seen her and found nothing wrong with her physically. Through the aid of a trained translator and Mr. S., the neurologist suspected some psychiatric difficulties. Aware that the finer nuances of a good mental status examination could not be assessed by the translator, he referred her to the psychiatrist on call.

Dr. R., a bilingual, bicultural psychiatrist, addressed the couple as Mr. and Mrs. S. (a sign of *respeto*) and introduced himself as a doctor who understood not only physical symptoms but those caused by *nervios*. He asked the couple where they came from, and before proceeding with the interview, he informed the patient he knew a family in a nearby town in Puerto Rico where his own family was from. He himself had been in New York 10 years. Dr. R. made a personal comment, thus addressing the cultural mode of *personalismo* and at the same time opened the interview for future questions about networking. As the couple relaxed they informed the doctor they had a *compadre* in that town. . . . Did the doctor know him? They then spoke spontaneously about their children and the multiple difficulties they had in school. Mrs. S. felt overwhelmed. She could not help them with their homework because of her poor English skills, and she felt they not only disrespected her but also were too outspoken and independent. They had acculturated much faster than her and were acting like her husband.

Mrs. S. missed her extended family and had few supports in New York. Her role as a mother was changing as her children grew older, and she felt useless and lonely. She then described symptoms of dysthymia. Dr. R., aware of the frequency of somatic complaints that often accompanies depressive symptoms in this population, asked her about this. Mrs. S. stated she had frequent pains in the back of her neck, body aches, and muscle pains often accompanied by feeling anxious and tense. Her family doctor had treated her with medication, to no avail. She had never seen a psychiatrist, because she thought they only treated "crazy" people. Dr. R. assured her that she was not "crazy" but that she certainly had been under a lot of stress and that her *nervios* could certainly be treated by a combination of the appropriate medication and by the active involvement of her and her family in order to better understand how to relieve her distress.

At this point in the interview, Dr. R. addressed Mr. S. and shared with him that it is not easy for men either. Mr. S. stated, "Well, you know, Doctor, men drown their pain through drinking." Following this metaphor, Dr. R. stated that drinking could drown the pain, but at times it drowned strong men with it. He then respectfully asked him how much and how frequently was he drinking. Mr. S. stated that during the last year it had increased, because he was having severe financial problems and lacked job security. Mrs. S. then stated that her husband always drank on "social Fridays" but that recently he was drinking every day and it was affecting his personality. He had changed to such a degree that she had decided to consult an *espiritista* who had told her that there were serious problems in their marriage. Dr. R. explored this further and suggested that perhaps he could find some resources for Mr. S. to help him with the finances as well as with his job situation. If things did not get better, he wanted to talk with him further about the drinking.

Dr. R., aware of the cultural sexual role of *machismo*, decided to discuss issues in the marriage only after Mr. S. fully trusted him and did not perceive him as a threat by talking about things that are "private to a couple." As the interview came to an end, Dr. R. assessed the strengths of the family as well. Mr. S. had a network of old friends in his community and was sociable and well-liked, and Mrs. S. was known to be an excellent cook and seamstress. Many people sought out her counsel for various health problems. Dr. R. ended the session by underlining these strengths and giving them an appointment. He gave them a phone number were he could be reached and promised to give them a personal call in the next few days to see how they were doing. He then stated that if he heard from his relative in Puerto Rico, he would ask him if he knew their *compadre.*

Because the process of departure is often prolonged in this culture, Dr. R. gave himself ample time to say goodbye in order to avoid being offensive and abrupt. The interview ended with a respectful handshake to Mr. S. and a comment to Mrs. S. that he wished her and her family the best. Perhaps in the next session she could bring a picture of her family in Puerto Rico and further discuss her experience of migration. Dr. R., after he completed the evaluation and had made a diagnosis, decided to implement a trial of medication mixed with supportive and family therapy and environmental interventions for Mrs. S. He eventually referred Mr. S. to a Hispanic Alcoholics Anonymous group in his community.

Conclusion

Puerto Ricans have a long history of exposure to different cultures. Their historical development combines the Indo-Caribbean, African, and Spanish value systems and physical characteristics. As their history evolved, they were exposed to the mainstream culture of the United States and the cultures of a host of other ethnic groups whose members settled in the large urban mainland centers.

Puerto Ricans are a people whose national identity evolved and solidified in the face of a long history of colonial rule, first by the Spanish and later in modified form by the United States. They have weathered major shifts in their cultural values and their language, have undergone an unusually intense industrial revolution, and have been strengthened by large waves of back-and-forth migration.

Epidemiologic research has offered some preliminary findings that suggest important mental health profiles for different Puerto Rican subgroups. The frequency of substance abuse in Puerto Rican males and of dysthymia in Puerto Rican females, and the frequency of somatic symptoms in the Puerto Rican population as a whole, should alert clinicians to the close relationship between culture and symptom expression. Service utilization patterns and the impact of sociocultural values and socioeconomic stressors such as migration, poverty, and acculturation are added factors that have to be considered in the assessment and treatment of this population.

Clearly, research has to be done in terms of specific biological or familial risk factors of the Puerto Rican population. There is a need for more transcultural studies comparing different racial and ethnic groups to assess the real impact of specific cultures on symptom expression. These studies must utilize a standardized and culturally sensitive methodology and instrumentation. Finally, conclusive research on the very difficult arena of treatment efficacy and specificity is still lacking.

While we wait for these research initiatives, social policies can reduce the environmental stress factors that certainly exacerbate symptom expression and may precipitate mental illness in vulnerable populations. Programs that are culturally and socially sensitive can be reinstituted to offer not only treatment services but also prevention and education programs. It is only then that Puerto Ricans with mental illnesses or who are experiencing extreme social stressors can be fully integrated as members of their culture and of society in general.

References

Abad V, Boyce E: Issues in the psychiatric evaluation of Puerto Ricans. Journal of Operational Psychiatry 10:28–39, 1979

Abad V, Ramos J, Boyce E: A model for delivery of mental health services to Spanish speaking minorities. Am J Orthopsychiatry 44(4):584–595, 1974

Achenbach TM, Edelbrock CS: Manual for the Child Behavior Checklist and Revised Child Behavior Profile. Burlington, VT, University of Vermont, Department of Psychiatry, 1983

Alegria M, Robles R, Freeman D, et al: Patterns of mental health utilization among island Puerto Rican poor. Am J Public Health 81(7):875–879, 1991

American Psychiatric Association: Diagnostic and Statistical Manual of Mental Disorders, 3rd Edition. Washington, DC, American Psychiatric Association, 1980

Bird HR, Canino I: The sociopsychiatry of espiritismo: findings of a study on psychiatric populations of Puerto Ricans and other Hispanic children. Journal of the American Academy of Child Psychiatry 20:725–740, 1981

Bird H, Canino G, Rubio-Stipec M, et al: Estimates of the prevalence of childhood maladjustment in a community survey in Puerto Rico. Arch Gen Psychiatry 45:1120–1126, 1988

Bird HR, Gould MS, Yager T, et al: Risk factors of maladjustment in Puerto Rican children. J Am Acad Child Adolesc Psychiatry 28:847–850, 1989

Bluestone H, Purdy B: Psychiatric services to Puerto Rican patients in the Bronx, in Transcultural Psychiatry: A Hispanic Perspective (Spanish Speaking Mental Health Research Center, Monograph No 4). Edited by Padilla ER, Padilla ER. Los Angeles, CA, University of California Press, 1977

Bluestone H, Vela RM: Transcultural aspects in the psychotherapy of the Puerto Rican poor in New York City. J Am Acad Psychoanal 10(2):269–282, 1982

Canino G: Functional and dysfunctional families of Puerto Rican female adolescents:

acculturation and sex role expectation, in Work, Family, and Health: Latino Women in Transition (Hispanic Research Center, Monograph No 7). Edited by Zambrana R. New York, Fordham University Press, 1982a, pp 27–36

Canino G: The Hispanic woman: sociocultural influences on diagnoses and treatment, in Health and Hispanic Americans: Clinical Perspectives. Edited by Becerra R, Karno M, Escobar J. New York, Grune & Stratton, 1982b, pp 117–138

Canino G, Canino IA: Culturally syntonic family therapy for migrant Puerto Ricans. Hosp Community Psychiatry 33(4):299–303, 1982

Canino G, Rubio-Stipec M, Shrout P, et al: Sex differences and depression in Puerto Rico. Psychology of Women Quarterly 11:443–459, 1987a

Canino G, Bird H, Rubio-Stipec M, et al: The prevalence of specific psychiatric disorders in Puerto Rico. Arch Gen Psychiatry 44:127–133, 1987b

Canino G, Gournam A, Caetano R: The prevalence of alcohol abuse and or dependence in two Hispanic communities, in Alcoholism—North America, Europe, and Asia: A Coordinated Analysis of Population From Ten Regions. Edited by Helzer J, Canino G. New York, Oxford University Press, 1992, pp 289–308

Canino I: Taking a history, in The Clinical Guide to Child Psychiatry. Edited by Shaffer D, Ehrhardt A, Greenhill L. New York, Free Press, 1985, pp 393–408

Canino IA, Canino G: Impact of stress on the Puerto Rican family: treatment considerations. Am J Orthopsychiatry 50(3):535–541, 1980

Canino IA, Velez CN, Canino G: Research and clinical issues in studying Hispanics: an overview with an emphasis on Puerto Rican children, in Health and Behavior: Research Agenda for Hispanics. Edited by Gaviria M, Arana JD. Champaign/Urbana, IL, University of Illinois Press, 1987, pp 219–232

Canino I, Early B, Rogler L: The Puerto Rican Child in New York City: Stress and Mental Health, 2nd Edition (Hispanic Research Center, Monograph No 4).New York, Fordham University Press, 1988

Canino IA, Rubio Stipec MA, Canino G, et al: Functional somatic symptoms: a cross-ethnic comparison. Am J Orthopsychiatry (in press)

Caplow T, Styker S, Wallace SE: The Urban Ambience. Totowa, NJ, Bedminster Press, 1964

Cobb C: Community mental health services in the lower socioeconomic classes: a summary of research literature on outpatient treatment (1963–1969). Am J Orthopsychiatry 42(3):404–14, 1972

Comas-Diaz L, Jacobsen FM: Ethnocultural identification in psychotherapy. Psychiatry 50(3):232–241, 1987

Current Population Report: Population Characteristics (Series P-20, No. 903). Washington, DC, U.S. Bureau of the Census, December 1985

De La Cancela V, Guarnaccia P, Carrillo E: Psychosocial distress among latinos: a critical analysis of ataques de nervios. Humanity and Society 10:431–447, 1986

Departamento de Educación: Informe Anual, División de Estadísticas. [Department of Education: Annual Report, Statistics Division.] San Juan, Puerto Rico, Departamento de Educación, 1987–1988

Departamento de Educación: Tazas de Deserción Escolar. [Department of Education: Dropout Rates (Statistics Division).] San Juan, Puerto Rico, Departamento de Educación, División de Estadísticas, 1988–1989

Departamento de Salud: Informe Anual de Estadísticas Vitales, División de Estadísticas. [Department of Health: Annual Report of Vital Statistics, Statistics Division.] San Juan, Puerto Rico, Departamento de Salud, 1988

Departamento de Salud: Oficina de Planificación, Evaluación e Informes—Boletín Informativo (Serie D-6: 2). [Department of Health: Planning Board, Evaluation and Information—Informational Bulletin.] Santurce, Puerto Rico, Departamento de Salud, Febrero 1989

Departamento de Trabajo: Encuesta de Vivienda. [Department of Labor: Life-Style Survey.] San Juan, Puerto Rico, Departamento de Trabajo, 1989

Departamento Servicios Sociales: Informe Social, Junta de Planificación. [Department of Social Services: Division Report, Planning Board.] San Juan, Puerto Rico, Departamento Servicios Sociales, 1988

Dohrenwend BP: Social status and psychological disorder: an issue of substance, an issue of method. American Sociology Review 31:14–34, 1966

Dohrenwend BP, Dohrenwend BS: Social Status and Psychological Disorder: A Causal Inquiry. New York, Wiley, 1969

English Proficiency of Latinos (Public Use Microdata Sample, 5% Sample)—New York City. Washington, DC, U.S. Bureau of the Census, 1980

Escobar J, Rubio-Stipec M, Canino G, et al: Unfounded physical complaints in the community: further validation of an abridged somatization construct. J Nerv Ment Dis 117:140–146, 1989

Fernandez-Marina R: The Puerto Rican syndrome. Psychiatry 24:79–82, 1961

Fitzpatrick JP: Puerto Rican Americans: The Meaning of Migration to the Mainland. Englewood Cliffs, NJ, Prentice-Hall, 1971

Garrison V: Supporting structures in a disorganized Puerto Rican migrant community. Paper presented at the 70th annual meeting of the American Anthropological Association, New York, December 1971

Garrison V: Doctor, espiritista, or psychiatrist? help seeking behavior in a Puerto Rican neighborhood in New York City. Med Anthropol 1:64–185, 1977a

Garrison V: The Puerto Rican syndrome, in Psychiatry and Spiritism: Case Studies in Spirit Possession. Edited by Crapanzano V, Garrison V. New York, Wiley, 1977b, pp 383–448

Gomez AG: The Puerto Rican American, in Cross-Cultural Psychiatry. Edited by Gaw A. Littleton, MA, John Wright-PSG Pub Co, 1982, pp 109–136

Gonzalez LG: Relación entre visión hacia los roles sexuales, actualización personal y problemas de salud mental en tres grupos de mujeres. [Relationship among view of sex roles, personal actualization, and mental health problems in three groups of mothers.] Tesis de Maestría, Universidad de Puerto Rico, Departamento de Psicología [Master's Thesis, University of Puerto Rico, Psychology Department], 1978

Graffagnino PH, Buchnam F, Orgun I, et al: Psychotherapy for latency age children in an inner city therapeutic school. Am J Psychiatry 127:626–634, 1970

Griffith MS: The influences of race on the psychotherapeutic relationship. Psychiatry 40:27–40, 1977

Guarnaccia P, Rubio-Stipec M, Canino G: Ataques de Nervios in the Puerto Rico Diagnostic Interview Schedule: the impact of cultural categories on psychiatric epidemiology. Cult Med Psychiatry 13:275–295, 1989

Guarnaccia P, Canino, G, Rubio Stipec M, et al: The prevalence of Ataques de Nervios in Puerto Rico: the role of culture in psychiatric epidemiology. J Nerv Ment Dis (in press)

Haberman PW: Ethnic differences in psychiatric symptoms reported in community surveys. Public Health Rep 85:495–502, 1970

Haberman PW: Psychiatric symptoms among Puerto Ricans in Puerto Rico and New York City. Ethnicity 3:133–144, 1976

Harwood A: Rx: Spiritist as Needed. New York, Wiley, 1977

Helzer JE, Canino G, Hwo HG, et al: Alcoholism: a cross-national comparison of population surveys with the DIS, in Alcoholism: Origins and Outcome. Edited by Rose RM, Barret J. New York, Raven Press, 1988, pp

Hohmann A, Richeport M, Marriott B, et al: Spiritism in Puerto Rico: results of an island-wide community study. Br J Psychiatry 156:328–335, 1990

Kardec A: El Libro de los Espíritus [The Book of the Spirits] (1869). Mexico City, Orion, 1951

Krause N, Carr LG: The effects of response bias in the survey assessment of the mental health of Puerto Rican migrants. Social Psychiatry 13:167–173, 1978

Leavitt RR: The Puerto Ricans: Culture Change and Language Deviance. Tucson, AZ, University of Arizona Press, 1974

Lubchanski I, Egri G, Stokes J: Puerto Rican spiritualists view mental illness; the faith healer as a paraprofessional. Am J Psychiatry 127:312–331, 1970

Mann E, Salvo J: Appendix: characteristics of new Hispanic immigrants to New York City: a comparison of Puerto Rican and non-Puerto Rican Hispanics, in The Puerto Rican Child in New York City: Stress and Mental Health. Edited by Canino I, Early B, Rogler L. New York, Fordham University Press, 1988, pp 123–141

Marcos LR: Bilinguals in psychotherapy: language as an emotional barrier. Am J Psychother 30:552–560, 1976

Marcos LR: Effects of interpreters on the evaluation of psychopathology in non-English speaking patients. Am J Psychiatry 2:171–174, 1979

Marcos LR, Urcuyo L: Dynamic psychotherapy with the bilingual patient. Am J Psychother 33:331–338, 1979

Marcos LR, Eisma JE, Guiman J: Bilingualism and sense of self. Am J Psychoanal 37:285–290, 1977

Martinez R, Sessman M, Bravo M, et al: Utilización de servicios de salud en Puerto Rico por personas con trastornos mentales. [Utilization of health services in Puerto Rico by people with mental disturbances.] P R Health Sci J 10:38–42, 1991

Meers DR: Psychoanalytic research and intellectual functioning of ghetto reared Black children. Psychoanal Study Child 28:395–417, 1973

Munoz M: The effects of role expectations on the marital status of urban Puerto Rican women, in The Puerto Rican Woman. Edited by Acosta B. New York, Praeger, 1979

Murphy LB, Moriarty AE: Vulnerability, Coping and Growth: From Infancy to Adolescence, 2nd Edition. New Haven, CT, Yale University Press, 1978

Oficina del Gobernador: Informe Económico al Gobernador (Junta de Planificación de Puerto Rico, Estado Libre Asociado de Puerto Rico). [Governor's Office: Governor's Economic Report, Planning Board of Puerto Rico, Commonwealth of Puerto Rico.] San Juan, Puerto Rico, Oficina del Gobernador, 1988

Offord DR, Boyle MH, Szatmari P, et al: The Ontario Child Health Study: prevalence of disorder and rates of service utilization. Arch Gen Psychiatry 44:832–836, 1987

Phillipus MJ: Successful and unsuccessful approaches to mental health services for an urban Hispanic American population. Am J Public Health 61(4):820–830, 1971

Pitta P, Marcos LR, Alpert M: Language switching as a treatment strategy with bilingual patients. Am J Psychiatry 38:255–258, 1978

Price CS, Cuellar I: Effects of language and related variables on the expression of psychopathology in Mexican-American psychiatric patients. Hispanic Journal of Behavioral Sciences 3:145–160, 1981

Ramos HA, Morales MM: U.S. immigration and the Hispanic community: a historical overview and sociological perspective. Journal of Hispanic Politics 1(1):1–17, 1985

Ramos-McKay JM, Comas-Diaz L, Rivera LA: Puerto Ricans, in Clinical Guidelines in Cross Cultural Mental Health. Edited by Comas-Diaz L, Griffith EH. New York, Wiley, 1988, pp 204–232

Robins LN, Regier O: Psychiatric Disorders in America. New York, Free Press, 1991

Robins LN, Helzer JE, Croughan J, et al: National Institute of Mental Health Diagnostic Interview Schedule: its history, characteristics, and validity. Arch Gen Psychiatry 38:381–389, 1981

Robins LN, Helzer JE, Weissman MM, et al: Lifetime prevalence of specific psychiatric disorders in three sites. Arch Gen Psychiatry 41:949–958, 1984

Robles R, Martinez, R, Moscoso M: A study of Puerto Rican return migration: impact on the migrant and the island (unpublished). Río Piedras, Puerto Rico, University of Puerto Rico, School of Public Health, 1980

Rodriguez CE: Puerto Ricans Born in the U.S.A. Boston, MA, Unwin Hyman, 1989

Rodriguez O: Hispanics and Human Services: Help Seeking in the Inner City (Hispanic Research Center, Monograph No 14). New York, Fordham University Press, 1987

Rogler LH, Cooney RS: Puerto Rican Families in New York City: Intergenerational Processes. Maplewood, NJ, Waterfront Press, 1984

Rogler L, Hollingshead A: The Puerto Rican spiritualist as psychiatrist. Am J Psychiatry 67:17–22, 1961

Rogler L, Hollingshead A: Trapped Families and Schizophrenia. New York, Wiley,

1965

Rogler LH, Hollingshead A: Trapped: Puerto Rican Families and Schizophrenia. Maplewood, NJ, Waterfront Press, 1975

Rogler LH, Cooney RS, Costantino G, et al: A Conceptual Framework for Mental Health Research on Hispanic Populations (Hispanic Research Center, Monograph No 10). New York, Fordham University Press, 1983

Rogler LH, Malgady RG, Rodriguez O: Hispanics and Mental Health: A Framework for Research. Melbourne, FL, Robert E Krieger Publishing Co, 1989

Rozensky RH, Gomez MY: Language switching in psychotherapy with bilinguals: two problems, two models, and case examples. Psychotherapy: Theory, Research and Practice 20:152–160, 1983

Ruiz P, Langrod J: The role of folk healers in community mental health services. Community Ment Health J 12(4):392–398, 1976

Salgado RM: The role of the Puerto Rican spiritist in helping Puerto Ricans with problems of family relations (DAI #ADG74-26616). Doctoral dissertation, Columbia University Teachers College, 1974

Shrout P, Canino G, Bird HI, et al: Mental disorders among Los Angeles Anglos and two Hispanic groups, island Puerto Ricans and Los Angeles Mexican Americans. Journal of Community Psychology (in press)

Sluzki CE: Migrations and family conflict. Fam Process 19(4):379–390, 1979

Srole L, Fisher AK: Mental Health in the Metropolis: The Midtown Manhattan Study. New York, McGraw-Hill, 1962

Sue DW: Counselling the Culturally Different: Theory and Practice. New York, Wiley, 1981

Torres-Matrullo CM: Acculturation and psychopathology among Puerto Rican women in the mainland United States. Am J Orthopsychiatry 46(4):710–719, 1976

Uriarte-Gaston M: Organizing for survival: the emergence of a Puerto Rican community (DAI #ADG88-02803). Doctoral dissertation, Boston University, 1987

Verhulst FC, Berde GFMG, Sanders-Woudstra JAR, et al: Mental health in Dutch children, II: the prevalence of psychiatric disorder and relationship between measures. Acta Psychiatr Scand 72:324, 1985

Weissman M, Livingston BM, Leaf P, et al: Affective disorders, in Psychiatric Disorders in America. Edited by Robins L, Regier E. New York, Free Press, 1991, pp 53–80

17   Culture and Psychiatric Care of Women

Carol C. Nadelson, M.D.
Veva Zimmerman, M.D.

C an the clinician approach patients simply as individuals, or do we all carry the baggage of our own cultures and gender-related subcultures?

Cultural stereotypes intermingle issues of culture and gender. Tannen (1990), for example, remarks on Barbara Bush's characterization of Geraldine Ferraro as "bitchy" (p. 209). She also notes that women from African, Mediterranean, Caribbean, and Eastern European cultures and backgrounds often are perceived by other Americans of northern European extraction as being aggressive, pushy, and domineering. In what is—or at least was—the dominant American culture, these traits are disparaged in women, though they may be highly praised in men.

All people are seen through others' lenses. What is more, these stereotypes are almost always based on gender as well as on cultural values. This is not likely to be apparent to the dominant groups—white males, for example—who create or inspire the stereotypes. But these factors are of critical concern, at all times, to members of so-called minority groups, because it is these values that perpetuate their disadvantage and the pain they often experience because of it.

The dominant idea of woman conjures up images of softness, nurturance, an affinity for relationships, and traits of moodiness and vulnerability. Women are also manipulative, according to the prevailing stereotype, and they require emotional support. These depictions cannot help but linger in the culturally derived preconscious of male physicians when they are evaluating a female patient, just as they color their relationships with all other women in their lives. Likewise, it may be internalized by women. The cost may be anxiety, and perhaps more depressive symptomatology when relational bonds are disrupted. Instead of being able to express anger, culturally approved personality constellations inhibit women's expression of aggressivity whether they are betrayed or wish to project themselves onto the larger world. The "virtues" of self-sacrifice, and service to others, may lead many women to decision making and behavior that simply is not in their own best interests.

Men, and masculinity, by contrast, carry expectations of muscularity, strength, dominance, and independence. They must project individuality and authority. The juxtaposition of these and other stereotypes with reality are the source of much confusion when men try to understand women, and when women try to understand men.

These stereotypic associations influence the questions we ask in research, and even our scientific formulations (Bleier 1984; Keller 1985). Eichler and her colleagues at the Ontario Institute for Studies in Education have elucidated three specific and troubling problems of bias in research: *androcentricity,* which they define as viewing the world from the male perspective; *overgeneralization,* which means that data obtained from only one of the sexes are applied to them both; and *gender insensitivity,* which means ignoring gender as a socially or medically important variable (Eichler et al. 1990).

The distortions that result are rife. When alcoholism is the subject of research, for example, the study populations selected or defined tend to be male (Eichler et al. 1990). The women looked at in these studies tend to be predefined as the *wives* of alcoholics. The ravages of suburban alcoholism in women thus remain hidden to the casual reader of these investigations. Even in studies completed within the last decade, men who suffer from alcoholism are depicted as victims of their wives' personalities and behavior. For years, coronary heart disease (CHD) was studied and presented as predominantly a male health problem. Recent studies and consciousness-raising have driven home the point that CHD is the principal killer of women as well. Yet, the studies have been done and the treatment recommendations that have been made are based solely on data from male populations ("Heart research efforts aim at fairness to women" 1990).

Women and Health

Women continue to be the ones who identify and deliver health care in families. Even in the postfeminist modern household, the woman tends to be the central caretaker. It is she who determines the marketing success of pharmaceutical products. More often than not, she is the one who calls the doctor and delivers children to the pediatrician when they are in need of care. Women, too, are greater consumers of health care services than men:

they average 25% more doctor visits per annum than men. These economic parameters define demographic findings about health care ("From the Alcohol, Drug Abuse, and Mental Health Administration" 1991).

Women's role in society has almost always been defined in terms of a social mandate to bear children. Improved neonatal survival on the one hand, and the ability to control reproduction on the other, both have demographic consequences and reveal women's strong influence on population dynamics.

Gender differences come to the fore in obstetrical care, particularly when the provider of care is a male. Pregnancy reopens a bridge back to a primitivism that all of us share. It also is a wordless reminder of Nature's ultimate control over our lives. A new mother quickly becomes caught up in the mysterious privilege of physically creating human life. The masculine experience of the male obstetrician is strikingly different. He may experience feelings of exclusion, rivalry, and competitiveness or may see the primitive process of gestation and birth as something that needs to be controlled or modified. This may be translated into excessive intervention.

Pediatricians are also subject to similar differences in experience and affect. In the past, they discouraged breast-feeding based on their conviction that bottle-feeding was better, because it facilitated regimentation of infants into their adult caretakers' schedules. The basis in science for this intervention was not identified, yet the change profoundly affected several generations of children in the United States and other countries. In the Third World, millions were persuaded by advertising and detailing campaigns to forswear the breast for the bottle. It seems clear that one factor in this switch, which many experts now view as highly misguided, was the differing perceptions and expectations of women and men.

Societal Change

Women's biological roles (like men's) subject them to experiences and grant them entitlements that are codified by the cultures in which they live. They may experience these attitudes and events as sources of distinction or of confusion, or as perquisites of femininity. Cultures vary when they define "normal" roles or behaviors, and each is affected differently by context.

The significant social changes that have occurred in the United States and other developed nations in the last several decades have changed the roles, lives, and stresses of both sexes. Concepts of normality and gender-related social roles and expectations have changed, and expanded, particularly for women. In many areas of life, the boundaries between masculine and feminine roles have broken down (Nadelson and Notman 1991).

The definition of "family" and its legal underpinnings have also changed to include nonbiologically or nonmaritally related partners. Who works and who earns is changing too, and the one-breadwinner family seems to be headed for extinction. Half of American mothers of preschool children work outside the home; by the time the children are in school all day, almost two-thirds of their mothers now work. What is more, it is economic need and not career ambitions that send most women into the workplace (Kahne 1990).

The results may not be wholly felicitous. On the one hand, a host of "problems" have been identified around the so-called "latchkey children," who face each late afternoon and many evenings without parental supervision. More important, because many of their mothers preside over single-parent families, which they cannot adequately support, poverty is a major part of women's new social role, and this may be the most salient factor in the "problems."

Men traditionally have society's approval for their roles outside the household. But their response to women's new roles, and to their rewards, even when they are major beneficiaries of their wives' employment, is ambivalent at best, and it may be a factor in the increasing rates of divorce and mental distress.

It is essential for us to understand these new disharmonies between men and women in any effort to assess contemporary women's emotional and psychological disturbances. This understanding, however, will be only the latest chapter in the long history of what is called—somewhat disparagingly, we believe—women and mental illness. (We do not, after all, hear comparable discussions about *men* and mental illness!) The experiences of Mr. and Mrs. D. illustrate some of these points.

Case Study 1

The D.s met in professional school, and developed a friendship and then a deeply shared intimacy. But after 5 years, their marriage became dysfunctional.

Mr. D., a somewhat sadistic and distant man, lapsed into long periods of highly romanticized concern for and rejection of his wife's vulnerabilities. The onset of this pattern was preceded by their discovery of her inability to conceive children. To the therapeutic observer, the defensive nature of the husband's concern and its brittleness were clear. But among their families, business friends, and neighbors, this concern was regarded as a desirable character resource. Mrs. D. responded to these periods of stereotyped concern with fear, marked inhibition, and a clinical depression. Casual observers of this family, however, did not perceive the relationship between her behavioral pattern and her husband's.

This dysfunctional relationship appeared to serve both partners: Mr. D. was able to contain his emergent aggression and shore up his threatened self-esteem by denying the kind of vulnerability he caustically projected onto his wife. Mrs. D., on the other hand, submitted to the role he assigned her with assumed passivity and a major suicidal depression in order to deal with her terror of her own aggression. This served as a protection from the imagined dire consequences if she were to successfully conquer the external world—which, professionally, she was well able to do. The relationship remained intact as long as Mrs. D. was capable of absorbing Mr. D's projected vulnerability. The stereotypes here were cleverly contrived to conceal each partner's core personality.

Gender Differences in Psychiatric Disorders

The effect of gender on psychiatric diagnoses has been well-established. Careful analysis in the Epidemiologic Catchment Area (ECA) study indicates that eating disorders, depression, and also some phobias occur more frequently in women, whereas antisocial behavior, alcoholism, and drug addiction are more common in men (Regier et al. 1984). Several hypotheses have been put forward through the years to explain these gender differences in the prevalence of mental disorders (Weissman and Klerman 1977). In a recent report, McGrath and colleagues (1990) proposed that the higher rate of depression in women is not the direct result of biological differences between the sexes. Rather, they attribute this extra burden of depressive illness to a "biopsychosocial" combination of risk factors that operate to women's detriment in the contemporary social setting. Historically sanctioned passive dependent behavioral patterns, physical or sexual abuse, and women's greater vulnerability to depression in their marriages all are implicated by McGrath and colleagues as constituents of women's greater mental health burden (McGrath et al. 1990). Women who are unhappily married are three times more likely to be depressed than are unhappily married men or single women. Mothers of young children are at higher risk of depression than older women whose children are grown.

Agoraphobia has been reported to be more prevalent in women. This phobia has been attributed, at least in part, to fear of object loss, separation anxiety, and self-punitive efforts to control aggressivity (Ginsberg et al. 1972; Regier et al. 1984). Reproductive events, including menstruation, pregnancy, childbirth, and menopause, are often linked to mental illness in women. For example, we diagnose premenstrual syndrome and postpartum psychoses, and we have only recently abandoned the concept of menopausal or "involutional" depression. Parenting and single parenthood are stressors that also appear to increase women's vulnerability to mental illness (McGrath et al. 1990). Women who belong to minority groups or who have problems of chemical dependency are at significantly greater risk for mental illness than white middle-class women (Frezza et al. 1990).

The gender gap in mental diagnoses begins to be apparent by late adolescence. It is not present earlier in childhood (McGrath et al. 1990). One reason may be because young women are much more likely to be victims of sexual abuse than are young men of the same age. Women tend to be less pleased with pubertal changes than young men. They face relational and intrapsychic conflicts between their abilities and the perception that continues to prevail that intelligence, competence, and other such attributes are a liability in the dating and mating game.

Ideas about women's vulnerability are often internalized and, when coupled with real-life events, may be inhibiting to women, in whom they can be a source of conflict. The case of A. H. illustrates this point.

Case Study 2

A. H. is a 36-year-old junior partner in a law firm, an outdoors person who is comfortable with the risks of injury, natural catastrophe, and encounters with wild animals that are part of the outdoors experience. She usually feels secure enough in her skills to master her fears in the wilderness.

On a hiking trip in the Canadian Rockies, however, A. H. found herself to be unusually fearful. Thinking back, she realized that she recently had read an account of a serial murderer who attacked women in the West. She realized that, for the first time in her life, she felt intensely vulnerable as a woman, and she changed her plans as a result.

The attribution of vulnerability to women appears to serve as a differentiating or isolating factor between the sexes. The woman is isolated in her weakness; the man can deny or ignore his own vulnerabilities by projecting it onto his spouse or other sexual partner, or onto women in general.

Another way to read the effects of gender differences in vulnerability to mental illness is to look at women's presenting complaints in the psychiatric consulting room. These complaints have changed as society has become more concerned about open sexual expression, and as it has become aware of the greater freedom of choice that women have claimed for themselves.

During the 1960s and 1970s, for example, college-age women began to appear in practitioners' offices complaining about their inability to reach orgasmic climax in their sex lives. When this phenomenon was studied, it became clear that their inhibitions reflected men's fears of the assertive expressiveness of women's emerging new attitudes about sexual intercourse as well as their own ambivalence about the new pressures they experienced (Kaplan 1983).

Differences in skin color or ethnicity based on nationality, cultural, or religious identifiers compound many clinical problems. Physicians, many of whom have not been well-trained in the nuances of racial and sexual politics, may fail to recognize the stereotypes that they apply to minority women—stereotypes that these women in turn may reinforce and encourage because they do not know how to escape them. These biases can seriously interfere with medical and psychiatric diagnosis and treatment and may even impinge on our research findings about these sensitive issues.

Aggressivity, for example, may be particularly difficult. For minority women, it may be even more misunderstood.

Case Study 3

T. F. is a 30-year-old assistant professor at a major university in the East. She is African American and has had to overcome many social and economic difficulties to reach this level of professional achievement. She understood, what is more, that many of her colleagues felt that she had arrived there because of affirmative action, not because of her talents.

Over the course of a semester, to prove herself T. F. began to seek and accept more and more work and responsibility. She increased the number of her student advisees, committing herself to participate in several research and writing projects on short deadline. Students complained that they could not understand her because she spoke too rapidly and moved too quickly from topic to topic.

Meanwhile, T. F. became more and more intense and aggressive in her dealings with colleagues, whom she frequently telephoned in the middle of the night during bouts of wakefulness. She lost weight rapidly, because she was not eating. But her colleagues, nevertheless, were slow in coming to the realization that she was hypomanic.

Looking back, after she had recovered, T. F. thought that cultural stereotypes had delayed recognition of her illness. She believed that her colleagues did not take her seriously and had excused her poor work performance in their own minds on the grounds that it perhaps is okay for African Americans not to perform well—a demeaning and humiliating point of view.

Cases like this underscore the urgency of wide professional—and we believe also societal—reassessment of both cultural- and gender-related stereotypes.

Gender issues play a role in our therapeutic efforts, even in such seemingly objective areas as psychopharmacology. We do not clearly know, for many psychotropic agents, the interactions of estrogen, progesterone, and other hormones with the drugs' absorption, kinetics, metabolism, and other parameters. Although these factors are sometimes studied in terms of women's specific reproductive events (e.g., pregnancy), they are not a routine part of all research and postmarketing studies of drugs.

One research area where this information has recently been collected with important gender-related results is in studies of substance abuse, particularly alcoholism. There now is evidence that sexually determined differences in alcohol metabolism lead to different patterns of alcohol consumption and alcoholism symptomatology (Broverman et al. 1970).

The delivery of mental health services is also influenced by the recipients's gender. Kaplan attributes these differences to masculine perceptions of healthy and unhealthy behavior, which now have been codified in DSM categories (Zeldow 1978). Another, perhaps not incompatible view is that the higher treatment rate for women reflects women's greater willingness to display their symptomatology. On the other hand, women may be at a disadvantage and at higher risk for mental illness.

Gender and Psychotherapy

Gender values influence psychotherapy in both clearly evident and subtle ways. These values can affect perceptions, diagnoses, and treatment of mental illness. When a patient's behavior is labeled "deviant" rather than "sick," for example, an assumption is made about what is and what is not normal. This judgment, in turn, may determine whether treatment is offered, the type of such treatment, and the outcome (Ginsberg et al. 1972).

As a chilling example of this, one of us recalls hearing from a highly regarded teacher of psychodynamics the view that hysterical features are highly desirable when they occur in women! He said this with affection and admiration, seemingly unmoved by the psychic pain and duress generated by the neurotic processes underlying hysteria in women, as well as in men.

Some of these issues have been explored in the literature but are often not incorporated into the teaching of psychotherapy. In a classic study, Broverman and colleagues (1970) showed that both male and female psychotherapists tended to use masculine descriptors in defining mental health in women, as well as in men (Ginsberg et al. 1972). Zeldow (1978) has shown that psychopathologic diagnoses continue to reflect traditional, male-oriented norms, rather than objective criteria of mental health. (Many other investigators have presented evidence that mental health definitions and diagnostic criteria continue to reflect traditional views to a greater extent than one might like to imagine [Loring and Powell 1988; Nadelson et al. 1982; Slavney and Chase 1985].) On the other hand, Slavney and Chase, who used videotapes of male and female actors depicting various behaviors, found that psychiatrists who viewed these tapes reported no diagnostic differences based on gender (Gilligan 1982; Warner 1978).

An opposite finding was reported by Loring and Powell (1988), who asked psychiatrists to assess case reports of patients with either an undifferentiated schizophrenic Axis I diagnosis or a dependent personality disorder Axis II diagnosis. They varied the gender and skin color of the "patients" in this study and in some cases did not stipulate their gender or race. The researchers found that the gender of the psychiatrist and of the "patient" influenced the psychiatrist's diagnosis.

In a somewhat similar study, Warner (1978) handed therapists a clinical profile of patients that contained both histrionic and antisocial behaviors (King 1989). The patient's gender was varied. If the profile identified the patient as a man, the therapists tended to diagnose antisocial personality. But if the patient was identified as a woman, the clinicians favored a diagnosis of hysterical personality. In Warner's view, *hysterical personality* and *antisocial personality* are sex-stereotyped diagnoses of the same mental condition.

The therapist's gender values cannot help but be communicated to patients. One indicator of these values is the type of questions the therapist asks and the type of comments he or she then makes. The timing of interpretations and the therapist's affective response to the clinical material also are freighted with these values. The therapist's responses to patient material on menstruation, substance abuse, and provocative or dangerous sexual behavior all can carry the message of the therapist's gender values. A therapist who is more responsive to work-related problems in male patients and to love-related problems in women is expressing gender values in his or her interactions with patients of both sexes. The therapist's prioritizing of these issues may be different than the patient's; thus, the therapist may fail to accommodate the patient's needs in treatment (Nadelson and Notman 1977, 1991; Nadelson et al. 1982; Person 1983).

Many patients say that their therapists fail to recognize or appreciate their life-styles (Nadelson and Notman 1977, 1991; Nadelson et al. 1982). This complaint is frequently heard from female patients working with male therapists, but this behavior can also occur frequently in male patients' treatment by female therapists. Dyadic relationships across social, cultural, and economic lines may cause similar problems. Although women have taken prominent roles as psychotherapists or psychoanalysts, most theoretical and even clinical literature is from the male perspective. Gilligan has remarked on the need for greater participation of the "female voice" (Gilligan 1982). Cross-cultural voices must also be heard.

The classical view has been that these values would not affect the process in the consulting room, because the transference was the primary therapeutic tool and the therapist's real personality, traits, and values were less relevant. Recent work suggests that the therapist's age, race, gender, and other specific traits are important therapeutic considerations (Nadelson and Notman 1991). These traits affect the order in which treatment issues come to the fore as well as the pace of therapeutic progress.

An African American patient may be inhibited about describing behavior(s) that he or she fears may reinforce a white therapist's stereotyped views. Details of sexual abuse or other sexual behavior may be withheld for the same reason. By the same token, women patients frequently tell female therapists that they do not discuss menstrual issues candidly or in detail with their male therapists. They also may shade or omit discussions about rape, hysterectomy, abortion, or other strongly feminine concerns (Nadelson and Notman 1991). This filtering of information can have serious negative consequences for therapy, and inappropriate treatment may be the result. A depressed woman who withholds information on earlier child abuse may not be treated in the same way as she might if she were able to be candid.

Patients' requests for therapists of a particular gender, race, or sexual orientation are based on values, attitudes, and stereotypes—just like therapists' referrals. For each, the reasons may be *political* (e.g., to a therapist who holds or professes certain beliefs), *social* (e.g., if there is a perceived need for the patient to have a strong role model), or *unconscious* (e.g., the patient's wish for a different mother). These conscious and unconscious choices by patient, referring therapist, and treatment therapist always should be explored in the treatment. The initial values and expectations may significantly affect the patient's therapeutic progress (Nadelson et al. 1982).

Some women seek a female therapist in the belief that a woman will be more supportive of their wishes for self-actualization, or more empathetic because, presumably, the therapist has faced some of the same problems these women have (Nadelson and Notman 1977, 1991; Nadelson et al. 1982). This may or may not be true. It may help solidify a working therapeutic alliance.

But these bonds cannot resolve the patient's problems—and it is important that the therapist keeps this in mind and conveys it to the patient in an appropriate manner.

Patients may seek a therapist of the same race or ethnic background for essentially similar reasons of (anticipated) shared values and understanding. Here, too, the "honeymoon" feelings may be enhanced by the patient's sense of having successfully established a good working relationship with his or her therapist. It also can be dangerously deceptive: if unexplored, it can help the patient avoid confrontation with pathologic feelings and maladaptive behaviors.

These same considerations apply in group and family therapy. Ethnic and cultural variables are, in a sense, real-life experiences. Instead of being seen categorically as transference phenomena or as resistances in therapeutic work, they must be analyzed in terms of their context within the patient's life.

When woman patients are also members of minority ethnic or social groups, there are special issues involved. These patients must be seen in a context, as representatives of what might be called "double minorities."

The dynamics at play here have been described by feminist sociologist Deborah King, who elucidates what she calls a "both/or" orientation that pervades African American women's relationships with their own group and, simultaneously, the wider world (King 1989). They are at once members of their group and, as professionals or patients, they stand apart from the group; they are outside of it. This in turn promotes the development of a "multiple consciousness," a sometimes inescapable sense of belonging yet not quite being there.

Because of their double-minority status, King (1989) explains, African American women are careful to avoid being taken as "fools of any type." They feel—she believes—that because of their devalued status, African American women lack the culturally sanctioned (indeed, culturally defined) protection that white skin, maleness, and wealth confer on the majority of the men whom they encounter professionally, in either role in the dyadic relationship.

There also are life-cycle considerations that can confound the therapist. In a study comparing Japanese American and white families in the United States, McDermott and colleagues (1983) found male/female differences in attitude during adolescence much more dramatic than ethnic differences between the two groups. Women in both groups expressed firmer connections regarding "strong interrelationships and obligations within the family, affectional ties, and open expression of emotion" (p. 1320). These gender differences, across cultural lines, certainly have strong implications for therapeutic process and perhaps also for the outcome of treatment.

Although there is a substantial emerging literature in this area, there are some shortcomings in the available data on gender and therapy. Most studies are of short-term individual psychotherapy, using simple therapeutic paradigms to facilitate data collection and analysis. Perforce, these studies do not look at psychoanalysis or long, complex forms of psychotherapy, where different findings might result (Nadelson and Notman 1991). Nonetheless, the available literature contains some useful information. Women, for example, are more likely to be referred for individual therapy than men; men are more likely to be referred to a male therapist. There also is the suggestion that male therapists choose more "feminine" therapeutic goals for female patients, whereas female therapists choose more "masculine" goals for their female patients (Brodey and Detgre 1972).

When therapists do not know the patients well, as when reviewing case records, gender differences do not appear to be important. But in the context of therapy, male therapists tend to prolong, and female therapists to foreshorten, those treatment situations deemed likely to arouse sexual attraction (Abramowitz et al. 1976a, 1976b).

In one study, Kirshner and colleagues (1978) looked at therapeutic process and outcomes in male:male, male:female, female:male, and female:female dyads. They found greater response to therapy among women treated by female therapists, and greater patient satisfaction, compared with women treated by men. The women in female:female treatment had the highest scores on self-rated improvement scales. Their self-esteem was better, too, as expressed in their attitudes toward academics, careers, and familial relations. The authors of this study suggest that female therapists have an advantage, which they share with their patients, based on women's greater interpersonal skills, compared with men's. Other investigators, however, do not find women to have greater sensitivity to interpersonal behavior than their male counterparts (Mendelsohn and Rankin 1969).

In another study, Orlinsky and Howard (1976) reported that depressed women feel more supported and satisfied with female therapists than with male ones. But no objective data could be generated to show that the female:female treatment outcomes were better than male:female. Similarly, Blase (1979) found that matched genders in the dyad increased satisfaction, but not overall treatment success. Others have buttressed the conclusion that the sex of the therapist does not play a significant or differential role in treatment outcomes, but the final word is not in on this complex topic (Goldenholz 1979; Gurri 1977; Malloy 1979).

The view has been expressed that American men's frequent reluctance to express their feelings—because to do so would seem unmanly—implies they may suffer more in therapy than women do. Men may get pushed into treatment because they perform badly before bosses or peers or find themselves in crises (Gove and Tudor 1973; Phillips and Siegel 1969). But they may have less inner motivation for *change* than women. Although women are said to suffer more from their feelings, symptoms, and events in their lives, they are perhaps not sicker than the men who seek psychotherapy, but only more sensitive and aware of their distress—and perhaps also less constricted about expressing it (Nadelson and Notman 1991).

When the therapist's clinical experience is taken into account, along with his or her gender, more experienced practitioners report better results and are less hindered by gender factors, whatever their sex and the sex of their patients, than are young and less-experienced therapists (Kirshner et al. 1978). Not surprisingly, a similar situation prevails among patients: younger, unmarried, less experienced patients are more vulnerable to gender differences and gender-related values and attitudes than are older, more experienced patients.

Gender differences may vary in importance depending on the type of therapy that is being offered. One suggestion is that the therapist's gender may be of greater importance in, say, short-term supportive psychotherapy, where the therapist may also act as a role model, than in psychoanalysis or psychoanalytically oriented psychotherapy, where transference plays the more significant role (Cavenar and Werman 1983; Mogul 1982).

Conclusion

Our growing perception of the ways that gender and ethnicity influence patients and therapists adds a new level of awareness to our knowledge of psychotherapy. Gender differences and gender issues must be taken into account and explored in the context of therapy.

References

Abramowitz SI, Abramowitz CV, Roback HB, et al: Sex-role related countertransference in psychotherapy. Arch Gen Psychiatry 33(1):71–73, 1976a

Abramowitz S, Roback H, Schwartz J, et al: Sex bias in psychotherapy: a failure to confirm. Am J Psychiatry 133:706–709, 1976b

Blase J: A study on the effects of sex of the client and sex of the therapist on client's
    satisfaction with psychotherapy (abstract). Dissertation Abstracts International
    49:6107–6107-B, 1979

Bleier R: Science and Gender: A Critique of Biology and Its Thesis on Women. New
    York, Pergamon, 1984

Brodey JF, Detgre T: Criteria used by clinicians in referring patients to individual or
    group therapy. Am J Psychother 26:176–184, 1972

Broverman I, Broverman D, Clarkson F, et al: Sex role stereotypes and clinical judg-
    ments of mental health. J Consult Clin Psychol 34:1–7, 1970

Cavenar JO Jr, Werman DS: The sex of the psychotherapist. Am J Psychiatry 140:85–
    87, 1983

Eichler M, Reisman AL, Borins G: Gender bias in medical research. Psychiatric News,
    January 5, 1990

Frezza M, Padova C, Pozzato G, et al: High blood alcohol levels in women: the role of
    decreased gastric alcohol dehydrogenase activity and first-pass metabolism. New
    Engl J Med 322:95–99, 1990

From the Alcohol, Drug Abuse, and Mental Health Administration. JAMA
    265(8):956, 1991

Gilligan C: In a Different Voice. Cambridge, MA, Harvard University Press, 1982

Ginsberg G, Frosch W, Shapiro T: The new impotence. Arch Gen Psychiatry 26:218–
    220, 1972

Goldenholz N: The effect of the sex of therapist-client dyad upon outcome of psycho-
    therapy (abstract). Dissertation Abstracts International 40:492-B, 1979

Gove WR, Tudor JF: Adult sex roles and mental illness, in Changing Women in a
    Changing Society. Edited by Huber J. Chicago, IL, University of Chicago Press,
    1973, pp 50–73

Gurri IM: The influence of therapist sex, client sex, and client sex bias on therapy
    outcome (abstract). Dissertation Abstracts International 38:898–899-B, 1977

Heart research efforts aim at fairness to women in terms of causes, care of cardiac
    disorders. JAMA 264(24):3112–3113, 1990

Kahne H: Economic perspectives on work and family issues, in Women and Men:
    New Perspectives on Gender Differences. Edited by Notman MT, Nadelson CC.
    Washington, DC, American Psychiatric Press, 1990, pp 9–22

Kaplan M: A woman's view of DSM-III. Am Psychol 38:786–792, 1983

Keller EF: Gender and Science. New Haven, CT, Yale University Press, 1985

King D, in Collins TH: The Social Construction of Black Feminist Thought. SIGNS
    14(4):745–773, 1989

Kirshner LA, Genack A, Hauser ST: Effects of gender on short-term psychotherapy.
    Psychotherapy: Theory, Research and Practice 15:158–167, 1978

Loring M, Powell BJ: Gender, race and DSM-III: a study of the objectivity of psychiat-
    ric diagnostic behavior. J Health Soc Behav 29:1–22, 1988

Malloy TE: The relationship between therapist-client interpersonal compatibility, sex
    of therapist, and psychotherapeutic outcome (abstract). Dissertation Abstracts In-

ternational 40:456-B, 1979

McDermott JF Jr, Robillard AB, Char WF, et al: Reexamining the concept of adolescence: differences between adolescent boys and girls in the context of their families. Am J Psychiatry 140(10):1318–1322, 1983

McGrath E, Keith GP, Strickland B, et al: Women and Depression. Washington, DC, American Psychological Association, 1990

Mendelsohn GA, Rankin NO: Client-counselor compatibility and the outcome of counseling. J Abnorm Psychol 74:157–163, 1969

Mogul K: Overview: The sex of the therapist. Am J Psychiatry 139:1–11, 1982

Nadelson CC, Notman MT: Psychotherapy supervision: the problem of conflicting values. Am J Psychother 31:275–283, 1977

Nadelson CC, Notman MT: The impact of the new psychology of men and women on psychotherapy, in American Psychiatric Press Review of Psychiatry, Vol 10. Edited by Tasman A, Goldfinger SM. Washington, DC, American Psychiatric Press, 1991, pp 608–626

Nadelson CC, Notman MT, Baker-Miller J, et al: Aggression in women: conceptual issues and clinical impressions, in The Woman Patient, Vol 3. Edited by Notman MT, Nadelson CC. New York, Plenum, 1982, pp 17–28

Orlinsky DE, Howard KI: The effects of sex of therapist on the therapeutic experiences of women. Psychotherapy: Theory, Research and Practice 13:82–88, 1976

Person ES: The influence of values in psychoanalysis: the case of female psychology, in Psychiatry Update: The American Psychiatric Association Annual Review, Vol 2. Edited by Grinspoon L. Washington, DC, American Psychiatric Press, 1983, pp 36–49

Phillips D, Siegel B: Sexual status and psychiatric symptoms. American Sociological Review 34:58–72 1969

Regier DA, Myers JK, Kramer M, et.al: The NIMH Epidemiologic Catchment Area Program. Arch Gen Psychiatry 41:934–941, 1984

Slavney PR, Chase GA: Clinical judgments of self-dramatization: A test of the sexist hypothesis. Br J Psychiatry 146:614–617, 1985

Tannen D: You Just Don't Understand. New York, William Morrow, 1990, p 209

Warner R: The diagnosis of antisocial and hysterical personality disorders: an example of sex bias. J Nerv Ment Dis 166:839–845, 1978

Weissman MM, Klerman GL: Gender and depression. Trends Neurosci 8:416–420, 1977

Zeldow PB: Sex differences in psychiatric evaluation and treatment. Arch Gen Psychiatry 35:89–93, 1978

18 Psychiatric Care of Ethnic Elders

F. M. Baker, M.D., M.P.H.
Orlando B. Lightfoot, M.D.

Four major populations within the United States have been identified as ethnic minorities: African Americans, Asian Americans and Pacific Islanders, American Indians and Alaska Natives, and Hispanic Americans. Although these groups were called ethnic minorities in the 1970s, demographic projections suggest that their combined populations will make them a majority of the United States population by 2010 (Angel and Hogan 1991; Gibson 1986; Manuel 1988). As we discuss the elders of these groups, we use the term "ethnic elder" to reflect changes in the composition of the American population and to recognize the unique place that these individuals usually hold in their families and cultures of origin.

Ethnic elders age 85 and over are the fastest growing segment of these populations (Angel and Hogan 1991). By the year 2030, 15.3% of people age 65 and older will be members of these four groups. In 2050, ethnic elders will make up 21.3% of the U.S. population (Angel and Hogan 1991). Each population of ethnic elders is composed of several groups with diverse cultural and ethnic backgrounds. The black population of the United States is composed of Africans, African Americans, and Afro-Caribbeans. These Americans of African origin are predominantly African American. Table 18–4 details their unique history in America (Baker 1982; Yeo 1991), and Table 18–5 lists cohort experience of African American elders. African Americans are 12% of the total United States population. Eleven percent of this population is aged 65 and older (Table 18–1). The educational level varies for those ages 65–74, 75–84, and over 85. Among what we have called the young old, of African American elders aged 65–74, 19% have completed high school (Table 18–2). The percentage of ethnic elders living below the poverty level as well as households living below the poverty level are shown in Table 18–3.

American Indians and Alaska Natives account for 1% of the total population in the United States (U.S. Bureau of the Census 1990). There are over

400 recognized tribes and over 250 languages (Manson and Callaway 1988). Table 18–6 details the unique experience of these first Americans within the United States. Fifty-four percent of American Indians and Alaska Natives live in predominantly urban areas, with less than 24% living on reservations (John 1991). People age 65 and over represent 6% of the American Indian and Alaska Native population. Twenty-five percent of these ethnic elders completed high school (Table 18–2), and 39% are rural residents. Twenty-five percent of individual elders were living below the poverty level (Table 18–3); data were not available for households living below the poverty level.

Although they are now 3% of the total U.S. population, Asian Americans and Pacific Islanders include more than 20 different ethnic groups, with origins in East Asia, Southeast Asia, the Indian subcontinent, Polynesia, Melanesia, and Micronesia. Six percent of this population is aged 65 and older (Table 18–1), and 64% of these ethnic elders live in California, Hawaii, and Washington, in declining order of population. Ninety percent live in urban areas (Morioka-Douglas and Yeo 1990). Tables 18–7 through 18–10 provide an overview of the history in the United States of two of the largest groups, Chinese and Pilipinos. Only recently included in U.S. Bureau of the Census data, 37% of these elders completed high school (Table 18–2) and 14% of individuals were living below the poverty level, the lowest percentage for all groups of ethnic elders (Table 18–3). Data are not available for these groups on the percentage of households that are living below the poverty level.

The population of Hispanic Americans is diverse, ranging from native-born American citizens to documented political-economic refugees from certain Latin American socialist governments (i.e., Cubans and Nicaraguans; Cuellar 1990b). Making up 8% of the total population, the three largest groups of Hispanic Americans are Mexican Americans, Cubans, and Puerto Ricans. Varying percentages of these groups are aged 65 and older: Cubans

Table 18–1.   Ethnic elders—percentage of U.S. population and percentage of ethnic elders aged 65 and over

Ethnic Elder Group (EEG)	% of Total U.S. Population	% of EEG Age 65+
African American	12	11
American Indian and Alaska Native	1	6
Asian American	3	6
Hispanic American	8	3

Source.   U.S. Bureau of the Census 1990.

11.7%, Mexican Americans 4.2%, and Puerto Ricans 3.6%. For Hispanic Americans from Central or South America, some 2.8% are aged 65 and over (Cuellar 1990b). Tables 18–11 and 18–12 detail the experience of Hispanic Americans in the United States. Twenty percent of these elders completed high school (Table 18–2). Twenty-six percent of Hispanic American individuals (Table 18–3) are living below the poverty level, and 21% of households are living below the poverty level.

Although hypertension, diabetes, and cancer are medical problems of concern to the four groups of ethnic elders, there are differences among the groups in the types of medical problems. Osteoarthritis, asthma, glaucoma, and goiter are the medical problems seen among African American elders (Baker et al., in press; Richardson 1990). Tuberculosis, liver and kidney disease, psychiatric and medical disorders related to substance abuse, and accidents are of primary concern in American Indian and Alaska Native elders (Angel and Hogan 1991; Cuellar 1990a; John 1991). Within the Asian American and Pacific Islander group, a higher incidence of liver and esophageal cancers are noted, as well as multi-infarct dementia in Japanese populations. Among ethnic elders, Japanese and Chinese elders have the highest rates of completed suicide (Sakauye et al., in press). Among Hispanic Americans, the prevalence of medical conditions other than hypertension and diabetes mellitus varies. Mexican-born Americans have twice the rates of accidents in comparison to other groups of Hispanic Americans. Puerto Ricans have twice the mortality rates from liver disease and cirrhosis in comparison to Mexican Americans and Cuban Americans (Angel and Hogan 1991; Cuellar 1990b).

Other chapters in this book have provided information about the unique history, cultural diversity, strengths, and problems of these groups that can ameliorate or exacerbate psychiatric symptoms. The preceding paragraphs

Table 18–2.   Education attainment of ethnic elders

	Ages 65–74			
Ethnic Elder Group	Completed College (%)	Completed High School (%)	Completed 5th and 6th Grade (%)	Without Any Formal Education (%)
African American	4	19	18	24
American Indian and Alaska Native	4	25	11	23
Asian American	10	37	13	21
Hispanic American	4	20	18	35

Source. U.S. Bureau of the Census 1981.

have provided some detailed information about ethnic elders to provide a context for the following discussion of their evaluation and treatment. Although little literature on ethnic elders exists, this is changing. In order to enable the reader to identify key resources on this topic, the four volumes by the Stanford Geriatric Education Center (Cuellar 1990a, 1990b; Morioka-Douglas and Yeo 1990; Richardson 1990) are included in the reference list, as well as the work of Sakauye and colleagues (in press); the texts edited by Gaw (1982b), Harper (1990), and Harootyan (1991); and a chapter on rehabilitation (Baker et al. 1990). The reader is encouraged to use these resources to obtain a better conceptualization of patients from a specific culture.

The historical experience and cultural context of ethnic elders is important because these factors influence:

1. The elders' definition of illness (medical and psychiatric);
2. Their expectation of the health care delivery system;
3. The time at which the decision to enter treatment is made; and
4. The person and/or system from which treatment is sought.

The biopsychosocial perspective on mental illness was first delineated by Engel (1977), and the clinical application of Engel's model was illustrated in 1980. Engel conceptualized his model as a Venn diagram of three overlapping circles representing three areas that either ameliorated or contributed to the development of mental disorders and their expression: biological, psychological, and social factors. Although this model is important for all age cohorts, it has particular pertinence for ethnic elders.

Relevant to the biological factors that contribute to mental disorders, the

Table 18–3. Economic status of ethnic elders: percentage of individuals and households below the poverty level

Ethnic Elder Group	Individuals Below the Poverty Level (%)	Households Below the Poverty Level (%)
African American	35	26
American Indian and Alaska Native rural residents	25 39	—
Asian American rural residents	14 10	—
Hispanic American	26	21

Source. U.S. Bureau of the Census 1990.

Task Force on Black and Minority Health (1985) documented the fact that minority groups have poorer health status throughout the life cycle than whites do. Regarding the psychological factors that are implicated in mental illness, the Task Force pointed out that ethnic elders and their families do not define mental disorders as "illnesses" to be treated by Western medicine with diagnostic tests and medications, but rather as conditions that bring shame upon the family (Baker 1982, 1988; Clevenger 1982; Gaw 1982a; Manson et al. 1987; Martinez 1977; Martinez and Martin 1966; Yamamoto 1982). People with psychiatric illnesses are managed within the family until it is no longer possible to contain their symptoms (Baker 1988; EchoHawk 1982; Li et al. 1972; Martinez 1988). The Task Force also indicated a social factor that is key in the diagnosis and treatment of ethnic elders: they continue to be involved actively in three-generational families and/or the extended family or kinship networks (Markides et al. 1986; Martin and Martin 1978; National Indian Council on Aging 1981; Sue and McKinney 1975). Social groups (possibly focused around games) and religion remain important and vital activities for ethnic elders (Clevenger 1982; Gaw 1982a; Martinez 1988; Taylor 1988). It is unclear whether the adult children of ethnic elders will change their familial and community participation pattern when they themselves reach their seventies.

The cultural dimensions of caring for a patient who is mentally ill and the impact of this illness on the patient's family are illustrated by the following case study.

Case Study 1

Mrs. A. is a 68-year-old married Puerto Rican woman, mother of three adult children, who is living with her husband of 45 years. She is fluently bilingual. She is an insulin-dependent diabetic and has a long history of bipolar disorder. Mrs. A. has been seen in the outpatient psychiatry clinic for manic and depressive symptoms. For these visits, she has been brought to the clinic by her daughter.

Mrs. A. arrived with her family for evaluation of increased irritability, forgetfulness, and inattention to her personal hygiene. These symptoms are not ones that the family usually associates with Mrs. A.'s bipolar disorder, but her chronic illness has presented in varied forms in the past. The family wants a review of Mrs. A.'s medications—lithium carbonate, 300 mg twice a day; NPH insulin, 40 units each morning; and Vasotec, 10 mg once a day. The family requested a general psychiatric evaluation.

The psychiatrist evaluating Mrs. A. had known her for some years and had not previously observed any symptoms of forgetfulness and inattention to per-

Table 18–4.   African Americans: Significant dates and periods in recent
history

Year	Periods and Events	U.S. Population (in Thousands)
Late 1800s	Chaos of Reconstruction Era in South; legal marriages, families reunited after emancipation; violence toward African Americans, Ku Klux Klan (KKK) founded, schools for freedmen burned; African American military units in Cavalry outposts in West and Spanish-American War; first African American graduate of West Point; "separate but equal" doctrine legalizes inequality, Jim Crow era begins; Tuskegee Institute founded by Booker T. Washington	
1909	National Association for the Advancement of Colored People (NAACP) founded by leading members of white and African American community, including W.E.B. DuBois	
1910–1920	Migration of 500,000 from South to urban North; continued violence and lynchings, KKK active	9,800
1917–1919	100,000 African American soldiers go overseas; "Red Summer," with African American GIs and civilians the target of bloody anti-African American rioting	
1920s	KKK claimed 5 million members in all parts of the United States; 1 million African Americans migrated from South to North and West; rise of arts and music, especially jazz, centered in Harlem (the Harlem Renaissance); Marcus Garvey preached racial pride and "Back to Africa"; labor and radical political movement emerged	
1930s	Great Depression; thousands lost jobs and sharecroppers destitute; Labor and Tenant Farm Unions developed as integrated organizations; some African American political leaders played leading roles in New Deal; poll tax, segregated schools and cities by law; antimiscegenation laws still exist in most Southern states; de facto segregation in North; Jessie Owen's victory in Berlin Olympics refutes Hitler's racism; Marian Anderson denied right to give concert in Constitution Hall, and 75,000 come to hear her sing outside Lincoln Memorial	11,800

Year	Periods and Events	U.S. Population (in Thousands)
1941–1946	1 million African Americans served in World War II, all in segregated units until 1945; veterans came home to segregation and continued discrimination; 369th Colored Infantry honored with New York City parade for its valor; Presidential proclamation bans discrimination in defense plants, heavy migration to work in plants in North and West	12,900
1948–1951	Armed forces officially desegregated, which worked well in Korean War	
1954	*Brown v. Board of Education* Supreme Court ruling ending "separate but equal" doctrine in education; Rosa Parks refuses to give up her seat to a white man, which started the Montgomery, Alabama, bus boycott	
1955	Rev. Martin Luther King's nonviolent resistance movement grow as African Americans demand civil rights	
1960s	Civil Rights Act, Black Power Movement emphasizing African American pride in African American history, Vietnam War, assassination of Rev. Martin Luther King triggers rioting in African American communities across the nation	28,900 (1985 est.)
1970s–1990s	Affirmative action implemented gradually; increasing number of elected African American officials; increasing conservatism and white backlash; *Bakke v. Regents of the University of California* decision; Supreme Court decisions on search and seizure; racist violence toward African Americans; Rodney King's beating by Los Angeles police officers triggers riots in African American community in Los Angeles	

sonal hygiene. She decided to involve an internist, a neurologist, a neuropsychologist, a nurse, and a social worker in the evaluation. This expanded, multidisciplinary team began a comprehensive review of Mrs. A.'s medical, psychological, functional, and social status. The contribution from each team member was additive and contributed to an understanding of Mrs. A.'s illness and its impact within her social network.

The completed assessment revealed that Mrs. A. had a dementing disorder in its early stages. Her internist confirmed a history of hypertension as well as a history of a fluctuating pattern of symptoms. Data from the psychiatrist, neurologist, and neuropsychologist resulted in a diagnosis of multi-infarct dementia.

The evaluation process also helped to review the impact on the family of Mrs. A.'s additional symptoms. Always an independent person, Mrs. A. was, according to information obtained by the nurse, not as attentive to her basic needs of toileting, grooming, bathing, food preparation, feeding, and compliance with her medication regimen as she had been in recent years. Her declining attention to these basic functions caused distress to her family.

As a strong Puerto Rican man, Mr. A. prided himself on taking the leadership role in the family, being responsible for problem solving as well as negotiating interactions between society at large and his family. He had required a good deal of counseling and support over the years to adjust to Mrs. A's psychiatric illness, which brought shame to the family. He understood more readily the medical concepts of pancreatic failure causing diabetes and blood-vessel inadequacy resulting in hypertension. When the idea of a biological switch in the brain was emphasized to explain the change in Mrs. A.'s mood, the psychiatric illness was more readily understood by Mr. A. and could be accepted. Therefore, Mr. A. was relatively comfortable in accepting brain failure as the cause of his wife's forgetfulness and relative loss of function.

However, it was very distressing for Mr. A. to monitor his wife's basic toileting, grooming, and bathing. He felt that this level of daily attention to her personal activities was demeaning and humiliating. The couple's daughter was of great assistance in completing these tasks for her mother. Though responsible for her own family and living in a separate household, the couple's daughter was thoroughly committed to supporting her parents in this time of need.

When cultural misunderstandings and language posed a potential barrier to the most appropriate care, the daughter who was very comfortable with the mores and customs of the majority culture helped both the family and other caregivers. She worked closely with the social worker in organizing a system of additional community caregivers, including a home health aide and a visiting nurse. These caregivers relieved Mr. A. of some of the burden of care for Mrs. A. and helped shore up his psychological resources for the future. In addition, Mr. A. was able to request an evaluation for some medical problems he was experiencing.

Lessons From Mrs. A.'s Case Study

There are many lessons to be learned from this case. These include the need for a multidisciplinary evaluation team, including internal medicine (preferably an internist with geriatric training), neurology, neuropsychology, nursing, and social work. This core team can be expanded as necessary to include a therapeutic recreation and/or occupational therapist, a physical therapist, a communication disorders specialist (speech and language therapist), and a nutritionist. A second lesson is that the psychiatrist, functioning alone without this group of professionals, is at a distinct disadvantage in accurately and effectively diagnosing and treating this kind of culturally complex problem. A third lesson is that the impact of the new symptoms and illness on the family system, resulting in a possible shift of roles and relationships, must be considered and, if indicated, addressed.

While Mr. A. negotiated the external boundary between the family and the community, Mrs. A. provided the nurture and support of family members (internal boundary). Mr. A. now had to become and assume the role of nurturant caregiver. Cultural and ethnic nuances must be appreciated thoroughly by the multidisciplinary team and the consultants, such as home health aides and visiting nurses—specifically, the attitude of the family toward a "stranger" entering their home and providing personal services to a family member. Learning about the culture and seeking advice from those more knowledgeable about the specific ethnic issues (Bernal 1982; Falicov 1982; Garcia-Preto 1982) will expand, modify, and enrich the evaluation and treatment process for the patient as well as the therapist. Such sensitivity to cultural issues will also facilitate the family's implementation of the treatment plan.

Culture and Medical Care

A patient's cultural context will partly determine the designation of specific symptoms as referable to illness, kind of treatment given, and person(s) or system(s) contacted to provide care. As the adult children of ethnic elders have moved into the American middle class, some of these children no longer live near their parents. However, in the 1990s, most ethnic elders are involved in three-generational families or extended families (Broudy and May 1983; Hines and Boyd-Franklin 1982; Markides and Vernon 1984; Stack 1971; Yamamoto 1982). These families provide social, emotional, and financial support for their elders.

The unique role of ethnic elders, as the senior or elder in the family as well as the elder in the church or clan, provides an ongoing source of self-esteem as well as an important, productive role after retirement from the formal work role. The lower rates of completed suicide in ethnic elders may be

Table 18–5. Cohort experiences—African American elders

Current Age Cohorts	Age at Historical Experiences			
	1900–1920	1920–1940	1940–1960	1960–Present
	Ku Klux Klan	"Red Summer"	World War II: segregated units and factory work in North and West	Civil Rights Movement
	Lynchings	W.E.B. Dubois	Return to segregated society	Dr. Martin L. King's nonviolent protests
	NAACP	Marcus Garvey's "Back to Africa" Movement	1954: Supreme Court ruling desegregating education	Black Pride
	Participation in World War II	Harlem Renaissance		Desegregation and affirmative action
		Great Depression		Vietnam War
				Crack epidemic
85+	Children and adolescents	Young adults	Middle-aged	Elders
75–85	Children	Adolescents and young adults	Young adults to middle-aged	Middle-aged to old
65–75		Children and adolescents	Adolescents and young adults	Adults to young old
55–65		Children	Children to young adults	Young adults to middle-aged

Sources. Baker 1982; Yeo 1991.

partially related to the fact that important roles in the family and in the community continue. National data that suggest an increase of completed suicide in African American men over age 75 remain unexplained (Baker 1989; Griffith and Bell 1989; Manuel 1988) and may be an artifact of reporting (Baker 1989).

Medical Characteristics of Ethnic Elders

More ethnic elders have medical illnesses than their mainstream cohorts. The health status of ethnic elders has been compromised by inadequate or poor health care over the years as well as multiple medical problems (usually a minimum of five chronic conditions). Therefore, any psychiatric symptoms observed must be evaluated thoroughly, because the etiology may be a medical problem that needs to be identified and stabilized. As a physician, the psychiatrist has an important perspective.

More so than other populations of older patients, ethnic elders require a comprehensive differential diagnostic assessment and a thorough review of their current medications. The possibility of complex pharmacologic interactions must be considered, because medications from several sources are ingested. These sources include medications prescribed by a physician, medications borrowed from a neighbor, and medications saved from 6 years back because "they worked very well for that symptom and they were expensive." The following may interact to potentiate or negate the effects of physician-prescribed medications or out-of-date medications: the prescription of herbs by traditional Chinese healers (Gaw 1982a), by an American Indian medicine man (Clevenger 1982), or by Mexican American *curanderos* (Martinez 1977); or the prescription of teas made from roots, bark, or herbs by an African American worker of roots (Baker 1988; Richardson 1990) or by a woman from the Caribbean who has knowledge of voodoo (Jordan 1975). It is important for the evaluating psychiatrist to be aware that ethnic elders may seek care and be receiving treatment from cultural healers. Whether from drug-drug interactions, outdated medications, or the interaction of Western and traditional medicines, the potential for drug-drug interactions producing altered cognitive or mood states exits in ethnic elders.

Requesting that the elder bring in "all" his or her medications (prescribed, purchased over-the-counter, borrowed from a friend or neighbor, prescribed by a native healer) is an important initial step in the evaluation process. Such a request demonstrates an understanding of how the ethnic elder may mobilize resources (Baker 1982; Richardson 1990). It also acknowledges the indigenous healer, who may be the primary health provider for the ethnic elder.

Table 18–6.   American Indians and Alaska Natives: Significant dates and periods in recent history

Year	Periods and Events	U.S. Population (in Thousands)
Before 1492	Precontact period began at least 20,000 years ago. Approximately 300 tribal groups with many subdivisions within tribal groups. Indian peoples of the Americas spoke more than 1,000 unique languages, derived from 56 language families.	Several million
1492– mid-1800s	Some early contacts between American Indians and Europeans were positive, but these were the exception. Exploitation of Indians and their lands shaped the Indian/European relationship from the beginning of contact. The introduction of alcohol was used to take advantage of American Indians (e.g., in order to more easily "buy" land—a concept that was very foreign to Indians).	
1500–1890	Epidemics era. Whites brought infectious diseases for which Indian people were not prepared immunologically. Five-sixths of some populations were killed by early epidemics. Leaders and other elders also died, leaving many communities without leadership. Also known as the Manifest Destiny era, a term coined in the mid-1800s to describe the desire of many Americans to possess a country that was larger than Europe and reached from coast to coast. Led to destruction of American Indians, not only by epidemics and alcohol, but also by war, massive forced migrations, and the formation of reservations. Forced suppression of American Indian cultures and religions, and education of children to be "white," also were important factors.	
Early 1800s	The Bureau of Indian Affairs (BIA), a portion of the War Department, took responsibility for Indian health care.	
Late 1800s	Revitalization movement. Religious movements were begun by American Indian people to try to regain lost culture. Heavily influenced by Christianity but with many traditional Indian practices.	
1849	The BIA, along with Indian health care, became part of the Interior Department.	

1887	The Dawes Act stipulated that communally owned (Indian) lands be divided into individual "allotments" of land to own and farm. As was the case many times before, much of this land found its way into white hands, often by fraud.	
1890–1970	Assimilation era. Following the Wounded Knee Massacre (1890), depression, alcoholism, and violence had reached their peak on reservations. The overt extermination policy of the United States changed to a more subtle one of "assimilating" Indians into white culture. Many Indians agreed to assimilation in an attempt to escape reservation life.	
1924	Citizenship and reorganization period. American Indians in 1924 became the last people given full citizenship and voting rights in the United States.	
1934	The Indian Reorganization Bill gave American Indians the right to self-government, but stipulated a discontinuation of land allotments. Established provisions for education and training of American Indians.	
1950–1960	Termination movement. An effort to end, tribe by tribe, any responsibility of the U.S. government for American Indian people, including health care. Accompanied by "relocation" of Indians from reservations to cities, where many became a part of the urban poor. Basically a new label for destruction of Indian communities and culture.	
1955	American Indian health care is transferred to the Indian Health Service, a part of the Department of Health, Education, and Welfare.	
1970	Indian Self Determination Act. Allowed American Indian people to have more control over their govenmental affairs.	
1976	Indian Health Care Improvement Act. Intended to increase tribal input into health care; met with mixed results. It was administratively oriented and did not address such topics as traditional healing.	
1980	The number of urban American Indian people surpasses the number of reservation and rural American Indian people.	1,400
1990	Staffing of the small Indian Health Service Mental Health Program slated for increases. No specific programs for the elderly.	1,900

Sources. Walker and LaDue 1986. Also see Chapter 8 in this book.

Table 18–7. Chinese Americans: Significant dates and periods in
immigration history

Year	Periods and Events	U.S. Population (in Thousands)*	Ratio of Males to Females
1850–1860	Sojourner male immigration from Southern China to *Jiujinshan* (Old Gold Mountain—San Francisco)		
1870s	Brutality and violence; discriminatory legislation	60	
1879	California Constitution adopted with anti-Chinese provisions		
1880		100	
1882	Chinese Exclusion Act banning immigration of Chinese laborers		
1882–1920	Declining immigration; decline of agriculture, mining, and railroad occupations; rise of urban service occupations; immigration of "paper sons" and "treaty merchants" through "the Shed"		
1890		101	27:1
1900		90	
1900–1930	Rise of family associations and "tongs" (secret societies)		
1910		72	
1920		62	7:1
1924	Immigration restrictions eased slightly		
1930s	Pearl Buck novels portray Chinese peasants as heros resisting Japanese invasion; "mutilated families"	75	
1940–1946	16,000 Chinese Americans served in Armed Forces	78	
1943	Repeal of all 15 Chinese Exclusion Acts; quota set at 105 per year		
1946	Law passed allowing "alien" wives to immigrate		
1947–1952	More than 9,000 wives immigrated; increased educational attainment; continued discrimination; high birthrates		

Year	Periods and Events	*U.S. Population (in Thousands)	Ratio of Males to Females
1950s	Cold War, two Chinas; fear of Communist threat from Chinese Americans; half of Chinese Americans are American born; increased acculturation	107	
1953	Refugee status available for 2,000 if approved by Taiwan government		
1960s	Continued discrimination in unionized employment	237	1.1:1
1965	New Immigration Act passed, persons with kin in U.S. favored		
1970s	Two Chinese American communities: one suburban, well-educated, the other with little education and low income; immigration of Chinese from Vietnam	436	
1980s	Image of "model minority;" heavy immigration from Hong Kong and Taiwan, including older adults	812	
1985 (est.)		1,079	

Source. Morioka-Douglas and Yeo 1990.
* Not counting Hawaii until after its statehood in 1959, when there were 38,000.

Therapeutic Alliance

A delineation of the unique cultural context of the four groups of ethnic elders is beyond the scope of this chapter. In addition to the initial chapters of this text, there are various texts that provide a historical overview for these populations and provide detailed information about each ethnic group (Bass et al. 1982; Chunn et al. 1983; Comas-Diaz and Griffith 1988; Coner-Edwards and Spurlock 1988; Favazza and Oman 1978; Foulks 1980; Gaw 1982b; Haldipur 1980; Jackson 1988; Lefley 1984; Lewis and Looney 1983; McGoldrick et al. 1982; Moffic 1983; Pinderhughes 1989; Singer 1977; Task Force on Black and Minority Health 1985; Thernstrom 1980; Willie et al. 1973). The reader is referred to this expanding body of literature for information specific to a particular group.

It is important to emphasize here that each group of ethnic elders has experienced direct exclusion from American society, because they are visibly different from whites of northern European extraction in physical features and/or skin color (Tables 18–4 to 18–12). Legalized segregation (African Americans), exclusionary immigration laws (Chinese), internment of American citizens during World War II (Japanese), the backlash against immigration in the 1960s (Puerto Ricans), ongoing tensions over border crossings (Mexican Americans), and genocidal acts during and after the U.S. Indian Wars (Native Americans) are parts of American history that ethnic elders recall (Baker 1987; Brown 1970; Garcia-Preto 1982; Sung 1970). Their attitudes toward therapists and the health care system are influenced by the experiences of their adolescent and young adult years, which occurred before World War II, as well as the oral histories they heard from their parents and grandparents. Becoming familiar with the history of the ethnic elders will help clinicians to understand their patients and will increase the ability to form a therapeutic alliance. The following case serves as an example of the importance of culturally based transference issues in establishing a strong therapeutic alliance with a patient.

Case Study 2

Mr. B. is a 73-year-old African American man who is a widower. He is a successful retired accountant who is not followed regularly by an internist. He lives alone. Since the death of his wife 18 months ago, his family has visited frequently and has noticed the following alterations in Mr. B.: continued acute mourning, sadness, depression, forgetfulness, and a mild gait disturbance. Another disturbing change was Mr. B.'s becoming disoriented and lost during a visit to a familiar foreign country. Although each of these changes caused concern, the family did not seek professional help until Mr. B.'s son observed that the patient was incontinent of urine. This particular symptom stimulated the family to seek help.

Mr. B. requested an African American physician; ethnicity and culture were pivotal factors in this case. As he considered revealing material about his mental functioning and intimate feelings, Mr. B. stated his belief that an African American would "really understand" and be more sensitive to his complaints and feelings.

His request for an African American evaluator was related to Mr. B.'s issues of transference and influenced the formation of the therapeutic alliance. The transference issues centered around his fears, anxieties, and fantasies about the intolerable changes in his intellectual function. Any threat to Mr. B.'s identity as a successful, capable, competent, articulate person who was important in the community caused him great anxiety. The request for an African American physician was partially an attempt to maintain his status and role in the community by finding someone whom he believed would know of his ability, his

Table 18–8. Cohort experiences—Chinese American elders

Current Age Cohorts	Age at Historical Experiences			
	1900–1920	1920–1940	1940–1960	1960–Present
	Exclusion Act in effect	Family Associations	Chinese in World War II	Increased education for some
	Urbanization	Tong Societies	Repeal of Exclusion Acts	"Model minority"
	Immigration of "paper sons"	Pearl Buck novels	Immigration of wives	Immigration from Hong Kong and Taiwan
	Heavily male	"Mutilated families"	Fear of Chinese Communists	
85+	Children and adolescents	Young adults	Middle-aged	Elders
75–85	Children	Adolescents and young adults	Young adults to middle-aged	Middle-aged to old
65–75		Children and adolescents	Adolescents and young adults	Adults to young old
55–65		Children	Children to young adults	Young adults to middle-aged

Source. Morioka-Douglas and Yeo 1990.

Table 18–9.   Pilipino Americans: Significant dates and periods in immigration and history

Year	Periods and Events	U.S. Population (in Thousands)	Hawaiian Population (in Thousands)
18th century	Tiny group of immigrants to Louisiana		
1898	After Spanish-American War, U.S. takes possession of the Philippine Islands but Pilipinos not eligible for U.S. citizenship		
1903–1930s	Students ("Pensionados") come to U.S. (First Wave)		
1910		3	2
1908–1920s	Heavy recruitment for Hawaii plantations		
1920		27	21
1920–1934	Male laborers ("Pinoys") to West Coast (Second Wave); discrimination and violence against Pinoys; antimiscegenation laws; land ownership not allowed; economic depression		
1930		108	63
1934	Tydings-McDuffie Act setting quota of 50 immigrants per year		
1934–1946	Very low immigration		
1940		99	53
1941–1946	Pilipino participation in U.S. Army and Navy		
1946	The Philippines becomes an independent nation; U.S. citizenship becomes available for Pilipino residents in U.S. and World War I veterans		
1946–1965	Family members of residents and veterans immigrate in large numbers		

Year	Periods and Events	U.S. Population (in Thousands)	Hawaiian Population (in Thousands)
1950		123	61
1960		181	69
1965	Immigration quotas relaxed		
1965–present	Increased immigration; most are professionals (Third Wave)		
1970	National data bases do not include separate category for Pilipino Americans	337	95
1980		774	109
1985 (est.)		1,051	

Source. Yeo 1991.

Number of older Pilipinos by age groups and percentage of males in the United States in 1980

	Age groups						
	50–54	55–59	60–64	65–69	70–74	75+	Total
Number	28,730	23,633	18,858	21,837	19,523	15,898	128,479
Percentage male	45.4	43.3	43.0	58.6	71.0	73.7	

Source. Adapted from Pido 1986.

competence, and his value and appreciate the distress he experienced with the changes in himself. If the therapist could appreciate Mr. B. and his assets, then Mr. B. would feel less humiliated and minimized by exposing his recently developed areas of difficulty.

Mr. B.'s fears of being judged, reviewed, and dehumanized were articulated partially through his request for a therapist who he anticipated would understand the underlying message in his request. He hoped his "evaluator," the African American psychiatrist, would be less negatively influenced by his blackness than someone who was not African American. Also, Mr. B. hoped that an African American psychiatrist would identify positively with him and see in him a part of himself or herself, a part that was valuable and that could function again.

Mr. B. had no prior psychiatric history. Following a detailed evaluation by the Geriatric Team, it was established that his cognitive deficits resulted from a major depressive disorder that was due to a pathological grief reaction. Neuropsychological testing revealed no fixed deficits and the uneven performance of a depressed person. Mr. B.'s neurologic examination had no focal findings, and his physical examination and laboratory studies were all normal.

In excellent physical health with only mild arthritic changes, Mr. B. responded to a trial of 100 mg of desipramine (Norpramin) a day; all of his presenting symptoms resolved within 3 months. He was able to verbalize his fears about his declining stamina, loss of the cognitive ability that he had at age 40, concern with becoming dependent on his adult children, and fear of loss of his leadership role within his community. With the resolution of his major depressive disorder, Mr. B. resumed his role in the community, and with the support of his adult children, began to consider the option of dating again. In addition to returning to active participation as an elder in his church, Mr. B. resumed his roles as a leader in his lodge, secretary of a national association of accountants, and an avid golfer. His total treatment lasted 14 months.

The therapeutic alliance issues involved a realistic concern about not knowing the medical referral network well enough to obtain competent advice and counsel about available practitioners and their relative expertise (Lightfoot 1988). Mr. B. justifiably wanted to put himself in the care of a competent clinician who would appreciate the devastating effects of his depressive symptoms on him. He needed to feel that the problems could be diagnosed and treated by an empathic therapist who could identify with him. Although Mr. B. had requested an African American therapist, these abilities are also found in clinicians who have developed cross-cultural sensitivities. Mr. B. wanted to ally himself with the healing powers and abilities of the physician. He undertook the psychiatric evaluation to get well and willingly engaged with an African American psychiatrist in the necessary effort to improve his condition.

Lessons From Mr. B.'s Case Study

The first lesson to be remembered from this case is the fact that many symptoms and functional changes in elders may be mistakenly accepted by caregivers as a "natural" part of the aging process. Two symptoms that affect activities of daily living (ADL) are often less well tolerated: incontinence of urine or feces and an inability to walk independently. A second lesson is that ethnic and/or cultural similarity between the patient and the therapist are, in some instances, vitally necessary before the transference concerns can be modified and a therapeutic alliance forged. Once an alliance is formed and engagement occurs, a patient can often widen his or her horizons beyond a specific ethnic or cultural similarity and allow other members of the medical team and professional caregivers to become involved. Finally, the extent to which a major depressive disorder can precipitate significant changes in cognitive ability, ADLs, and personal hygiene is underscored by Mr. B.'s case study. Although the possibility of his having adult-onset diabetes, hypothyroidism with an associated urinary tract infection, or an intracerebral event (stroke or hemorrhage) needed to be ruled out, the workup for these disorders was negative.

The Functional Status of Ethnic Elders

The assessment of elders should include information about their functional status (American Geriatric Society Public Policy Committee 1989; Brummel-Smith 1988; Kane et al. 1989; Lightfoot 1982). Functional status in elders can often be generally assessed by the question, How well are they able to complete the basic ADLs: bathing, toileting, dressing, and feeding? Some other specific questions might also be asked: Are they able to shop for food, prepare it, and eat it without special devices or the assistance of others? Are they able to complete the unfastening or repositioning of clothing, but unable to clean themselves after voiding or defecating? Have they become reluctant to bathe? Is this because of a fear of water or a loss of understanding of what the water is and its purpose? Although these questions are not routinely considered in other age cohorts (except children), they should be a routine part of an assessment of the older patient.

People with dementia have a change in ADLs as their disease progresses. Patients recovering after a stroke may have some residual deficits in ADLs as well as speech and cognitive or affective changes. Severe deforming rheumatoid arthritis may also result in impairments requiring assistance with ADLs.

For ethnic elders, the revelation of deficits in these areas may be profoundly disturbing, knowledge to be kept within the family, a "shame not be broadcast." Recognizing the potential sensitivity about deficits in these areas as well as resistance to acknowledging mental illness, a therapist needs a skillful and sensitive approach to an exploration of these deficits. Acknowledging that people change in their abilities because of illnesses that affect the body is an initial contextual framework that can facilitate the family's and patient's acceptance of and acknowledgement of a problem that the elder did not "cause."

Table 18–10. Cohort experiences—Pilipino American elders

Current Age Cohorts	Age at Historical Experiences			
	1900–1920	1920–1940	1940–1960	1960–Present
	Pensionados	Pinoys to California and Alaska	World War II enlistment	Immigration of professionals after quota system abolished
	Workers to Hawaii	Discrimination	Citizenship possible	Elders immigrate
		Great Depression	Immigration increase in spite of quota	
		Immigration cut		
		Antimiscegenation laws		
85+	Children and adolescents	Young adults	Middle-aged	Elders
75–85	Children	Adolescents and young adults	Young adults to middle-aged	Middle-aged to old
65–75		Children and adolescents	Adolescents and young adults	Adults to young old
55–65		Children	Children to young adults	Young adults to middle-aged

Source. Pido 1986.

Emphasizing that physical illness can produce changes in the mind as well as the body and that these changes can affect an individual's ability to care for him- or herself is a desensitizing approach to begin with in the exploration of symptoms and their effect on ADLs. Such approaches enable therapists to collect the needed information with minimum distress to the patient and his or her family. Following the initial interview, seeing the patient first alone and then seeing the accompanying family member(s) will facilitate the clarification of the functional status of the ethnic elder. Emphasizing the psychiatrist's role as physician by taking vital signs, checking the oral cavity, checking whether the skin tents when pinched (a clinical sign of dehydration), and listening to the content of the words and the nonverbal communication of an ethnic elder patient will facilitate the therapeutic alliance and make it easier for the patient to gradually reveal "embarrassing changes" in function.

It is important to be aware that the ethnic elder may have a bias toward taking responsibility for symptoms and/or disease states that he or she cannot control. Any explanations and facilitating comments should emphasize that system failure within the elder's body has caused the symptoms. It will be important for the psychiatrist to understand that in the belief system of some ethnic elders (i.e., Mexican Americans, Navajo, Chinese), disease occurs because of a disharmony with the environment caused by an external force, which might be a malevolent individual.

The following case study illustrates the great importance of functional status for the ethnic elder, even the possible etiology of some mental disorders.

Case Study 3

Ms. C. is a 68-year-old widowed Navajo woman who has been hearing voices and seeing figures wrapped in yellow robes for approximately 2 months. This had been happening with increasing frequency. As an elder with second sight, she has been an important figure in her community as well as in her clan. When she was unable to sleep for 3 days, paced incessantly, and accused her daughter's family of trying to harm her, Ms. C. was brought to the regional hospital for evaluation. Because of her symptoms, she was referred to the psychiatry service.

The psychiatrist began by taking a detailed history of her symptoms, her medical illnesses, and her current medication. She established that Ms. C. had had non-insulin-dependent diabetes for several years and had mild "heart problems" that were treated successfully with digoxin. Within the previous year, she had developed symptoms of asthma that had necessitated treatment with theo-

Table 18–11. Mexican Americans: Significant dates and periods in immigration history

Year	Periods and events	U.S. Population (in Thousands)*
Late 1500s– early 1800s	Gradual colonization of Northern provinces of "New Spain"	
1821	Mexico's Independence from Spain	
1845–1854	Conquest of Northern Mexico by U.S. and annexation of territories of U.S. Southwest	80
1850–1900	Increased immigration to California for Gold Rush and to Texas and Arizona ranching and farming; anti-Mexican laws, wage discrimination, segregation, and invalidation of title for many Mexican land-grant holders	
1900		381 to 562
1910	Mexican Revolution followed by political and economic chaos, spurring immigration to U.S.	
1920–1928	500,000 entered on permanent visas, and thousands more informally; "coyote" industry; establishment of the Border Patrol; increased employment in railroads and manufacturing, some in Midwest; development of urban barrios	
1928–1942	Immigration reversed dramatically due to Great Depression and Dust Bowl; forced repatriation of 500,000 residents to Mexico; family-oriented migrant farming; segregated housing and social organizations, including labor unions	
1942–1947	350,000 Mexican Americans served in World War II; increased immigration to fill war-related industrial labor shortage; first Bracero program; anti-Mexican press coverage of conflict between "zoot-suiters" and servicemen and police	
1947–1960	Ex-GIs organize for civil rights; declining agricultural jobs, increasing urbanization and education in highly segregated communities; documented immigration of 273,000 in the 1950s; periodic raids and mass deportations of undocumented residents	
1965	Immigration and Nationality Act setting 20,000 ceiling on annual immigration and favoring family members of U.S. permanent residents	

Year	Periods and events	U.S. Population (in Thousands)*
1960s	Chicano Movement; increased immigration of women	
1970s	85% urban; migration from Texas to Midwest, and West; greater political organization and power; greater recognition of Mexican Americans in U.S. Catholic Church; bilingual education; widescale deportation of undocumented workers	6,000
1980s	Emphasis on education; continuation of Mexican heritage and Spanish language through arts and media; amnesty program; continued deportations	
1990 (est.)	Increased interest in Mexican American elderly; beginning studies of cognitive impairment, medical illnesses (diabetes, heart disease), and functional status	13,300

Source. Yeo 1991.
*Estimated; these census data are highly unreliable in most years.

phylline. There was no prior psychiatric history. In view of the sudden onset of symptoms, a thorough evaluation by the Geriatric Team was instituted.

As a result of the evaluation of Ms. C., the following data were obtained. The internist documented the presence of bilateral cataracts that were mature enough to require surgical intervention. The neurologist found no focal findings and confirmed the internist's report of diabetic retinopathy and only mild evidence of diabetic neuropathy.

The nurse, a Navajo and a member of the patient's clan, provided insight into the family's understanding of Ms. C.'s symptoms. It was their belief that a witch had placed a spell on her 2 months before. As her symptoms worsened, a medicine man had been consulted. A special cleansing ceremony, a sing, was being organized when her symptoms worsened and a consultation with a practitioner of Western medicine was obtained. The clan was concerned because of the role of Ms. C. in this large extended family and her importance in its religious belief system. Following a home visit by the social worker, who was trusted and well known to the Navajo community, it was established that Ms. C. had been responsible for the administration of her own medication in her daughter's home and had resisted the assistance of "those youngsters" in her family (i.e., relatives who were in their early 50s). Her medication bottles, which should have contained prescriptions for 2 months, only had enough medication for a few days. Neuropsychological testing revealed problems with attention, registration, and recall that were consistent with a toxic delirium. When laboratory tests came in, Ms. C. was found to have toxic levels of digoxin and theophylline, which explained her symptoms.

A family meeting was held to review the findings and to discuss Ms. C.'s care. The family requested that the medicine man be a part of this meeting, which the Geriatric Team welcomed. The results of the evaluation were shared and the following recommendations were made: stopping all medications, observation in the hospital for a few days to confirm the absence of complications and to remove Ms. C.'s bilateral cataracts. Her vision was so impaired at this point that she was at risk of confusing her medications again and/or harming herself while cooking or walking.

The medicine man had worked with the Geriatric Team over several years. He confirmed that it would be helpful to reestablish the balance of Ms. C. with her environment and supported her hospitalization and the cataract surgery. He recommended specific ceremonies and a tea, known to be nontoxic, to be used only after her symptoms of delirium had resolved. To remove the influence of the witch who the family believed had precipitated the sequence of events, a sing was planned, which was to be completed at the time Ms. C. was released from the hospital. Counteracting the influence of the witch would return her to harmony with nature and prevent another cycle of deterioration.

During the 3-week hospitalization, several members of her clan visited Ms. C. and were supportive. The Geriatric Team nurse introduced Ms. C. to several Navajo elders who had had cataract surgery, and they discussed the procedure and its effects together. With insight from other elders in her clan regarding the procedure and its outcome, Ms. C. consented to the surgery and had an uneventful course. She returned to her clan and allowed a visiting nurse to organize her medications in a weekly medicine box.

The sing had been carefully planned. The 3-day ceremony began on the day of her discharge from the hospital. With the combined efforts of a native healer and a Western-medicine treatment team, Ms. C. was returned to harmony with nature. She continued to be well 18 months after her hospitalization and to describe her adult children as too young to be responsible for full initiation into the Navajo way.

Lessons From Ms. C.'s Case Study

This case study illustrates the effective way in which the belief system of the ethnic elder can be respected and incorporated into an effective treatment of the presenting symptoms. Also, the importance of not making a precipitous psychiatric diagnosis of late-onset schizophrenia or delusional disorder is underscored. Again, in Ms. C.'s case, a thorough evaluation by the multidisciplinary Geriatric Team was critically important, because the team identified the vision impairment that had led to the patient's toxic delirium from polypharmacy. A further point emphasized by this case is the importance of involving other ethnic elders in the clarification of the proposed Western-style treatment. If there has been no prior experience with a proposed treatment, multiple explanations are indicated. For the ethnic elder, explanations from others who are "like themselves" are particularly meaningful in obtaining truly informed consent.

Finally, the effective liaison between the native healer and the Western-medicine treatment team is illustrated. Working effectively with a native healer is possible, but it does require a willingness to acknowledge and attempt to understand a different conceptual model of illness than that taught in medical school.

Rehabilitation

Public health emphasizes three levels of prevention: primary, secondary, and tertiary (Langsley 1985; Mausner and Kramer 1985). Primary prevention is illustrated by immunization programs that decrease the prevalence of disease. Secondary prevention involves the treatment of illness to arrest its course and return the person to health, and tertiary prevention focuses on rehabilitation. In psychiatry, primary prevention may be illustrated by programs in elementary and junior high schools to discourage substance abuse. The hospitalization of patients for treatment of psychiatric disorders illustrates secondary prevention. The work with the survivors of a person who has completed a suicide is an example of psychiatric tertiary prevention, as are rehabilitation programs for people with chronic mental illness.

The concept of tertiary prevention in elders was expanded by Rubenstein and colleagues (1989). The expanded concept includes all of the ADLs that are usually described—basic grooming, toileting, feeding, and dressing—and adds ambulation with and without assistance, holding objects, opening doors, and maneuvering in the home. This expanded definition of ADLs has pertinence for the elder, particularly if moving from his or her home of several decades to live either in a senior residence or with an adult child, or (as is rare for an ethnic elder) in a nursing home. Elders who have difficulty with ADLs are likely to come to the attention of social workers or visiting nurses often, because their social network is concerned about the elder's obvious difficulty in managing. A progressive deterioration in physical health that results for the first time in dependency on others to complete ADLs may precipitate a major depressive disorder in an ethnic elder. Although most ethnic elders have the resources of the extended family

Table 18–12. Cohort experiences—Mexican American elders

Current Age Cohorts	Age at Historical Experiences			
	1900–1920	1920–1940	1940–1960	1960–Present
	Heritage of loss of land	Massive immigration	World War II participation	Chicano Movement
	Mexican Revolution	Great Depression	Immigration	Deportations
		Repatriation	Urbanization	
			GI Forum	
85+	Children and adolescents	Young adults	Middle-aged	Elders
75–85	Children	Adolescents and young adults	Young adults to middle-aged	Middle-aged to old
65–75		Children and adolescents	Adolescents and young adults	Adults to young old
55–65		Children	Children to young adults	Young adults to middle-aged

Source. Yeo 1991.

(Markides and Vernon 1984; Markides et al. 1986), this may not be true for some, as the following case study shows.

Case Study 4

Mr. D. is a 92-year-old widowed Chinese man who resides in a small apartment in an urban center. Since his arrival in the United States, he has lived alone. Because of the Chinese Exclusion Act, he was unable to bring his wife and son to the United States at the time of his initial immigration. When the laws were finally changed in the 1960s, his son had died in war and his wife had died of cancer. Having focused during his working life on saving money for his family and sending it "back home," Mr. D. had little savings for himself. Initially immigrating to work on the railroad, he later worked in a Chinese laundry. Subsequently, he worked in a Chinese restaurant as a waiter and retired from this position.

Because Mr. D. was devastated by the death of the family he had not seen in over 40 years, he had made few friends and had not become involved in the Chinese American community. When he retired, he moved into housing that he could afford on his meager Social Security benefits. When he was ill, Mr. D. sought help from a Chinese herbalist.

After not seeing Mr. D. for 3 weeks, his landlord found him sitting in his apartment without food and with evidence that he had been doubly incontinent. Mr. D. was brought to the local emergency room. He was mute and refused to talk with either an internist or a psychiatrist. Because of the absence of information, Mr. D.'s refusal to cooperate with an evaluation, and a social worker's confirmation on a home visit that Mr. D.'s environment was deteriorated, he was admitted to a Geriatric Psychiatric Unit for evaluation.

Mr. D. cooperated with the taking of vital signs, and a physical examination was completed with his cooperation. Through the hospital, a medically trained Chinese interpreter was obtained. After several visits with Mr. D., the interpreter was able to communicate with him. Another medically trained interpreter conversant with his particular dialect was identified and met with Mr. D. over several days. When a relationship was established between them, it was possible to complete an assessment over a period of 2 weeks.

Although he had completed only 6 years of formal education, Mr. D. demonstrated a bright, quick mind that readily grasped concepts. He stated that he was ready to die because he had lived a long life. In the absence of family, he did not have the valued role of elder and had not become actively involved in the Chinese community. Mr. D. stated that he "had nothing to live for." He was extremely isolated and had no connections with any social network.

Because of his small income, Mr. D. ate an inadequate diet of starches and infrequent sources of protein. He had nutritional deficiencies of vitamins B_{12}

and folate, and there was evidence of muscle wasting. He was unable to turn knobs to open his clothing closet on the unit and required help to rise from a low chair.

Mr. D. had not maintained an interest or belief in Confucianism and had no other religious beliefs. His only social contact was the herbalist that he had visited for management of cold symptoms or muscle aches over the years. When the herbalist had died a month ago, Mr. D. had withdrawn to his room.

When a detailed interview was completed with the assistance of an interpreter, it was established that Mr. D. had an acute grief reaction, which was complicated by his nutritional deficiencies. His neurologic examination was remarkable only for decreased muscle strength and muscle wasting that was symmetrical. His neuropsychological evaluation, completed by an Asian neuropsychologist with testing adjusted to nonwhite norms, revealed normal cognitive functioning, with some impairment in ability to attend and slowing of cognition that was related to Mr. D.'s cachectic state. When he was retested at discharge, there were no deficits.

Occupational and rehabilitation therapy were involved actively in the remobilization of Mr. D. as his nutritional status improved and his energy level was regained. The nursing evaluation identified a community setting where his weight would be monitored and a complete meal provided. Although the community facility was attended by a mixture of ethnic elders, there were a significant number of Chinese elders there.

The social work assessment focused on the identification of additional community resources that could be mobilized to reengage Mr. D. so that his overall quality of life would be improved. An outreach program from the Asian community that focused on Asian elders was identified, and the program director visited Mr. D. in the hospital and described the program. Program participants visited Mr. D. in the hospital. Two Chinese elders who had a similar background to that of Mr. D. became regular visitors. The three regularly got together to play a board game that they had played in their youth in China.

As his weight increased and his nutritional status improved, Mr. D. had increased energy. The occupational and rehabilitation therapy were also effective. At discharge, he was ambulatory and completed all his ADLs. He was discharged on no medications and referred to a day hospital program for social contact. From noon until 4:00 P.M. each day, Mr. D. participated in the Asian elder program. On weekends, he was visited by his two new friends, and Meals on Wheels were provided.

Lessons From Mr. D.'s Case Study

This case study illustrated the consequences of earlier national policy on the life course of an ethnic elder in the United States. The importance of using a medically trained interviewer is underscored. Everyone involved in the treatment program for an ethnic elder should be clear on what the task of the interaction will be. The interviewer should be comfortable with asking what would be "insensitive" or "intrusive" questions in his or her culture of origin. The role of rehabilitation and occupational therapy in the habilitation of a debilitated elder is also emphasized. Finally, Mr. D.'s case illustrates the mobilization of community resources by nursing and social work interventions to provide services for an ethnic elder (Baker et al. 1990).

Conclusion

Ethnic minority elders for the most part are survivors of great difficulties. The majority of these elders have experienced significant economic hardships, had inadequate health care throughout their lives, and been faced with the resultant multiple health problems. Therefore, those ethnic elders who survive into their eighth decade possess significant physical and constitutional strengths. Although their cultures of origin may have viewed psychiatric illnesses as "shameful" or "not to be discussed," increasing understanding of mental disorders by the greater society, as well as increasing discussion in the media, have modified this attitude to some extent. The referral of an ethnic elder to a psychiatrist by his or her internist or family practice physician usually results in a successful engagement if the psychiatrist is culturally sensitive, respects the elder's macrohistory (i.e., his or her history in the context of world and national events), and is empathic as he or she explores the elder's microhistory (i.e., personal history; Asnes 1983; Baker 1982). The support of an elder's adult children also facilitates the acceptance of a psychiatric assessment.

We have used case studies to illustrate key concepts in working with ethnic elders. Specific references have been cited to enable the reader to develop or expand his or her knowledge of a specific ethnic group or groups. The successful outcome of treatment with these elders has been illustrated. The opportunity to work with families and involved friends is an additional dimension of this fulfilling work (Sakauye et al., in press). The reader is referred to several publications that address issues of cultural and psychiatry in general (Baker 1990; Favazza and Oman 1978; Foulks 1980; Haldipur 1980; Lefley 1984; Markides and Mindel 1987; Moffic 1983; Moffic et al. 1988).

References

American Geriatric Society Public Policy Committee: Comprehensive geriatric assessment. J Am Geriatr Soc 37:473–474, 1989

Angel JL, Hogan DP: The demography of minority aging populations, in Minority Elders: Longevity, Economics, and Health—Building a Public Policy Base. Edited by Harootyan LK. Washington, DC, Gerontological Society of America, 1991, pp 1–13

Asnes DP: Psychotherapy of the elderly: the life validation approach in psychotherapy with elderly patients. J Geriatr Psychiatry 16:87–97, 1983

Baker FM: The black elderly: biopsychosocial perspectives within an age cohort and adult development context. J Geriatr Psychiatry 15:225–237, 1982

Baker FM: The Afro-American life cycle: success, failure, and mental health. J Natl Med Assoc 79:625–633, 1987

Baker FM: Afro-Americans, in Clinical Guidelines in Cross-Cultural Mental Health. Edited by Comas-Diaz L, Griffith EEH. New York, Wiley, 1988, pp 151–181

Baker FM: Black youth suicide: literature review with a focus on prevention, in Report of the Secretary's Task Force on Youth Suicide—Vol 3: Prevention and Intervention in Youth Suicide. Washington, DC, U.S. Department of Health and Human Services, 1989, pp 3-177–3-195

Baker FM: Ethnic minority elders: differential diagnosis, medication, treatment, and outcomes, in Minority Aging: Essential Curricula Content for Selected Health and Allied Health Professionals. Edited by Harper MS. Baltimore, MD, Williams & Wilkins, 1990, pp 549–577

Baker FM, Kamikawa LM, Espine DS, et al: Rehabilitation in ethnic minority elderly, in Aging and Rehabilitation II—The State of Practice. Edited by Brody SJ, Pawlson LG. New York, Springer, 1990, pp 186–207

Baker FM, Lavizzo-Mourey R, Jones BE: Acute care of the African American elder. J Geriatr Psychiatry Neurol (in press)

Bass BA, Wyatt GE, Powell GJ: The Afro-American Family: Assessment, Treatment, and Research Issues. New York, Grune & Stratton, 1982

Bernal G: Cuban families, in Ethnicity and Family Therapy. Edited by McGoldrick M, Pearce JK, Giordano J. New York, Guilford, 1982, pp 187–207

Broudy DW, May PA: Demographic and epidemiologic transitions among the Navajo Indians. Social Biology 30:1–16, 1983

Brown D: Bury My Heart at Wounded Knee—An Indian History of the American West. New York, Holt, Rinehart and Winston, 1970

Brummel-Smith K: Geriatric rehabilitation. J Am Geriatr Soc 2:15–18, 1988

Chunn ZC, Dunstun PS, Ross-Sherrif F (eds): Mental Health in People of Color: Curriculum Development and Change. Washington DC, Howard University Press, 1983

Clevenger J: Native Americans, in Cross-Cultural Psychiatry. Edited by Gaw A. Littleton, MA, John Wright-PSG Pub Co, 1982, pp 149–161

Comas-Diaz L, Griffith EEH (eds): Clinical Guidelines in Cross-Cultural Mental Health. New York, Wiley, 1988

Coner-Edwards AF, Spurlock J: Black Families in Crisis: The Middle Class. New York, Brunner/Mazel, 1988

Cuellar J: Aging and Health: American Indian/Alaska Native Elders (SGEC Working Paper Series, No 6, Ethnogeriatric Reviews). Stanford, CA, Stanford Geriatric Education Center of Stanford University Medical School, 1990a

Cuellar J: Aging and Health: Hispanic American Elders (SGEC Working Paper Series, No 5, Ethnogeriatric Reviews). Stanford, CA, Stanford Geriatric Education Center of Stanford University Medical School, 1990b

EchoHawk M: Discussion: cultural aspects of mental health care for Native Americans, in Cross-Cultural Psychiatry. Edited by Gaw A. Littleton, MA, John Wright-PSG Pub Co, 1982, pp 159–161

Engel GL: The need for a new medical model: a challenge for biomedicine. Science 196:129–136, 1977

Engel GL: The clinical application of the biopsychosocial model. Am J Psychiatry 137:535–544, 1980

Falicov CJ: Mexican families, in Ethnicity and Family Therapy. Edited by McGoldrick, M, Pearce JK, Giordano J. New York, Guilford, 1982, pp 134–163

Favazza AR, Oman M: Overview: foundations of cultural psychiatry. Am J Psychiatry 135:811–835, 1978

Foulks EF: The concept of culture in psychiatry residency education. Am J Psychiatry 137:811–816, 1980

Garcia-Preto N: Puerto-Rican families, in Ethnicity and Family Therapy. Edited by McGoldrick M, Pearce JK, Giordano J. New York, Guilford, 1982, pp 164–186

Gaw A: Chinese Americans, in Cross-Cultural Psychiatry. Edited by Gaw A. Littleton, MA, John Wright-PSG Pub Co, 1982a, pp 1–29

Gaw A (ed): Cross-Cultural Psychiatry. Littleton, MA, John Wright-PSG Pub Co, 1982b

Gibson RC: Blacks in an Aging Society. New York, Carnegie Corporation, 1986

Griffith EEH, Bell CC: Recent trends in suicide and homicide among blacks. JAMA 262:2265–2269, 1989

Haldipur CV: The idea of "cultural" psychiatry—a comment on the foundations of cultural psychiatry. Compr Psychiatry 21:206–211, 1980

Harootyan LK (ed): Minority Elders: Longevity, Economics, and Health—Building a Public Policy Base. Washington, DC, Gerontological Society of America, 1991

Harper MS (ed): Minority Aging: Essential Curricular Content for Selected Health and Allied Health Professionals. Washington, DC, U.S. Government Printing Office, 1990

Hines PM, Boyd-Franklin N: Black families, in Ethnicity and Family Therapy. Edited by McGoldrick M, Pearce JK, Giordano J. New York, Guilford, 1982, pp 84–107

Jackson JS (ed): The Black American Elderly—Research on Physical and Psychosocial Health. New York, Springer, 1988

John R: The state of research on American Indian elders' health, income security, and social support networks, in Minority Elders: Longevity, Economics, and Health—Building a Public Policy Base. Edited by Harootyan LK. Washington, DC, Gerontological Society of America, 1991, pp 38–50

Jordan WC: Voodoo medicine, in Textbook of Black-Related Diseases. Edited by Williams RA. New York, McGraw-Hill, 1975, pp 716–738

Kane RL, Ouslander JG, Abrass IB: Developing clinical expectations, in Essentials of Clinical Geriatrics—Second Edition. New York, McGraw-Hill, 1989, pp 373–395

Langsley DG: Prevention in psychiatry: primary, secondary, and tertiary, in Comprehensive Textbook of Psychiatry/IV—Fourth Edition. Edited by Kapan HI, Sadock BJ. Baltimore, MD, Williams & Wilkins, 1985, pp 1885–1888

Lefley HP: Cross-cultural training for mental health professionals: effects in the delivery of services. Hosp Community Psychiatry 35:1227–1229, 1984

Lewis JM, Looney JC: The Long Struggle: Well-Functioning Working Class Black Families. New York, Brunner/Mazel, 1983

Li FP, Schlief NY, Chang CJ, et al: Health care for the Chinese community in Boston. Am J Public Health 62:536–539, 1972

Lightfoot OB: Psychiatric intervention with blacks: the elderly—a case in point. J Geriatr Psychiatry 15:209–223, 1982

Lightfoot OB: Personality disorder and outcome in the treatment of late-life depression. J Geriatr Psychiatry 21:147–153, 1988

Manson SM, Callaway: Health and aging among American Indians: issues and challenges for the biobehavior sciences, in Health and Behavior: A Research Agenda for American Indians. Edited by Manson SM, Dinges N. Denver, CO, University of Colorado Health Sciences Center, 1988, pp 160–210

Manson SM, Walker RD, Kivlahan DR: Psychiatric assessment and treatment of American Indians and Alaskin Natives. Hosp Community Psychiatry 38:165–173, 1987

Manuel RC: The demography of older blacks in the United States, in the Black American Elderly—Research on Physical and Psychosocial Health. Edited by Jackson JS. New York, Springer, 1988, pp 25–49

Markides KS, Mindel CH: Aging and Ethnicity. Newbury Park, CA, Sage, 1987

Markides KS, Vernon SW: Aging, sex-role orientation and adjustment: a three-generations study of Mexican Americans. J Gerontol 39:586–591, 1984

Markides KS, Boldt JS, Ray LA: Sources of helping and intergenerational solidarity: a three-generational study of Mexican-Americans. J Gerontol 41:506–511, 1986

Martin EP, Martin JM: The Black Extended Family. Chicago, IL, University of Chicago Press, 1978

Martinez C: Curanderos: clinical aspects. Journal of Operational Psychiatry 8:35–38, 1977

Martinez C: Mexican Americans, in Clinical Guidelines in Cross-Cultural Mental Health. Edited by Comas-Diaz L, Griffith EEH. New York, Wiley, 1988, pp 182–203

Martinez C, Martin HW: Folk diseases among urban Mexican-Americans. JAMA

196:161–164, 1966

Mausner JS, Kramer S: Levels of prevention, in Epidemiology—An Introductory Text. Philadelphia, PA, WB Saunders, 1985, pp 9–13

McGoldrick M, Pearce JK, Giordano J. Ethnicity and Family Therapy. New York, Guilford, 1982

Moffic HS: Sociocultural guidelines for clinicians in multicultural settings. Psychiatr Q 55:47–54, 1983

Moffic HS: Kendrick EA, Reid K, et al: Cultural psychiatry during psychiatric residency. Journal of Psychiatric Education 12:91–101, 1988

Morioka-Douglas N, Yeo G: Aging and Health: Asian/Pacific Island American Elders (SGEC Working Paper Series, No 3, Ethnogeriatric Reviews). Stanford, CA, Stanford Geriatric Education Center of Stanford University Medical School, 1990

National Indian Council on Aging: American Indian Elderly: A National Profile. Albuquerque NM, National Indian Council on Aging, 1981

Pido AJA: The Pilipinos in America. New York, Center for Migration Studies, 1986

Pinderhughes E: Understanding Race, Ethnicity, and Power. New York, Free Press, 1989

Richardson J: Aging and Health: Black American Elders (SGEC Working Paper Series, No 6, Ethnogeriatric Reviews). Stanford, CA, Stanford Geriatric Education Center of Stanford University Medical School, 1990

Rubenstein LZ, Calkins DR, Greenfield S, et al: Health assessment for elderly patients. J Am Geriatr Soc 37:562–569, 1989

Sakauye KM, Baker FM, Chacko RC, et al: Report of the Task Force on Ethnic Minority Elderly. Washington, DC, American Psychiatric Association (in press)

Singer BP: Racial Factors in Psychiatric Intervention. San Francisco, CA, R and E Research Associates, 1977

Stack C: All Our Kin. New York, Emerson Hall, 1971

Sue S, McKinney H. Asian Americans in the community mental health care system. Am J Orthopsychiatry 45:111–118, 1975

Sung BL: Mountain of Gold: The Story of the Chinese America. New York, MacMillan, 1970

Task Force on Black and Minority Health: Report on the Secretary's Task Force on Black and Minority Health—Vol I: Executive Summary. Washington DC, U.S. Department of Health and Human Services, 1985

Taylor RJ: Aging and supportive relationships among black Americans, in The Black American Elderly—Research on Physical and Psychosocial Health. Edited by Jackson JS. New York, Springer, 1988, pp 259–281

Thernstrom S (ed): Harvard Encyclopedia of American Ethnic Groups. Cambridge, MA, Harvard University Press, 1980

U.S. Bureau of the Census: Years of school completed for persons 15 years old and over by age, sex, race, and Spanish origin: 1980 (Table 262), in 1980 Census of the U.S. Population, Vol 1: Detailed Population Characteristics (United States Summary Section A: United States—PC80-1-D1-A). Washington, DC, U.S. Government Printing Office, 1981, pp 1-40–1-51

U.S. Bureau of the Census: United States Population Estimates by Age, Sex, Race, and Hispanic Origin: 1980 to 1988 (Series P-25, No 1045). Washington, DC, U.S. Government Printing Office, 1990

Walker RD, LaDue R: An integrated approach to American Indian mental health, in Ethnic Psychiatry. Edited by Wilkinson CB. New York, Plenum Medical, 1986, pp 143–194

Willie CV, Kramer BM, Brown BS (eds): Racism and Mental Health. Pittsburgh, PA, University of Pittsburgh Press, 1973

Yamamoto J: Japanese Americans, in Cross-Cultural Psychiatry. Edited by Gaw A. Littleton, MA, John Wright-PSG Pub Co, 1982, pp 31–54

Yeo G: Cohort experiences of minority elderly. Paper presented at conference on "Ethnicity: Impacts on Mental Health Care for Older Adults," Stanford Geriatric Education Center, Forest City, CA, 6 June 1991

19   Cultural Considerations in the Psychiatric Care of Gay Men and Lesbians

James P. Krajeski, M.D.

P roviding quality psychiatric care to gay men and lesbians is not possible without understanding the cultural issues that affect their lives. This understanding requires an examination of the cultures that gay men and lesbians have evolved for themselves and the cultural environment in which they live.

The terms "gay men" and "lesbians" ordinarily evoke certain mental images or stereotypes that may or may not be accurate. However, an understanding of gay men and lesbians requires a recognition of the inherent diversity within these groups of individuals.

Definitions

Labels such as "gay man," "lesbian," or "homosexual" tell very little about an individual. Homosexuality is only one part of an individual's identity, and, furthermore, only one element of an individual's sexual identity. Shively and De Cecco (1977) describe four components of sexual identity: biological sex, gender identity, social sex-role, and sexual orientation. Gender identity is defined as an individual's conviction of being either male or female. This sense of self may or may not be consistent with an individual's biological sex. The term "social sex-role" refers to behaviors and characteristics that are ordinarily associated with concepts of masculinity or femininity. Finally, sexual orientation refers to an individual's physical or affectional sexual preference. Sexual orientation itself may be conceptualized as being made up of several facets (e.g., sexual attraction, behavior, fantasy, and emotional or social preference; Klein et al. 1985).

For the most part, someone is labeled homosexual if his or her sexual behavior and emotional interest are directed toward the same sex. The affectional aspect of homosexuality is sometimes not well appreciated, but it is this strong emotional attraction to individuals of the same gender that characterizes gay men and lesbians (i.e, they fall in love with persons of their own gender).

Certainly, there is a continuum between homosexuality and heterosexuality; many individuals do not readily fit into either one of these categories. For example, some individuals may regularly engage in opposite-gender sexual relationships but may have significant emotional or fantasy attractions to members of the same gender. Moreover, awareness of sexual orientation may change. For example, it is not unusual for individuals to report that they were relatively unaware of their attraction to the same gender until they reached a certain age. Recognizing that sexual orientation may be viewed as existing on a continuum is important because the labels "gay men" and "lesbians" may obscure this diversity.

Demographics

Although precise population statistics do not exist, there are at least several million gay men and lesbians in the United States. The exact size of the gay male and lesbian population is uncertain because of self-reporting bias and inconsistent definitions of homosexuality used in studies. In a world in which they face discrimination and ostracism, individuals may not readily identify themselves as gay men or lesbians. A National Institute of Mental Health task force on homosexuality (Gebhard 1972) estimated that about 4% of white college-educated adult males were predominantly homosexual; about 1%–2% of women were estimated to be homosexual. Marmor (1980) estimated that ranges of more or less exclusive homosexual behavior in Western culture are 3%–5% for women and 5%–10% for men.

A more recent analysis of survey data from 1970 suggests that 3.3% of the adult male population had homosexual contacts "occasionally" or "fairly often" (Fay et al. 1989, p. 346). (No statistics were given for female homosexuality.) Because of problems with presumed reporting bias, Fay and colleagues caution that this figure is likely to be the lower bound of the estimate and that the figure could well be twice as high. Also, this estimate was based on sexual behavior and did not encompass a larger group of individuals who would be identified if a broader definition of homosexuality had been used.

Psychiatry and Homosexuality

The history of the relationship between psychiatry and homosexuality is intriguing. A psychoanalyst writing in the 1950s says that "homosexuals are essentially disagreeable people. . . . They are subservient when confronted with a stronger person, merciless when in power, unscrupulous about trampling on a weaker person" (Bergler 1956, p. 26). The common view of psychiatrists was once that homosexuality represented a mental disorder. The evidence for this was largely based on theoretical considerations that presumed that homosexuality was a bad outcome and, therefore, there must be a pathological origin for it. Early research on the origins of homosexuality was particularly notable for its poor quality and bias. Sweeping generalizations about all gay men and women were made based on patient populations. Much of the early research ignored women and their issues. Even today, a focus on male homosexuality typifies research on and discussions of homosexuality.

However, since the early 1970s, there has been a remarkable shift in views of psychiatrists about homosexuality. Initially, the American Psychiatric Association (APA) found itself embroiled in challenges to the notion of homosexuality as a mental illness. In San Francisco in 1970, gay activists confronted psychiatrists at an APA meeting and threatened confrontations at future meetings. The process of change in response to challenges both within and outside the APA is detailed by Bayer (1981). The decision to remove homosexuality from the official *Diagnostic and Statistical Manual of Mental Disorders, Second Edition* (American Psychiatric Association 1968) was reached after a review of the issue by various components of the APA. The decision was ratified by the Assembly of District Branches and the Board of Trustees in 1973. This process is the same as that followed within the APA today in making decisions on scientific matters, and similar processes exist in other medical organizations.

The unusual aspect of the APA's decision was the subsequent gathering of signatures to force a referendum of the entire APA membership on the issue. The vote of the membership ultimately upheld the decision of the Board of Trustees to remove homosexuality from the diagnostic nomenclature. This vote has had its political cost, because it has made it possible to present the removal of homosexuality as a decision based on a popular vote rather than one based on science. However, this argument is disingenuous; it ignores the readily apparent fact that the decision to remove homosexuality was made as all decisions in the APA are made. Furthermore, the decision was ratified by the membership of the organization, a process that should lend greater authority to the decision, not less.

After 1973, a category remained in the diagnostic nomenclature that referred to homosexual individuals who were dissatisfied with their sexual orientation. This category, which was most recently named "ego-dystonic homosexuality" was eliminated from the APA's *Diagnostic and Statistical Manual of Mental Disorders, Third Edition, Revised* (DSM-III-R) in 1987 (American Psychiatric Association 1987). The explanation in DSM-III-R for removing the diagnosis is as follows:

1. It suggested that homosexuality was a mental disorder;
2. Gay men and lesbians typically go through an "ego-dystonic" phase in our culture;
3. The diagnosis was rarely used clinically or in the scientific literature; and
4. Even "treatment" programs attempting to change sexual behavior have not used the diagnosis.

The elimination of "ego-dystonic homosexuality" marked the removal of the last vestige of the official stigmatization of homosexuality as a mental disorder.

Gay Culture and Subcultures

In everyday conversation, references are commonly made to the "gay community." There may be a tendency to view this community as a monolithic, homogeneous group. However, this view is inaccurate. Although the "gay community" may be generally united on certain issues, such as the elimination of bias against gay men and lesbians, the community is really a collection of diverse individuals. There is no reason to believe that homosexual men and women are any less diverse than their heterosexual counterparts. Gay men and lesbians are in all social strata. They are members of all minority and ethnic groups, they work in all occupations, they live in small and large towns, and they hold diverse views on virtually any issue.

The concept of community in relation to gay men and lesbians would be more precisely expressed as one of a plurality of communities. The lesbian or gay man living in a rural area may have little in common with the lesbian or gay man living in a large city and may or may not perceive her- or himself to be part of a larger gay community. Or the individual may identify with the gay rural community versus the gay urban community. The needs and issues of different individuals may define different gay communities. In large cities, there may be a readily definable gay community, but not all gay men and lesbians see themselves as a part of the community, nor do they necessarily share common views on a variety of issues. This concept is seemingly little different from the way members of racial or ethnic minorities view their "communities." The common bond of sexual orientation may be overridden by other concerns.

The experiences of gay men and lesbians who also are members of other minority groups may be quite different from those of the predominant white American culture in the United States. Unfortunately, there is little research available on these communities and the ways in which gay/lesbian identity and minority group status interact or clash. Members of various groups may share certain experiences and face similar obstacles. One writer (Navarro 1989) notes that a common experience of gays who are also members of other minority groups is a feeling of being pressured to choose between two worlds (e.g., the gay community and the Latino community) and not feeling truly at home in either. Prejudice and discrimination within the gay community is another obstacle for many minority group members who attempt to find validation within the gay and lesbian community (Loiacano 1989).

Although there is value in attempting to understand the common characteristics or experiences of gay men and lesbians who are also members of minority groups, there is also the inherent danger of perpetuating stereotypes. Obviously, minority group members do not all perceive issues or problems in the same way. For example, Asian American gay men and lesbians may disagree whether it is easier or more difficult to "come out" to fellow Asian Americans (Chan 1989). Just because gay men or lesbians share a certain ethnic or racial background does not mean that they also share the same experiences, feelings, or opinions.

Myths and Realities

It is difficult to make generalizations about gay men and lesbians because of their inherent diversity and because the research data about gay men and women are limited. One major problem with data gathering has been the lack of representative samples of gay men and lesbians, which limits the conclusions that can be made. Still, there has been research on sufficient numbers of gay men and lesbians to show that certain common stereotypes are unwarranted.

One widespread stereotype suggests that homosexual men and women lead unhappy lives. This view is exemplified by the following quotation:

A therapist asks a gay patient, "Do you want to lead the kind of life they lead? . . . Can you see yourself as a sad aging homosexual? I'm sure you've heard as many dreary tales about the shallowness of such people's lives and how very lonely they are" (Hatterer 1970, p. 116). But people acquainted with gay men and women find that such a stereotype is not true. Reporting on one of the largest research samples of gay men and women, Bell and Weinberg (1978) concluded, "Many [gay men and lesbians] could very well serve as models of social comportment and psychological maturity. Most are indistinguishable from the heterosexual majority with respect to most of the nonsexual aspects of their lives. . . . " (p. 230).

Another common stereotype holds that gay men and lesbians are unable to develop and maintain satisfactory relationships. The Bell and Weinberg (1978) study found that more than half of the males and nearly three quarters of the women were involved in a "relatively steady relationship." The actual numbers and length of relationships of gay men and lesbians as compared with heterosexual men and women are unknown. However, it is obvious to those who are acquainted with gay men and lesbians that many of their relationships last as long as heterosexual relationships and appear to be similar in quality.

However, the issue of relationships must ultimately be considered in the context of the dominant culture. Support for relationships from family members is often not present. Raising children in a gay or lesbian relationship can be difficult because of society's attitudes. It is problematic for gay men or lesbians to adopt children. Legal incentives such as marriage or laws formally recognizing gay relationships in matters of joint property ownership and inheritance are absent. The availability of spousal benefits for partners of gay men and lesbians is rare. Thus, not only is there virtually no reinforcement for homosexual relationships; there is actually considerable disincentive for establishing gay relationships because of the visibility they create and the potential for discrimination that can follow. Therefore, it would indeed be surprising if homosexual relationships in general were found to be as permanent or trouble-free as heterosexual relationships.

Men and Women

Just as there are significant differences between heterosexual men and heterosexual women, there are important differences between homosexual men and lesbians. As mentioned earlier, it is common for discussions of homosexuality to make no reference to lesbians; the research literature has likewise focused much more on gay men than on lesbians. Perhaps the relative lack of attention to lesbians is derived from general societal attitudes toward or disregard for women. Whatever the reasons for the lack of attention to lesbians, it is important to conceptualize the homosexual population as consisting of both women and men and to recognize that this is one more aspect of its diversity.

Adolescents

Frequently ignored as a segment of the gay population are young men and women. Adolescents who are gay or who may be developing an awareness of being gay may be particularly vulnerable to stresses associated with societal and family attitudes about homosexuality. A small study of self-described gay or bisexual male teenagers found that discrimination, verbal and physical assaults, and strong negative attitudes from parents and friends were common occurrences in their lives (Remafedi 1987). For gay teenagers, other problems cited in the literature include:

1. Isolation and fear of disclosure of their sexual orientation;
2. Problems related to the teenagers' need to hide or deceive others about their sexual orientation (Martin 1982); and
3. The lack of certain common social developmental experiences of adolescence such as social involvements and interpersonal attachments (Malyon 1981).

Stigma

One of the most significant aspect of the lives of gay men and lesbians is the stigma that has been attached to homosexuality in our society. The pervasive dislike and hatred of gay men and lesbians have profound influences on how gay men and lesbians view themselves and how they interact with each other and the heterosexual world. The examples of bias against gay men and lesbians are evident in society's major institutions such as organized religion, the judicial system, and the educational system. The United States Supreme Court has held that homosexual acts between consenting adults are not constitutionally protected (*Bowers v. Hardwick* 1986), and homosexual acts are illegal in 25 states and the District of Columbia (O'Neill 1989). This criminalization of homosexual behavior is often used as a justification for the views of those who otherwise abhor homosexuality.

Heterosexual Bias

Heterosexual bias is defined as "a belief system that values heterosexuality as superior to and/or more natural than homosexuality" (Morin 1977, p. 629). The influence of this concept on psychological research was demonstrated in Morin's review of research reported between 1967 and 1974 on lesbianism and male homosexuality. Examples of heterosexual bias included a research emphasis on what causes homosexuality and how it might be prevented, a focus on whether homosexuals are "sick," and methods for "diagnosing" homosexuality. In other words, the emphasis was on looking at the "pathology" of homosexuality.

The problem of heterosexual bias continues to affect far more than the social science research establishment. What is considered acceptable sexuality in American society is based on heterosexuality, and bias against homosexuality is endemic. Remarks by a member of Congress in the *Congressional Record* vividly illustrate the fervor that supports and perpetuates such bias:

> As long as I have the pleasure to serve in the U.S. Congress, I will continue to affirm the heterosexual ethic at every turn, with every subtly [sic], with every bit of imagery I can conjure, with the help of good people across this Nation, as well as with the help of a majority of my colleagues in Congress, and also by the grace of God. (Dannemeyer 1989, p. 3514)

Homophobia

The term "homophobia" has become entrenched in our language in recent years. The concept is used in various ways to refer to antihomosexual attitudes or feelings and is closely akin to concepts of sexism or racism. Fyfe (1983) notes that this term has been used to describe various cultural, attitudinal, and personal biases against gay men and lesbians. He points out that homophobia is not truly a phobia in the clinical sense; as an alternative, he proposes the use of the term "homosexual bias." Though this term may be more precise clinically than homophobia, the concept of homophobia has not been replaced. In fact, it generally carries with it the connotation of a more deep-seated, emotionally based dislike or fear of gay men and lesbians than does the word "bias."

American society is rife with antihomosexual feelings that intrude in the lives of gay men and lesbians. Although there has been a significant shift in attitudes within the past two decades, many societal institutions continue to foster antihomosexual attitudes. Homosexuality is regularly condemned by organized religions. Because acquired immunodeficiency syndrome (AIDS) has heavily affected gay men, it is viewed by many as a punishment for sin. Even a major medical journal carried an editorial asking whether in AIDS we might be witnessing "a fulfillment of St. Paul's pronouncement: 'the due penalty of their error'?" (Fletcher 1984, p. 150). Our school systems are regularly prohibited from teaching about homosexuality. Gay men and lesbians have been denied security clearances and are still prohibited from joining the military. Legislation banning discrimination against gay men and lesbians in such areas as employment and housing is very rare, which leaves almost no legal recourse against acts of discrimination.

Homophobia is sufficiently pervasive that it is impossible for a gay man or lesbian to grow up in American society without being faced with some ramification of it. Commonly, gay men and lesbians incorporate some of society's negative attitudes in their own concepts of themselves. This internalized homophobia may lead to problems with self-esteem and may profoundly influence virtually all aspects of people's lives, including careers, relationships, and overall personal satisfaction.

Mental Illness in Gay Men and Lesbians

It has been commonly suggested that gay men and lesbians are less well adjusted than heterosexual men and women. It would not be surprising if this were so because of the oppression and discrimination that gay men and women face. However, an examination of the literature on the psychological functioning of gay men and lesbians reveals no inherent relationship between sexual orientation and psychopathology.

Meredith and Riester (1980) summarized the findings of 18 research studies that compared gay men or lesbians with other groups. They reviewed studies that used various means of examining psychological functioning, including psychiatric interviews, self-report questionnaires such as the Minnesota Multiphasic Personality Inventory (MMPI; Hathaway and McKinley 1970), and projective tests. The results of these studies were consistent in challenging the concept that homosexuality is pathological.

Another review of a large number of psychological studies of homosexual men and women who were not patients reached a similar conclusion: gay male and lesbian subjects were no less well adjusted psychologically than their heterosexual counterparts (Hart et al. 1978). Although studies may find differences between heterosexual and homosexual groups on various measures, one review of numerous studies concludes that "homosexuality in and of itself bears no necessary relationship to psychological adjustment" (Gonsiorek 1982, p. 79). All of these reviews contradict the conclusions of earlier, poorly designed studies involving patient populations. What is surprising is that the findings of research on the psychological well-being of *patient* populations would even be considered to be valid for *nonpatient* populations and that these findings would be generalized from such research to the population at large.

Whether there is a higher or lower incidence of mental illness among gay men and lesbians compared with their heterosexual counterparts is essentially an unanswered question. One might anticipate a higher prevalence of certain problems in a stigmatized population (e.g., depression, suicide, and drug use). However, although there are frequent assertions that one or another condition is more common in gay men or lesbians, the literature does not provide definitive evidence relating incidence and prevalence of mental illness to sexual orientation. Typifying the state of research on the relationship between sexual orientation and mental disorders is a review of studies of alcohol and substance abuse among lesbians. The review concludes that the research is both qualitatively and quantitatively limited and that additional research is necessary (Mosbacher 1988).

Treatment of Mental Illness

The problems for which gay men and lesbians seek treatment in most instances are the same kinds of problems for which other individuals seek treatment. What is unique to the gay man or lesbian is his or her own experience in dealing with sexual orientation. For many individuals, the impact of being gay has a powerful influence, directly or indirectly, on nearly all facets of their lives. The therapist must be aware of the pervasive way that sexual orientation and society's reaction to it can influence the lives of gay men and lesbians.

Gay men and lesbians may seek treatment because of specific issues related to their sexual orientation. Some may be dissatisfied with being gay, whereas others may experience stress dealing with their sexual orientation. Still others may seek treatment for problems associated with everyday living, such as difficulties with a relationship or career in which their sexual orientation is a factor. No matter what the problem, therapists should have an understanding of the basic process by which gay men and lesbians become aware of and deal with their sexual orientation.

"Gay Identity Development" and "Coming Out"

The process by which gay men and lesbians become aware of their sexual orientation and adjust to it is frequently referred to as "gay identity development." The term "coming out" commonly has various meanings. It may mean a personal recognition of being gay or a public acknowledgment of being gay; or it may refer to the entire process of personal acknowledgment and adjustment to sexual orientation. In this chapter, the terms "coming out" and "gay identity development" refer to this latter concept and are used interchangeably.

Various models have been developed to explain the coming-out process (Cass 1979; Hanley-Hackenbruck 1989; McDonald 1982; Troiden 1979). They generally share the same concepts but may apply different terms to different parts of the process. It is appropriate to conceptualize the coming-out or identity development process as a psychological journey beginning with an emerging awareness of a individual's sexual orientation and ending with an integration of gay identity into his or her entire life. The journey may begin and end at different ages; it may take different amounts of time; it may be filled with roadblocks, or starts and stops; or it may never be fully completed.

Identity development begins with some kind of awareness of being different. This awareness may be directly connected to sexuality, or it may be a more vague awareness of difference. As the awareness of same-sex attraction or interest develops and increases, the individual begins to make an association between his or her self-concept and homosexuality. At the same time, the individual may incorporate many of society's negative views of homosexuality, resulting in guilt and significant problems in self-esteem. He or she may develop different strategies to deal with the increasing recognition of the homosexual orientation. These may include denial, reaction formation, or suppression of impulses (e.g., attempts at developing heterosexual relationships, violence against gays, or immersion in school or work).

As individuals come to acknowledge more fully the homosexual aspect of themselves, they may have different reactions, depending on their personal experiences. Having positive gay role models may be tremendously helpful in easing discomfort about sexual orientation. Negative role models and the incorporation of negative images of being gay may lead to increased distress.

Contacts with gay men or lesbians may significantly influence how the person feels. Clandestine contacts and furtive relationships may hinder personal development, but positive role models and relationships may lead to a greater sense of satisfaction. The attitudes of parents, families, friends, and ministers may significantly influence the individual's attitude toward his or her emerging homosexuality. Meeting a wide range of individuals and recognizing the diversity of the gay community as a whole may help the individual to incorporate positive psychological images.

The final step in coming out involves the integration of gay identity into other aspects of identity. As the person develops a more positive self-image, he or she experiences an increasing sense of self-esteem and, eventually, pride in being gay. If the person gains a sense of comfort with a gay identity, greater openness about sexual orientation may result. With the acceptance of his or her orientation by family, friends, and co-workers, a complete integration of sexual orientation into the individual's life may occur. If this integration is achieved, then sexual orientation is placed in perspective as a valued and respected characteristic, but nevertheless only one of many characteristics that defines the individual.

A multitude of factors may influence the process of coming out or identity development. Hanley-Hackenbruck (1989) notes that the identity process is related to variables such as an individual's personality, age at first awareness of "difference," overall psychological functioning, family rigidity, religious upbringing, and negative or traumatic experiences involving sexual orientation. Identity development is also likely to be influenced by changes in societal attitudes toward homosexuality. The process is likely to be different for someone who grew up in the 1950s than for someone growing up in the 1990s.

Human immunodeficiency virus (HIV) infection is a relatively new influence on the process of identity development, because HIV infection and AIDS markedly altered the lives of gay men and lesbians during the last decade. HIV infection has certainly forced gay men to reassess their own values and their sexuality. Some elements of society have been quick to use HIV infection as a rationale for condemning homosexuality. On the other hand, the response to HIV infection within gay communities has been largely exemplary. It has unleashed a tremendous visible effort of compassion, caring, and mutual support that was never before so evident. For many, it has strengthened their view of themselves and their community as worthwhile, loving, and caring individuals.

Ultimately, for any particular individual, the influence of specific factors on identity development is difficult to predict. As a result of various factors, some individuals spend their lives tormented by their inability to resolve the negative images of homosexuality they have incorporated. Others seem to have little difficulty adjusting to the idea of being gay.

Therapeutic Responses to Patients

Therapists should always assess where the patient is in the coming-out process. For example, is the patient stuck in an early turmoil-ridden phase? To what extent has the patient incorporated negative images? Has the patient been able to integrate his or her gay identity with other aspects of personal identity? The answers to these and similar questions will help the therapist to make sound interventions consistent with the patient's ability to accept and integrate these interventions into his or her life.

Specific Issues

Frequently, in working with gay men and lesbians, there is a need for therapists to help overcome stereotypes that limit these patients' options in life. It is not uncommon to hear in therapy phrases such as "gay men are only interested in sex," "gay or lesbian relationships never last," or "the only place to meet someone is in a gay bar." The therapist must be sufficiently knowledgeable about the gay community to recognize complaints that are distortions and that may actually mask the patient's psychological problems. If the therapist agrees with the patient's assertion that gay men or lesbians cannot form stable relationships, the therapist reinforces a false stereotype and hinders the patient from looking at why he or she has trouble forming relationships.

> J., who is 25 years old, seeks therapy because he is dissatisfied with "gay life." He has few friends and has had a series of short-term stormy relationships, which he attributes to his belief that "gay men just aren't cut out for relationships."

In assessing such a patient, the focus should shift from generalizations about gay men to the specific traits that result in the development of stormy relationships. Part of the assessment should determine to what extent J.'s attitudes about homosexuality or internalized homophobia may complicate his relationships. However, the therapist should not automatically assume that the relationship problems are primarily related to some aspect of J.'s homosexuality. Just as with heterosexual individuals, a patient's problems may result from any number of factors.

Therapists must be able to deal with the realities of the world as they exist for the individual gay man or lesbian. For example, the necessity for some individuals to keep sexual orientation hidden takes a significant emotional toll on the individual. Issues frequently arise in therapy of whether the patient should inform a friend or an employer of his or her sexual orientation.

There are good reasons for disclosing sexual orientation under some circumstances. In the workplace, being open about sexual orientation can relieve the stress of maintaining a veil of secrecy and deceit about one's personal life that is necessitated by hiding sexual orientation. It can open the way to support from colleagues in times of personal stress (e.g., the illness of a lover). It can make a person feel an integral part of the workplace. On the other hand, depending on the particular employer, being open about sexual orientation can lead to discrimination, ostracism, or being fired. These kinds of issues must be carefully analyzed to determine the extent to which fear of disclosure represents reality and the extent to which it represents internalized homophobia and a problem in gay identity development.

> E. is a 35-year-old physician. She complains of depression and finds no meaning in life except for her work. She is a lesbian, but her only friends are heterosexual men and women, with whom she does not discuss her sexual orientation. She is concerned that if people find out about her homosexuality, her career will suffer.

An assessment of E.'s situation should explore her attitudes and feelings about her sexual orientation. To what extent is she psychologically stuck in an early phase of her development as a lesbian? How much is homophobia contributing to her social isolation from other gay men and lesbians and precluding her being open with her friends? What is the reality of her concern about her career? Answers to these kinds of questions will guide the direction of therapy and help to determine the relationship between her sexual orientation and her presenting complaints, if there is a relationship. Of course, it is possible that E. has a condition, such as a biologically based depression, that is entirely unrelated to any issues about sexual orientation. The therapist must be careful to avoid jumping to conclusions based solely on a patient's sexual orientation.

Therapists must be alert to countertransference issues and must always be careful to avoid inserting their own judgments into the therapy. For example, the therapist who says, "I don't see why you would want to tell people what you do in bed" in response to a discussion of disclosure in the workplace displays a lack of understanding of the issues. This view more likely reflects the therapist's discomfort with the patient's sexual orientation. Moreover, the therapist has failed to recognize the potential all-encompassing nature and influence of sexual orientation on an individual's life.

It is essential that a therapist be knowledgeable about the diverse factors that come into play when treating the gay man or lesbian who also has a major identity with another group (e.g., a particular racial, ethnic, or religious identification). One of the unique goals of working with a gay man or lesbian often is to help integrate the gay identity with other aspects of the individual's identity. The problem for the therapist is to be sufficiently knowledgeable about the patient's cultures or identities to avoid reinforcing the patient's own homophobia, racism, prejudice, or misconceptions that may be associated with one of the identities. The therapist will need to help resolve conflicts where values of different identities clash. He or she must be sensitive to differing cultural views of homosexuality but at the same time must respect and value the patient's gay or lesbian identity.

Occasionally, patients will ask for therapeutic assistance in changing their sexual orientation. Although there have been claims that sexual orientation can be changed through therapy, in fact, the claims are largely unsupported. An analysis of one such study reveals serious flaws, including imprecise definitions of homosexuality, imprecise measures of change, and particularly inadequate follow-up of the study subjects (Krajeski 1984).

Similar criticisms apply to virtually all studies reporting on attempts to change sexual orientation. Such attempts should not be regarded as innocuous. Common sense would indicate that concerted and persistent attempts by therapists to reinforce negative images of homosexuality and positive images of heterosexuality will lead to problems for those patients who do not change. Isay (1989) gives case examples of individuals harmed by attempts to change sexual orientation. Some of the resulting problems include low self-esteem, depression, apathy, and a lack of zest in living. In fact, attempts to change orientation need to be looked at from a cultural standpoint. Therapists must be careful to avoid unwittingly serving as an agent of social control and potentiating the victimization and stigmatization of gay men and lesbians.

Gay Affirmative Therapy

The term "gay affirmative therapy" has come to be frequently applied to therapy that equally values homosexuality and heterosexuality. Coleman (1978) outlines the development of a new model of treatment for gay men and lesbians that assists individuals in accepting and valuing their sexual orientation. The model of gay affirmative therapy has been developing over the years and has been applied to various situations and populations, including men, women, adolescents, and couples (Krajeski 1986). Any therapist working with gay men and lesbians should be conversant with the concepts of gay affirmative therapy.

Cohen and Stein (1986) offer several recurrent clinical themes that should be considered in this context. Their work is based on the following premises:

1. Homosexuality is not per se associated with psychopathology;
2. Sexuality has great clinical relevance to psychotherapy; and
3. Men and women experience their homosexuality in very different ways within American society.

Stein (1988) suggests several topics that therapists should explore in order to work effectively with gay men and lesbians. These include attitudes about homosexuality and sexual acts, awareness of the effects of stigmatization, familiarity with gay life-styles, knowledge of coming out, and the meaning of homosexual identity. Therapists must also be able to adapt principles and methods used for heterosexual individuals to gay populations (e.g., couples therapy, family therapy, and sexual dysfunction therapy).

Support Groups

The gay community has frequently developed its own support groups, which may be useful as an adjunct to therapy or as an alternative to it. In larger cities, there are many kinds of groups available that may be directed to specific populations. Examples of these include groups specifically for men, women, gay fathers, lesbian mothers, couples, and gays who are members of minorities. Such groups may help individuals to learn the strategies other gay individuals use to cope with various situations and to gain assistance through mutual help and support. Information about these groups can usually be obtained from local gay telephone hotlines or local gay publications.

Gay Organizations

The multitude of gay organizations that have arisen in the past few years may also be very useful to individuals. There are organizations suitable for almost any interest—from various activity groups such as sports, photography, travel, and politics, to occupationally oriented groups such as those for gay physicians or gay federal workers, to community-service groups, such as those providing AIDS support services. All of these organizations are particularly helpful in providing activities that are meaningful to the people involved.

Ethics

In the last few years, there has been increasing attention to ethical issues in the treatment of gay men and lesbians. The ethics of attempts to change sexual orientation have been widely discussed in the literature (Davison 1977, 1978; McConaghy 1977; Silverstein 1977). More recently, there have been efforts to ensure that psychiatrists are not using their expertise inappropriately in a variety of situations such as job screening, court evaluations, and military proceedings.

Because homosexuality is not a mental disorder, psychiatrists should have no role in attempting to diagnose homosexuality. The "Principles of Medical Ethics With Annotations Especially Applicable to Psychiatry" (American Psychiatric Association 1985) have been amended to make specific reference to sexual orientation in a statement that now reads: "A psychiatrist should not be a party to any type of policy that excludes, segregates, or demeans the dignity of any patient because of ethnic origin, race, sex, creed, age, socioeconomic status, or sexual orientation" (p. 3). As with the many instances in our society of institutional discrimination against gay men and lesbians, ethical violations may not immediately be perceived as such because actions of psychiatrists are in accord with "traditional" discrimination. However, to ensure that they are not violating ethical standards, psychiatrists must review their role carefully in situations where gay men or lesbians may be discriminated against.

Conclusion

Gay men and lesbians are a diverse group of individuals faced with significant discrimination in our society. Lack of societal support and criminalization of homosexual behavior have significant negative effects on the lives of gay men and women. Research does not reveal any inherent connection between sexual orientation and psychopathology. However, homophobia and its consequences significantly affect gay men and lesbians. Treatment for issues specifically related to sexual orientation should follow gay affirmative models. Therapists who work with gay men and lesbians should be nonhomophobic, should understand the coming-out process, should be knowledgeable about the gay community and its diversity, and should be well acquainted with community resources.

References

American Psychiatric Association: Diagnostic and Statistical Manual of Mental Disorders, 2nd Edition, Revised. Washington, DC, American Psychiatric Association, 1968

American Psychiatric Association: The Principles of Medical Ethics With Annotations Especially Applicable to Psychiatry. Washington, DC, American Psychiatric Association, 1985

American Psychiatric Association: Diagnostic and Statistical Manual of Mental Disorders, 3rd Edition, Revised. Washington, DC, American Psychiatric Association, 1987

Bayer R: Homosexuality and American Psychiatry: The Politics of Diagnosis. New York, Basic Books, 1981

Bell AP, Weinberg MS: Homosexualities. New York, Simon & Schuster, New York, 1978

Bergler E: Homosexuality: Disease or Way of Life? New York, Collier Books, 1956

Bowers v Hardwick et al. 106 S. Ct. 2841 (1986)

Cass VC: Homosexual identity formation: a theoretical model. J Homosex 4:219–235, 1979

Chan CS: Issues of identity development among Asian-American lesbians and gay men. Journal of Counseling and Development 68:16–20, 1989

Cohen CJ, Stein TS: Reconceptualizing individual psychotherapy with gay men and lesbians, in Contemporary Perspectives on Psychotherapy With Lesbians and Gay Men. Edited by Stein TS, Cohen CJ. New York, Plenum, 1986

Coleman E: Toward a new model of treatment of homosexuality: a review. J Homosex 3(4):345–359, 1978

Dannemeyer W: Homosexuality (Congressional Record—House). Bethesda, MD, Congressional Information Service, June 29, 1989, pp 3511–3514

Davison GC: Homosexuality and the ethics of behavioral intervention, Paper 1: homosexuality, the ethical challenge. J Homosex 2(3):195–204, 1977

Davison GC: Not can but ought: the treatment of homosexuality. J Consult Clin Psychol 46:170–172, 1978

Fay RE, Turner CF, Klassen AD, et al: Prevalence and patterns of same-gender sexual contact among men. Science 243:338–348, 1989

Fletcher JL: Homosexuality: kick and kickback. South Med J 77:149–150, 1984

Fyfe B: "Homophobia" or homosexual bias reconsidered. Arch Sex Behav 12:549–554, 1983

Gebhard PH: Incidence of overt homosexuality in the United States and Western Europe, in National Institute of Mental Health Task Force on Homosexuality: Final Report and Background Papers (DHEW Publ No ADM-76-357). Edited by Livingood JM. Washington, DC, U.S. Department of Health, Education and Welfare, 1972

Gonsiorek JC: Results of psychological testing on homosexual populations, in Homosexuality: Social, Psychological, and Biological Issues. Edited by Paul W, Weinrich JD, Gonsiorek JC, et al. Beverly Hills, CA, Sage, 1982

Hanley-Hackenbruck P: Psychotherapy and the "coming out" process. Journal of Gay and Lesbian Psychotherapy 1:21–39, 1989

Hart M, Roback H, Tittler B, et al: Psychological adjustment of nonpatient homosexuals: critical review of the research literature. J Clin Psychiatry 39:604–608, 1978

Hathaway SR, McKinley JC: Minnesota Multiphasic Personality Inventory, Revised. Minneapolis, MN, University of Minnesota, 1970

Hatterer LJ: Changing Homosexuality in the Male: Treatment for Men Troubled by Homosexuality. New York, McGraw-Hill, 1970

Isay RA: Being Homosexual: Gay Men and Their Development. New York, Farrar Straus & Giroux, 1989

Klein F, Sepekoff B, Wolf TJ: Sexual orientation: a multi-variable dynamic process. J Homosex 11(1/2):35–49, 1985

Krajeski JP: Masters and Johnson article "seriously flawed." Am J Psychiatry 141:1131, 1984

Krajeski JP: Psychotherapy with gay men and lesbians: a history of controversy, in Contemporary Perspectives on Psychotherapy With Lesbians and Gay Men. Edited by Stein TS, Cohen CJ. New York, Plenum, 1986

Loiacano DK: Gay identity issues among Black Americans: racism, homophobia, and the need for validation. Journal of Counseling and Development 68:21–25, 1989

Malyon AK: The homosexual adolescent: developmental issues and social bias. Child Welfare 60:321–330, 1981

Marmor J: Overview: the multiple roots of homosexual behavior, in Homosexual Behavior. Edited by Marmor J. New York, Basic Books, 1980

Martin AD: Learning to hide: the socialization of the gay adolescent, in Adolescent Psychiatry Developmental and Clinical Studies, Vol 10 (Annals of the American Society for Adolescent Psychiatry). Edited by Feinstein SC, Looney JG, Schwartzberg AZ, et al. Chicago, IL, University of Chicago Press, 1982

McConaghy N: Behavioral intervention in homosexuality. J Homosex 2:221–227, 1977

McDonald GJ: Individual differences in the coming out process for gay men: implications for theoretical models. J Homosex 8(1):47–60, 1982

Meredith RL, Riester RW: Psychotherapy, responsibility, and homosexuality: clinical examination of socially deviant behavior. Professional Psychology 11:174–193, 1980

Morin SF: Heterosexual bias in psychological research on lesbianism and male homosexuality. Am Psychol 32:629–637, 1977

Mosbacher D: Lesbian alcohol and substance abuse. Psychiatric Annals 18:47–50, 1988

Navarro M: Special problems for gays of color (Gay in America, Part 3). San Francisco Examiner, June 6, 1989, p A-17

O'Neill C: Battle "state" lines drawn—life after Hardwick ruling. Bay Area Reporter,

September 7, 1989, pp 12–13

Remafedi G: Male homosexuality: the adolescent's perspective. Pediatrics 79:326–330, 1987

Shively MA, De Cecco JP: Components of sexual identity. J Homosex 3(1):41–48, 1977

Silverstein C: Homosexuality and the ethics of behavioral intervention, Paper 2. J Homosex 2(3):205–211, 1977

Stein TS: Theoretical considerations in psychotherapy with gay men and lesbians. J Homosex 15(1/2):75–95, 1988

Troiden RR: Becoming homosexual: a model of gay identity acquisition. Psychiatry 42:362–373, 1979

20 The Mental Health Impact of AIDS on Ethnic Minorities

Francisco Fernandez, M.D.
Pedro Ruiz, M.D.
Eric G. Bing, M.D.

A cure for acquired immunodeficiency syndrome (AIDS) is far from being found. Despite recent advances in the management of its complications, specifically with the use of zidovudine (AZT), the most valuable course of action for combating AIDS is prevention through education of noninfected individuals. Education concerning the importance of early medical intervention and assistance in coping for infected individuals and their social support networks is also essential. In order to maximize the probability that these strategies will be successful, it is imperative that mental health care deliverers consider the culturally relevant issues and adapt strategies to the ethnically diverse communities affected by human immunodeficiency virus (HIV) infection.

Epidemiology

HIV is not transmitted by casual contact. HIV and AIDS are transmitted by sexual contact, through exposure to infected blood and blood components, and perinatally from mother to child. People from ethnic minorities are found among every risk group related to HIV disease: gay and bisexual men with and without a history of intravenous drug use (IVDU), heterosexual intravenous drug users (IVDUs), heterosexual contacts of people with AIDS (PWA), people with hemophilia, infants of women with AIDS, and recipients of blood products. There are also large numbers of ethnic minority individuals among the growing potential risk groups that have not yet been delineated in the statistics, such as prison inmates, homeless people, and migrant workers.

It may be surprising to learn that, despite the public perception of AIDS as a disease of white gay males. Forty percent of Americans diagnosed with AIDS are from ethnic minority groups (Centers for Disease Control [CDC] 1990). To emphasize the disparity of proportionality, it is important to note that African Americans constitute less than 12% of the population of the United States (Goldfinger 1990) but make up 30% of the AIDS cases (CDC 1990); Hispanics constitute only 6.4% of the population of the United States but nearly 16% of AIDS cases (CDC 1990). The disproportional representation among AIDS patients of minority women and children is even more pronounced (Mays and Cochran 1988), African American women being 13 times more likely and Hispanic women being 9 times more likely than are white women to contract AIDS (Mays and Cochran 1988). Consequently, high rates of pediatric AIDS result from infected women who are of child-bearing age and have no access to quality health care. Among pediatric cases of AIDS, 77% of the patients are African American or Hispanic (CDC 1990). Ninety percent of these children were infected perinatally, and 67% of those perinatally infected have at least one IVDU as a parent (Brooks-Gunn et al. 1988; CDC 1986, 1987, 1988, 1990).

It is startling to realize that AIDS is the leading cause of death among African Americans and Hispanics ages 25–45. To some extent, this may be due to the fact that most information and risk-reduction educational programs have been targeted toward white gay males, a population that has had the highest overall number of AIDS cases. As a consequence, ethnic minorities and IVDUs (especially women) have been far less likely to have proper information about HIV infection or progression, available treatment options, and the importance of early detection and medical intervention (Evans 1988; Reed and Freireich 1988). For this reason, individuals in minority communities may not be aware that they are infected until late in the course of the disease, when they may have already infected many unsuspecting partners and may have missed essential opportunities to delay the progression of their own disease.

Epidemiological differences must be considered when developing effective AIDS risk and reduction and educational programs aimed at ethnic minorities. Demographic information is helpful and essential to realistic assessment of risk for a specific community. For example, among Hispanics, New York has the highest cumulative incidence of AIDS in the country (Sumaya and Porto 1989). In New York, Hispanic adults are nine times more likely to contract AIDS than are non-Hispanic adults in the same geographical area. Nearly 50% of these cases are related to IVDU. However, for example, the proportional rates of AIDS among Hispanics in California and Texas are considerably lower, as are the rates of cases involving IVDU, which is roughly 4% in Texas (National Coalition of Hispanic Health and Human Services Organization [COSSMHO] 1987). Therefore, the 40% overall increase reported by the CDC and the number of AIDS cases among Hispanics in the United States most accurately reflect the high rate of IVDU among Hispanics with AIDS in the Northeastern United States.

In view of the specific regional breakdown, it would certainly be unfair to assign a high IVDU risk category to Hispanic groups other than to those in areas where IVDU is a special concern. Hispanic communities in other regions of the country have different risk factors that are responsible for higher cumulative incidences for ethnic minorities than for whites (Sumaya and Porto 1989). Education and treatment programs must make use of specific pertinent cultural factors for each minority community rather than relying on broad-based statistical information that may inaccurately reflect the health-related behaviors and attitudes of various specific subpopulations identified as one larger minority group.

Psychosocial and Cultural Risk Factors

Being infected with HIV or having AIDS elicits social stigma and practical liabilities, regardless of a person's race and socioeconomic status (Fernandez and Ruiz 1989). AIDS frequently forces significant social changes including loss of job, denial of insurance, denial of public services, loss of social and financial support systems, denial or delay of health care services, and effects of adverse legislation and employer regulations (such as mandatory HIV screening, quarantine, and other restrictions). For ethnic minorities who may already face ostracism and social and economic limitations (Kessler and Neighbors 1986; Kessler et al. 1985), these social changes can be particularly catastrophic.

A variety of sociocultural factors have made minority groups particularly vulnerable to HIV infection and its ravaging effects. Let us compare some of the different cultural aspects of African Americans and Hispanics, the two minority groups with the most AIDS cases among them, and relate these to HIV infection.

African Americans

AIDS has a devastating effect on the impoverished portion of the African American community that, prior to AIDS, was already under siege from the

effects of unemployment, poverty, substance abuse, and crime. The preponderance of AIDS cases among African Americans is among those who
are the poorest. It is estimated that up to 50% of African Americans are
living below the poverty level in the United States (U.S. Department of
Health and Human Services 1985), and it is a well-known fact that there is
a huge disparity in the quality of the American health care delivery system
that benefits whites and persons of means and that which benefits poor
African American populations. As one might expect, the mortality and
morbidity rates between these two subgroups is widening (Johnson 1989).
Unfortunately, the survival time for African Americans infected with AIDS
is the shortest of any population subgroup. Poor African Americans must
be afforded access to quality medical care and counseling, or the epidemic
of AIDS among this population will never be fully controlled.

In addition to the lack of medical attention, which is of paramount importance, certain attitudinal influences related to low socioeconomic conditions may be detrimental to the control of AIDS among poor African
Americans (Carrillo 1987). These attitudes tend to be cross-cultural within
poverty-ridden inner-city communities and may affect an individual's vulnerability to high-risk behavior (Mays and Cochran 1987). Conditions of poverty often destroy an individual's self-esteem and self-efficacy, invoking a
fatalistic sense of powerlessness. High crime rates, drug and alcohol abuse,
violence, unemployment, overcrowding, and high infant, child, and adolescent mortality rates tend to produce a pervasive sense of denial, immediacy,
and hopelessness. Combined with a lack of knowledge about AIDS and a
perceived lack of self-determination and self-worth, many poor African
Americans may be unable to assimilate behaviors that can reduce AIDS risk.

As a result, there are a variety of cultural and social factors that must be
taken into account to understand the responses of the African American
community to AIDS. First of all, the family subsystem characteristic of the
African American community usually plays a considerable role in the emotional support network for the African American AIDS patient. African
Americans, particularly those with low incomes, often have extended networks of family and friends who provide a necessary and vital safety net.
These extended "kinship networks" may provide tangible assistance, such as
money, shelter, food, and child care, as well as much needed emotional support (Mays and Cochran 1987).

As a result of the reliance that many African Americans have on their
extended family and friends, those AIDS patients who are rejected (either
because of the life-style that precipitated the illness or the illness itself) experience an intense sense of loss that may be clinically significant, to the

extent that psychiatric treatment is required for either anxiety or depression. Too often, this treatment is inaccessible. Second, churches and their leaders are particularly powerful in the African American community; as a result, they also have a strong impact on poor African Americans (Mays and Cochran 1987). Because a conceptual system of opposites (such as good or evil, natural or unnatural) prevails in this culture, many poor African Americans may not accept the origin or chronic course of some diseases. However, those with strong religious beliefs may rely on God and their church as a significant support system. Third, psychological factors affecting poor African Americans also play an important role in dealing with the stress of HIV disease (Mays and Cochran 1987). In addition to those attitudinal factors, a poverty-stricken African American community may have other psychological needs that must first be addressed.

Among HIV-infected African Americans, an internalization of emotions may amplify the psychological and social withdrawal often experienced by patients with AIDS. The stigma of being associated with socially unacceptable conduct (e.g., homosexuality, a cultural taboo) can lead to deterioration of the necessary social and familiar support systems available within these groups (Bing et al. 1990). A loss of emotional support may serve to validate a sense of hopelessness and lack of self-determination. This particular coping style of emotional internalization and denial can lead to depression and a serious risk of suicide.

The following case studies may help to illustrate these issues among African Americans.

Case Study: Depression

Ms. A. is a 35-year-old African American woman who was in her normal state of good mental health until her husband of 7 years was hospitalized with *Pneumocystis carinii* pneumonia. She had not suspected that her husband could have AIDS. Though she knew her husband was an IVDU many years earlier, she had assumed that he was no longer at risk. She was advised by the hospital staff to get tested for HIV and discovered that she, too, was HIV positive.

Ms. A. said in retrospect that she did surprisingly well after finding out that she was infected with HIV and that her husband had AIDS. She continued working as an elementary school teacher and attending church and her twice-weekly Bible study classes. A deeply religious woman, Ms. A. sought strength in prayer. Though she was very well-liked and respected by the other church members, she kept her husband's illness and her condition to herself, fearing that she would be rejected by her church.

As her husband's illness progressed, Ms. A. was unable to cope with her husband's illness herself. She sought assistance at an AIDS service organization that was started by an African American minister and his church. When she was referred to the staff psychiatrist, Ms. A. was experiencing severe insomnia, had lost 15 pounds, and had difficulty concentrating. In addition, she said that she had lost faith in God and had contemplated ending her own life if her husband died.

Ms. A. was started on 20 mg of fluoxetine (Prozac) and referred to a local Christian counselor who was knowledgeable about AIDS. Within 5 months, she was able to function adequately at work, gained 5 pounds, slept well, and resumed her church activities. Ms. A. had a mild recurrence of depressive symptoms following the death of her husband. However, this time, she was able to confide about the nature of her husband's death and her own illness and get support from her church.

Case Study: Anxiety

Mr. B. is a 45-year-old African American gay man who is alcoholic and who describes himself as a lifelong "incessant worrier." He stated that he had relieved his anxiety with alcohol until he was forced to enter a drug and alcohol detoxification program 4 years ago as a condition of probation, following an arrest for driving under the influence of alcohol. Mr. B. said that he was able to control his anxiety by attending daily Alcoholics Anonymous (AA) meetings.

Mr. B. did reasonably well until he found out that he was infected with HIV. He learned this when he attempted to apply for life insurance. Mr. B. began to be increasingly worried and anxious much of the day, particularly in his job a grocery clerk. In addition, he began to have discrete episodes of panic characterized by flushing, trembling, tachycardia, and diaphoresis whenever he thought that someone suspected that he was sick. He was unable to disclose his serostatus even to people in AA, because many of them also worked with him. These fears compromised his ability to function at work, and his co-workers actually began suspecting that something might be wrong with him.

Mr. B. described his anxiety to his internist, who suggested that Mr. B. begin taking an anxiolytic. Mr. B. refused, fearing that he would get addicted to the drug. At the urging of his sister, Mr. B. sought psychiatric help. He expressed concern that he would lose his job if anyone knew that he was gay and/or infected with HIV. He knew that many of his co-workers were homophobic and were afraid of AIDS. In addition, he feared his anxiety would cause him to start drinking again and lose much of what he had gained since he had been sober.

Mr. B. was taught deep-breathing exercises and progressive muscle relaxation, which helped in reducing the level of his anxiety. He calmed down to the point where he could seek assistance from AIDS organizations. Mr. B. was referred to an AA group for HIV-infected men. he also received legal counseling from the local AIDS legal network on job protection, should he be fired because of his HIV-positive status. He continued to be mildly anxious, but his panic attacks ceased.

From the perspective of AIDS prevention and care, it is vital that clinicians become aware of the prevailing family, religious, and psychosocial network systems among African Americans, as illustrated in these two cases.

Hispanics

The influences of cultural factors also affect the prevention and treatment of AIDS among Hispanics. As we mentioned previously, HIV infection is disparately pervasive among various Hispanic subgroups. However, members of underprivileged Hispanic communities carry a proportionately higher risk of HIV infection than do whites. Therefore, we address some of the cultural factors that transcend subcultural boundaries.

In most Hispanic cultures, the role of a strongly traditional family is very important. The image of *machismo,* which has often been stereotyped, nonetheless has a significant impact on Hispanic males. Although women working outside the home have taken on some of the so-called male prerogatives in recent years, it is generally true that the idealized role of the father remains the "protector" of the family. The mother is considered to be in the "heart of the home," attending to the spiritual, emotional, and physical well-being of the family to the best of her capabilities. This role often entails self-sacrifice on the part of the woman. In general, Hispanic women have been reported to be less likely to know about HIV modes of transmission and prevention strategies, such as condom use, than women of other racial or ethnic groups (Aruffo et al. 1990). As a group, Hispanic women are likely to feel powerless regarding their individual risk for AIDS (Holmes and Fernandez 1988; Mays and Cochran 1988). For example, it may be more difficult to impose safe-sex practices (such as the use of condoms) on a reluctant sex partner, especially in a culture that may impose social or even physical sanctions against assertiveness in women.

Hispanic children are expected to behave in a fashion that reflects deference to these traditional roles and values. Because of the strength of the family unit, loyalty is expected from each member. As in the African American communities that are at risk for HIV infection, Hispanics, who may feel they have shamed their family through culturally unacceptable behavior (such as homosexuality and drug abuse), may express denial or internalize emotions and may face the loss of familial emotional and/or financial support. The family may also be psychologically torn between their cultural commitment to the family member with AIDS and their cultural commitment to stringent codes of acceptable behavior, which may have been transgressed by their relative. The family must often deal with their own emotional pain and social shame as they attempt to lend support to the AIDS patient.

Case Study: Dementia or Depression

Mr. C. is a bilingual Cuban American and a former IVDU who was being treated for AIDS over the past year at a community health clinic. He had a history of a mixed personality disorder but had become more unmanageable and had made multiple suicide attempts in the last 8 months. During a recent psychiatric inpatient admission, he was tested with a comprehensive neuropsychological testing battery and was discharged with the diagnosis of AIDS dementia complex. He was referred to an AIDS Neurobehavioral Rehabilitation Program for cognitive retraining.

During the evaluation phase, it became apparent that Mr. C. was markedly depressed. When he developed AIDS, he became noncompliant with his medical treatment and had discontinued his AZT months before his psychiatric admission. Estranged from his family of origin, Mr. C. could not see himself going home "to die." He had felt his family was nonsupportive and distant and would not contact them for fear of rejection over his HIV status.

Mr. C. agreed to be treated for his depression with 300 mg/day of bupropion (Wellbutrin). He also attended a dedicated day care program for people with HIV disease. A case manager was assigned to Mr. C. Through the case manager, Mr. C.'s family was brought into the treatment loop, and they eventually took over some of the management of Mr. C.'s care.

This case illustrates various points regarding the care of Hispanics with HIV. Mr. C.'s diagnosis of AIDS dementia was made in the context of cognitive inefficiencies secondary to depression. Even nondepressed Hispanic patients who are bilingual and whose preferred language is English may score significantly worse on standardized neuropsychological tests than their white counterparts. Thus, norms of commonly used tests of neuropsychological function may not be generalizable to ethnic minorities, even after controlling for the effects of age and education (Bing et al. 1991). Moreover, the importance of the case-management model in integrating the various aspects of caring for this population is highlighted. The emotional strength enabling the family to provide care for the HIV patient may, in part, be affected by the number of demands placed on them and by their ability to obtain support and psychosocial services for themselves. This unique interplay of family dynamics should be considered when developing treatment programs for Hispanics. The case manager cannot only consult the patient; instead, he or she must often consult with caregivers and families as well as community boards, city councils, schools, courts, and other community agencies and institutions.

There may be additional serious and as yet unexplored ramifications for the Hispanic AIDS patient, his or her primary caregivers, and the support network of family members, all of whom are subject to great stress. This stress may affect not only their relationship with the HIV-infected individual. In addition, it may have the potential to compromise the patient's immune strength and to increase the risk of impairing the physical, social, and psychological functioning of his or her significant others. It is of great importance that mental health professionals provide not only culturally individual care to HIV-infected Hispanics and their families, but that they also act as advocates for their patients' needs in the political, legal, and sociocultural milieu of their communities of origin.

Clinical Aspects

In addition to understanding the epidemiological, cultural, and psychosocial factors related to HIV infection and AIDS in ethnic minorities, all mental health professionals should be aware of the modes of transmission and possible modes of infection in their own treatment settings. It must be reemphasized that HIV infection is transmitted by sexual contact, through exposure to infected body fluids and secretions, and perinatally from mother to child. The most significant modes of transmission in ethnic minorities are drug abuse and unprotected sexual contact. An unlikely but possible mode of transmission in the health care setting is contact with infected blood through a needle stick or through skin or mucous membranes that are not intact. There is also a minimal risk of transmitting HIV infection from person to person by using contaminated instruments.

A medical history taken as part of a comprehensive psychiatric examination cannot always reliably identify those patients infected with HIV, partly because this infection can be asymptomatic for up to 8 years (Forstein 1989). Moreover, psychiatric evaluations may inaccurately interpret symptoms of HIV infection that mimic psychiatric disturbances unrelated to HIV (Fernandez 1989).

The primary forms of psychological distress for HIV patients are adjustment reactions to a variety of illness-related events and social stressors, grief and bereavement reactions, and emotional strains from dramatic changes in life-style. In addition, HIV can directly infect the central nervous system, causing neuropsychological impairment and dementia and creating a tremendous burden for the patient and his or her family and primary caregivers.

It is important that all health care professionals recognize and understand the psychiatric manifestations of HIV infection in all members of our society. Increasing amounts of evidence point to the fact that HIV is neurotropic and infects the brain tissue (Gabuzda and Hirsch 1987) as well as the body's immune system.

Whenever HIV-infected individuals show abnormal mental or emotional states, the various medical causes of disordered brain function must systematically be reviewed. Psychiatrists and other mental health care providers must collaborate closely in dealing with the psychiatric complications of HIV infection. For instance, in diagnosing anxiety or depression, clinicians must be aware that these conditions may also be the direct result of HIV's involvement of the central nervous system. Changes in a person's mental or emotional state can potentially be related to the direct infection of the brain by HIV, a secondary brain infection from an opportunistic organism, the individual's emotional reaction to his or her illness, or an unrelated psychiatric disorder previously or newly diagnosed. Because HIV infection can present initially as a neurobehavioral disturbance (Beckett et al. 1987), all mental health care providers should be knowledgeable about the medical aspects of AIDS and the psychiatric disturbances that may be present. Specific knowledge about the effects of HIV disease on brain-behavioral relationships allows for more accurate diagnosis and, therefore, more effective treatment of the psychiatric presentations of people with HIV disease or AIDS.

Clinicians should also note that people of all ages and backgrounds may be infected with HIV and thus be carriers. Therefore, measures that may protect against the transmission of the disease should be undertaken and followed routinely for all patients with mental illness, including the growing population of mentally ill homeless people who are HIV positive.

AIDS Prevention and Public Policy Regarding Ethnic Minorities

Education concerning AIDS prevention is among the most effective ways to encourage and achieve risk-reducing behaviors (Ostrow 1989a, 1989b). However, although it is true that accurate knowledge of high-risk behaviors for HIV transmission may motivate a person's initial changes in behavior, knowledge alone is insufficient for his or her permanent behavior change. The factors that motivate initial behavioral changes may be very different from those that sustain a beneficial change. Therefore, once it has been established that education about AIDS transmission and prevention is the keystone of any effective prevention program, clinicians must then address ways to maintain low-risk behaviors and shore up people's knowledge.

In the case of ethnic minority groups, supporting the practice of low-risk behaviors is complex and must be done in culturally and linguistically sensitive ways that are appropriate to the particular target group. Often, there are significant environmental barriers that potentially interfere with an individual's ability to translate knowledge about AIDS risk into effective changes in his or her behavior (Ostrow 1989a). Attempts to increase an individual's personal motivation for behavioral change without providing assistance to overcome external barriers to change can have serious adverse consequences for both the physical and mental health of the individual.

There is a relative paucity of reliable reports on the serious issues of AIDS among ethnic minority communities. A significant vacuum also exists within the literature regarding processes and procedures for initiating and developing culturally sensitive programs in public health AIDS education and risk reduction. The time has come to replace the impractical general prescriptive formulas currently prevalent among the few published reports on AIDS programs for minority groups. Simplistic urging of the use of culturally and linguistically sensitive information is inadequate for the development, promotion, and enhancement of AIDS-related public health programming aimed at ethnic minority groups. Rather, mental health professionals must have a detailed understanding of the factors that will affect the adoption of low-risk behaviors by a particular subgroup. These basic factors include family structure and values; religion; community and leadership structure, beliefs, and values; language preferences; and knowledge about and attitudes toward sexual behavior, beliefs, and practices (Ostrow 1989b).

Within the framework of a culturally and linguistically sensitive AIDS prevention program and health promotion model, more extensive criteria can be applied to meeting the needs of each individual. All of us in the profession must make sure that the information being presented is simple and culturally and linguistically unambiguous; that the behaviors to be modified are clearly identified; and that substitute behaviors, pleasures, and social activities are presented that are supported by the community and its leaders. We must also make sure that adequate facilities, services, and resources are available for people who need assistance in adopting these behavioral changes and that all possible cultural, ethnic, economic, and geographic barriers to positive behavior changes are recognized and remedied. Finally, there must be adequate follow-up procedures and reinforcements to ensure that appropriate changes have been adopted and will be maintained.

Such a comprehensive AIDS prevention and health promotion program for ethnic minorities will work for the community by working *with* the community and its individual members with genuine concern, respect, and determination.

Conclusion

In this chapter, we have attempted to call attention to the current status of AIDS among various ethnic minorities in the United States. Particular attention was focused on African Americans and Hispanics, because the epidemiologic data clearly indicate a disproportionately high incidence of HIV-positive individuals and PWA among African Americans and Hispanics. The unique psychosocial and cultural risk factors of these ethnic minority groups were discussed as well as the role these important factors play in determining AIDS-related behaviors and health maintenance procedures among African Americans and Hispanics. From a clinical perspective, we focused on specific diagnostic and therapeutic issues that need to be emphasized with this disease. A public policy perspective was advanced, with emphasis on education and prevention.

Finally, we have called for an adequate response to the need for current and relevant epidemiological studies on AIDS and ethnic minorities. Additional research efforts on the sexual behavior patterns of ethnic minorities in this country, as well as research on substance abuse patterns in these populations, are sorely needed. Only then can appropriate public policy plans be effectively devised with appropriate psychocultural and psychosocial influences in mind. Our ultimate goal should be optimal procedures of care and prevention of AIDS among ethnic minorities in the United States, and worldwide, by means of accurate and culturally sensitive education and medical intervention.

References

Aruffo JF, Coverdale JH, Chacko RC, et al: Knowledge about AIDS among women psychiatric outpatients. Hosp Community Psychiatry 41(3):326–328, 1990

Beckett A, Manschrek T, Vitagliano H: Symptomatic HIV infection of the CNS in a patient without clinical evidence of immune deficiency. Am J Psychiatry 44:1342–1344, 1987

Bing EG, Nichols SE, Goldfinger SM, et al: The many faces of AIDS: opportunities for intervention. New Dir Ment Health Serv 48:69–81, 1990

Bing EG, Miller EN, Satz P, et al: The effect of immunologic and demographic factors on neuropsychological test performance: the Multicenter AIDS Cohort Study. Proceedings of the VII International Conference on AIDS, Florence, Italy, June 16–20, 1991, 2:9

Brooks-Gunn J, Boyer CB, Hein K: Preventing HIV infection and AIDS in children and adolescents: behavioral research and intervention strategies. Am Psychol 43(11):958–964, 1988

Carrillo JE: A rationale for effective smoking prevention and cessation interventions in minority communities (Smoking Behavior and Policy Discussion Paper Series). Cambridge, MA, Harvard University Institute for the Study of Smoking Behavior and Policy, 1987

Centers for Disease Control: Acquired immunodeficiency syndrome (AIDS) among blacks and Hispanics—United States. MMWR 35:655–666, 1986

Centers for Disease Control: Human immunodeficiency virus infection in the United States: a review of current knowledge. MMWR 36(56):1–48, 1987

Centers for Disease Control: Reports on selected racial/ethnic groups. MMWR 37(SS–3):1–10, 1988

Centers for Disease Control: HIV/AIDS Surveillance Report. Atlanta, GA, Centers for Disease Control, July 1990

Evans LA: Cancer prevention and detection programs among minorities, II: cultural communication problems. Cancer Bulletin 40(2):89–90, 1988

Fernandez F: Psychiatric complications in HIV-related illnesses, in The American Psychiatric Association AIDS Education Project AIDS Primer. Washington, DC, American Psychiatric Association, 1989, pp 6-1, 6-27

Fernandez F, Ruiz P: Psychiatric aspects of HIV disease. South Med J 82(8):999–1004, 1989

Forstein M: MV Testing, in The American Psychiatric Association AIDS Education Project AIDS Primer. Washington, DC, American Psychiatric Association, 1989, pp 8-1, 8-7

Gabuzda DH, Hirsch MS: Neurologic manifestations of infection with human immunodeficiency virus: clinical features and pathogenesis. Ann Intern Med 107:383–391, 1987

Goldfinger SM: Psychiatric Aspects of AIDS and HIV Infection. San Francisco, CA, Jossey-Bass, 1990, p 70

Holmes VF, Fernandez F: HIV in women: current impact and future implications. The Female Patient 13:47–54, 1988

Johnson J: The AIDS epidemic, in The American Psychiatric Association AIDS Education Project AIDS Primer. Washington, DC, American Psychiatric Association,

1989, pp 2-1, 2-3

Kessler RC, Neighbors HW: A new perspective on the relationships among race, social class, and psychological distress. J Health Soc Behav 27:107–115, 1986

Kessler RC, Price RH, Wortman BC: Social factors in psychopathology: stress, social support and coping processes. Annu Rev Psychol 36:531–572, 1985

Mays VM, Cochran SD: Acquired immunodeficiency syndrome and Black Americans: special psychosocial issues. Public Health Rep 702(2):224–231, 1987

Mays VM, Cochran SD: Issues in the perception of AIDS risk and risk reduction activities by Black and Hispanic/Latin Women. Am Psychol 43(11):949–957, 1988

National Coalition of Hispanic Health and Human Services Organizations: AIDS: the impact on Hispanics in selected states. Washington, DC, National Coalition of Hispanic Health and Human Services Organizations, 1987

Ostrow DG: Prevention of HIV infection and disease, in The American Psychiatric Association AIDS Education Project AIDS Primer. Washington, DC, American Psychiatric Association, 1989a, pp 7-1, 7-13

Ostrow DG: AIDS prevention through effective education. Daedalus 118(3):229–254, 1989b

Reed E, Freireich EJ: Cancer treatment and support programs for minorities, I: treatment. Cancer Bulletin 40(2):92–93, 1988

Sumaya CV, Porto MD: AIDS in Hispanics. South Med J 82(8):943–945, 1989

U.S. Department of Health and Human Services: Report of the Secretary's Task Force on Black and Minority Health, Vol 1. Washington, DC, U.S. Government Printing Office, 1985

Glossaries of
Ethnic Terms

Glossary of Chinese Terms

The romanization system used for Chinese terms in this book is the Wade-Giles system. In Wade-Giles romanization, consonants are not always pronounced as English speakers might sound them out. That is, the consonants in words romanized with apostrophes are pronounced as written (e.g., *k'uei* is pronounced "kway"). Romanized words without apostrophes are pronounced differently, as shown in other terms defined in this glossary (e.g., *kuei* is pronounced "gway").

The dialect used here is the most prevalent one—Beijing (Peking) dialect, or Mandarin Chinese. Chinese is a language in which tones, or changes in pitch, can affect the meaning of a syllable. In this glossary, the four tones of spoken Chinese are denoted by superscripts 1 to 4. In the example below, diacritical marks (which are not used in Wade-Giles romanization) have been added to the syllable *ma* to help show how each tone would be pronounced:

1. High tone (pitch is high and even, almost sung): *mā*
2. High rising tone (pitch rises to high): *má*
3. Low rising tone (pitch falls and then rises): *mǎ*
4. High falling tone (pitch falls abruptly): *mà*

The characters in this glossary are to be read from left to right.

氣   Ch'i [chee[4]]
Literally means breath or vapor but is used to connote vitality. In Chinese metaphysics, *ch'i* is conceived as an all-pervasive dynamic force that permeates the whole macrocosm and the human body and is regulated by *yin-yang* and the Five Evolutive Phases (see *wu-hsing*).

精   Ching [jing[1]]
A concept closely related to *ch'i*, this term means "essence," as in the idea of "vital essence" thought to be contained in semen.

清　明   Ch'ing-ming [ching[1]-ming[2]]
Chinese festival to commemorate the dead and past ancestors; All Saint's Day.

中 醫 師 **Chung-i-shih** [jong[1]-ee[1]-sher[1]]
Traditional Chinese medical doctor.

邪 氣 **Hsieh-ch'i** [shyeh[2]-chee[4]]
Free-floating energy force (*ch'i*) that may invade
the human body to cause illnesses.

邪 病 **Hsieh-ping** [shyeh[2]-bing[4]]
A possession illness, caused by the invasion of
hsieh-ch'i.

仁 **Jen** [ren[2]]
Confucian concept of goodness and benevolence
in interpersonal relationships.

觀 音 **Kuan-yin** [gwan[1]-yin[1]]
The Buddhist Goddess of Mercy.

狂 **K'uang** [kwang[2]]
A Chinese folk mental illness characterized by
an excited state. The term is used in Chinese
vernacular to denote insanity and a loosening
of self-control. It suggests a state of hypomania
or mania and is thought to be related to a
preponderance of *yang* forces in the body.
(See *tien*.)

鬼 **Kuei** [gway[3]]
Demons originating from *yin*; opposite of *shen*.

國 語 **Kuo-yü** [gwo[2]-yeu[3]]
Mandarin Chinese, adopted as the Chinese
national language.

禮 **Li** [lee[3]]
Confucian concept of deportment meaning
propriety in interpersonal relationships. A person
is thought to exhibit *li* when his or her behavior
conforms to the prescribed social role.

怕 冷 **P'a-leng** [pah[4]-lung[3]]
Literally, "afraid of cold"; frigophobia.

神 **Shen** [shern²]
Benevolent gods arising from *yang*; opposite of *kuei*.

腎 虧 **Shen-k'uei** [shenn⁴-kway¹]
A state of kidney deficiency or weakness. "A psychological condition popularly associated with excessive semen loss owing to frequent intercourse, masturbation, nocturnal emission or passing of 'white turbid urine,' which is believed to contain semen" (Wen JK, Wong CL: Shen k'uei syndrome: a culture-specific sexual neurosis in Taiwan, in Normal and Abnormal Behavior in Chinese Culture. Edited by Kleinman A, Lin T. Dordrecht, Netherlands, D Reidel, 1980, p. 357)

道 士 **Tao-shih** [dao⁴-sherh⁴]
A Taoist priest.

癲 **Tien** [dian¹]
A Chinese folk illness characterized by withdrawal and/or seizure phenomena and suggestive of schizophrenia or epilepsy. The condition is thought to be related to a preponderance of *yin* forces within the human body. (See *k'uang*.)

財 神 **Ts'ai-shen** [tsai²-shern²]
The god of wealth.

土 地 **T'u-ti** [too³-dee⁴]
The tutelary god in charge of everyday affairs in a Chinese village.

巫 **Wu** [woo¹]
A shaman who possesses special power to exorcise.

五 行 **Wu-hsing** [woo³-shing²]
A system of correspondences that further elaborate *yin-yang* and *ch'i*. "The Five Evolutive

Phases . . . constitute stretches of time, temporal segments of exactly defined qualities that succeed each other in cyclical order at reference positions defined in space . . . the Five [Phases] define conventionally and unequivocally energetic qualities changing in the course of time. They typify the qualities of energy by the use of five concepts (wood, fire, earth, metal, water) which, because of the richness of their associations, are ideally suited to serve as the crystallizing core for an inductive system of relations and correspondences." (Porkert M: The Theoretical Foundation of Chinese Medicine. Cambridge, MA, MIT Press, 1974, pp. 45–56)

陰　　陽

Yin-yang [in^1-yahng^2]
A Chinese bipolarity metaphysical concept that is simultaneously both opposite and complementary. "Yin and yang are the elementary terms used to express a fundamental premise of Chinese thought: they convey the idea of the polar quality of all effects. . . . Some of the primary correspondences of *yin* are: Earth, moon, autumn, winter, things female, cold, the inside or interior, darkness, the lower part, quiescence, night, the right side. Of *yang*: Heaven, sun, spring, summer, things male, heat, the outside or surface, brightness, the upper part, movement, day, the left side." (Porkert 1974, pp. 9, 24)

Glossary of Japanese Terms

The characters in this glossary are to be read from left to right.

甘　え **Amae** [ah-mae']
"Passive love" (*doi*).

甘　え　る **Amaeru** [ah-mae'-ru]
To depend and presume upon another's benevolence (*doi*).

甘　い **Amai** [ah-maee']
Sweet.

甘　や　か　す **Amayakasu** [ah-mah₁-ya-ka'-su]
To accept another's *amae*.

武　士　道 **Bushido** [boo-shee'-do]
Ethical code of the Japanese military class.

出　稼　ぎ **Dekasegi** [day-₁kah-say'-gee]
Dekasegi immigration involved Japanese laborers who left their native land to temporarily work elsewhere. These individuals always maintained the eventual goal of returning home to Japan.

五　世 **Gosei** [go'-say]
Fifth generation away from Japan.

腹　切　リ **Hara-kiri** [ha₁-ra-kee'-ree]
Ritual disembowelment/suicide/*seppuku*.

一　世 **Issei** [ee'-say]
First generation away from Japan.

帰　米　二　世 **Kibei nisei** [kee₁-bay-nee'-say]
Second generation away from Japan who were born in the United States but sent back to Japan for schooling and who later returned to the United States as adults.

気違い　**Kichigai** [kee'-chee-guy]
"Crazy."

森田　**Morita** therapy [mo-ree'-ta]
A Japanese therapy developed by Shoma
Morita in order to treat *shinkeishitsu* neurosis.
Based in Zen Buddhism, the therapy is aimed
at liberating the patient from excessive
self-preoccupation and intellectualization.

内観　**Naikan** therapy [naee'-kan]
A Japanese therapy aimed at building moral
constraints into the individual based on a
sense of obligation; developed by Ishin
Yoshimoto in 1954 during his work with
penitentiary inmates.

日本学校　**Nihon-gakko** [nee₁-hon-gak'-ko]
Japanese school.

二世　**Nisei** [nee'-say]
Second generation away from Japan.

三世　**Sansei** [san'-say]
Third generation away from Japan.

切腹　**Seppuku** [seh'-poo-koo]
Ritual suicide/*hara-kiri*.

神経質　**Shinkeishitsu** [shin₁-kai-shee'-tsu]
"Nervousness," a Japanese form of neurosis
treated by Morita therapy.

四世　**Yonsei** [yon'-say]
Fourth generation away from Japan.

Glossary of Korean Terms

The Korean and Chinese characters in this glossary are to be read from left to right. (Chinese characters for Korean terms appear underneath the Korean characters.)

체
体
면
面

Che-myun [cheh-myun]
An ethos of face-saving. Maintaining *che-myun* is important in protecting the dignity, honor, and self-respect of the individual and the family.

天
巫
舞

Goot [g͞oot]
Shamanistic ceremony involving dancing, jumping, and drumbeating, and invoking shamanistic gods during a ceremonial ritual of healing.

한
恨

Haan [hän]
An individual and collective subconscious emotional complex among Korean people, involving suppressed feelings of anger, rage, despair, frustration, holding grudges, indignation, and revenge. It is a syndrome believed to result from victimization of a Korean person both as an individual and as a Korean and is thought to be an important contributing factor to the development of *hwa-byung* ("anger disease").

화
火
병
病

Hwa-byung [whä-byuŋ]
A syndrome of mixed depressive and anxiety disorders, with characteristic symptoms of a feeling of mass or heavy and oppressive feelings in the chest or abdomen. It is thought to be a unique Korean culture-bound syndrome. Feelings of *haan* are thought to contribute to *hwa-byung*.

정
情

Jeong [juŋ]
A human emotion that brings people together and connects them emotionally in mutual affection and attachment. *Jeong* embraces such concepts as

595

feeling, empathy, compassion, attachment, pathos, sentiment, and love. The word frequently combines with another word to define or modify the affective relationship, such as *mo-jeong* (motherly love), *woo-jeong* (brotherly love between two friends), and so on.

무
巫

당
黨

Mudang [mōo-daŋ]
A shaman who performs shamanistic ceremony.

멋
風

流
味

Muht [mut]
Exquisite, beautiful, splendid, and elegant. *Muht* refers to an ethos of exquisite artistic and cultural taste among Korean people.

눈
目

치
尺

Noonchi [nōon-chee]
"Measuring with eyes," referring to a capacity for mind reading through sight, or an intuitive, sixth-sense perception of another person's gestures, facial expression, and other nonverbal cues.

팔
八

자
字

Palja [päl-jä]
Fate; destiny. In traditional Korean society, accepting *palja* with a stoical attitude was often the only way of coping with the woes of life and difficulties over which people had no control.

Glossary of Pilipino and Related Terms

Amok [a-muck']
Malayan term for a dissociative state in which people act out violent impulses and attack others indiscriminately.

Amor propio [a-mor pro'-pi-o]
An exaggerated sense of self-importance and oversensitivity to slights.

Anitos [a-ni'-tos]
Spirits of animate and inanimate objects in one's environment as opposed to *diwata*, or higher spirits or godheads.

Arbolarios [Herbalarios] [ar-bo-lar'-ios]
Herbalist; one who treats with the use of herbs.

Atake ng nerbyos [a-ta₁-ke nang ner'-byos]
Attack of "nerves" similar to the Puerto Rican *ataques de nervios*.

Ataques de nervios [ah-tah'-kays deh-nerr'-ve-os]
Nervous episodes or "attacks," a Puerto Rican syndrome characterized by altered consciousness and combative and/or demanding behavior. Known as *atake ng nerbyos* in the Philippines.

Bahala na [ba-ha'-la-na]
Literally "will of God"; an attitude of optimistic fatalism that enables acceptance of adverse fate because of the anticipation that God will eventually order everything toward a righteous and beneficial end.

Bah tschi [bah'-see]
A Thai word for "easy startle" syndrome.

Bangungut [bang-ung'-ut]
Nightmare death syndrome in which a person after a heavy meal develops nightmares wherein he or she panics and tries to awaken. Failure to awaken results in death.

Bayanihan [ba-ya-ni'-han]
Communality; community working together.

Bilat [be-lat']
Visayan word for vulva. Equivalent Tagalog word is *po-ki*.

Bisa [be'-sa']
Psychic forces within the body.

Bulo-bulo [bu'-lo bu-lo]
Healing by magic. Magicians practice *bulo-bulo* to effect healing.

Delicadeza [del-e-ca-day'-sa]
Nonconfrontational communication and style of relating.

Dwendes [dwen'-des]
Tiny beings or spirits (similar to leprechauns).

Enkantos [eng-kan'-tos]
Enchanted, usually unseen seductive spirits or beings, generally
represented as white, rich, and powerful, who can cause suffering upon
those they seduce.

Espiritista [es₁-pi-ri-tis'-ta]
Member of spiritist sects that believes in and practice mediumship, an
espiritista believes in reincarnation and spirit intervention. Psychic healers
and psychic surgeons belong to this sect.

Gaba [ga'-ba]
Curse for misdeeds, imminent retribution resulting in illness, or
misfortune for past misdeeds of an individual or his or her family.

Haan tao [ha-an ta-o]
Supernatural entities. Literally means "beyond human."

Hangin [ha'-ngin]
"Wind." A wind that causes illness or illness produced by object intrusion
by sorcery or spirits through distances. (Presumed to be carried by the
wind.)

Hija [hi'-ya]
"Shame" associated with a devastating sense of social inacceptability.

Hika [hi'-ka]
Asthma believed to be triggered by moods.

Hiwit [he'-wit]
Visayan term for sorcerer. *Gin hiwitan:* to be victimized by sorcery.

Hupa [hu'-pa]
Bad dreams.

Ikota [i-ko'-ta]
Siberian word for "easy startle" syndrome.

Illustrados [i-lus-tra'-dos]
The elite social class in the Philippines, usually of Spanish or Chinese
extraction.

Imu [e'-moo]
Japanese (Ainu) word for "easy startle" syndrome.

Juramentado [hu₁-ra-men-ta'-do]
Pilipino term for *amok,* usually referring to the Muslim and Moro *amok.*

Kabuhi [ka-bu'-hi]
Illnesses caused by fright (exemplified by posttraumatic stress disorders).

Kapre [ka'-pre]
Malevolent supernatural being depicted as a dark giant.

Katipunan [ka-ti-pu'-nan]
To gather together; togetherness, solidarity.

Lanti [lan'-ti]
A childhood illness caused by fright, as may occur when a child witnesses conflict between parents. (Similar to Mexican *susto.*)

Latah [law'-taaw]
Malayan term for an illness characterized by hyperstartle, associated with compulsive repitition of words or phrases, echolalia, and/or coprolalia.

Liget [li'-get]
Life force.

Mahinhin [ma'-hin-hin]
Gentle and self-effacing, or subtle charm.

Mali-mali [ma-li ma'-li]
Visayan term for *latah* or hyperstartle reaction, with echolalia and coprolalia.

Manghihilot [mang-hi-hi'-lot]
A bonesetter who corrects dislocations or realigns broken bones by manipulation and massage.

Mankukulam (or **mancocalam**) [man-ku-ku'-lam]
Tagalog term for sorcerer.

Multo [mul'-to]
A ghost or "soul of the dead."

Myriachit [mee-ryeh'-cheet]
Siberian equivalent of *latah.*

Na sa dugo [na-sa-du-go']
"In the blood"; a hereditary disease.

Pakikisama [pa₁-ki-ki-sa'-ma]
Sense of deep comaraderie; conceding to group wishes; smooth interpersonal relationahips.

Pasma [pas'-ma]
Spasm; illness from exposure to excessive heat/cold.

Pasma sa kaon [pas,-ma sa ka'-on]
Ilness resulting from exposure to prolonged hunger that may manifest physical as well as behavioral changes.

Patrón [pa-tron']
A benefactor, usually wealthy and/or powerful.

Pilay [pi-lay']
To be lame; lameness.

Pilay looming [pi-lay, loo'-ming]
Muscle pain limiting motion.

Querida [ke-ri'-da]
Spanish word for sweetheart, mistress, loved one.

Sakit [sa-kit']
Illness or pain.

Santermos [san-ter'-mos]
Natural spirits that participate in the function of social and ecological systems.

Silok [si'-lok]
Tagalog term for *latah*.

Singaw [sing'-auo]
Illness caused by vapors, often manifested as skin or mucosal erruptions.

Singaw ng lupa [sing,-auo nang lu'-pa]
"Earth vapors or smells" that cause illness.

Susto [sus'-to]
Mexican "fright disease."

Tampal-tampal [tam-pal, tam-pal']
Hives or urticarial rashes or wheals.

Tomawo [to-ma-wo]
Ghosts.

Tomay [to-may]
Ilokano term for sorcery.

Uget [u-get]
"Bad feelings in the heart"; to feel despondent, to have heartache with loss of appetite.

Usug [u-sug']
An infant illness manifested by crying fits, abdominal pains, and vomiting believed to be caused by contact with a person of strong willpower (*dugan*) or life force (*liget*).

Utang nang loob [oo-tang, nang lo'-ob]
Debt of gratitude that obligates a person to reciprocate a favor.

Yuan [yu-an]
A Burmese word to describe a hyperstartle reaction similar to *latah*.

Glossary of Mexican Terms

Agringado [ah₁-green-gah'-do]
Americanized.

Barrio [bah'-ree-oh]
Neighborhood.

Carro [cah'-ro]
Anglicized Spanish word for automobile; word was originally used in the United States by Mexican Americans and is now used in Latin America.

Curanderismo [coo-rahn-dey'-rees-mo]
A system of folk beliefs in Latin America and the Southwestern United States.

Curandero [koo₁-rahn-dey'-roh]
A folk healer.

Dame el chart (dame el expediente) [dah-mey el ex₁-pay-dee-en'-tay]
"Give me the chart."

Gringo [green'-go]
Pejorative term used by many Latin Americans to refer to Americans.

Haciendas [hah-see-yen'-das]
Large, self-sufficient ranches. In Mexico, the breakup of the *haciendas* and the distribution of lands was one of the objectives of the Revolution of 1910.

La Llorona [la yoh-roh'-na]
The crying woman—a Mexican legend of a woman who killed her children then went about wailing at night.

Macho [mah'-cho]
Usually an exaggerated manliness, but may also connote the masculine sense of family responsibility.

Mal puesto [mal pooey'-stoh]
A folk illness involving the belief that a hex (*mal*) has been placed on someone by a friend or lover with the assistance of a witch and usually with a jealous motive.

Mestizo [me-stee'-zoh]
Someone of mixed blood (e.g., the offspring of Spanish and Indian parents).

Peón [pay-ohn']
Unskilled laborer.

Personalismo [per-so-nah'-lees-mo]
Personalism; the Latin emphasis on personal relations in social dealings.

Señor(a) [say-neor'[a]]
Mister (or Mrs.).

Señorita [say-neor-ee'-tah]
Miss.

Susto [soo'-stoh]
A Latin American folk illness characterized by various symptoms of
anxiety and depression and thought to be caused by loss of the soul
following a fright.

Usted [oo-stayd']
The formal "you" (informal is *tú* [too]).

Watchar [wah-char']
Hispanicized version of "to watch."

Glossary of Puerto Rican Terms

Ahijados [ah-e-hah'-dos]
Godchildren.

Ataques de nervios [ah-tah'-kays deh-nerr'-ve-os]
Nervous episodes.

Centros [then'-tros]
Places in which spiritualist practices are held.

Compadrazgo [com-pah-drath'-go]
Copaternity, the connection contracted by a godfather with the parents of a child for which he stands sponsor.

Compadre [com-pah'-dray]
The word by which the godfather and godmother address the father of their godson or goddaughter and by which the father and mother address the child.

Confianza [con-fe-ahn'-thah]
Confidence, trust, reliance, assurance.

Curanderismo [coo-ran-day-rees'-mo]
A belief system based on the healing power of indigenous plants and herbs.

Espiriteros [es-pee-ree-teh'-ros]
People who believe that the spirits of the dead communicate in various ways to human beings. They are considered less knowledgeable than *espiritistas*.

Espiritismo [es-pee-ree-tees'-mo]
The belief that the spirits of the dead communicate in various ways to human beings, usually through a medium.

Espiritistas [es-pee-ree-tees'-tahs]
People who believe that the spirits of the dead communicate in various ways to human beings, usually through a medium.

Facultades [fah-cool-tahd'-es]
A belief that the spirit has special powers that need to be developed.

Fraternidad Surcos [frah-ter-nee-dahd soor'-cos]
A brotherhood that studies the writings and meanings of *espiritismo*.

Orgullo [or-gool'-lyo]
Pride.

605

Padrinos [pah-dree'-nos]
Godparents.

Personalismo [per-so-nah-lees'-mo]
From the verb *personificar* [per-so-nee-fee-car']: to personify, to take things personally.

Repartimiento [ray-par-te-me-en'-to]
Portion of territory that was given as a fief to the conquerors of Spanish America.

Respeto [res-pay'-to]
Respect, consideration, observance.

Santerismo [san-tay-rees'-moh]
A belief system based on the syncretization of African and Catholic religions in which Catholic saints represent African deities.

Verguenza [ver-goo-en'-thah]
Shame.

Index

*Page numbers in **boldface** type refer to tables.*